EMS: A Practical Global Guidebook

EMS: A Practical Global Guidebook

Judith E. Tintinalli, MD, MS, FACEP
Professor and Chair Emeritus
Department of Emergency Medicine, School of Medicine
Adjunct Professor
Department of Health Policy and Management, School of Public Health
Lecturer, Medical Journalism, School of Journalism and Mass Communications
University of North Carolina at Chapel Hill
Chapel Hill, North Carolina

Peter Cameron, MBBS, FACEM, MD, FIFEM
Professor of Emergency Medicine,
Department of Epidemiology and Preventive Medicine
Monash University
Director of Research
Emergency & Trauma Centre
The Alfred Hospital
Melbourne, Australia
President, International Federation for Emergency Medicine

C. James Holliman, MD, FACEP
Program Manager, Afghanistan Healthcare Sector Reachback Project
Professor of Military and Emergency Medicine
Center for Disaster and Humanitarian Assistance Medicine
Uniformed Services University of the Health Sciences
Clinical Professor of Emergency Medicine
The George Washington University School of Medicine and Health Sciences
National Naval Medical Center, Bethesda, Maryland

2010
PEOPLE'S MEDICAL PUBLISHING HOUSE—USA
SHELTON, CONNECTICUT

People's Medical Publishing House–USA
2 Enterprise Drive, Suite 509
Shelton, CT 06484
Tel: 203-402-0646
Fax: 203-402-0854
E-mail: info@pmph-usa.com

PMPH-USA

09 10 11 12 13/PMPH/9 8 7 6 5 4 3 2 1

13-digit ISBN: 978-1-60795-043-1
10-digit ISBN: 1-60795-043-X
Printed in China by People's Medical Publishing House of China
Copyeditor/Typesetter: Spearhead Global, Inc.
Project Manager: Barbara Steckler, BS, EMT-P
Editor: Jason Malley
Cover Designer: Mary McKeon

Notice: The authors and publisher have made every effort to ensure that the patient care recommended herein, including choice of drugs and drug dosages, is in accord with the accepted standard and practice at the time of publication. However, since research and regulation constantly change clinical standards, the reader is urged to check the product information sheet included in the package of each drug, which includes recommended doses, warnings, and contraindications. This is particularly important with new or infrequently used drugs. Any treatment regimen, particularly one involving medication, involves inherent risk that must be weighed on a case-by-case basis against the benefits anticipated. The reader is cautioned that the purpose of this book is to inform and enlighten; the information contained herein is not intended as, and should not be employed as, a substitute for individual diagnosis and treatment.

Sales and Distribution

Canada
McGraw-Hill Ryerson Education
Customer Care
300 Water St
Whitby, Ontario L1N 9B6
Canada
Tel: 1-800-565-5758
Fax: 1-800-463-5885
www.mcgrawhill.ca

Foreign Rights
People's Medical Publishing House
Suzanne Robidoux
Copyright Sales Manager
International Trade Department
www.pmph.com/en/

Japan
United Publishers Services Limited
1-32-5 Higashi-Shinagawa
Shinagawa-ku, Tokyo 140-0002
Japan
Tel: 03-5479-7251
Fax: 03-5479-7307
Email: kakimoto@ups.co.jp

United Kingdom, Europe, Middle East, Africa
McGraw Hill Education
Shoppenhangers Road
Maidenhead
Berkshire, SL6 2QL
England
Tel: 44-0-1628-502500
Fax: 44-0-1628-635895
www.mcgraw-hill.co.uk

Singapore, Thailand, Philippines, Indonesia,
Vietnam, Pacific Rim, Korea
McGraw-Hill Education
60 Tuas Basin Link
Singapore 638775
Tel: 65-6863-1580
Fax: 65-6862-3354
www.mcgraw-hill.com.sg

Australia, New Zealand
Elsevier Australia
Locked Bag 7500
Chatswood DC NSW 2067
Australia
Tel: +61 (2) 9422-8500
Fax: +61 (2) 9422-8562
www.elsevier.com.au

Brazil
Tecmedd Importadora e Distribuidora
de Livros Ltda.
Avenida Maurilio Biagi 2850
City Ribeirao, Rebeirao, Preto SP
Brazil
CEP: 14021-000
Tel: 0800-992236
Fax: 16-3993-9000
Email: tecmedd@tecmedd.com.br

India, Bangladesh, Pakistan, Sri Lanka, Malaysia
CBS Publishers
4819/X1 Prahlad Street 24
Ansari Road, Daryaganj, New Delhi-110002
India
Tel: 91-11-23266861/67
Fax: 91-11-23266818
Email:cbspubs@vsnl.com

People's Republic of China
People's Medical Publishing House
No.19, Pan Jia Yuan Nan Li
Chaoyang District
Beijing 100021
P.R. China
www.pmph.com

Contributors

Silvio L. Aguilera, MD, MBA
Medical Director
Vittal Socorro Medico Privado S.A.
Buenos Aires, Argentina

Kumar Alagappan, MD, FACEP
Professor of Clinical Emergency Medicine,
    Senior Associate, Chairman
Department of Emergency Medicine
Albert Einstein College of Medicine
Long Island Jewish Medical Center
New York, New York

Mohammed Al-Mogbil, MD
Consultant
Pediatric Emergency Medicine
King Faisal Specialist Hospital & Research
    Centre
Riyadh, Saudi Arabia

Lisa Diane Amir, MD, MPH
Instructor in Pediatrics
Department of Emergency Medicine
Tel Aviv University, Sackler School of Medicine
Petah Tikva, Israel

**Bill Barger, AssocDipHealthScience
(amb), MICA Cert**
Operations Manager
Operational Quality & Improvement
Ambulance Victoria
Doncaster, Victoria, Australia

Rick Bissell, PhD, MS, MA
Professor
Department of Emergency Health Services
University of Maryland, Baltimore County
Baltimore, Maryland

Scotty Bolleter, BS, EMT-P
Director of Education
San Antonio AirLife
San Antonio, Texas

William J. Brady, MD, FACEP, FAAEM
Professor & Vice Chair
Emergency Medicine
Departments of Emergency Medicine and
    Medicine
Unviersity of Virginia Medical Center
Operational Medical Director
Charlottesville-Albemarle Rescue Squad
Charlottesville, Virginia

Ian Brennan, HdipEMT, MScEMS
Advanced Paramedic, Leading EMT
Emegency Medical Service
Health Service Executive National Ambulance
    Service
Wicklow Town, Co. Wicklow, Ireland

Jane H. Brice, MD, MPH
Associate Professor
Department of Emergency Medicine, School of
    Medicine
University of North Carolina at Chapel Hill
Medical Director, Orange County Emergency
    Medical Services
Chapel Hill, North Carolina

Lawrence H. Brown, MPH, TM
Sr. Principal Research Officer
Tropical Medicine & Rehabilitation Services
Anton Breini Centre, School of Public Health
James Cook University
Townsville, Queensland, Australia

Kenneth H. Butler, DO
Associate Professor
Associate Director Residency Program
Department of Emergency Medicine
University of Maryland
Baltimore, Maryland

José Cabañas, MD, EMT-P
Adjunct Assistant Professor, Associate Medical
    Director
Clinical Research Unit
Medical Director Special Operations
Emergency Services Institute
Department of Emergency Medicine
Wake Emergency Physicians
Deputy Medical Director
Wake County EMS
Raleigh, North Carolina

Giles N. Cattermole, MA, BM, BCh, FCEM
Assistant Professor
Accident & Emergency Medicine Academic Unit
Chinese University of Hong Kong
Montacute, Somerset, England

**Jimmy Tak-shing Chan, MBBS, FRCS(Ed),
FCSHK, FHKAM, FHKCEM, FHKAM,
FFAEM**
President
Hong Kong Association for Conflict &
    Catastrophic Medicine, EMS Faculty
 Regional Director
Advanced HazMat Life Support
International Medical Advisor
Hong Kong Police College
Clinical Associate Professor
Accident and Emergency Medicine Academic
    Unit
Alice Ho Miu Ling Nethersole Hospital
NTE Cluster Hospital Authority
New Territories, Hong Kong Special
    Administrative Region

**Yuk-Yin Chow, MBBS, FRCS, FRACS,
FHKCOS, FHKAM**
Honorary Clinical Associate Professor, Chief of
    Service
Department of Orthopedics & Traumatology
Tuen Mun Hospital
New Territories, Hong Kong Special
    Administrative Region

**Robert A. Cocks, MD, FRCS, Dip
Aviation Medicine**
Honorary Professor of Accident & Emergency
    Medicine
Sr. Medical Officer-Aviation Medicine
Aviation Office, Cathay Pacific
Lantau, New Territories, Hong Kong Special
    Administrative Region

Alex Currell, BA, BE, MEng Sci
General Manager, Strategy & Planning
Ambulance Victoria
Doncaster, Victoria, Australia

**Col. Robert A. De Lorenzo, MD,
MSM, FACEP**
Professor of Military & Emergency Medicine
Uniformed Services
University of the Health Sciences
Chief, Department of Clinical Investigation
Brooke Army Medical Center
San Antonio, Texas

Conor Deasy, FCEM
Department of Epidemiology & Preventive
    Medicine
Monash University
The Alfred Emergency & Trauma Centre
Melbourne, Victoria, Australia

Mazen J. El Sayed, MD
Clinical Instructor, EMS Fellow
Deptarment of Emergency Medicine
Boston Medical Center, Boston EMS
Boston, Massachusetts

Mark Fitzgerald, MB, BS, FACEM
Associate Professor, Director of Trauma
    Services
The Alfred Emergency & Trauma Centre
Melbourne, Victoria, Australia

**Colin A. Graham, MD, MPH, FRCS,
FCCP, FCEM, FHKCEM, FHKAM**
Professor, Honorary Consultant
Accident & Emergency Medicine Academic
    Unit
Chinese University of Hong Kong
Prince of Wales Hospital
New Territories, Hong Kong Special
    Administrative Region

Khalid Abu Haimed, MBBS,
FAAEM, FRCPC
Assistant Professor, Chair
Department of Emergency Medicine
King Faisal Specialist Hospital & Research Centre
Riyadh, Saudi Arabia

Pinchas Halpern, MD
Assistant Professor
Departments of Emergency Medicine,
   Anesthesiology, and Critical Care Medicine
Sackler Faculty of Medicine, Tel Aviv University
Chair of Emergency Medicine, Tel Aviv Medical
   Center
Tel Aviv, Israel

Manuel Hernandez, MD, MBA, FACEP
Director of Clinical Intelligence
Emergency Medicine, Business Planning
Sg2 Health Care Intelligence
Chicago, Illinois

Kim Hinshaw, MB, BS, FRCOG
Consultant
Department of Obstetrics & Gynecology
Sunderland Royal Hospital
Sunderland, United Kingdom

Jon Mark Hirshon, MD, MPH, FACEP
Associate Professor, Research Director
National Study Center for Trauma & EMS
University of Maryland School of Medicine
Baltimore, Maryland

Brian Horan, DO
Clinical Instructor
Emergency Department
University of California San Francisco at Fresno
Fresno, California

Shingo Hori, MD, DMSci
Professor and Chairman
Department of Emergency Medicine
Keio University
Tokyo, Japan

Nabih Jabr
EMS Instructor, EMS Training Manager
Emergency Medical Service
Lebanese Red Cross
Metn, Lebanon

Juliusz Jakubaszko, MD, PhD
Professor and Chairman
Department of Emergency Medicine
Wroclaw Medical University
Wroclaw, Poland

Paul A. Jennings, Paramedic, BN,
MClinEpi, FACAP
Intensive Care Paramedic and Research Fellow
Monash University
Ambulance Victoria
Melbourne, Victoria, Australia

Somchai Kanchanasut, MD
Thai Board of Emergency Medicine
Retirement Officer, Committee of National
   Board of Thai EMS
Ministry of Public Health
Bangkok, Thailand

Amin Antoine Kazzi, MD, FAAEM
Professor and Chair
Department of Emergency Medicine
American University of Beirut
President
Lebanese Society for Emergency Medicine
Beirut, Lebanon

Pairoj Khruekarnchana, MD
Thai Board of Emergency Medicine
Acting Chief, Department of Emergency
   Medicine
Rajavithi Hospital
Department of Medical Services, Ministry of
   Public Health
Bangkok, Thailand

A.J. Kirk, MD, FF/EMT
Assistant Professor
Disaster & Homeland Security
Assistant Medical Director
Dallas Fire Rescue, American Airlines Center
Tactical Physician, Carrollton Police
   Department
University of Texas-Southwestern
Dallas, Texas

David J. Krieger, MD
Department of Family Medicine
Terem Emergency Medical Center
Jerusalem, Israel

Douglas F. Kupas, MD, FACEP
Commonwealth EMS Medical Director
Pennsylvania Department of Health
Harrisburg, Pennsylvania
Associate Chief Academic Officer
Geisinger Health System, Bureau of EMS
Danville, Pennsylvania

Major Julio R. Lairet, DO, FACEP
Assistant Professor of Military & Emergency
  Medicine
Director of Enroute Care Research Center
Uniformed Services University of Health Sciences
Volunteer Assistant Professor of Clinical
  Emergency Medicine
Indiana University School of Medicine
Helotes, Texas

Benjamin J. Lawner, DO, EMT-P
Clinical Instructor
Department of Emergency Medicine
University of Maryland School of Medicine
Deputy EMS Medical Director
Baltimore City Fire Department
Baltimore, Maryland

Daniel L. Lemkin, MD, MS, FACEP
Assistant Professor
Department of Emergency Medicine
University of Maryland School of Medicine
Baltimore, Maryland

Alberto J. Machado, MD
Residency Director, Chair of the Emergency
  Center
Departmentof Emergency Medicine
Hospital Alemán
Buenos Aires, Argentina

Francis Mencl, MD, MS, FACEP, FAAEM
Associate Professor
Department of Emergency Medicine
Summa Health System-Akron
Akron, Ohio

**David Menzies, MCEM, Dip Med Tox, Dip
IMC (RCSEd), DMMD**
Specialist Registrar in Emergency Medicine
Emergency Department
St. Vincent's University Hospital
Dublin 4, Ireland

Larry J. Miller, MD
Chief Medical Officer
Vidacare, Inc.
Shavano Park, Texas

Jerry Mothershead, MD
Commander (ret), Assistant Professor
  Emergency Medicine
Program Manager and Senior Scientist
Center for Disaster and Humanitarian
  Assistance Medicine
Uniformed Services University of the Health
  Sciences
Williamsburg, Virginia

Sergey M. Motov, MD, FAAEM
Assistant Professor Clinical Emergency
  Medicine
Assistant Residency Program Director
Department of Emergency Medicine
SUNY Downstate Medical Center
Maimonides Medical Center
Brooklyn, New York

**Terrence Mulligan, DO, MPH, HPF,
FACOEP, FNVSHA, FACEP, FAAEM**
Co-Director Emergency Medicine Residency /
  Plv. Opleider Spoedeisende Geneeskunde
University Medical Center Utrecht
Utrecht, The Netherlands
Assistant Professor and Faculty
Department of Emergency Medicine
University of Maryland School of Medicine
 Chair, ACEP Section for International
  Emergency Medicine
ACEP Ambassador to the Netherlands
ACEP Ambassador to EuSEM

Marcus E. H. Ong, MBBS, MPH, FAMS
Associate Professor
Consultant, Emergency Medicine, Office of
  Research, Graduate Medical School
Singapore General Hospital
Duke-National University of Singapore
Republic of Singapore

Ricardo Ong, MD, MBA, DMO, FS
Command Surgeon
Special Operations Command-Africa
United States Army

Gerald O'Reilly, MBBS, FACEM, MPH Int'l Health
Hon. Lecturer, PhD Student, Emergency Physician
    & International Operations Manager
School of Public Health & Preventive Medicine
Monash University
Emergency & Trauma Centre
The Alfred Emergency & Trauma Centre
Melbourne, Victoria, Australia

Gürkan Özel, BS, EMT-P, MS, FP-C
Chief Flight Paramedic, Clinical Training &
    Quality Coordinator
Aeromedical Program
Koçoğlu Air Ambulance, Ankara Turkey
Tunceli, Turkey

Ian Patrick, ASM, B. of Paramedic Studies, MICA, Associate Diploma Genl. Adm.
Adjunct Professor, Consultant
University Sunshine Coast, IC Paramedic,
National President
Australian College of Ambulance Professionals
Diamond Creek, Victoria, Australia

Devin T. Price, EMT-P, MS
Adjunct Faculty
Southwestern Community College
Chula Vista, California

Neha Puppala, BS, MD
Department of Emergency Medicine
Summa Health Systems
Akron City Hospital
Cuyahoga Falls, Ohio

Nadeemuddin Qureshi, MD, FAAP, FCCM
Consultant in Pediatric Emergency Medicine
Director of Research
Department of Emergency Medicine
Chair, International Emergency Medicine
King Faisal Specialist Hospital & Research Centre
Riyadh, Saudi Arabia

Timothy H. Rainer, MD
Professor, Chinese University of Hong Kong
Director, Trauma & Emergency Centre
Prince of Wales Hospital
Shatin, New Territories, Hong Kong Special
    Administrative Region

Christoph Redelsteiner, PhDr, MSW, MSc, EMT-P
Lecturer, Scientic Director
Emergency Health Services Management
    Program
University of Applied Sciences, School of
    Social Work
Danube University
Vienna, Austria

Gilberto Salazar, MD
Clinical Assistant Professor
Department of Emergency Medicine
University of Texas Southwestern Medical Center
Assistant Medical Director
Farmers Branch Texas Fire & Rescue
Dallas, Texas

Ehud C. Sarlin, MD
Department of Emergency Medicine
Long Island Jewish Medical Center
New York, New York

Eric Schmitt, MD, MPH
Department of Emergency Medicine
University of California San Francisco at Fresno
Fresno, California

Dagan Schwartz, MD
Department Head
Department of Emergency Medicine
Ben Gurion University
Kiryat-Ono, Israel

Helen Simpson, BM, BS, E Med Sci, MRCOG
Consultant Obstetrican, Clincal Director
    Obstetrics
Department of Obstetrics & Gynecology
James Cook University Hospital
Middlesbrough, North Yorkshire, United
    Kingdom

Karen Smith, BSc, PhD
Honorary Senior Lecturer
Monash University
Manager Research & Evaluation
Department of Research & Evaluation
Ambulance Victoria
Doncaster, Victoria, Australia

Helen A. Snooks, BsC
Professor of Health Services Research
Institute of Life Science, School of Medicine,
    Swansee University
Centre for Health Information, Research &
    Evaluation (CHIRAL)
Swansee, Wales, United Kingdom

Mark R. Sochor, MD
Associate Professor
Department of Emergency Medicine
University of Virginia Medical Center
Charlottesville, Virginia

Benjamin Sojka, NREMT-P
Assistant Chief of Operations
Charlottesville-Albemarle Rescue Squad
Charlottesville, Virginia

Susanne J. Spano, MD
Wilderness Medicine Fellow
Department of Emergency Medicine
University of California San Francisco at Frenso
Fresno, California

Robert E. Suter, DO, MHA, FACEP, FIFEM
Past President, American College of Emergency
    Physicians
Professor of Emergency Medicine
University of Texas-Southwestern
Dallas, Texas

Harm van de Pas, MD, FNVSHA
Medical Director
Midden-West-Noord Regional Ambulance Service
St. Elizabeth Hospital
Tilburg, The Netherlands

Yehezkel Waisman, MD
Associate Professor, Director
Department of Emergency Medicine
Schneider Children's Medical Center of
    Israel
Petah Tiqva, Israel

Lori Weichenthal, MD, FACEP
Associate Clinical Professor, Associate Residency
    Director
Director Wilderness Health Science Services
University of California San Francisco at Fresno
Fresno, California

Garry John Wilkes, MBBS, FACEM
Clinical Associate Professor, Medical Director
St. John Ambulance
Belmont, Western Australia, Australia

**Malcolm Woollard, MPH, MBA, MA(Ed)
Dip IMC(RCSEd), RN, MCPara, FACAPI**
Professor in Pre-hospital & Emergency Care
Coventry University and Charles Stuart
    University
Chair, College of Paramedics
Director, Prehospital Emergency & Cardiac
    Care Applied Research Group
Honarary Consultant Paramedic
West Midlands & South East Coast Ambulance
    Service, NHS Trust
Powys, United Kingdom
Adjunct Senior Research Fellow
Monash University, Victoria, Australia

Foreword

The first ever professional organisation of doctors working in emergency departments, the Casualty Surgeons Association, was established in the United Kingdom (UK) in 1967. This created increased awareness in emergency medical care eventually to an extent where the exchange of the science and art of Emergency Medicine (EM) was thought to be necessary. The first International Conference on Emergency Medicine was held in London in 1986 and that gathering of physicians, either trained in EM or interested in providing emergency care, led to understanding the importance of organised emergency care, recognition of EM as a specialty in many countries and the formation of the International Federation for Emergency Medicine (IFEM).

IFEM believes that society has a right to expect immediate care in an emergency situation. This justifies the increased awareness in providing and receiving emergency health care. But quality care can only be delivered when there is an organised Emergency Medical Service (EMS). The Sixtieth World Health Assembly in 2007 also recommended the development of 'techniques for reviewing policy and legislation related to provision of emergency care' and that 'additional efforts should be made to strengthen provision of trauma and emergency care so as to ensure timely and effective delivery'.

Whilst there are two prominent models of EMS, i.e. Anglo-American and Franco-German, there has been a trend towards increasing acceptance of the Anglo-American model. After recognition of EM (then Accident and Emergency Medicine) as a specialty in the UK in 1975, the USA, Australasia, and Canada also took early positive steps towards that as well. Organised EMS became more important as technology improved and early intervention by skilled personnel began to make a difference. This technological advancement helped realise the importance of more organised EMS and training and has led to delivering a quality care through early intervention by skilled personnel.

Professor Judith Tintinalli, Professor Peter Cameron, and Professor Jim Holliman are internationally known leaders in EM who have edited this book. Many prominent authors from around the world have contributed to this book to make it unique and first of its kind. The topics covered will lead to a better understanding of the subject, organising an efficient EMS, and creating competence in those who deliver emergency care.

Being the president of the IFEM, I am honored to have been asked to write a foreword for this book, as it is an official book of IFEM. IFEM is pleased to be associated with this project as it believes that all those who require emergency care should have it by skilled personnel. This can only be achieved by having an efficient EMS. This book will help achieve that goal.

Gautam G. Bodiwala, CBE, DL, D Sc (Hon), MS, FRCS, FRCP, FCEM, FIFEM
President
International Federation for Emergency Medicine

Contents

Part 1

Foundations

Part 1

Standard EMS Terms and Definitions

C. James Holliman

This chapter presents definitions of the most important and common terms used in this book. A number of common EMS terms have very different meanings in different countries; therefore to make the information offered in this book clear and unambiguous to all readers, we have established precise definitions of these common terms. The terms used throughout the book are in accord with the definitions set in this first chapter. The definitions chosen in this chapter are not meant to slight or ignore alternative word meanings used in other countries but instead are intended to provide consistency of terminology.

LIST OF TERMS AND DEFINITIONS

Advance Directives: official written documents that denote a person's wishes to receive or refuse certain specified types of medical care (such as CPR or endotracheal intubation).

Advanced Life Support (ALS): the level of care provided by an Emergency Medical Technician-Paramedic (EMT-P) or even more highly trained EMS personnel such as nurses or physicians. ALS level care includes advanced airway management such as endotracheal intubation, defibrillation, use of parenteral medications, and cardiac monitoring. Note that the mere presence of a physician does not define ALS; the presence of advanced medical equipment would also be required.

Air ambulance: an aircraft, either fixed-wing or rotary wing (helicopter), which has been fitted with medical equipment for patient transport.

Air Medical Services: the systems or use of aircraft to transport patients for medical care or evaluation. Generally Air Medical Services would provide at least some degree of medical care during transport.

Ambulance: a vehicle dedicated to patient transport and fitted with at least some medical equipment.

Ambulance attendant: Ambulance personnel who usually have had at least a few hours of first aid training and can assist the more highly trained ambulance personnel (such as EMTs or doctors) with initial patient care and movement. They may also serve as the ambulance driver and are usually not involved with patient care during transport to a medical facility.

Ambulance driver: The person who operates the ambulance vehicle; usually this term would apply to a driver who has not had medical training and is not responsible for patient care.

Basic Life Support (BLS): the level of care provided by the EMT-Basic (or EMT-Ambulance). See the definition of EMT-B below for a listing of BLS care components.

Bypass: the situation where EMS personnel do not transport the patient to the closest medical facility but instead to a medical facility farther away, either because of the relative care capabilities of the facilities or the request by a facility that it not be brought any new patients (usually due to overcrowding).

Bystander (also called **passerby**): a person who happens to be in the vicinity of a medical emergency but who is not part of the local organized EMS system. Generally, this is a member of the general public without advanced medical training. Individuals in the vicinity of a medical emergency who happen to have medical training but who are not part of the EMS system are also called bystanders.

Cardiopulmonary resuscitation (CPR): the provision of basic resuscitation efforts for a patient in cardiac or cardiopulmonary arrest, to include at least chest compressions and artificial ventilation (either mouth to mouth or using equipment adjuncts) and also including advanced care if available (such as parenteral medications and defibrillation).

Clinic: a medical facility providing mainly outpatient nonemergency care. Generally a clinic would not have inpatient beds. A clinic may treat emergencies if needed, but its primary role is to provide nonemergency care.

Clinical practice guideline: synonym for "protocol" (see below)

Continuing Medical Education (CME): medically related education for health care personnel after completion of their basic or required initial training. This can also be termed **Continuing Professional Development (CPD)**, which would then apply to education programs not just for healthcare workers but also for other types of workers or professionals.

Dispatch: notification of EMS personnel about an incident and mobilization of EMS unit(s) to the location of the incident. Notification is usually done by a communications center and would include information about the type, severity, and location of the incident.

Dispatcher: the person responsible for notifying EMS personnel that an emergency has occurred and that response is needed; usually this person would be in a communications center and notify the EMS personnel electronically by telephone, radio, or intercom.

(Ambulance) Diversion: request by a medical facility to refuse to receive any new patients in transport by the EMS system for a specified period of time (usually due to overcrowding).

Emergency Department (ED): the area of a medical facility devoted to providing emergency medical care; usually this would be staffed at least part time by an emergency physician.

Emergency Medical Care: patient care for an acute condition; this care can be given by a variety of different medical practitioners, including technicians, nurses, paramedics, physician assistants, and/or physicians.

Emergency Medical Services (EMS): the system that organizes all aspects of care provided to patients in the prehospital or out-of-hospital environment. The term "EMS" in context may encompass or refer to local, regional, national, or international systems for delivery of patient care.

EMS notification: the notification to a receiving medical facility (usually by radio or telephone) of a patient transport by an EMS service. This would normally not include any request for orders or interventions by the staff of the receiving facility.

Emergency Medical Technician (EMT): . A person who has completed a specific training program in prehospital emergency care and who has achieved formal certification for such training. Worldwide there are different levels of EMTs, but the two general types are **EMT-Basic** and **EMT-Paramedic**. Typical duties (or "scope of practice") of the **EMT-Basic** include: perform CPR; lift and move patients; extricate patients from vehicles or confined spaces; perform patient assessment and evaluation; administer oxygen by mask, cannula, collar, or bag-valve-mask; use oral or nasal airways, pocket masks, and bag-valve ventilation; perform oropharyngeal suctioning; provide emergency first aid treatment for bleeding, shock, burns, heat or cold illness, trauma, and medical emergencies; stabilize or splint suspected fractures; assist in emergency childbirth; use an automated external defibrillator; and perform other noninvasive emergency care measures. In some EMS systems EMT-Basics are authorized to administer a limited number of medications, such as an albuterol metered dose inhaler for acute asthma and/or subcutaneous epinephrine for anaphylactic reactions. **EMT-Paramedics (EMT-P)** typically have all of the skills of the EMT-Basic with the addition of recognition of cardiac dysrhythmias and acute ST-segment elevation myocardial infarction, defibrillation, intravenous and/or intraosseous line placement, use of parenteral medications, endotracheal intubation, and other advanced airway management techniques. **EMT-P** is generally the most advanced EMT level and involves training times of at least 300 additional hours. (Note that in some countries such as Australia the training time for paramedics is several years and may include the equivalent of a postgraduate university degree.) In some countries such as the US there are several

Table 1–1	Comparison of Training Times for Different EMS Personnel	
Personnel Type	**Usual Training Time**	
Ambulance attendant	1 to 20 hours	
First responder	40 hours	
EMT-A	110 to 140 hours	
EMT-B	110 to 140 hours	
EMT-I	180 to 500 hours	
EMT-P	450 to 1,500 hours	
Physician Assistant	2 to 4 years	
Nurse Practitioner	4 to 6 years	
Emergency Physician	6 to 13 years	

"levels" of EMT: **EMT-A** ("EMT-Ambulance") or **EMT-B** ("EMT-Basic") have completed at least 110 hours of training, **EMT-I** ("EMT-Intermediate") have completed a longer training course (usually several hundred hours in addition to the EMT-B training) and have additional clinical skills, including defibrillation (**EMT-D**) and intravenous line placement (**EMT-IV**). Table 1–1 contains a comparison of the different "levels" of EMTs.

Emergency Medicine (EM): this medical specialty involves providing unscheduled evaluation of acute illness and injury, care for the acute phase of illness or injury, and referral of patients to other medical practitioners for either nonemergent, definitive, or follow-up care. An excellent definition of EM is the official definition from the International Federation for Emergency Medicine (IFEM): "EM is a field of practice based on the knowledge and skills required for the prevention, diagnosis, and management of acute and urgent aspects of illness and injury affecting patients of all age groups, with a full spectrum of episodic undifferentiated physical and behavioral disorders; it further encompasses an understanding of the development of prehospital and inhospital emergency medical systems and the skills necessary for this development." EM is generally practiced in fixed medical facilities but can refer to care provided in the prehospital or out-of-hospital environment. Note that EM encompasses all types of illness and injury and all age groups of patients.

Emergency Physician (EP): a physician who has graduated from a medical school and whose main work involves the clinical practice of providing emergency care. Note that an EP may not have received specialty postgraduate training in Emergency Medicine (EM). So the term "EP" refers to any physician whose main practice is in EM whether or not he/she is specialty-trained or board certified.

First Aid: initial emergency care provided early at the scene of an emergency usually by medically untrained people until more advanced health care personnel reach the scene. First aid consists of simple techniques that can be applied with improvised tools or equipment.

First Responder: a nonmedical professional (usually a fireman and/or a policeman) who has received limited training in first aid or basic elements of emergency care. For example, the standard training program for first responders in the US is about 40 hours' duration. As a further example, the scope of practice (duties) of the first responder in the US include: perform patient assessment and evaluation, perform CPR (ventilations and chest compressions), administer oxygen using a mask, nasal cannula, demand valve unit, or bag-valve mask, use oropharyngeal airways and pocket masks, perform oropharyngeal suctioning, provide emergency first aid for bleeding, shock, burns, poisoning, heat and cold emergencies, medical emergencies, suspected fractures, and emergency childbirth, and call for dispatch of more advanced prehospital care units (such as ambulances) after initial patient assessment.

Hazmat (Hazardous Materials): Hazardous materials are dangerous chemicals, explosives, biologicals, or radioactive materials that are toxic to people or the environment.

Hazmat Teams: personnel (who may not necessarily be EMS personnel) who are specially trained in the management of and utilization of special equipment for incidents involving exposure to hazardous materials.

Hospital: a medical facility providing a range of ambulatory and inpatient services and possibly operative services. Generally this would be a fixed medical facility but could be a temporary facility such as a tent. Generally a hospital provides medical services with physicians and nurses and has the capability to admit patients for inpatient (overnight or longer) care.

Inpatient: a patient who stays for care or evaluation in a medical facility overnight or longer.

Medic: Military personnel responsible for the provision of first aid or other immediate life-saving procedures on the battlefield.

Medical Control: the administrative supervision and medical direction of an EMS organization or system.

Military EMS: Organizational or operational aspects of the EMS system used by a national armed force (such as an army, navy, air force, or marines).

Mutual Aid: the agreement of different EMS organizations to help each other. Usually this would constitute an agreement that if one EMS organization was too busy or occupied to be able to handle a new patient, the other organization would take care of the patient even if located outside the organization's normal geographic area of responsibility. Mutual aid agreements also encompass EMS organizations cooperating in managing mass casualty events and disasters.

Nurse Practitioner (NP): a nurse with more advanced training and capable of semi-independent medical practice to include performing a medical history and physical examination and prescribing medical treatments. Note that in some countries the duties and scope of practice of the NP are very similar to that of the physician assistant.

Off-Line Medical Control: the components of medical supervision and administration of an EMS organization or system that do not involve the direct management of care of a patient. This would include clinical care protocol development, standing orders, review of written reports of care provided, and required Continuing Medical Education. Off-line medical control includes prospective elements (relevant legislation, policy and procedure manuals, protocol development, and research) and retrospective elements (review of ambulance transport reports, statistical reviews, education conferences, quality improvement programs, and counseling "feedback" sessions by management personnel for the patient-care EMS personnel).

On-Line Medical Control (also known as on-line medical direction): the direct (either in person or by electronic communication such as telephone or radio) supervision and direction of prehospital medical care by a physician.

Outpatient: a patient who receives medical care at a medical facility but does not stay overnight for further care or evaluation.

Out-of-hospital care: medical care provided to patients who are located in settings other than a hospital; generally this term applies to patients who are not planned or intended to be transported to a hospital. (see "prehospital care" below to note the slight difference in meaning of this term set).

Overcrowding: A situation where ED resources are insufficient to provide adequate emergency care in a timely fashion in the ED (note that some prefer to use the term "crowding" instead to emphasize the unacceptability of this situation). Also in some countries such as Australia the term "**Access Block**" is preferred to "overcrowding" to emphasize the key difficulty in getting patients in the emergency department physically moved to inpatient care after the decision has been reached that the patient requires inpatient care.

Paramedic (EMT-P, see earlier): a person with advanced medical training and certification. Skills generally would include the ability to provide defibrillation, use parenteral medications, and perform endotracheal intubation or other advanced airway management techniques.

Patient Care Record (also called "run sheet" or "run report"): the paper or electronic document that provides information on a patient care event handled by EMS personnel.

Pediatric: refers to patients less than 18 years of age.

Physician Assistant (PA): a person who has received advanced medical training and is able to perform some, but not all, of the skills and duties of a physician, usually including performing a complete history and physical exam, prescribing treatments and medications, and performing advanced wound repair. As an example, the usual training duration for PAs in the US is two years, and they often take many of the same classroom courses and clinical rotations (clerkships) as medical students enrolled in Doctor of Medicine programs.

Prearrival Instructions: Advice given by the EMS dispatcher or communications center to a bystander or a person who has telephoned about an emergency. Prearrival instructions may include simple airway maneuvers or applying direct pressure to bleeding areas.

Prehospital care: medical care provided to patients in settings other than a hospital and who are planned or intended to be transported to a hospital for further care or evaluation. (note that this term has a slightly different meaning than "out-of-hospital care" above).

Protocols: The overall steps for patient care or the sequence of prehospital care measures pre-approved for use by EMS personnel. Protocols include standing orders, (see below) that are followed in the absence of on-line medical control or direction and additional medical care steps that require communication with medical control before implementation. Protocols can be considered synonymous with the term "clinical practice guidelines."

Quality Improvement (QI): the efforts or programs by an EMS organization to review, monitor, and improve the patient care it offers. This term implies efforts by EMS organizations to try to continuously improve rather than just reach a particular benchmark and then stop efforts. The term "**Quality Assurance**" has also been used but implies a care review system that centers around attainment or delivery of certain specific parameters without necessarily having continued ongoing efforts at constant improvement.

Ramping: the situation where ambulance patients are at least temporarily not allowed to be off-loaded from ambulances due to overcrowding or access block in the ED (i.e., patient transfer from the ambulance is delayed by the ED staff until a bed or treatment space becomes open and available).

Rescue: the removal of a patient from an unsafe environment; examples are extrication of patients from wrecked vehicles and dangerous environments such as cliffs. Rescue may involve nonmedical personnel and personnel with specialized nonmedical training.

Rescue vehicle: a vehicle with special equipment for rescue, to include, for example, power tools for dismantling of vehicles.

Run Report: the written or electronic report of an EMS patient encounter. A run report may be required whenever an EMS unit is dispatched or mobilized to the scene, even if no care is provided, if the patient refuses care, or if the patient has left the scene.

Standing Orders: The preestablished list of steps that prehospital personnel perform in the absence of on-line medical control or direction. Standing orders are a part of EMS protocols.

Tactical EMS: the provision of prehospital or out-of-hospital care in unsafe situations such as riots, areas with ongoing gunfire, or where the situation requires police presence.

Tiered Dispatch: the ability of the dispatcher or communications facility to mobilize EMS units with different care capability levels, depending on the incident. An example is the dispatch of a BLS ambulance for an isolated leg injury, or the dispatch of an ALS unit for a possible acute myocardial infarction.

Trauma Center: a receiving medical facility capable of providing comprehensive trauma care, including acute emergency care, operative care, access to subspecialties, and rehabilitation. Note that in a number of countries trauma centers are categorized into different "levels" or capabilities of care (ranging from the highest level trauma center with full trauma care capability to the basic or "lowest" level of trauma center such as might be found at a small rural facility) based on the staffing and infrastructure of each facility.

Triage: the categorization of patients by severity or priority for care and/or transport to a medical facility. One simple triage system is to class patients as "emergent" (need to be evaluated and treated very rapidly), "urgent" (need to be evaluated and treated "soon"), and "nonurgent" (evaluation and treatment can be safely delayed). Note that there is variation in the specific time intervals that would be recommended or required for each of these three examples of triage categories in different EMS systems. Also note that there are many different triage categories and systems in use, and many of these have more than three triage categories.

Universal precautions: the protective measures used by medical personnel to prevent their own exposure to potentially contaminated or infectious body fluids or aerosols. This usually includes at a minimum the routine use of waterproof gloves, goggles or eye shields, and facemasks before undertaking patient care when there is the possibility of body fluid or aerosol exposure.

CHAPTER 2

International EMS Development

Ehud Sarlin, Kumar Alagappan

KEY LEARNING POINTS

■ EMS systems are needed on a worldwide basis, and there is support from the World Health Organization for development of EMS systems in countries where this service is lacking.

■ Different structures of EMS systems exist in different countries; some utilize physicians as the main or supervisory prehospital care providers and others utilize nonphysicians.

■ EMS system development in any country needs to be coordinated with other components of the national health care system.

It is estimated that by the year 2010, 60% of the world's population will live in urban settings. The increased population density in these areas often leads to a rise in violent crime, traumatic injuries and motor vehicle accidents, and cardiorespiratory illnesses. This creates a need for prehospital care and often spurs the development of this care in areas where it is rudimentary or nonexistent.

Approximately 5 million people die every year from injuries of various sorts, and millions more are permanently disabled.[1] The economic burden of such deaths and injuries is staggering. The impact of intentional and accidental injury is highest in the developing world due largely to hazardous and poorly regulated work environments, unsafe roads and motor vehicles, and lack of well-trained emergency medical personnel. The World Health Organization (WHO) in its landmark 2005 treatise on EMS and prehospital trauma care systems has established the importance of EMS and prehospital trauma care systems in reducing morbidity and mortality from injury and violence and therefore the need and priority for development of EMS systems worldwide.[1]

To underscore this importance, the WHO drafted a document outlining the key concepts for developing prehospital trauma care systems. Minimally, according to the WHO, an effective prehospital care system should contain the following elements: "prompt communication and activation of the system, the prompt response of the system, and the assessment, treatment and transport of injured people to formal health care facilities, when necessary." The WHO believes that such care can, and should, be provided to all injured patients regardless of country or terrain in which their injuries occur and regardless of the economic status of the country or municipality rendering care and treatment.

This chapter will review some important principles of EMS system development applicable to any new system and present the structure of a number of different national EMS systems from around the world to highlight the current status of these national systems and to provide options for newly developing systems to consider.

THE ROLE OF PREHOSPITAL CARE

While the old adage "prevention is the best medicine" most aptly applies to traumatic injury, minimizing the poor outcomes, mortality, and long-term morbidity of traumatic injuries can be achieved with a well-organized EMS system. Proper wound care, immobilization of fractures, availability of oxygen, intravenous fluids, prompt recognition of life-threatening conditions, and transport to definitive care can all reduce morbidity and mortality. Unfortunately, in much of the developing world, such services are unavailable and care and transport of the sick and injured patient are carried out by lay people, if at all.[1] Let us examine, then, how EMS systems can be effectively organized to provide lifesaving services to the sick and injured.

KEY COMPONENTS OF AN EMS SYSTEM

The WHO recommends using preexisting EMS systems as the cornerstone of any attempt to improve upon prehospital services as opposed to trying to build a new system from scratch. It also recommends engaging local community leaders in efforts to develop any EMS system as a way of ensuring buy-in and increasing the likelihood that systems will succeed in their missions once developed. Several sectors of a society, starting with the government, domestic organizations, both private and public, and health care institutions are but a few of the stakeholders that must work together to create an organized plan, develop a needs assessment, and coordinate the creation of a modern EMS system for their environment.

A "lead organization," as the WHO calls it, should be responsible for oversight of any EMS system to supervise its financing and development. This agency should have the legal power to implement changes that will improve the EMS system it oversees. In some countries these responsibilities will be assumed by the ministry or department of health, while in others they will be assumed by the interior or transportation ministry.

EMS SYSTEM MODELS

There are various models of development and regulation of prehospital care systems.[1] These include:

1. National systems — EMS systems administered by national governmental agencies or ministries.
2. Local or regional systems — EMS systems administered by local or regional governments, often as part of local or regional police or fire departments.
3. Private systems — Systems in which private EMS companies contract with local, regional, or national governments to provide prehospital care.
4. Hospital-based systems — EMS systems based at and/or run by central or referral hospitals.
5. Volunteer systems — Common in smaller, rural areas, volunteer systems rely on community volunteers who donate their time to provide local prehospital care.
6. Hybrid systems — EMS systems that combine features of some or all of the above systems.

In order to properly run an effective EMS system that provides safe and current therapies and treatment for the sick and injured, an EMS organization must have a well-qualified medical director responsible for accruing appropriate resources and funding, for providing training and establishment of clinical protocols, and for providing evaluation ("audit" or review) of the operation and performance of the EMS system. Additionally, EMS agencies must plan and prepare for management of large-scale disasters and mass casualty events.

There are numerous levels of prehospital care providers with different levels of training, skills, and certification (see Chapter 1 for definitions and descriptions of these different provider levels). While training standards and certifications vary based on country, regions, and municipalities, the WHO outlines a few general categories of prehospital medical training.

The First Responder

First responders are often lay people or nonmedical public service professionals (such as fire or police personnel) who provide basic medical care and call for additional help once an emergency is recognized (see **Chapter 9, First Responders & Bystanders** for more information). Within this category there are two subcategories. "Basic first-aid providers" take a short training course and are taught to recognize medical emergencies and call for help. "Advanced first-aid providers" receive additional training, usually lasting anywhere from one day to several weeks (e.g., the standard US "first responder" training course is 40 hours' duration), and are generally more likely to encounter medical emergencies based on their occupation. These individuals provide basic first aid, such as stopping bleeding, cleansing wounds, and splinting extremity fractures until more advanced personnel arrive on the scene of an emergency.

Basic Prehospital Trauma Care

Called EMTs in the US and elsewhere, these responders undergo even more extensive training in courses lasting between 100 and 400 hours and learn to provide additional care such as extrication, immobilization, administration of oxygen, and safe transport of the sick and injured patient to hospitals for definitive care.

Advanced Prehospital Trauma Care

In some locales advanced level prehospital care is provided by physicians or nonphysician paramedics who typically undergo thousands of hours of training. These rescuers possess the skills and equipment to provide all the basic care outlined above as well as more advanced therapies such as electrocardiographic monitoring, intravenous and intraosseous access, administration of medications, endotracheal intubation, needle decompression of tension pneumothorax, and needle cricothyroidotomy.

With the advancement of medicine and improved treatments for myriad diseases and medical conditions, life expectancy has increased dramatically in developed and even developing countries. Trauma and accidental deaths, however, continue to be a major cause of mortality worldwide, and because trauma deaths tend to affect young victims, the years of life lost to such injuries is staggering. EMS then plays an important role in prevention of deaths from traumatic causes by delivering essential prehospital care and by providing safe and expeditious transport of the injured patient to hospitals that can provide definitive care.

CATEGORIES OF TYPES OF PREHOSPITAL CARE

In this chapter we provide an overview of EMS systems in different parts of the world and we compare and contrast how prehospital care is delivered worldwide. Some basic similarities do exist. There are four main categories of prehospital care. In much of the developing world there is "unorganized prehospital care" in which injured patients are transported in a somewhat haphazard fashion to the hospital by medically untrained individuals, such as law enforcement personnel, or by lay bystanders in vehicles that are not specifically designed to transport sick or injured patients. In Basic Life Support (BLS) EMS systems, EMTs provide basic, "noninvasive" care to patients

such as providing oxygen, splinting fractures, dressing wounds, and safe transportation of patients to the hospital for treatment. In some locales advanced level care is supplied by paramedic Advanced Life Support (ALS) providers who typically undergo hundreds to thousands of hours of training. These rescuers possess the skills and equipment to provide all the basic care outlined above as well as more advanced care skills. Finally, there are so called Doc-ALS EMS systems in which physicians respond to emergencies in the prehospital setting. In a time when globalization is at the core of every industry and field of specialty, including medicine in general and emergency medicine in particular, it is instructive to take a brief survey of EMS systems throughout the world. In doing so, strengths of various systems can be compared and contrasted and EMS systems throughout the world can learn from each other in the common goal of providing the best possible prehospital medical care no matter where patients are in need of such care.

Franco-German Model

The Franco-German model of EMS is based upon a "field treat and stabilize" concept. This approach means the health care provider (often a physician) stays at the scene and stabilizes the patient by bringing a (near) hospital level of care to the patient at the scene. This service is usually run by physicians who have an extensive scope of practice with very advanced technology. In many European countries, the specialty of "emergency medicine" mainly relates to prehospital care and is considered a supraspecialty. A core specialty training must first be obtained, and then emergency medicine training and certification can be obtained. As an example, a specialist in surgery can move on to become further trained in emergency medicine or an anesthesiologist can move on to study emergency medicine as a second "add-on" discipline. Most emergency physicians in Franco-German systems provide advanced medical care on the scene and en route to a health care facility. Some of the transported patients are often directly admitted to the hospital units bypassing the hospital ED. In this model, patients are frequently escorted directly to the appropriate hospital floor as opposed to the ED. This decision is determined by the attending prehospital physician. Countries that utilize this model include Germany, France, Greece, Switzerland, Malta, and Austria.[2]

Anglo-American Model

In contrast to the Franco-German model, the Anglo-American model is largely based around a "scoop and run" philosophy. This approach brings the patient to the hospital quickly with limited stabilization and treatment time in the field, and definitive care is then rendered by emergency physicians in hospital-based EDs. This operational philosophy, however, is not universally fully applied even in countries that subscribe to the Anglo-American model and may be more applicable to the trauma scenario, where scoop and run is used more often than in medical emergencies, where crews sometimes tend to stay on the scene for longer periods of time, stabilizing the patient prior to transport. Many of the EMS programs are run or allied with a public service such as the police or fire department. The Anglo-American system is usually conducted with trained paramedics and/or EMTs. In countries following this model, emergency medicine is generally recognized as a separate, independent medical specialty and is mainly hospital-based. Training programs in emergency medicine are hospital-based rather than field-based as in the Franco-German model. All patients within the Anglo-American model are transported by EMS personnel to hospital EDs rather than directly to hospital inpatient units. Countries that have this type of model include the United Kingdom, United States, Canada, New Zealand, Australia, and Iran.[2]

EMS in Australia

Ambulance services in Australia operate on the Anglo-American (as opposed to the Franco-German) EMS service delivery model. The services are divided into two basic groups: the statutory services and volunteer groups. Statutory ambulance services are provided by the state/territorial government, as a single-entity, third-service model, government department. In Western Australia and in the Northern Territory, all statutory ambulance service is provided by St. John Ambulance Australia, under contract to the state/territorial government. In the other states and territories, the activities of St. John Ambulance are limited to first-aid training and special events support, with the occasional disaster response. In most of Australia ambulance service is provided by the Ambulance Service of the state and is government-funded. Because of its vast territory, Australian EMS services rely heavily on aeromedical transport, including both helicopter and fixed-wing transport to cover much of the sparsely populated regions. Aeromedical transport is provided by the state as well as by the Royal Flying Doctor Service.[3]

EMS in China

Chinese EMS systems are absent in most rural areas of this country. This has led to the development of a few emergency service centers (stations) in both rural and urban areas. With the vast territory of China and the marked differences in size of cities and needs of the population, there are five different models of prehospital emergency service that have been adopted: (1) independent emergency service centers, (2) prehospital emergency service centers without beds, (3) prehospital emergency services supported by a general hospital, (4) unified communications command centers with prehospital emergency care to be handled by different hospitals, and (5) three-level emergency service networks in small cities.

In the cities, there is an urban ambulance dispatch or "rescue" center to provide both transport and inpatient care. Ambulances are staffed with a physician and a driver. The physicians are from the hospital or the center. Access to EMS is accomplished by simply dialing "120." Emergency calls go directly to the nearest rescue center/hospital and a physician is dispatched. There is no on-line radio communication between hospitals and ambulances at this time (late 2009).

The "prehospital emergency service" is an integral and important part of the Chinese EMS system in some areas. China is now attempting to unify its various systems. Although the Chinese EMS system development began in the 1980s with the "importing" of EMS principles from other systems, China has assimilated both traditional and unique EMS components. As it is undergoing development it remains unclear whether a systematized and standardized national EMS structure will emerge soon.[4]

EMS in South Africa

EMS is provided by each South African provincial government. The government operated ambulance is often referred to as "Metro." In addition to the paid responders, the government system is supplemented in numerous areas by unpaid volunteers. In cases where volunteers are used, the standards for operation are set by the provincial Health Department, which also provides vehicles, equipment, and operating expenses. Operations are administered at the local level through the Emergency Management Service, which also oversees police and fire protection. The co-location of ambulances with fire services is common in South Africa, even though they are two independent services. The national emergency number for ambulances in South Africa is "10 177."

The publicly operated ambulance services are supplemented by private-for-profit ambulance services. The government services and private companies are further supplemented by voluntary ambulance services, including the South African Red Cross. All are required to meet the same sets of standards as the public services with respect to staff qualifications. These services are self-dispatching and do not participate in the national emergency number scheme.

EMS in Japan

Emergency medical services are provided by the "fire defense" headquarters of the local government in Japan. Ambulances are allocated to each region based on population, with approximately one ambulance being allocated for every 50,000 people. There is a one-tiered EMS system. Ambulances are staffed by three crew members trained in rescue, stabilization, transport, and advanced care of traumatic and medical emergencies. There are three levels of care provided by ambulance personnel, including a basic-level ambulance crew (First Aid Class One, FAC-1), a second level (Standard First Aid Class, SFAC), and the highest level (Emergency Life Saving Technician, ELST). ELSTs are trained in all aspects of BLS and some ALS procedures relevant to prehospital emergency care.

The medical control system requires further development as the activities of ambulance crews become more sophisticated and hectic. This concern has been compounded by the marked recent increase in the volume of emergency calls. Currently, private services for transportation of nonacute or minor injury/illness have been introduced in some areas, and dispatch protocols to triage "119" emergency calls are being developed.[5]

EMS in Canada

In Canada, each province or territory is responsible for its own EMS, including both ambulance and paramedic services. These services may be contracted to a private provider or may be delegated to the local government level, which may in turn create its own service delivery arrangements with municipal departments, hospitals, or private providers. The approach and the standards all vary considerably among provinces and territories.

Typically, the provincial/territorial government provides enabling legislation, standards, accreditation or licensing, and oversight to a variety of potential system operators, including municipalities, hospitals, or private companies. Municipalities or hospitals may in turn elect to provide EMS service directly, as a branch of another municipal department, such as the fire department or health department, or may contract out this responsibility to a private company. The approaches used for service delivery are governed by what is permitted under the local legislation of the individual province or territory or under the by-laws of the local municipality when that municipality accepts responsibility for EMS service.[6,7]

EMS in the Netherlands

A number of private carriers provide EMS in the Netherlands. They are under contract to the Dutch government. The system consists of a number of private ambulance companies, each with its own designated service area and with standards of operation that are provided by the government contract. All contracts stipulate that the contractor is required to meet all standards published for vehicles, equipment, training, and performance by the Dutch Ambulance Institute. All contracts for EMS in the Netherlands are sent to tender every four years, with the contract being awarded to the most successful applicants. Netherlands law forbids EMS systems to earn any profit. Any surplus revenue is required to be directed to additional improvements to the system, including training, equipment, and vehicles. The Dutch system is a rare exception to the rule in Europe in that it operates on a variation of the Anglo-American model of EMS care and not on the Franco-German model.

Since 1992, Dutch law mandated that at least one nurse must be on every ambulance in the country. These nurses have all completed the training required for a registered nurse in the Netherlands and have completed additional training and certification in anesthesia, cardiac care, or operating room before they can apply for an additional year of training to qualify as a Registered Ambulance Nurse. All "paramedics" in the Netherlands are nurses and this term refers to a nurse with the appropriate additional EMS-related training.

As a result of this advanced training, all Dutch ambulances and rapid response vehicles are capable of providing Advanced Life Support (ALS) without online medical control. Protocol compliance is conducted by a physician who is known as the medical manager. In situations where the patient's condition is more complicated and beyond the scope of the paramedic, the medical manager can be called for support. Additional help can also be requested of a mobile medical team.

All of the ambulances in the Netherlands have two crew members, one paramedic and one driver. The medical training of the driver is minimal, and that individual can only assist with lifting the patient and equipment. The Netherlands is also well covered by government-operated aeromedical services nationwide.

EMS in India

The Indian subcontinent is now undergoing a transformation of the EMS services provided. Initially almost all private enterprise, there is now an attempt to standardize what used to be a potpourri of prehospital responders from trained ambulance personnel to partially trained auto rickshaw drivers. A study from Chennai found the most common mode of transportation to the ED was via the auto rickshaw. This led to on-site training these drivers with basic first aid skills.

In 2005, a non-governmental organization (NGO) founded the Emergency Research Institute (EMRI). This organization sought to develop prehospital care in India. EMRI has developed its own standards for the ambulances and the equipment it uses. It also trains its own prehospital workers. EMRI initially started in the city of Hyderabad but now has been adopted by numerous states in India.[8]

India has an excellent mobile telephone service that reaches into most rural areas. In order to provide a single access number, there has been extensive political and financial maneuvering and squabbling in many states and territories for one access number. EMRI has introduced "108" and this number is now being accepted by many Indian states and territories.

EMS in Singapore and Hong Kong

Both are island cities that can sometimes have major traffic snarls delaying the arrival of an ambulance. Therefore the EMS system on both islands is supplemented by trained prehospital personnel who can ride motorized two-wheel motorbikes and get to the scene of an injury or illness very quickly. Basic first-aid kits and often a defibrillator are carried by each of these units. The patient is stabilized, and an ambulance is summoned if the patient needs to go to the hospital. Both Hong Kong and Singapore utilize the Anglo-American EMS model and have well-established hospital EDs and physician training programs in emergency medicine. In Singapore, which is very densely populated and has many high-rise buildings that contain narrow hallways and stairwell landings, delays exist in the oft-neglected "on-scene arrival time to patient contact" time-frame. Singapore's current EMS system is under the auspices of the Singapore Civil Defense Force (SCDF) but was formerly overseen by various agencies including the Emergency Ambulance Services (EAS), the Singapore Fire Brigade, and the Central Ambulance Service, which was coordinated by the ED at Singapore General Hospital. Singapore utilizes the universal emergency access number "995",

through which calls are directed to Central Dispatch Control Rooms. This is staffed by former firefighters who have undergone specialized training to become EMS dispatchers.

EMS in New Zealand

In New Zealand EMS is provided by two major groups: Wellington Free Ambulance (WFA) and St. John Ambulance. St. John Ambulance of New Zealand is a charitable organization providing health care services to the New Zealand public. Services include emergency and nonemergency ambulance treatment and transport, first-aid training, and first-aid supplies. The organization is funded by the Ministry of Health and District Health Board funds (via ambulance service contracts), Accident Compensation Corporation (ACC) levies, part and full charges to patients, plus donations and fundraising. EMS training in this country is run primarily by St. John Ambulance, a charitable organization that works independently of the government.

The WFA serves the Wellington region of New Zealand with a system staffed by both professional and volunteer personnel. Approximately three quarters of the cost of these services is covered by the Ministry of Health and the Accident Compensation Corporation, while the rest is covered by public donations and funds raised from training courses. Emergency medical calls throughout New Zealand are answered by certified Emergency Medical Dispatchers (EMDs) at the national access number: "111." Using state-of-the-art technology, dispatchers can easily see the location of each ambulance and can dispatch the closest available vehicle using GPS technology. New Zealand has an ALS EMS system that responds to about 800,000 calls per year and about 30% of EMS runs are for trauma.

EMS in Israel

The Magen David Adom (MDA) is Israel's national emergency medical, disaster, ambulance and blood bank service. There are approximately 1,200 emergency medical technicians, paramedics, and emergency physicians who are employed by MDA. However, Israel still relies on over 10,000 volunteers who serve in both operational and administrative capacities for the EMS. The organization has over 700 ambulances and operates about 95 stations.[9]

The majority of the ambulance fleet is BLS ambulances. These units are supplemented by ALS ambulances and a variety of first responders. The ALS ambulances are further classified into two types:

Mobile Intensive Care Units (MICUs) and Intensive Care Ambulances. The former include a physician among its crew members, while the latter do not and therefore requires medical control approval for performance of certain procedures and administration of certain medications. An unusual feature in Israel is that there are also armored ambulances present nationwide.[9] The system is highly dependent on volunteers, many of whom are from outside of Israel. As a recognized national aid society, according to the Geneva Conventions MDA may become an auxiliary arm of the Israeli Defense Force during wartime. Young people holding dual citizenship, often from the US, are permitted to fulfill their national service obligations by serving in MDA instead of in the regular military. Many of the major ambulance stations have special units for responding to mass-casualty incidents like natural disasters or terrorist attacks. The system, for the most part, conforms to the Franco-German (as opposed to the Anglo-American) model of EMS care (although Israel has full-service hospital EDs and well-established emergency medicine residency training), and the presence of physicians at highly acute emergencies is common. In addition, emergency ambulance service is supplemented by a variety of private carriers who are often tasked with interfacility transfers only. Given the frequently challenging environments in which MDA ambulances operate, the service is equipped with a number of specialized response vehicles.[9]

There is a fleet of motorcycles designed to reduce response times in busy cities by easily negotiating traffic-congested areas. The motorcycles are equipped with sirens and emergency medical equipment carrying devices so that responders can begin administering emergency care prior to ambulance arrival. "Tractor" ambulances are a unique feature and are used in the Old City section of Jerusalem where the streets are often impassible by standard vehicles. These tractors are essentially modified All Terrain Vehicles (ATVs) that enable rescuers to reach patients, administer advanced treatment, and transport a patient to larger streets where a standard ambulance awaits to complete the transfer of care to a hospital ED. Many ambulances utilized by MDA have four-wheel drive transmission, allowing for easy transport in inclement weather or on uneven terrain, such as beaches.[9]

MDA can be accessed nation-wide via a single access number, "101." As of February 14, 2008, and in order to accommodate the approximately 650,000 hearing-impaired citizens of the country, Magen David Adom instituted an SMS (text message) service that allows emergency help to be summoned by sending an SMS message from any cellular phone. The message is received by MDA dispatchers via a plasma screen, and ambulance crews are then dispatched.[9]

EMS in Greece

In 1987 the two previous providers of EMS in Greece, the Hellenic Red Cross and the Social Insurance Institute (IKA), merged to become the Ethniko Kentro Amesis Boitheias (EKAB), the current provider of EMS in Greece which uses both the European emergency access telephone number "112" and the older Greek number "166." There are about a dozen EKAB stations throughout Greece, each with its own dispatch center, that provide EMS coverage to more than 95% of the population. Each substation is staffed by its own EMTs and physicians.[10]

Greece employs a two-tier EMS system consisting of BLS ambulances (staffed by EMTs) and advanced Mobile Intensive Care Units (staffed by a physician and EMTs). Physicians wishing to participate in prehospital care can attend a course, free of charge, that prepares them for ambulance work. In addition to ground transportation EKAB also operates a number of helicopters for aeromedical transport. As it is a relatively young system, EKAB is recruiting more EMTs and physicians to staff its ambulances and is introducing motorcycles into its fleet in order to improve response times in busy cities with congested roadways.[10]

EMS in South Korea

EMS on a national basis in Korea is still undergoing development. The universal number "119" is used as the access number through the country and was created in response to a number of tragic events in the 1990s, including the collapse of the Sung-Su bridge in 1994, the collapse of the Sampoong Department Store in 1995, and a natural gas explosion in Daegu in that same year. The national access number was created after a government advertisement campaign in 1999, and the call volume then increased dramatically.[11,12]

The paramedic training program in Korea is intensive and comparable to US standards. Even though ACLS training, interpretation of electrocardiograms (ECGs), and advanced airway techniques are required, the Korean paramedics operate essentially as BLS crews with limited physician support, protocols, and medications. EMS care is currently overseen by the Korean Fire Department. According to their level of training the paramedics in Korea are underutilized, and prehospital protocols that would allow these highly trained medics to implement care at the scene of an emergency are lacking. They are discouraged from formally assessing patients, performing procedures, and providing medication until they reach a hospital setting. There may be numerous cultural and other prevailing beliefs that nonphysician personnel cannot perform prehospital care competently.[11,12]

EMS in the United Kingdom

In the UK, EMS is provided through local ambulance services that are known as trusts. Each service is specific to one or more local authorities similar to the police. In England there are 12 ambulance trusts, with boundaries generally following those of the regional government offices. Since 2006, the number of ambulance trusts fell from 29 to 13. The reduction can be seen as part of a trend dating back to 1974, when local authorities ceased to be providers of ambulance services. Emergency medical calls in the UK are received via the "999" national access number. There are also private ambulance services that have their own telephone numbers. Ambulances in the UK provide basic as well as advanced life support. Those EMS personnel wishing to further their education have the option of enrolling in one of a number of university-based programs to earn a degree in Paramedic Science.[13-15]

EMS in Lithuania

The history of EMS in Lithuania dates back to the 19th century with the establishment of the Vilnius Society of Ambulances.[16] Funded by charities, the aim of the society was to provide free medical assistance in case of accident. Three years later the country's first ambulance station was established and was among the first in Europe. Between 1945 and 1990 Lithuania had a unique system of specialized ambulances with teams of specialists in fields as varied as neurology, psychiatry, cardiology, and critical care staffing ambulances. This system was largely abandoned in 1990, and the country now uses a more standard model of EMS with ambulances staffed by prehospital personnel of various levels of training. Some ambulances have physicians on board, but others do not and often don't have well-established protocols, making standardization one of the biggest problems of the Lithuanian EMS system. Another prevalent problem is the use of ambulance services for nonemergent conditions. In fact, some general practitioners have contracts with ambulance services to provide nonemergent primary care to their patients during nonoffice hours. The EMS situation in Lithuania is mirrored in most of the other ("ex-Communist") countries of eastern and central

Europe. Of note, lay people in Lithuania are required to pass a 12-hour first aid course in order to obtain a driver's license.[16]

EMS in Portugal

Since 1980 EMS in Portugal has been run by the National Institute for Emergency Medicine (INEM) of the government's ministry of health and serves about 75% of the population. Activated through the national access number "112", a two-person, mostly volunteer, BLS crew responds to the emergency call. If ALS-level care is required, a hospital-based rapid intervention vehicle is dispatched carrying on it a physician (usually an anesthesiologist) and a nurse. INEM also has at its disposal a small number of helicopters.[17]

EMS in the United States

Given its vast size and multitude of private, volunteer, and government-run EMS agencies, it is nearly impossible to neatly categorize EMS and prehospital trauma care delivery in the US. As an example, the US employs the following types of EMS systems in different areas throughout the country:

1. Local or regional systems — EMS systems administered by local or regional governments, often as part of local police or fire departments.
2. Private systems — Systems in which private EMS companies contract with local governments to provide prehospital care.
3. Hospital-based systems — EMS systems based out of and run by central or referral hospitals.
4. Volunteer systems — Common in smaller, rural areas, volunteer systems rely on community volunteers who donate their time to provide local prehospital care. Volunteer EMTs and paramedics are often held in high regard by members of the communities in which they serve. Volunteer responders need to be available from home and, sometimes from work. Employers must be understanding of workers who may need to leave their place of work at a moment's notice to respond to an emergency call, and families must be accepting of the fact that their relatives may need to leave a family dinner, religious service, or special event if they are called upon to do so.
5. Hybrid systems —EMS systems that combine features of some or all of the above systems.

   The main regulation of most EMS systems in the US is at the state government level, and the structure and operation of state EMS systems vary widely.

Given the differing systems, differing terrain, and varied populations in different parts of the country, the percentage of traumatic compared to medical EMS calls varies widely. In most of the US. EMS is provided by either BLS or ALS systems. There are very few Doc-ALS systems, although there are some volunteer and even nonvolunteer EMS systems that have physicians responding to calls in the prehospital setting, often for mass casualty events when on-site medical direction and supervision of prolonged extrication are required.

INTERNATIONAL EMS ORGANIZATIONS

A variety of EMS organizations exist, many of them with websites on the worldwide web, whose mission it is to support, provide continuing education, and promote the goals and activities of their members. What follows is a survey of some of these organizations.

The International Association of Emergency Medical Services Chiefs (IAEMSC)[18] provides position papers on topics relevant to EMS workers worldwide, such as operational safety guidelines given the threat of mass casualty events, seasonal infectious diseases, or major disasters. It also provides news updates on issues that may interest EMS and fire department personnel. According to its website, the IAEMSC leadership is elected by its voting membership.

The International Association of Fire Chiefs (IAFC)[19] represents, according to its website, "the leadership of over 1.2 million firefighters and emergency responders...[s]ince 1873, the IAFC has provided a forum for its members to exchange ideas and uncover the latest products and services available to first responders." Guided by its motto of "lead, educate, serve," the organization provides discussion forums for its members to voice concerns and communicate with each other, up-to-date news items of interest to first responders, job and career information, and information about conferences and expos. It also provides panels of experts for the press to contact for comment on issues related to fire safety and fire codes, hazardous materials, and staffing. The association's website provides an extensive list of links to organizations, both private and governmental, for further inquiry.

The International Association of EMTs and Paramedics (IAEP)[20] is a "7,000-member-strong EMS union working for EMS professionals." The IAEP engages in collective bargaining for its members, takes part in political action to promote its agenda, and boasts a "powerful voice" on the political scene. The association provides legal expertise to its members through attorneys working full time for them.

The Paramedic Association of Canada (PAC)[6] has 14,000 members according to its website and "exists to promote quality and professional patient care through working relationships among organizations with similar interests." The British Paramedic Association (BPA) represents EMS workers in Britain and has set for itself the goals of self-regulation of prehospital care in Britain, upholding standards of proficiency, continuing medical education, and professional support and advice. It, too, provides an extensive discussion forum for members on its website and proposes cutting-edge ideas for advancing prehospital care.

The Ontario Paramedic Association (OPA)[7] has worked since the mid-1990s to "enhance the professional image of paramedics, to improve communications between paramedics, and to lobby for improvements to the standards of patient care." The OPA uses a listserv to communicate with its members and to provide a forum for sharing of ideas about EMS and its advancement in Ontario; it also mails a bimonthly newsletter to its members. The OPA is composed of more than ten local chapters and on its website provides information regarding EMS news, upcoming conferences, and information about becoming a paramedic for those interested. It also maintains an extensive listing of job openings and career opportunities.

UniMed First Aid, an Australian-based organization, is a nonprofit group that promotes and teaches first aid and prehospital care. Its website includes information for the public regarding basic first-aid treatment, provides a link to a wholesaler of first-aid equipment, and promotes safety and mitigation of illness and injury.

SUMMARY

As much of the world rapidly urbanizes, EMS has had to advance in order to keep up with the acute illnesses and injuries that occur in these populations. EMS systems need to be flexible enough to respond to temporary or permanent changes in terrain or political climate as these and other factors impact upon the kind of emergencies that arise and how care is rendered. EMS contributes to the overall function and well-being of health care systems by providing the first health care responder to the acutely ill or injured patient. As the portal of entry to the health system for so many people, EMS needs to be robust and strongly supported by government and by the population it serves. Depending on where patients find themselves, their EMS will either "scoop and run" to a healthcare facility (Anglo-American model) or they may "stay and resuscitate" (Franco-German model) and then transport these patients to healthcare facilities. Although there has been a debate as to which system/model is better, outcome studies have been inconclusive. The best model for many areas may be a hybrid model encompassing features of both types of systems. Each country should adopt a system best suited for its needs.

References

1. World Health Organization, Injury Prevention, http://whqlibdoc.who.int/publications/2005/924159294X_chap2.pdf.
2. The Lancet Student: Models of International EMS systems, http://www.thelancetstudent.com/2009/09/17/models-of-international-emergency-medical-service-ems-systems/ (accessed 11/15/09).
3. Trevithick S, Flabouris A, Tall G, Webber CF. International EMS systems: New South Wales, Australia: *Resuscitation* Nov;59(2):165, 2003. International EMS systems: New South Wales, Australia.
4. Thomas TL, Clem KJ. Emergency medical services in China. *Acad Emerg Med* Feb;6(2):150, 1999.
5. Tanigawa K, Tanaka K. Emergency medical service systems in Japan: past, present, and future. *Resuscitation* Jun;69(3):365, 2006.
6. Paramedic Association of Canada, http://www.paramedic.ca/ (accessed 11/21/09).
7. Ontario Paramedic Association, http://www.ontarioparamedic.ca/ (accessed 11/21/09).
8. Asian Hospital & Healthcare management: Emergency Services in India, http://www.asianhhm.com/healthcare_management/emergency_services_india.htm (accessed 11/15/09).
9. Magen David Adom in Israel, http://www.mdais.org (accessed 11/21/09).
10. Papaspyrou E, Setzis D, Grosomanidis V, Manikis, Boutlis D, Ressos C. International EMS systems: Greece; *Resuscitation*, 63(3):255, 2004.
11. Christopher C, Lee M I, Gil-Joon Suh. Time for change: The state of emergency medical services in South Korea, *Yonsei Med J* 47(4):587, 2006.
12. Sung-Hyuk Choi, Yun-Sik Hong, Sung-Woo Lee, In-Chul Jung, Chul-Su Kim. Prehospital and emergency department care in South Korea. CJEM 9(3): 171, 2007.
13. British Paramedic Association, College of Paramedics, http://www.britishparamedic.org/ (accessed 11/21/09).
14. London Ambulance Service (NHS) http://www.londonambulance.nhs.uk/working_for_us/paramedic_science_degrees.aspx (accessed 11/21/09).
15. BBC News, 21 June 2007 http://news.bbc.co.uk/2/hi/health/6227034.stm (accessed 11/21/09).
16. Vaitkaitis D. EMS systems in Lithuania. *Resuscitation* 769(3):329, 2007.
17. Gomes E, E Gomes, R Araújo, M Soares-Oliveira, N Pereira, International EMS Systems: Portugal. *Resuscitation* 62(3) p.257-60, Sept.2004.
18. International Association of Emergency Medical Services Chiefs, Position Statement Recommended EMS Agency Operational Security Measures, http://www.iaemsc.org/ (accessed 11/22/09).
19. International Association of Fire Chiefs, http://www.iafc.org/ (accessed 11/21/09).
20. International Association of EMTs and Paramedics, http://www.iaep.org/ (accessed 11/21/09).

CHAPTER 3

Historical Timeline of International Events

Francis Mencl, Neha Puppala

KEY LEARNING POINTS

- True civilian EMS services first developed in Europe and North America in the 1800s after earlier military battlefield evacuation of casualties was started.

- EMS system development needs to be coordinated with development of hospital-based emergency care.

- Effective EMS system development often requires support from the government.

Fundamentally the goal of all EMS systems is the same: to stabilize and treat the injured or ill patient in the prehospital setting and deliver the patient to the proper location for definitive medical care. How this is accomplished and how much gets done in the "field" and by whom varies throughout the world, depending on needs, cultural norms, and the availability of resources. In all countries the initial efforts historically have been to simply transport the patient to the hospital, and aside from rare in-the-field amputations, often very little on-the-scene care has been provided to the patient. Consequently, many of the earliest ambulance services were hospital-based and much of early EMS was driven by the need to care for injuries and/or by military adventures or retrieval and isolation of individuals with suspected contagious diseases. Realistically, given the state of medicine and available medical interventions in the remote past, there was not much else to be offered to patients prehospital except for first aid for injuries.

A comprehensive detailed timeline of the evolution of EMS throughout the world could itself fill an entire book. Nevertheless, there are certain common trends that can be identified and will be highlighted in this chapter using the timeline of EMS development in selected countries and regions.

EARLY HISTORY

It is tempting to consider the Old Testament biblical Good Samaritan as the world's first EMS provider, and in searching the history of EMS it is interesting to look for other evidence of EMS-like activities in ancient history. There is no doubt that this is where EMS has its roots, especially in times of armed conflict. In ancient Rome older military centurions were sometimes assigned the task of removing wounded soldiers from the battlefield and then caring for them, reflecting a degree of organization and purpose beyond a simple clean-up after the fracas. During the Crusades, the Knights Hospitaller of the Order of St John, the precursor to today's St. John Ambulance Service, performed a similar function, including providing care in the hospital for injured soldiers. Other ancient conflicts likely saw the organized evacuation of wounded from the battlefield as well, although these are not always well documented.

However, it is likely that much of this early battlefield activity was haphazard at best, and in the absence of any field care, organized transport, and/or coordination with subsequent in-hospital treatment, the simple and isolated act of caring for the wounded is not enough to constitute an EMS system. True EMS is a much more recent phenomenon. Conflicts such as Napoleon's military adventures (1792–1815), the American Civil War (1861–1865), as well as the First World War (1914–1918) saw field evacuations become more organized and purposeful, with delivery of patients to aid stations and field hospitals. Larrey, one of Napoleon's surgeons, definitively established the role of the ambulance in military conflict. In March of 1864 the US Congress passed legislation entitled "An Act to Establish a Uniform System of Ambulances in the United States," creating a single system of ambulances for the armies of the nation.[1]

Different urban areas around the world began to organize their rescue services in the mid to late 1800s. New York City's Bellevue Hospital established a hospital-based emergency ambulance service in 1869 under the leadership of a Dr. Dalton, who had served during the Civil War as the director of a field ambulance corps.[1] In 1892 Boston City Hospital Ambulance Service, the forerunner of today's Boston EMS, began serving the citizens of that city with 11 horses and 2 ambulance carriages whose only function was to deliver patients to the hospital; they provided no prehospital care except for field amputations by surgeons.[2] In 1883 the city of Toronto, Canada, acquired two ambulances to transport those with infectious disease to the local sanitarium.[3] Predating the North American developments, in Europe the Prague (Czech Republic) EMS had already been established in 1857, Vienna's (Austria) EMS in 1881, Krakow's (Poland) in 1891 and London's (UK) in 1897.[4,5] In Melbourne, Australia, a horse-drawn ambulance service began operation in 1899.[6] Elsewhere in Asia, Africa, and South America, EMS did not arrive until much later.

HISTORY OF EMS IN COUNTRIES USING EMT/PARAMEDIC-BASED SYSTEMS

Canada

Canada has evolved an EMT and paramedic-based EMS system similar to that in the US, the UK, Australia, New Zealand, Hong Kong, Singapore, South Africa, and a handful of other mostly English-speaking countries. Canada's most populous city, Toronto, has a daytime population of 3.5 million in an area of 650 square km (246 square miles)[7]. Toronto's EMS operates as a third (separate) city government service, independent of fire and police and is the sole provider of emergency medical response for the city.[8] A timeline for Toronto EMS is presented below to illustrate the evolution of a paramedic-based EMS system. Selected major medical breakthroughs and events in prehospital care elsewhere (in italics) have been included as well.

1832	The Toronto Board of Health organizes a horse-drawn ambulance service to transport victims of cholera.[8]
1863	*Red Cross is established in Europe.[9]*
1865	*The first known US civilian hospital–based ambulance service is started out of Commercial (now the Cincinnati General) Hospital in Cincinnati, Ohio.[10]*
1881	Toronto General Hospital starts a hospital-based ambulance service.[8]
1883	The City of Toronto acquires two ambulances to transport those with infectious disease to the local sanitarium.[7]
1888	The Toronto Police Force begins to operate full-time emergency ambulance service using four horse-drawn vehicles.[8]
1889	St. John's Ambulance Brigade begins to offer formal training for ambulance attendants.[8]
1889	The city of Toronto's Department of Public Health (DPH) takes over the responsibility of transporting contagious patients. The DPH continues to provide ambulance service for the citizens of Toronto until 1967.[8]
1897	*The London Metropolitan Asylums Board (MAB) establishes the first permanent ambulance service in London, England, to transport patients to its hospitals.[11,13]*
1899	*Michael Reese Hospital in Chicago, Illinois (US), begins to operate an automobile ambulance capable of speeds up to 16 mph.[12]*

1911   The first motorized ambulance is purchased by a Toronto funeral home.[3,8]

1913   Toronto Police Ambulance Service begins converting from horse-drawn to motorized vehicles. The process is completed by 1918.[8]

1928   *The first US rescue squad (Roanoke Life Saving Crew) is started in Roanoke, VA.[12]*

1930   *London City Council takes over all ambulance services in London.[11,13]*

1933   The Toronto Police Department ends its involvement in the city's ambulance service and turns the operation of their ambulances over to the Department of Public Health. [3,8]

1947   *A 14-year-old child's heart is successfully defibrillated during open heart surgery in Cleveland, Ohio.[12]*

1948   *In the US 40,000 citizens are trained in first aid by the American Red Cross as part of nation-wide civil defense.[12]*

1951   *Helicopters are used for medical evacuations during the Korean war.[12]*

1952   *Dr. Paul Zoll, Chief of the Cardiac Clinic at Beth Israel Hospital in Boston, performs successful external electrical stimulation of a patient's heart during cardiac arrest.[14]*

1953   The Metropolitan Toronto municipality is created, which dramatically increases the service area. Nonetheless ambulance operations remain fragmented, with sporadic and often delayed service.[3,8]

1956   *Dr. Elan and Dr. Peter Safar develop mouth-to-mouth resuscitation, challenging the widely accepted pressure-arm lift technique.[12]*

1959   *Johns Hopkins Hospital researchers in Baltimore, Maryland, develop the first portable defibrillator.[12]*

1960   *Dr. Zoll demonstrates that external electrical counter-shock is effective in terminating supraventricular tachycardia and ventricular tachycardia.[14]*

1960   *Closed cardiac massage is described by Dr. Kouwenhoven and colleagues in JAMA. Dr. Kouwenhowen is also heavily involved in the development of early defibrillators.[15]*

1960   *Captain Martin McMahon, commander of the Baltimore (Maryland) City Fire Department Ambulance Division, experiments with various types of artificial respiration by paralyzing firefighters to determine which method works best.[12]*

1960   *Los Angeles County Fire Department in California equips every engine, ladder, and*

rescue company with a resuscitator and is the first large department to uniformly adopt medical emergency responsibility.[12]

1965   *More people in the US died in auto accidents (50,000) than in 8 years of the Vietnam War.[12]*

1965   *President Lyndon Johnson signs into law the National Highway Safety Act. This begins the National Highway Traffic Safety Administration.[12]*

1966   *"Accidental Death & Disability — The Neglected Disease of Modern Society" is published by The National Research Council. Also known as "The White Paper," it was the catalyst for improving the delivery of prehospital care. An excerpt from the report states: "Expert consultants returning from both Korea and Vietnam have publicly asserted that, if seriously wounded, their chances for survival would be better in the zone of combat than on the average city street."[12]*

1966   *Dr. Pantridge in Belfast, Ireland, starts delivering prehospital coronary care using ambulances and demonstrates improved survival in out-of-hospital cardiac events.[12]*

1966   The Carl Goldenberg Report recommends that the Municipality of Metropolitan Toronto take over all remaining public ambulance services and set up a Central Ambulance Dispatch to coordinate all ambulance activity.[3,8]

1967   The amalgamated Toronto City's suburban fire departments surrender their ambulances, resulting in the evolution of the Dept. of Public Health Ambulance Service into the city-operated Department of Emergency Services (DES). DES provides centralized dispatch services to remaining private operators.[8]

1967   *The American Ambulance Association publishes an article that states that as many as 25,000 Americans are either crippled or left permanently disabled as a result of the efforts of untrained or poorly trained ambulance personnel.[12]*

1968   *Dr. Grace out of St. Vincent's Hospital in New York City starts the first mobile coronary care unit in the US Originally staffed with physicians, they are later replaced by paramedics.[12]*

1968   *The American Telephone and Telegraph (AT&T) begins to reserve the digits "911" for emergency use.[12]*

1968   *The Virginia Ambulance Law is passed in the state of Virginia, establishing the state's authority to regulate ambulances, verify first-aid training, and issue permits.[12]*

1968 *The American College of Emergency Physicians (ACEP) is formed.[12]*

1969 *The Miami, Florida Fire Department starts the nation's first paramedic program under Dr. Eugene Nagel. Shortly thereafter the very first out-of-hospital defibrillation occurs with the patient surviving and leaving the hospital neurologically intact.[12]*

1969 *In Seattle, Dr. Leonard Cobb at Harbor View Medical Center teams up with the Seattle Fire Department and creates Medic I using a recreational vehicle manned by firefighters based at the hospital and dispatched only on cardiac-related calls.[12]*

1969 Experiments in prehospital advanced life support begin in Toronto with the introduction of "Cardiac One," a unit staffed by a hospital intern (physician) that carries a large "portable" monitor.[3,8]

1969 *The Heartmobile, staffed by a physician and three firemen, is introduced in Columbus, Ohio, by Ohio State University Medical Center. Later it will become part of the Columbus Division of Fire and physicians will abandon their role in prehospital care in Columbus.[12]*

1969 *The Miami Florida Fire Department begins its paramedic program under the direction of Dr. Eugene Nagel. This includes radio transmission of ECGs and on-line direction of paramedics by physicians.[12]*

1970 *The Charlottesville-Albemarle Rescue Squad in Charlottesville, Virginia (US), starts the nation's first volunteer paramedic program under Dr. Richard Crampton. One of their first patients was President Lyndon Johnson, who suffered a heart attack while visiting his son-in-law Chuck Robb there.[12]*

1971 *The popular television program Emergency! debuts on television in the United States. At the start of the show, there were only 12 paramedic units in the entire country. Four years later at least 50% of the population of this country is within 10 minutes of a paramedic unit.[12]*

1972 The province of Ontario begins to train ambulance crews through the community colleges. Training consisted of 1,400 hours of classroom and field experience. Today's entry level training takes two years.[3,8]

1973 *St. Anthony's Hospital in Denver, Colorado, starts the nation's first civilian aeromedical transport service.[12]*

1973 *The Star of Life is published by the US DOT (Department of Transportation) as the official symbol of EMS.[12]*

1973 *The EMS Systems Act (public law 93-144) is passed by the US Congress, which funds 300 regional EMS systems.[12]*

1974 A number of tragic incidents involving the death of children and long ambulance times point out deficiencies in the Toronto system and result in calls for change.[3,8]

1975 *Emergency medicine is recognized as a specialty in the US.[12]*

1975 *The University of Pittsburgh (Pennsylvania, US) and Nancy Caroline, MD, are awarded a contract to develop the first nationwide paramedic training course. The National Association of EMTs is formed.[12]*

1975 The Metropolitan Toronto Department of Ambulance Services is created, absorbing the last five remaining private ambulance companies and single provincial service and providing a single, unified ambulance service in Metro Toronto, which operates until 1998.[8]

1977 Ontario is the first Canadian province to provide a helicopter-based air ambulance system. The Toronto-based air ambulance program begins to serve remote areas in Northern Ontario.[16]

1978 The Canadian Association of Emergency Physicians is established.[17]

1981 *The Australasian Society of Emergency Medicine is formed.[18]*

1980 The Royal College of Physicians and Surgeons of Canada (RCPSC) recognizes the specialty of emergency medicine in Canada.[19]

1982 911 emergency telephone service is introduced in Toronto.[3,8]

1984 The first paramedic teams are trained in ALS and introduced into the Toronto system. Some go on to become Advanced Care Paramedics (Level III).[3,8]

1985 *The National Association of EMS Physicians is formed in the US.[12]*

1991 *The Commission on Accreditation of Ambulance Services sets standards and benchmarks for ambulance services to obtain in the US.[12]*

1995 Paramedics begin to defibrillate patients in the field in Toronto.[3,8]

1995 Toronto Level II paramedics go into service. They are accredited a year later by the Canadian Medical Association.[3,8]

1996 Toronto EMS begins a mountain bike program.[3,8]

1995   *Los Angeles City Fire Department institutes EMT Assessment and Paramedic Engine companies.*[12]

1996   *New York City EMS is absorbed by the Fire Department of New York (FDNY).*[12]

1997   *The US cities of San Francisco and Chicago institute paramedic engine companies.*[12]

1998   Metropolitan Toronto is restructured from a regional government overseeing six member municipalities into a single, unified city. Metro Ambulance becomes Toronto Ambulance, and later adopts its current name to reflect its evolving role from primarily a provider of medical transportation to an actual provider of medical care.[3,8]

2003   Severe Acute Respiratory Syndrome (SARS) outbreak occurs in Toronto; five paramedics are infected and hundreds quarantined.[3,8]

Today (December 2009) the Toronto EMS service employs almost 1,200 individuals, including four levels of paramedics and over 100 dispatchers who work out of 41 dedicated EMS stations geographically distributed across the city. Toronto EMS operates about 250 vehicles, 150 of which are ALS ambulances.[7] It also operates 18 Emergency Response Units (ERUs). These are rapid response vehicles that are staffed by a single paramedic who can assess and treat but not transport. The ERUs supplement the approximately 90 ambulances in service during peak times.[3] Ornge, a privately held air ambulance contractor, provides air ambulance services under contract to the Government of Ontario.[16] Using computer-aided dispatch and the Advanced Medical Priority Dispatch System and aided by an automatic vehicle locating system, the Toronto EMS communications center processes about 425,700 calls per year and responds to approximately 265,000 requests for service, resulting in about 180,000 patient transports a year.[3] Pre-arrival instructions are routinely given and a translation service is available.[3,8]

Throughout the rest of Canada, the history of ambulance services has also been one of numerous local and individual initiatives, including volunteer ambulance brigades, private operators, and fire departments.[20,21] During the 1950s and 1960s ambulance services were often run by funeral homes, a model then also common in the US, presumably because they were the only vehicles configured to carry a stretcher, and they were used to interfacing with hospitals.

In the Montreal region of the province of Quebec, city-wide ambulance service was originally introduced by the city's police service (Service de Policie de la Ville de Montreal) in 1958. The surrounding suburbs initially copied this model, but when their police services were centralized under the Montreal Urban Community in 1970, so was their ambulance service.[22] In the 1980s and 1990s, changes to the prehospital system led to the creation of the Urgences-santé. Modeled somewhat after the French Service Mobile d'Urgence et de Réanimation (SAMU) and in sharp contrast to the rest of North America, this service used physicians in the field to provide advanced care until 2002.[21] Interestingly, the idea never really caught on in the rest of the province, which continued to evolve its EMS using EMTs, as did the rest of Canada.

On the other side of Canada, in the province of British Columbia (BC), ambulance services in the past were also largely uncoordinated, consisting of private operators, often funeral homes, as well as fire and municipal services. As a result of recommendations made by the Foulkes Commission's report on health care released in 1973, the Government of British Columbia created the Emergency Health Services Commission (EHSC), which in turn created the BC Ambulance Service on July 4, 1974. This agency now serves to standardize care throughout the entire province.[20]

United States of America

Following the city of Cincinnati and predating Toronto by a few years, New York City's Bellevue Hospital established a hospital-based emergency ambulance service in 1869 under the leadership of a Dr. Dalton, who had served during the Civil War as the director of a field ambulance corps.[1] Initially staffed by physicians and surgeons, these ambulances were dispatched by telegraph.[23] However, as call volumes rose, orderlies were frequently sent, in a move that presaged the evolution of EMS in the US. Other hospital and municipal ambulance services soon started up, much as they would do in Toronto. Meanwhile, this model began to be copied in other parts of the country.[1] Just up the coast from New York, in 1892 and at about the same time as Toronto, Boston City Hospital Ambulance Service, the forerunner of today's Boston EMS, began operations with 11 horses and 2 ambulance carriages. Their only function was to deliver patients to the hospital, and they provided no prehospital care except for field amputations by surgeons.[24] An ambulance "satellite" at the Boston City Hospital Relief Station in Haymarket Square opened a few years later in 1900. More ambulance stations followed as horse-drawn ambulances were gradually replaced by mechanized units. Eventually the Police Department's ambulances took over much of the work.

In time Bellevue was joined by a conglomeration of other private, hospital, and municipal services that were gradually merged into the New York City Health and Hospitals Corporation, which dispatched both its own ambulances and those of area hospitals.[23]

With the explosion of resuscitation research and mobile cardiac care units in the 1960s to the 1970s (see timeline) prehospital care in the US began to evolve rapidly. An influx of military medics from the Vietnam War provided a readily available supply of people who could become paramedics. Meanwhile Fire Departments faced with decreasing numbers of fires were looking to preserve their existence and many moved to assume the public safety function inherent in the EMT and paramedic. The acceptance of emergency medicine as a specialty in both Canada and the US helped as well, as the emergency physician was a natural EMS ally. At the same time the recognition that large numbers of people were dying on the highways and byways of America led to government action and money to promote improved ambulance services in the 1970s. Today EMTs and paramedics are found throughout the entire country, although with considerable variation in training and duties between different states. Physicians are seen only infrequently in the prehospital care role and are usually in an EMS prehospital advisory role.

United Kingdom

At about the same time as EMS systems were beginning to get organized on the European continent and across the ocean, the first permanent ambulance service in London was established by the Metropolitan Asylums Board (MAB) in 1897 to transport patients to its hospitals.[11] Their work would eventually be assumed by a municipal authority, when in 1930 it was taken over by the London City Council, a pattern that was often repeated in other countries as their systems matured. In 1946 the National Health Service (NHS) Act was passed, which made it a requirement for ambulances to be freely available for all who called them.[13] The present-day London Ambulance Service was established in 1965 by the fusion of nine other existing services in the London area. It has since grown from 156 ambulances in 1930 to over 400, with 100 rapid response cars, 10 motorcycles, and 14 bicycle units.[13] Prehospital care in the UK is provided by registered paramedics, most of whom work for the regional NHS trusts, of which there are 17 throughout the UK Physicians attend in the field as members of BASICS (British Association for Immediate Care) or as doctors employed by London HEMS (Helicopter EMS).[25,26] A number of private providers continue to exist.[27] This includes St. John Ambulance, which has over

40,000 volunteers and 1,000 ambulances throughout the country and was instrumental in the evolution of ambulance services throughout the UK, Australia, New Zealand, South Africa, and other Commonwealth countries.[28]

THE DOCTOR IN THE FIELD AND ON THE AMBULANCE

France

Possibly the earliest EMS effort in Europe was that of Larrey, one of Napoleon's surgeons, who organized a system of "flying ambulances" in 1792 which more or less definitively established the role of the ambulance in military conflict. A year later and following the 23-hour Austrian Embassy fire in Paris, the "Corps des Gardes-Pompes de la Ville de Paris" (fire department) was organized, which in 1819 by Imperial Decree of the Emperor Napoleon Bonaparte became a military organization. From its very beginning until the present day the fire department has had a role in providing emergency rescue and ambulance services to the citizens of Paris. Today the Paris Fire Department operates 69 ambulances, helping to back up the physician-staffed Paris SAMU.[29]

Physician involvement in French EMS began in earnest when the first SMUR (Service Mobile d'Urgence et de Réanimation) or "Emergency and Resuscitation Mobile Service" was created in Paris in 1956 by Professor Maurice Cara to transport critically ill patients from one hospital to another during a polio epidemic.[30] Gradually their responsibilties grew to include emergency response. However this concept of physican mobile intensive care units did not extend out to the rest of the country until 1965, when it was finally replicated throughout all of France. Today physicians play a major role in the assessment, treatment, and transport of many EMS patients in France. However the fire department continues to be involved as well, providing response, assessment, and transport for some of the less seriously injured. In fact a number of callers (~35%) to SAMU do not even receive an ambulance response.[31] Depending on the call, the physician-supervised dispatcher may elect to send a general practitioner to make a "house call" or simply refer the caller to their own doctor instead. Other response options include EMT-staffed ambulances, BLS trained firefighter first responders with AEDs, a physician-staffed mobile intensive care unit SMUR, or a physician-staffed rapid response car to rendezvous on the scene with other responding units. Pre-arrival instructions are routinely given to callers by dispatch.[31,32]

Germany

As in France, German physicians have long played a major role in their nation's EMS response. It was this observation that led to the concept of the Franco–German model of EMS in which physicians play a major role in the provision of out-of-hospital care.[33,34] In recent years, however, this paradigm is shifting as more and more often the prehospital doctors are being augmented and replaced by paramedics.

The development of ambulance services in Germany started the way it did in so many other countries in the late 19th century, mainly with untrained volunteer aid and rescue organizations.[35] Although the idea of sending the doctor to the patient in an emergency rather than bringing the patient to the doctor existed before the Second World War, it was not until after the war that this began to be realized on a large scale, when a number of university medical centers including those in Cologne, Frankfurt, Heidelberg, and Munich began to work on this. Additionally, the increasing motorized traffic beginning in the early 1950s saw increasing numbers of dead and injured on the roadways, and this was additional impetus to the professionalization of prehospital care. Meanwhile, in most rural areas the German Red Cross provided and continues to provide ambulance services, while in some cities and urban areas the fire department is the major EMS provider.[35]

In order to provide a higher standard of care among the volunteers and untrained responders and to help standardize care throughout the nation, the occupation of *Rettungssanitäter* was created in the 1970s. This position requires only three months of training and is uniform throughout Germany. Recognizing the limitations of this level of provider, an additional level of prehospital provider was introduced in 1989, that of the *Rettungsassistent*, which requires two years of training. In most cases these paramedics can perform assessments and some interventions on their own, although many ALS procedures are allowed to be done only under the direction and supervision of a physician. In some life-threatening situations paramedics can perform these actions in the absence of a physician.[35,36]

Physicians who work on the ambulances (*Notarzt*) are most often anesthesiologists. At this time emergency medicine is not yet recognized as an independent or distinct medical specialty. German general practitioners (GPs) are not formally affiliated with the EMS system; however, they both interact with and impact on the EMS system. Most cities and counties run a service called *Ärztlicher Hausbesuchsdienst* (Physician Home Call Service), which arranges for a GP to make house calls for all people in the specific area. This physician will see patients from his or her own practice but will also visit and treat patients all over the area when on call. This provides a better treatment option for those patients who, in other EMS systems, might generate low-acuity ambulance calls. Occasionally, the visiting GP will contact the EMS dispatcher and request an ambulance.[36]

Today the EMS service in Berlin is organized by the fire department as a two-tiered system. The first tier consists of numerous paramedic-staffed ambulances housed at fire stations. These paramedics are trained to perform CPR, including bag-mask ventilation, and to use semiautomated defibrillators. They are supported by a second tier of hospital-based mobile intensive care units (MICUs), each staffed by a paramedic and an "emergency physician."[37] In some communities the doctor rides in a rapid response vehicle or chase car. In most emergencies, only the ambulance is dispatched. However, if the situation at the scene is of a more severe nature, the ambulance crew can call the physician for assistance. In certain situations such as unconsciousness, cardiac arrest, respiratory distress, or chest pain, the physician will be dispatched simultaneously and rendezvous with the ambulance at the scene.[36]

The obvious advantage of this rendezvous system is that the physician is used sparingly for the most critical cases and therefore fewer are required to cover the service area. The paramedic ambulances can handle the more common but less serious cases as well as transport the stabilized critically ill patient, freeing up the physician for the next critical case. This arrangement has been copied by other agencies in other countries. Prague EMS has been operating its rendezvous system for years, and this model is being adopted by some of the other Czech and Slovak cities. In reality it is analogous to the two-tiered response systems seen in certain US cities in which a smaller number of paramedics back up a much larger number of BLS units.

Austria

Despite an early start with Vienna's EMS back in 1881 with the formation of the "Vienna Voluntary Rescue Society," well-organized EMS in Austria did not begin to occur until the 1970s, when motivated general practitioners started to cooperate with organizations responsible for patient care and transportation, mainly in rural areas.[9,38] In 1983 the Austrian Society for Emergency and Disaster was founded with the goal of educating and training physicians, paramedics, and nursing staff working in emergency medical systems and to coordinate research activities in prehospital medicine. In 1987, the Austrian Medical Association developed criteria for education and training of emergency physicians that became national law in 1998. Like France and Germany, Austria also uses EMTs. However, they are a much more recent phenomenon, having been legally recognized only since 2002. There are two levels of EMTs: The Basic EMT (*Rettungssanitater*), with 260 hours of training and an exam, can provide BLS care, CPR, and defibrillation, and the advanced EMT (*Notfallsanitater*) has the skill set of a US paramedic, although with much less independence and authority to act.[38]

Czech Republic and Poland

The first Polish EMS agencies started in Krakow in 1891 and developed tremendously throughout Poland after the Second World War when the local emergency departments, helicopter emergency services, and first responder ambulance services started to cooperate with the fire service. Currently, however, EMS is a separate service, although all firefighters are trained as EMTs.[5] Physicians continue to play a major prehospital role but paramedics are recognized and utilized. Emergency medicine is a recognized specialty; consequently many resuscitation ambulances previously staffed by anesthesiologists are being staffed by trained emergency physicians. The physician is accompanied by two additional personnel who may be nurses or paramedics. Other primary response ambulances, although staffed by a physician, may contain only one paramedic or nurse. Since 2007 transport ambulances for patients not requiring ongoing invasive care or blood transfusion are staffed by paramedics. In some urban areas, paramedics on motorcycles are also used to provide a more rapid response.[5,39]

Northern Europe

The EMS systems in Northern Europe exhibit variable structures, with mainly prehospital physicians used in the Scandinavian countries and mixed paramedic or physician rendezvous systems used in most other areas.[39] In the Netherlands paramedics are highly trained professionals who must first complete nurse training and then have critical care experience; they then can go to paramedic school. There is no regular on-the-scene physician back-up, and the nurse-paramedics operate independently using protocols. This situation arose in part because there were no certified emergency physicians until recently (EM was approved as an independent specialty in 2007) who

could provide medical direction or a comprehensive level of care for the undifferentiated patient in the ED.

In contrast, Denmark is mostly covered by a two-tiered system with three levels of paramedics (basic, intermediate, and advanced) backed up by physicians in a rendezvous system. Only physicians are allowed to intubate. In Copenhagen, the Copenhagen Fire Brigade provides ambulance service and does its own dispatch. In the remainder of the country dispatch is handled by the police, and ambulance services are provided by Falck, a Danish company that bought its first ambulance in 1908 and also provides 60% of the Danish fire protection services.[40-42]

Elsewhere in Europe, despite the role that untrained volunteers played in the early days of prehospital care, physicians play a major role in the EMS systems in the countries of the former Soviet bloc as well as in most of the Mediterranean countries. The decision to use physicians has been driven by many factors in these countries. In part the decision has been economic because physicians have been abundant and often not paid much more than nurses or paramedics. In theory this enabled the system to provide a higher level of provider, although in reality because of poor pay and without specialized training for many, this was never a profession or career but rather a "stepping stone" to something else. As professionalism has crept in, standards and expectations are changing, and this is impacting the models for the delivery of prehospital care. In many countries, however, a physician was also required because there were no true EDs in any of the hospitals, most of which were organized on a pavilion model with different buildings (pavilions) housing different divisions or specialties. Thus ambulance patients required a high level of triage to determine which ward they were to be transferred to, and this decision was best made by a physician.[39]

ASIA

Prehospital care systems in Asia are a relatively recent phenomenon and vary tremendously from extremely sophisticated to nonexistent, often in the same region or area. Growth and development have been slow, in part paralleling the slow recognition of Emergency Medicine as a specialty as well as from a lack of financial resources that are often concentrated in urban pockets. On rare occasions, progress has been rapid, usually surrounding major national events such as the Olympics or following major natural disasters such as the 2004 tsunami affecting Thailand and surrounding regions, or the 2008 Sichuan Province earthquake in China. While tragic in terms of injury and loss of life, these events have revealed system deficiencies and illustrate the importance of prehospital care. There are also societal changes as this part of the world moves from a predominantly agrarian and family-centered society with strong cultural beliefs about destiny and the value of life to a more mobile consumerist and urban-based society with altogether different expectations. Coincident with this there are also changing patterns of disease and injury wrought by increasing roadway traffic, urbanization and changing lifestyles, and extended life expectancy.

Industrialized and "developed" countries such as Japan have long faced difficulties in providing efficient prehospital care in a densely populated and sophisticated urban environment. This issue now faces providers in many Asian nations experiencing rapidly growing urban areas, most notably China. Nonetheless, rural settings remain challenging for EMS in all countries as health care providers must design systems that can disperse sparse resources to the farthest rural areas, which then compete for resources in crowded, rapidly growing cities.

This situation is frequently found in India, where lack of funds and equipment and the poor rural road conditions are among the obstacles to the advancement of prehospital systems. Even when prehospital care exists at a local level, inefficient organization at the regional and national levels becomes a barrier to further progress and encourages the development of multiple systems. China is an example of a country with several different prehospital systems in place without true national standardization or effective enforcement of government prehospital protocols. The inadequacies of China's existing prehospital systems have become starkly evident during recent national disasters. Thailand has experienced similar difficulties. While a few of Thailand's prehospital systems are advanced, these successes are not replicated nationally. Recent events in that country have demonstrated how unforeseen events can overwhelm even prehospital systems that have disaster plans in place as well as those with only superficial organization of services.

The next section will focus on the timelines of EMS development in India, Japan, China, and Thailand to illustrate how EMS systems have developed to address unique environments or situations relevant to Asia.

India

With about 1.3 billion people, India has become the most populous country ahead of China but is only seventh in terms of land area.[43,44] Although most of the population is still rural (72% in 2001), this percentage has been steadily dropping. In recent years there has been a great increase in industry, mobility, and urbanization, which in turn has led to a higher incidence of injury related to accidents.[45] Densely populated and congested urban centers coexist with remote rural areas with limited resources, which creates a challenging environment for the provision of homogeneous or standardized prehospital care. This position puts a unique strain on the already limited resources of a rapidly developing nation in which prehospital systems are in their infancy.

Given its size and the diversity of its population, it is perhaps no surprise that prehospital care is grossly different among different states in India. In most areas there is little organization of trauma care even at the local level. A few regions have made significant advances and stronger leadership has emerged recently, but there is still no cohesive national network in place. A significant obstacle, as in many other nations, has been the need for the populace and government to fully recognize the importance of organized, efficient systems of prehospital care.

Timeline History of Prehospital Care in India

1984 The city of Delhi develops a plan to create an ambulance service run by the local government. However, the Centralized Ambulance Transport Service (CATS) is not implemented until 16 years later.[46]

1997 In response to a large number of accidental injuries, the city of Bangalore creates an EMS system and designates "1062" as the access number for emergency services. The network now includes 40 hospitals and 45 ambulances.[46]

1998 Hyderabad city links together a network of emergency departments to develop an EMS system managed by the Apollo Group, which has since started similar networks in other regions of India. The emergency access number is "1066."[46]

1999 The Pune city EMS system is initiated at Sanjeevan Hospital and has since grown to include several area hospitals in the partnership. "1050" is selected as the emergency phone number.[47]

1999 The Society for Emergency Medicine India (SEMI) is formed.[48]

1999 The First National Conference of Emergency Medicine is held in Hyderabad and has been held annually ever since.[49]

2000   The Society for Emergency Medicine India (SEMI) is recognized.[48]

2000   The EMS council of Pune is formed.[47]

2000   Delhi's municipal Centralized Ambulance Transport Service (CATS) is finally implemented. It coexists along with several private ambulance services in the same city.[46]

1999-
2002   Pune EMS increases its supply of ambulances and equipment and incorporates additional hospitals into its system. The Indian Red Cross Society begins participating.[47]

2002   The Academy of Traumatology begins studying the various trauma systems throughout India.[50]

2002   The Lifeline Foundation, a private organization out of Vadodara, Gujurat, is formed to investigate the provision of free ambulance and emergency medical services in India. It has since initiated several projects in the states of Gujurat and Maharashtra.[51]

2002   The Highway Rescue Project is initiated by the Lifeline Foundation to provide emergency services on highways in the state of Gujarat. It incorporates a comprehensive rescue system of ambulances, police, fire services, and advanced rescue/extraction equipment. This program has since spread to highways in other states.[46]

2002   The group Ambulance Access for All (AAA) forms an EMS system in the city of Mumbai.[46]

2002   The first paramedic training program was started by Symbiosis International University, which offers a Post Graduate Diploma in Emergency Medical Services (PGDEMS). Similar programs have since started in six other locales in the state of Maharashtra.[47]

2003   The National Conference of Emergency Medicine (EMCON) is organized in Pune.[47]

2004   A group of eight hospitals in Ahmedebad, Gujurat, create an EMS council to coordinate EMS activities, including ambulance dispatch from a central command center. Its activities lasted until the state government contracted prehospital services to a nonprofit organization.[46]

2004   The Apollo group and Stanford University in California initiate a one-year Emergency Medical Technician Intermediate (EMT-I) training program in Hyderabad, Andhra Pradesh. A six-month paramedic education course is begun in Ahmedabad, Gujurat through the collaborative efforts of the Apollo group, the R Tolat Foundation, and New York Long Island Jewish Hospital.[46,49]

2004   The International Trauma Life Support (ITLS) program is introduced at Pune.[47]

2005   The Emergency Management Research Institute (EMRI) is created to organize emergency prehospital care with "108" as the official number to reach the EMRI emergency services (including police and fire departments) in the city of Hyderabad, Andhra Pradesh. Since then the project has spread to ten other states.[52]

2005   The Lifeline Foundation organizes a free ambulance service for a consortium of nine public and private hospitals in Vadodara, Gujarat.[51]

2005   The Indian Institute of Emergency Medical Services begins testing an EMS system in Kottayam, Kerala.[46]

2006   Vinayaka Mission University (VMU) in Salem, Tamil Nadu, offers a Bachelor of Science Emergency & Trauma Care Technology course.[46]

2007   EMS bill passes in Gujarat.[46]

2007   Delhi is the first city in the country to implement "ambulance standards" in response to a mandate from the high courts.[46]

2007   The Ministry of Road Transport and Highways forms a committee to provide recommendations for trauma care on highways.[46]

2007   The Central Health Ministry creates the Paramedical and Physiotherapy Central Councils bill. The Committee on Health and Family Welfare is given the responsibility for evaluating the effectiveness of creating standards for paramedic education and training.[46]

2007   The National Rural Health Mission (NRHM) begins providing funding to assist states in improving their rural prehospital care systems. These funds are supposed to be provided until 2011.[46]

2009   EM is officially recognized as the 30th specialty in India — 10 years after the founding of SEMI. (Note that EM was recognized in the US 11 years after the founding of the first emergency medicine society.)[49]

2009   Fifth Indo-US Emergency Medicine Summit is held at Coimbatore, Tamil Nadu.[49]

Current Prehospital Care System in India

Indian EMS has made several advances in recent years, often the result of local initiatives and supported by private funds and overseas agencies. As occurred in various "western" nations, numerous local government, hospitals, and private agencies run most of the existing services, which tend to be located in urban areas. Only recently has leadership at the national level begun to take a more active role.[50] However, there are few national standards in place, and with no institutions of learning aimed at paramedic education, national recognition of the EMS profession is still elusive.[53] Not surprisingly then, staffing of ambulances does not always include qualified personnel.[54] Only a few of the larger and well-funded healthcare institutions are able to provide formal training for their medical personnel. Education for ambulance personnel includes paramedic courses, but these are limited and again confined to urban areas, often near a large university. The goal of standardizing paramedic education remains elusive. The Academy of Traumatology offers physicians education in basic skills with the National Trauma Management Course (NTMC) and is accredited by the International Association of Trauma Surgery and Intensive Care (IATSIC).[50] Smaller institutions and those that are primarily supported through public funds are not yet able to offer this type of training, and nothing comparable is available for paramedics.

The local organization of EMS in most areas of India is deficient. There is usually no central dispatch to direct ambulance services. There are also no national EMS protocols for ambulance personnel to follow with regard to appropriate patient assessment, triage, transfer, and disposition to a medical facility. Patient disposition to a medical facility is usually based on the requests of patients or family or the patient's financial status.[50] This, rather than what is best for the patient's health, determines how and where a patient is transported.

The Future of Prehospital Care in India

Recent years have seen an emergence of greater leadership in Indian EMS, especially at local levels, often with the assistance of private organizations and a large overseas Indian community. Services are being consolidated and standards are being introduced, although locally. Emergency medicine was recently recognized as a specialty, and this will likely accelerate the evolution of prehospital care as well. However, there are still many obstacles facing Indian EMS systems. The low numbers of trained physicians, many of whom seek employment outside the country, create difficulties in staffing EDs. Therefore, it is unlikely that physicians will ever be employed in the prehospital setting to the extent seen in Europe, and it is likely that prehospital care will be heavily dependent on paramedics. This poses a major challenge, as there is the lack of any official recognition for EMTs or EMT-Ps. Prehospital care

also employs no guidelines to standardize ambulance equipment, staff, emergency facilities, and training. This leads to lack of organized patient triage and disposition. These issues must be addressed before Indian EMS systems can take the next steps in improving prehospital care.

Japan

Japan is a leading industrialized nation that, along with Hong Kong and Singapore, has one of the better developed EMS systems in Asia. It has several characteristics that set it apart from other systems in the area, mainly in the successes the national government has had in standardizing and organizing prehospital care. This may stem from its relatively compact land area (slightly smaller than California and slightly larger than Germany) as well as the fact that some form of prehospital care has existed since before the Second World War.[43,55]

Timeline History of Prehospital Care in Japan

1930s   Just prior to the Second World War the Tokyo Police begins organizing ambulance services for trauma victims.[55]

1947   The Fire Defense Agency is created to provide ambulance transport.[56]

1961   Hospitals begin providing round-the-clock emergency care.[55]

1964   Tokyo Olympic Games. The emergency notification system is created.[57]

1970   Osaka gas explosion.

1973   The Japanese Association for Acute Medicine (JAAM) is created in an effort to address issues in trauma medicine.[56]

1976   The Emergency Medical Care Consultation Committee (EMCCC) presents several recommendations for the improvement of emergency and prehospital care.[58]

1977   The Ministry of Health and Welfare acts on the EMCCC's recommendations and organizes a three-level system of emergency care.[56]

1977   Supplements to the emergency notification system are added.[57]

1987   An amendment to the Fire Protection Law makes fire departments responsible for medical emergencies such as stroke and heart attack and not just for trauma victims.[56]

1990   The Medical Study Group for Quality (EMSQ) forms to study the nation's trauma systems. Their research exposes weaknesses in the existing systems.[59]

1991	The paramedic profession is officially recognized, and paramedics are required to be nationally certified.[57]
1991	Japan's Lower House of Representatives makes the recommendation that prehospital systems use the European model of dispatching physicians in response to emergency calls.[57]
1991	The Emergency Life-Saving Technicians (ELST) Law is passed, creating the role of paramedics with advanced training.[56,60]
1995	Kobe (Hanshin-Awaji) earthquake.
1997	The National Emergency Medical System is established.[57]
1998	An amendment promoting helicopter transport of patients is added to the Existing Fire Service Law.[56]
1999	Initial efforts to set up prehospital helicopter transport systems serving eastern and western areas in Japan are made by the Ministry of Health and Welfare.[56]
2000	National protocols for field personnel are developed.[59]
2000	A report is published by the Ministry of Welfare about the medical care and transport provided by existing prehospital systems.[57]
2000	The Basic Trauma Life Support (BTLS) course and the Prehospital Trauma Care Japan (PTCJ) course are offered.[59]
2001	The Doctor-Heli program is started by the Ministry of Health, Labor, and Welfare, putting physicians on board helicopters.[59]
2001	Congress passes the Lifesaving Emergency Medical Technician (LEMT) Act.[59]
2003	The Japanese Association for Acute Medicine (JAAM) begins overseeing the BTLS and PTCJ courses.[59]
2003	The Japan Prehospital Trauma Evaluation and Care (JPTEC) council is created under the JAAM to standardize education for prehospital personnel, train course instructors, and develop national protocols for these prehospital providers.[59]
2003	The Japanese Society for Emergency Medicine (JSEM) recommends allowing paramedics to initiate procedures without waiting until an ambulance is on the scene to transport the patient.[57]
2004	The Japanese Association for the Surgery of Trauma and JAAM develop a national trauma registry database.[57]
2004	The Japan Foundation for Ambulance Service Development creates guidelines for pre-

hospital triage based on the presence of 10 possible chief complaints.[60]

2006	Paramedics are allowed to administer adrenaline for patients in cardiac arrest.[57]
2006	A committee is established by the Fire and Disaster Management Agency to evaluate the use and misuse of ambulance transport.[60]
2007	The helicopter service law is passed by Congress in an effort to combat prehospital care inefficiencies and shortages.[57]

The 1964 Tokyo Olympics were a major impetus to improve the quality of emergency care in Japan and resulted in the assignment of specific healthcare facilities to provide emergency care and also increased ambulance capabilities.[55] In the late 1960s, as Japanese industry grew and urbanization progressed, there was a sharp increase in the number of road traffic accidents.[58] With little to no coordination within the existing prehospital care systems, victims were often transported to facilities ill equipped to treat their injuries. Media coverage of this deficiency and subsequent pressure on the government prompted reform of the EMS system. The national government began to assume a greater responsibility for this area of health care.

In the late 1970s the government issued several major recommendations to improve emergency care that were put into effect by the Ministry of Health and Welfare in the ensuing years. The changes included the creation of a three-level classification scheme for medical facilities, the development of tertiary care centers (emergency and critical care centers), and finally the creation of an adequate number of emergency medical information centers for each region to organize prehospital care and handle dispatch.[58]

A major gas explosion in 1970 in Osaka brought to light several deficiencies in the EMS system, including the lack of interagency communication or triage protocols. Today, Osaka has a central dispatch center for its fire and ambulance services that employs Japan's advanced computer technology.[60] In addition to appropriately direct rescue efforts, prehospital guidelines now establish a command station at the site of any future disaster and utilize field tags to triage patients.[60,61]

Another major disaster to afflict Japan was the Kobe (Hanshin-Awaji) earthquake in 1995, which killed several thousand people and injured tens of thousands more.[56,61] The magnitude of the disaster completely overwhelmed the local EMS capabilities, again in part because there was no central organization directing citywide rescue efforts or triaging patients to appropriate destinations. Consequently each local transport service operated independently, without communicating with other agencies.[55,60] Aeromedical transport, while potentially very useful in this type of situation, was underutilized. This prompted the government to amend laws to promote helicopter transport and create prehospital helicopter transport systems.[56]

There are deficiencies and discrepancies between Japan's suburban and rural-based systems, many of which have inadequate staff and equipment according to national guidelines. The majority of prehospital transport is to secondary tier facilities under the national three-tiered system.[57] Other issues relate to the paramedics themselves, who have no requirements for recertification or continuing education.[57] Furthermore, they are still not employed to their full capacity. Prior to the 1990s all ambulance personnel were limited to providing only basic life support.[56] The ELST act of 1991 created a class of paramedic with an increased level of training compared to that of EMT-I and EMT-II. However, it is only recently that paramedics have been allowed to perform procedures that are considered standing orders in most US protocols, such as administering epinephrine or defibrillation in cardiac arrest. Several national organizations and sectors of the government are investigating giving Japanese paramedics more responsibility in the prehospital setting.

China

China's large size and a population exceeding 1.3 billion people pose immense challenges to its prehospital care system.[43,62] Additionally, China possesses some of the remotest, most inaccessible regions as well as many of the fastest growing cities in the world. In 2000 approximately 36% of the population lived in urban areas. This rose by approximately 10% from 1990 to 2000. Nonetheless for now the majority of the population still lives in rural areas where access to advanced emergency care is limited to nonexistent. These people often rely on the village "barefoot doctor," an individual with minimal medical training and usually no formal training at an educational institution.[63] Not surprisingly then, prehospital care is virtually nonexistent in these locales. Even in urban areas only 25% of these urban dwellers have medical insurance, and access to ambulance care is spotty.[64] While China's prehospital care is highly variable in terms of availability, existing systems are also diverse in terms of structure and organization, and national guidelines that have been formulated to standardize these systems are not enforced. As a result, the prehospital care a patient receives in Beijing can vary greatly from that received in Sichuan.

As is so often the case, China's prehospital care had its first beginnings out of necessity and as a result of war. The large numbers of wounded seen during the Second World War required emergency care and transport that was not available at the time.[65] This situation led to an awareness of the need for an organized EMS system.

Timeline History of Prehospital Care in China

1940s   During the Second World War Dr. Norman Bethune, a Canadian surgeon, joined China's army medical service. He instructed the Chinese on rapid prehospital transport, first-aid care, and trauma management. This serves as the basis for the beginnings of China's prehospital care.[65]

1950s   Emergency service stations form an early prehospital system in urban centers.[65]

1980s   The Ministry of Health develops policies on emergency medical care in the prehospital arena.[64,65]

1983   The Chinese Association of Emergency Medicine is founded to promote and support the growth of Emergency Medicine.[64]

1984   Project HOPE funds two emergency medicine nurses from the Second Affiliated Hospital of Zhejiang University College of Medicine to go to the US for a 6-month period of training in emergency medicine.[66]

1986   The emergency phone number designated by the Ministry of Health and the Ministry of Posts and Telecommunications is "120."[65]

1986   The first national emergency care residency program in China is set up at the Peking Union Medical College Hospital.[66]

1987   The Society of Emergency Medicine is established by the Chinese Medical Association and publishes the *Chinese Journal of Emergency Medicine*.[64]

1989   Project HOPE establishes the Emergency Medicine Guidance Center in Zhejiang Province. HOPE provides the center with advanced equipment and arrangements are made for an American-trained clinician to work there.[66]

1993   The Ministry of Health establishes the National Medical Emergency Training Center (NMETC) in Shanghai. The facility coordinates workshops in prehospital care instructing ambulance personnel, physicians, nurses, college students, as well as fire fighters and policemen.[63]

1995   The Ministry of Health formulates a list of requirements for the designation of an "Emergency Service Center" and guidelines for use in disaster situations.[65]

1997   The NMETC and Tongji University develop a trial course on prehospital care, covering disaster medicine, triage, first-aid skills, and CPR.[63]

2001   Leadership from emergency centers in multiple cities forms the Emergency Center Professional Committee (ECPC) as a branch of the Chinese Hospital Association (CHA). This brings the leadership together in an effort to address the lack of national organization and promotes information exchange and sharing in an effort to develop national standards.[67]

2002   The ECPC is replaced by the Emergency Medical Center Branch.[67]

2002   The Emergency Medical Center (First Aid Station) Branch meets with representatives from 32 emergency centers and from the Ministry of Health and the CHA, resulting in a number of proposals for prehospital care, diagnosis, treatment, and protocols. The Medical Department of the Ministry of Health reviews the proposals and begins conducting trials to evaluate the validity of these protocols.[67]

2002   Training for the specialty of Emergency Medicine (EM) is incorporated into the medical school curriculum. Nanjing Medical University begins offering a major in EM.[63]

2002-2003   The "Italy project:" the Italian government and health professionals conduct workshops in prehospital care at the NMETC. The workshops are considered a success and now serve as a model for training.[63]

2003   The Second Affiliated Hospital of Zhejiang University begins offering a doctoral degree in emergency medicine.[66]

2003   SARS outbreak.

2004   The Queensland Ambulance Service (QAS) and Queensland University of Technology (QUT) begin coordinating with the Chinese Hospital Association to develop prehospital training courses.[63]

2005   A workshop involving paramedics working through simulated disasters is held in Australia by the QAS and QUT to educate representatives of the CHA.[63]

2008   Beijing Olympic Games leads to increases in the supply and efficiency of prehospital systems.[67]

2008   The Sichuan earthquake kills 87,000 people and affects an additional 46 million. Significant deficiencies are seen, especially in the communications and command structure of prehospital care.

The prehospital system is largely government funded and overseen by the Ministry of Public Health. In the various provinces and cities the local bureaus of public health provide money for staffing and operation. Prehospital care is also incorporated into local fire and police departments.[64] However, there is no coordination between these local bureaus. This contributes to the vastly different forms of prehospital systems that are currently employed in different provinces. There are currently four main models of prehospital care as illustrated in the cities of Beijing, Shanghai, Chongqing, and Guangzhou. Beijing has an Emergency Medical Center (EMC) equipped with an ED, ambulance station, and dispatch. The EMC transports patients to its own ED or to other hospitals. The Shanghai Communications Center dispatches vehicles but transports patients to the closest available hospital. In Chongqing each hospital provides its own EMS, supplying staff and vehicles for a pure hospital-based EMS system. The city of Guanzhou has a central communication center that acts solely as a dispatch service and directs vehicles from the hospital closest to the patient.[63,66] Similar to the US "911" or the European "112," a national number, "120," is dialed to reach a prehospital emergency service institution (equivalent to the US dispatch service), which forwards calls to ambulance dispatch centers.[64] In China, the paramedic profession is not officially recognized, and physicians are found on board ambulances. Physicians are not required to have training in prehospital care or any emergency medicine specialization. There are only 30 to 50 hours of EM teaching in medical school.[64] Many of the prehospital physicians are newly graduated and once graduated there are no formal EMS protocols to follow. Some health organizations are beginning to require that physicians and nurses have two to three years of clinical practice before working in prehospital care.[63] However, this is not widespread, and there is no defined requirement for training in prehospital care. There are short courses in prehospital care, for example at the training center in Shanghai, but these are not widely available. Physicians and nurses also prefer not to work in prehospital care. This is probably because of lack of recognition of this area of medicine, limited availability of training opportunities, and lower compensation. Staff shortage is especially evident in rural areas, where there may not be any type of organized prehospital care. Often, the staff of the local

ED provides this service. A few provinces have enforced more stringent requirements for the qualifications of the prehospital team that is dispatched. In Henan province (the most populous province of China) the Highway Trauma Rescue Group consists of a surgeon, two medics, an orderly, and a driver. Internal medicine, surgery, anesthesia, and emergency physicians are employed in prehospital care throughout Guangzhou.

The city of Shenzhen requires prehospital care doctors and nurses to rotate every three months in the ED. They must also know how to perform vital procedures such as intubation, CPR, defibrillation, and basics including splint/dressing application.[64] Transportation is largely via ambulance. Mobile intensive care units (MICUs) are occasionally available. There is also a monitoring vehicle that holds more equipment and medications for resuscitation. Aeromedical transport is very rarely used.[64]

Thailand

With an estimated 67 million people in an area of 513,120 square kilometers, or roughly the same area as Spain, Thailand is a "small" country compared to China or India.[43] Its health care system, particularly emergency and prehospital care, is in its early developmental stages despite an early start with the Por Tek Tsung (see timeline below). In many areas prehospital care is still limited to a taxicab-type service or a pickup truck, which provides simple transport and no medical intervention. In select regions, Thailand has a reasonably well-organized system of prehospital care, such as the trauma system in the Khon Kaen province, and following the 2004 tsunami the number of hospitals with disaster plans has increased dramatically. The latter is an excellent example of how national disasters can catalyze change in a dramatic fashion. (For more information see **Chapter 5, Interactions with Governments.**)

Timeline History of Prehospital Care in Thailand

1909   The Por Tek Teung Foundation is established by Chinese immigrants and provides volunteers to collect and bury the bodies of the indigent populace. Today this volunteer organization still transports injured victims to local hospitals and the dead to the city morgues. Since then a number of similar foundations have emerged.[68-70]

1989   Khon Kaen Regional Hospital (KKRH) develops a trauma program that is now the

most developed prehospital/trauma system in the country.[69]

1993   A hotel collapses in the city of Nakorn Ratchisima (Korat Town), killing approximately 100 and injuring several hundred. Rescue efforts are disorganized and chaotic. After this event, the Korat hospital begins developing a regional disaster plan with the help of the KKRH.[69]

1995   Campaign to educate the public on the importance of wearing motorcycle helmets and to promote compliance with helmet laws begins. Increased helmet use and a significant reduction in head injuries are seen at the trauma center (KKRH).[69]

1996   A trial program providing two years of training in prehospital care to 16 students is begun. Relying on the Internet and with no true syllabus or text, it is nonetheless an important step toward formalized training.[69]

1996   KKRH communications center is assigned the responsibility of serving as a central command for several provinces in the event of a mass casualty incident. This designation plays a vital role in the events surrounding the 2004 tsunami.[69]

1996   The Ministry of Public Health (MPH) stations midwives on motorcycles around Bangkok in an effort to prevent the delivery of babies in motor vehicles due to traffic delays.[69]

1996   Vajira Hospital in Bangkok attempts to decrease transport time by bypassing roads using speedboats, a process only partially successful because delays occur in transporting the boats from the hospital to the river.[69]

2001   The Ministry of Public Health forms a division called Narenthorn to standardize prehospital care and implement a national system in all areas. This unit forms an EMS network in the Bangkok area with plans to have local systems in place throughout the rest of the country by 2006.[68,71]

2002   The Provincial Health Department develops a comprehensive plan for EMS in Chiang Mai Province. The plan enrolls 9 of its 23 hospitals and several volunteer/charity transport services in the project.[68]

2002   The local health department in Chiang Mai holds the first Basic Trauma Life Support (BTLS) course for area prehospital providers.[68]

2004   On December 26, 2004 a large earthquake in the Indian Ocean creates a tsunami that sweeps over the southern coast of Thailand and several surrounding countries. In Thailand, the majority of victims are received at Krabi Hospital, a large regional trauma center in the Krabi province. With a disaster plan anticipating no more than 40 victims, they receive 1,300 in the first few days, a number that does not include those treated in the field. Many of the smaller hospitals have no disaster plan. Lack of coordinated prehospital care overwhelms many hospitals.[72,73]

2005   The Sumatra earthquake tests hospital preparations. A massive earthquake off the coast of Sumatra triggers tsunami fears and activates disaster plans created after the December event three months earlier. Ultimately no tidal wave or additional earthquake occurs, and after 24 hours operations are allowed to resume as normal.[72]

2008   The Emergency Medical Institute of Thailand, overseen by the Ministry of Public Health, assumes the responsibilities of Narenthorn to develop EMS.[71]

2008   The Emergency Medical Service System Act comes into effect to regulate the emergency services and raise their standards, especially the numerous competing foundations. National Institute of Emergency Medical Service System (NIEMS) is created.

In Thailand, as in so many countries, initial "EMS" was a volunteer effort to simply get the wounded to the hospital and the dead off the streets. Remnants of this still exist, and the Por Tek Teun Foundation and the Ruamkatanyu Foundation often compete with each other for patients and bodies using ambulances and pick-ups to race around in a dangerous fashion.[68,70] They also compete with the government-run services in the city. The equipment and experience found on these designated rescue vehicles varies according to different published studies. Most vehicles carry oxygen tanks and first-aid kits, and some have crews experienced in using extrication equipment to remove victims from accident sites. Others have ALS units capable of defibrillation and intubation.[68] Communication occurs via radio command centers at a local hospital or the foundation's own facilities. In Bangkok the Bangkok Metropolitan Administration (BMA) also serves as a transport service and provides more formal training for its volunteers.[69] However, other provinces have less government-organized prehospital transport and therefore small charities continue to provide volunteers

and pick-up trucks to serve this function. The Ministry of Public Health (MPH) oversees national health care through a number of Provincial Health Offices that coordinate the activities of hospitals in their defined geographic region. The largest of these hospitals are regional centers with up to 1,000 beds with the capacity to provide training for medical and prehospital staff. Slightly smaller are provincial hospitals with up to 500 beds. Last are the small community hospitals with 10 to 60 beds and only 1 to 5 physicians.[69] However, there is no government oversight of the charity or volunteer transport services. The training or equipment found in these organizations is inconsistent and often limited.

The singular event that most moved the Thai system to change was the 2004 tsunami, which spotlighted the importance of prehospital care and an organized system to address mass casualty events. The fact that a limited plan even existed probably saved many lives. Krabi Hospital, a large regional trauma center, was able to activate protocols it already had in place. Many smaller hospitals had no such contingency plans.[72,73] The few volunteer and government ambulance agencies that were unable to cope with normal traffic were simply overwhelmed and could not keep up with the demand for evacuation. With numerous patients arriving by foot, boat, or other alternative transportation, patient flow was not well directed to the appropriate-level care facility or those with the capacity to handle additional victims.[72,73]

The response to the tsunami varied by region. In Phuket the focus of prehospital services was on rapid transport to a local hospital for care.[73] There was no organization in the transport of patients or determination of transport priorities. As a result some hospitals were quickly overwhelmed by the patient load. Better communication was needed to determine patient distribution and divert transportation if required. Had patients been appropriately triaged at the scene, some could have avoided or at least delayed transport to a medical facility. This would have relieved the strain on the limited number of medical transport vehicles. This type of field triage was done in Phang Nga and Krabi provinces. Medical teams were able to offset some of the burden on the local hospital by transporting only the critically ill. They provided the remaining majority with basic care and referred some of these to primary care centers.[73] Even after the majority of tsunami victims had been evacuated from the coastal areas, medical teams and mobile units provided a vital service. They were dispatched into the community to conduct house calls, where they assessed patients and transported them as needed for further care.[73] Despite considerable improvements there are still some densely populated coastal regions where there is virtually no prehospital care. Ambulances are staffed by attendants and a driver with little to no medical training who serve to "scoop and run."[74]

The most organized and advanced prehospital system is located in the region of Khon Kaen. The province has a designated telephone number allowing residents to contact the prehospital care communication command center directly, which then dispatches ambulances staffed by nurses from Khon Kaen Regional Hospital (KKRH). KKRH functions as the region's level-one trauma center and accepts patient transfers from other hospitals. There exists a trauma audit system that reviews patient outcomes and evaluates the current quality of care provided. The trauma registry collects information on trauma patients and has used the data to implement public health initiatives, including requiring motorcycle helmets. The success of this system has been recognized nationally, leading to the creation of a national trauma registry in the capital city of Bangkok.[69]

The level of training and availability of prehospital staff continue to pose a challenge in Thailand EMS. In the Khon Kaen Regional Hospital system ambulance staff consists of nurses who fill the role of emergency medical technicians.[69] Throughout the country few physicians function in this capacity. Without a recognized paramedic profession, physicians may actually have the best type of training to allow them to function in prehospital situations. Physicians complete six years of medical school and in their last year of training rotate through the ED. Resident physicians, no matter what their specialty, also work in the ED.[71] There is, however, no formal training program or residency in Emergency Medicine and thus there are no true EM physicians. Emergency Medicine is not yet an officially recognized specialty in Thailand.

SUMMARY

EMS has its historical origins in military battlefield casualty evacuation services followed by city ambulance systems that first developed in the late 1800s. Increasing government involvement in operating EMS systems has been a common pattern in many countries. Physician-based delivery of prehospital care has evolved to care delivery by nonphysicians in many countries. The European and North American timeline of the EMS system development has been compressed in many countries currently working on improving their EMS care delivery.

The Asian countries are now experiencing a period of economic growth and increasingly urban populations. As a result, the leading cause of death in Asian nations continues to be injury, usually due to traffic accidents. Initial efforts by EMS have been to get the injured to the hospital as quickly as possible. These efforts are often performed by volunteers. However, as lifestyles change other diseases are "catching up" and will change the focus of prehospital care. As more can be done for the patient, the training and competencies of the prehospital care providers will need to go up. Organized dispatch of prehospital services, efficient transport of patients, and appropriate prehospital interventions can reduce mortality and morbidity. These will require more competent prehospital providers. At the same time the numbers of doctors in most Asian countries is not adequate to meet current needs let alone afford the luxury of placing them on ambulances.

The major issues facing EMS in this region of the world are varied and complex. National standardization of EMS protocols and recognition of the paramedic profession are still elusive in most countries. These two goals should be prioritized. They may be more easily achieved if Emergency Medicine is officially recognized as a medical specialty. Thus far, in many countries, EM still struggles for or has only recently gained this distinction. Leadership efforts should be aimed in this direction.

While the above are goals for the federal governments, local officials can contribute to EMS development in several ways. Interagency cooperation to address traffic issues and limit competition or confusion in patient triage and transport is vital. Consolidation of services is often the easiest route to ensuring uniformity of care, and we see this play out around the world as EMS systems mature. Ensuring that adequate and well-trained personnel staff transport vehicles with at least basic equipment on board is an initial step to be taken. Providing funds for the required equipment or training workshops has posed and will continue to pose a challenge.

Although there are many obstacles to the advancement of Asian EMS systems, progress has been made. EM is increasingly becoming a recognized specialty and what often follows is the establishment of an EMS profession. Nations with highly developed prehospital systems are coordinating with and lending their expertise to those without such systems. This has led to improvements in training and education efforts. Research into improving prehospital care is also becoming more prominent. The course of prehospital development in Asia will be interesting to chart in the coming years.

References

1. Marshall J. Tells development of ambulance service: growth of modern city vehicles from war types described by A. Jackson Marshall – hospitals here answer many calls. *New York Times,* Sunday February 28, 1915, p. xii.
2. City of Boston (US) http://www.cityofboston.gov/EMS/about/
3. Toronto EMS: http://www.torontoems.ca/.
4. EMS in Prague: http://www.zzshmp.cz/data/documents/6/posterbarc.pdf.
5. Hladki W, Andres J, Trybus M, Drwila R. Emergency medicine in Poland. *Resuscitation* 75: 213; 2007.
6. Ambulance Victoria, Australia: http://www.ambulance.vic.gov.au/.
7. Toronto, Canada statistics: http://www.toronto.ca/demographics/index.htm
8. Toronto EMS, History: http://www.torontoems.ca/main-site/about/ems-overview.html.
9. Dara S, Ashton RW, Farmer JC, Carlton PK. Worldwide disaster medical response: An historical perspective. *Crit Care Med* 33(1):S2; 2005.
10. Cincinnati & Ohio History Information http://www.gifttree.com/Cincinnati/Cincinnati-history.html
11. London Ambulance Service, NHS: History: http://www.londonambulance.nhs.uk/about_us/who_we_are/our_story/a_brief_history.aspx
12. EMS History: www.angelfire.com/co/fantasyfigures/710history.html
13. London Ambulance Service, NHS: Chronology: http://www.londonambulance.nhs.uk/about_us/who_we_are/our_story/chronology.aspx
14. Zoll, Major Events & Corporate Milestones: http://www.zoll.com/about-zoll/corporate-milestones/.
15. Kouwenhoven WB, Jude JR, Knickerbocker GG. Closed-chest cardiac message. *JAMA* 173(10):1064; 1960.
16. Ontario EMS history: http://www.ornge.ca/About Ornge/Pages/History.aspx (accessed Dec. 2, 2009).
17. College of Emergency Medicine, UK & Ireland: Air ambulance: http://www.collemergencymed.ac.uk/asp/resourceview.asp?ID=22.(http://www.collemergencymed.ac.uk).
18. College of Emergency Medicine, UK & Ireland: History of the Specialty: http://www.collemergencymed.ac.uk/CEM/History%20of%20the%20specialty/Landmarks%20in%20the%20development%20of%20the%20specialty/default.asp (http://www.collemergencymed.ac.uk)
19. Emergency medicine practice and training in Canada http://www.cmaj.ca/cgi/reprint/168/12/1549.
20. British Columbia Ambulance Service http://www.bcas.ca/EN/main/about/537/history-1970-1980.html.
21. Agence d'évaluation des technologies et des modes d'intervention en santé (AETMIS). Introduction of advanced life support in pre-hospital emergency medical services in Québec. Report prepared by Reiner Banken, Brigitte Côté, François de Champlain and André Lavoie (AETMIS 05-01). Montréal: AETMIS, 2005. available at http://www.jephc.com/uploads/990202WebVersion4.pdf.
22. Urgences-Santé Quebec: history: http://www.urgences-sante.qc.ca/
23. Fire Department New York City EMS History: http://www.nyc.gov/html/fdny/html/ems_week/ems_history.shtml
24. City of Boston (US) http://www.cityofboston.gov/EMS/about/
25. The British Association for Immediate Care: http://www.basics.org.uk/index.
26. London's Air Ambulance: http://www.londonsairambulance.com.
27. Paramedic Resource Centre: http://www.paramedic-resource-centre.com/ambulance_services.htm
28. St. John Ambulance service worldwide: http://www.sja.org.uk/sja/about-us/st-john-ambulance-worldwide.aspx
29. Paris Fire Brigade: History:http://www.spiritus-temporis.com/paris-fire-brigade/history.html
30. Service Mobile d'Urgence et de Réanimation http://www.samu-de-france.fr/en
31. Nikkanen HE, Pouges C, Jacobs LM: Emergency medicine in France. *Ann Emerg Med* 31:116; 1998.
32. Adnet F, Lapostolle F. International EMS Systems: France. *Resuscitation* 2004; 63:7–9.
33. Dykstra EH. International models for the practice of emergency care. *Am J Emerg Med* 15(2): 208; 1997.
34. Dick WF. Anglo-American vs. Franco-German emergency medical services system. *Prehosp Disaster Med* 18(1):29; 2003.
35. Paramedics in Germany: http://en.allexperts.com/e/p/pa/paramedics_in_germany.htm
36. Emergency Medical Services in Germany: (2006) *Resuscitation,*68(1),pp.45–49.
37. Arntz HR, Agrawal R, Richter H, Schmidt S, et al. Phased chest and abdominal compression-decompression versus conventional cardiopulmonary resuscitation in out-of-hospital cardiac arrest. *Circulation* 104:768; 2001.
38. Weninger P, Hertz H, Walter M. International EMS: Austria. *Resuscitation* 65(3):249; 2005.
39. Mencl F. International EMS systems. Kuehl, AE (Ed), Prehospital Systems and Medical Oversight. Vol 2, ch 24, pp. 281–306 National Association of EMS Physicians, 2009.
40. Langhelle A, Lossius HM, Silfvast T, et al. International EMS systems: the Nordic countries. *Resuscitation* 61:9; 2004.
41. Andersen MS, Nielsen TT, Christensen EF. A study of police operated dispatch to acute coronary syndrome cases arising from 112 emergency calls in Aarhus County, Denmark. *Emerg Med J* 23:705; 2006.
42. Falck, http://www.falck.com/home/business_areas/_emergency. Accessed 12/15/09.
43. Central Intelligence Agency World Factbook https://www.cia.gov/library/publications/the-world-factbook/. Accessed December 12, 2009.
44. World Health Organization. India. World Health Statistics 2008. World Health Organization, 15 Oct. 2009. http://www.who.int/countries/ind/en/.
45. Joshipura M. Trauma care in India: current scenario. *World J Surg.* 32(8):1613; 2008.

46. EMS Pune. Development of EMS in India. EMS India. March 31 2009. EMS Pune. 15 Oct, 2009, http://www.emsindia.in/newsdetail.php?id=56&start=0&status=1

47. Rajhans P. EMS Pune: Retracting the First Steps. *EMS India.* 2009. EMS Pune. 15 Oct 2009. http://www.emsindia.in/subsectioncontent.php?id=48&catid=23.

48. Ramakrishnan TV. The Society for Emergency Medicine India: Home. 2007. Society for Emergency Medicine India. 15 Oct. 2009. http://www.semi.org.in/.

49. Subhan, I. Apollo Hospitals, Hyderabad. *Emerg Med* 2009. Apollo Hospital Group. 15 Oct 2009. http://www.emergencymedicine.in/.

50. Joshipura MK, Shah HS, Patel PR, Divatia PA. Trauma care systems in India – An overview. *Ind J Crit Care Med* 8(2):93; 2004.

51. Lifeline Foundation. Highway Rescue Project. Lifeline Foundation. 2006. (Vadodara, Gujarat, India). 15 Oct 2009. http://www.highwayrescue.org/.

52. Emergency Management and Research Institute. Emergency Management. 2009. GVK Industries. 15 Oct 2009. http://www.emri.in/.(India)

53. Academy of Traumatology India. EMT Course: Curriculum Development. 2009. Academy of Traumatology India. 25 Nov 2009. http://www.indiatrauma.org/EMT%20course.htm

54. Ramanujam P, Aschkenasy M. Identifying the need for pre-hospital and emergency care in the developing world: A case study in Chennai, India. *J Assoc Physicians India.* 2007 Jul;55:491–5.

55. Lewin M, Hori S, Aikawa N. Emergency Medical Services in Japan: An opportunity for the rational development of pre-hospital care and research, *J Emerg Med* 28(2):237; 2005.

56. Mashiko K., Trauma systems/centers: a Japanese perspective. *Trauma* 1999;1:285–289

57. Suzuki T, Nishida M, Suzuki Y, et al. Issues and solutions in introducing Western systems to the prehospital care system in Japan. *West J Emerg Med* 9(3):166; 2008.

58. Kobayashi K. Trauma care in Japan. Trauma Quart 14(3):249; 1999.

59. Mashiko K., Trauma systems in Japan: history: present status and future perspectives. *J Nippon Med Sch* 72(4):194; 2005.

60. Toyoda Y, Mastuo Y, Tanaka H, et al. Pre-hospital score for acute disease: a community based observational study in Japan. *BMC Emerg Med* 7:17; 2007.

61. Tanaka H, Iwai A, Oda J, et al. Overview of evacuation and transport of patients following the 1995 Hanshin – Awaji earthquake." *J Emerg Med* 16(3): 439; 1998.

62. World Health Organization. China. World Health Statistics 2008. 2008. World Health Organization. 15 Oct 2009. http://www.who.int/countries/chn/en/. (Accessed November 24, 2009.)

63. Hou X, Lu C. The current workforce status of pre-hospital care in China. *J Emerg Primary Health Care* Vol 3, Issue 3; 2005: 1–11

64. Hung KKC, Cheung CSK, Rainer TH, **Graham CA**. International EMS systems: EMS systems in China. *Resuscitation* 2009;**80**:732–735

65. Dai K. Trauma care systems in China. Injury 34(9): 664; 2003. (Accessed November 24, 2009.)

66. Shao JF, Shen HY, Shi XY. Current state of emergency medicine education in China. *Emerg Med J* 26: 573; 2009

67. China EMSS. China Emergency Medical Service System (EMSS): History. 2009. Emergency Medical Center (First Aid Station) Branch of Chinese Hospital Association. Sept 2009. http://www.emss.cn/english/emcbcha.asp (Accessed February 2010)

68. Brown, MD, Ted. (2003). Prehospital Care of Road Traffic Injuries in Chiang Mai, Thailand. UC Berkeley: Safe Transportation Research & Education Center. Retrieved from: http://escholarship.org/uc/item/7ng2k4c3

69. Church AL, Plitponkarnpim A. Emergency medicine in Thailand. *Ann Emerg Med* 32(1):93; 1998.

70. NY Times archives 2002: http://www.nytimes.com/2002/01/29/news/29iht-bodies_ed3_.html?pagewanted=1 (Accessed December 2, 2009)

71. Sinthavalai R, Memongkol N, Pattanaprechawong N, et al. A study of distinctive models for pre-hospital EMS in Thailand: knowledge capture. *World Acad Sci Engineering Technol* 55; July 2009. www.waset.org/journals/waset/v55/v55-24.pdf

72. Johnson L, Travis A. Trauma response to the Asian tsunami, Krabi Hospital, Southern Thailand. *Emerg Med Australasia* 18(2):196; 2005.

73. Schwartz D, Goldberg A, Ashkenasi I, et al. Prehospital care of tsunami victims in Thailand: description and analysis. *Prehospital Disaster Med* 21(3); 2005.

74. Smith G. Prehospital emergency care in South East Asia: Three cities. *J Emerg Primary Health Care* 6(2); 2008.

Structures of Different National EMS Systems

Gerard O'Reilly, Mark Fitzgerald

KEY LEARNING POINTS

- Most of the world's population does not have access to a formalized EMS.

- The common necessary domains of EMS system structure are responsible authority; agent(s) of EMS provision; EMS transport, equipment, and human resources; and triage and dispatch processes.

- Different nations have different approaches to the administrative authority and agents of EMS, from a centralized, government-run approach to EMS delivery by private companies.

- Many countries depend upon volunteer agencies to deliver EMS.

- The "Anglo-American" paramedic-based model of care is being increasingly adopted by developed EMS systems.

Countries have developed at different rates and in different sociopolitical directions. Similarly, the various national health systems, including EMS, have evolved differently across nations.

This chapter will provide a broad outline of the structures of different national EMS systems. It will first identify the features or *domains* of EMS organization common to *all* EMS systems; it will then consider each of these *domains* as headings by which different national EMS systems can be described and compared.

Clearly, a practical manual such as this cannot afford to focus on the structural details of each and every EMS at national and regional levels. Instead, the pattern of major variations in EMS structure, with examples, is used as the basis of this chapter.

OVERVIEW

In each nation, the structure of EMS sits at a point upon a spectrum for each of several structural domains (see below): no EMS structure can be described wholly by one end or extreme of the spectrum. The point on the spectrum at which a national EMS structure lies will depend upon, among other factors, the following contexts:

1. **Level of national development.**
   a. Developed.
   b. Developing.
   c. Undeveloped.
2. Factors *within* the **level of national development.**
   a. Sociopolitical framework.
   b. Health system priorities.
   c. Geography.

For each nation, the dominant characteristics – or point on the spectrum – of the different domains will generally depend, in a broadly predictable fashion, upon the nature of the contexts listed above. These domains will provide the framework headings of this chapter and are listed below:

A. **Administration.**
1. **Authority** The authority responsible for EMS may be adopted at one of the following levels:
   a. National.
   b. State or Province.
   c. Regional or District.
   d. Community.
   e. Individual.
2. **Agent** The *agents* of EMS provision will often represent all of the elements described below, the point upon the spectrum being determined by the *predominant* agent:
   a. Government.
   b. Volunteer.
   c. Not-for-profit agency (e.g., St. John Ambulance, Red Cross).
   d. Private contractor.
   e. None.
3. **Finance** Similarly, the funding of EMS will often depend upon the national characteristics in the previous domains:
   a. Government (public)-funded.
   b. Volunteer.
   c. Private.
   d. None.
   The matter of EMS financing, intimately linked to EMS structure, will be dealt with in **Chapter 20, Financing of EMS Services & Cost Effectiveness**
B. **Resources.**
1. **EMS transport:** Multiple forms of EMS transport exist, the principal modes being.
   a. Road.
   b. Air.
   c. None.
2. **Human Resources:** EMS staff skills, training, and credentialing will be covered in **Chapter 5, EMS Interactions with Governments.**
C. **Processes.**
1. **Operations:** Operational leadership and clinical direction depend upon, among other features, the predominant strategic model:
   a. Anglo-American.
   b. Franco-German.
   These will be further defined and summarized below.

2. **Triage:** The coordination of EMS dispatch will occur at one of the following levels:
   a. Central.
   b. Local.
   c. Hospital.
   d. Ad Hoc.
   e. None.

NATIONAL EMS SYSTEMS

Having considered the domains common to all EMS systems, we will compare the structures of different national EMS systems using these domains as headings.

Administration

Among developed countries the structural models (i.e., the point on the spectrum of the two domains: Authority and Agent) can be linked to, and often predicted by, the national sociopolitical model and approach to health care (Table 4-1 and Table 4-2).

As will be ascertained from the examples provided below, in countries that have a more socialized health system (e.g., the UK, New Zealand, France), the responsibility (and funding) for EMS is the central or regional government. At the other end of the spectrum, the approach to EMS administration across the US is variable. The administration and delivery of EMS may be state-based but is often regional; the funding model is largely independent of central government. Of the other developed nations, most countries of Western Europe are more likely to be administered along the

Table 4–1	Predominant EMS Authority in Selection of Developed Systems		
Nation	**National**	**State/ Province**	**Regional**
Australia		✓	
Canada		✓	
France	✓		
Hong Kong	✓		
Israel	✓		
Italy			✓
Netherlands	✓		
New Zealand	✓		
UK	✓		
US			✓

Table 4–2	Predominant EMS Agent(s) in Selection of Developed Systems					
Nation	**Government**	**Agency***				**Private**
		Red Cross	*St. John*	*Other*	*Voluntary**	
Australia	✓✓		✓		✓	
Canada	✓					✓
France	✓✓					
Hong Kong	✓✓					
Iceland		✓✓				
Israel				✓✓	✓✓	
Italy						✓
Netherlands						✓✓
New Zealand			✓✓		✓	
Norway						✓
UK	✓✓	✓	✓		✓	
US	✓					✓

*Where a nongovernment agency contributes to EMS provision, the *majority* of staff may be either paid or volunteers.

lines of the former approach. Australia has a centralized but state-based approach to EMS administration, while the model for Canada lies somewhere between Australia and the US.

Authority

Most developed countries now provide a government-funded EMS that can be run on a state or provincial level, or in some cases, at national level. In the UK, a national *network* of ambulance trusts operate the EMS.[1] In each of the four health care systems of England, Wales, Scotland, and Northern Ireland, EMS is provided through local ambulance services or "Trusts." Each Trust in England is linked to at least one area of local authority in a similar way to the police services.

A number of countries in Western Europe have a mixed model. In the Netherlands, for example, EMS is provided by the government in partnership with private companies. Similarly, EMS in Norway is operated both by the government, through each of the four Regional Health Authorities, and organizations such as the Red Cross. In Sweden, the regional health authority (the county) is responsible for EMS.[2] Although EMS in Poland is typically *provided* by the local, publicly operated hospital, it is *funded* by the government of Poland.

In Canada, responsibility for EMS has been allocated to the provincial and territorial levels of government. Except in the province of British Columbia, which operates its EMS directly, the authority for EMS

service delivery varies between jurisdictions *within* the provinces or territories. That is, the provincial or territorial government will usually provide enabling legislation, standards, accreditation, and oversight to a variety of potential EMS operators, These may include municipalities, hospitals, or private companies.[3,4]

In the US, EMS is run on a regional model, with individual authorities having the responsibility for providing these services. EMS is regulated at the most basic level by the federal government, which sets the minimum standards that EMS providers in all states must meet, but it is regulated more strictly by individual state governments, which often require higher standards from the services they oversee.[5]

In developing countries, there is widespread recognition at the central government level of the need for EMS. In Sri Lanka, for example, prehospital care is considered to be an essential, core component of the trauma system. The Pre-Hospital Care Committee, Trauma Secretariat, Sri Lanka, was established following the 2004 tsunami; its goals are that "everyone in Sri Lanka has access to trained prehospital medical personnel and ambulances are available."[6]

There remains, however, considerable variation in the public investment in EMS development. More than half of the people in the world do not have access to a dedicated EMS (including ambulances).[7] India has an embryonic and variable EMS system. EMS is frequently operated from private hospitals with little observable integration with local hospitals.[8]

Agent(s)

In general, the agent(s) of EMS delivery in each country or region match the national or state-based approach to EMS responsibility. As introduced previously, EMS delivery will occur through a predictable mix of government services; volunteers; agencies such as the Red Cross and St. John Ambulance; and private organizations (refer to Table 4-2).

Among those nations with a developed EMS, Australia delivers most EMS directly through a government-operated service. Canada and the US, on the other hand, provide EMS through a variety of elements, depending upon the approach of the state or provincial authority.

In addition to government-provided EMS, some charities or nonprofit companies also operate EMS, often alongside a patient transport function.[9] These are often dedicated to providing ambulances for the community or for cover at major events, including sports. The Red Cross provides this service in many countries, either on a volunteer basis or contracted by an authority such as the government. Other smaller organizations with a similar role include St. John Ambulance.[10] In many countries, these volunteer ambulances provide support to the full-time ambulance crews during a major incident or disaster.

EMS may be also be provided by private ambulance companies, with paid employees. These private organizations are often on contract with the local or national government authority. It is not uncommon for many private companies to limit their role to nonurgent patient transport, but occasionally these private services are contracted to provide emergency care and/or event-specific cover.

The range and combination of agent(s) of EMS delivery used by different developed nations are highlighted by the following examples:

In Australia, the agents of EMS can be divided into two basic groups: the statutory services and the volunteer groups. In most Australian states, statutory ambulance services are provided by the state government within a single-entity government department. In Western Australia, and in the Northern Territory, EMS is provided by St. John Ambulance Australia, under contract to the state government. In all other states and territories, the activities of St. John Ambulance are limited to first-aid training and special events support, with the occasional disaster response.[3]

In New Zealand, there are two main organizations providing EMS: St. John Ambulance and Wellington Free Ambulance. While both land ambulance service providers do have paid staff, they also rely heavily on a volunteer work force, especially in rural areas.

In Hong Kong, the statutory provider of EMS is the Hong Kong Fire Service. Again, the supplementary agencies, St. John Ambulance, and the Auxiliary Medical Service focus primarily on special event coverage and public education.

The varied role of organizations such as the Red Cross and St. John Ambulance as agents for the provision of national EMS, from central operators to more peripheral agents, can be illustrated in the history of EMS in the UK. Both organizations predated the existence of the government-organized service and remained the principal agents of EMS under contract to the UK government until the 1970s. Currently, the primary activity of both organizations is the provision of cover at events as an extension of their role in community first aid.

Perhaps surprisingly, private ambulance services are becoming more common in the UK, performing a number of roles. They provide event-based medical cover, often alongside the volunteer agencies described above. While the most common type of private ambulance provider is in the patient transport role, a quarter of the UK ambulance trusts contract private companies to do "front line work."[3]

EMS in the Netherlands is delivered by a number of private ambulance organizations, which are contracted to the government. Similarly, EMS in Norway is operated through one of the four regional health authorities, but typically is outsourced to private providers.

In South Africa, EMS is provided by each South African province. The system of government-operated ambulances is generally referred to as Metro.[11] In addition to the paid responders, the government system is supplemented in many areas by unpaid volunteers (South African Red Cross and St. John Ambulance). There are also several private-for-profit ambulance companies that operate nationally.

Israel is unique in having a well-developed, centralized, national government-run EMS, with the vast majority of EMS staff being volunteers. The predominant provider is Magen David Adom (MDA), supplemented in some areas by Hatzalah and the Palestinian Red Crescent Society. Approximately 90% of MDA staff work on a voluntary basis.[12]

Other countries have a relatively decentralized provision of EMS, with the main actors varying according to the state or province. EMS in Italy is provided from a variety of different sources and the agents of delivery can vary considerably from one location to another. Volunteer organizations, including the Italian Red Cross, are the primary EMS agencies.

In Canada, the approaches used for service delivery are variable depending upon the province or territory and even the local municipality. Provincial governments may contract directly with a single private company.

Outside of large cities in the US, EMS is often provided by volunteers. A feature of EMS in the US is that many colleges and universities now also have their own EMS agencies for their campuses. Most are staffed by student volunteers.

EMS can be provided by stand-alone organizations in developed countries, but in other cases it is operated by the local fire or police service. This is particularly common in rural areas, where maintaining a separate service may not be as cost-effective (see **Chapter 45, EMS in Rural & Wilderness Areas**).

In developing countries, the range of EMS agents is variable and often unpredictable. In many regions, especially rural, there are no identified agents of EMS provision. In this very common setting, the "agent" might include one or more of family, familiar or unfamiliar bystander(s), or the driver of a three- or four-wheel taxi. Where a dedicated EMS exists, the agent will often be a private hospital, with either on-site or remote dispatch. Some cities may have municipal EMS agents, while regional, state, or national EMS delivery is more the exception than the norm.

Countries such as Sri Lanka have an embryonic national *approach* to EMS delivery. The pattern of EMS delivery across India and China is variable; prehospital EMS is more likely to exist in large urban areas. Few countries in sub-Saharan Africa have a dedicated national agency for EMS.

Finance

EMS financing is covered in **Chapter 20, Financing of EMS Services & Cost Effectiveness.**

Resources

EMS Transport

The most basic EMS "system" is provided as a transport operation only. This is still the case in many developing countries, where operators as diverse as taxi drivers and undertakers may provide this service. This approach may be more ad hoc than organized.

In India, for example, most patients arrive at hospital by private transport or taxi. In one study of the access of stroke patients to a stroke unit in India, only 12% of patients arrived by ambulance.[13] Even where there is "dedicated" EMS transport, the vehicles that are used to carry patients to hospitals may be primarily designated as mortuary vans (Figure 4-1). In Ghana,

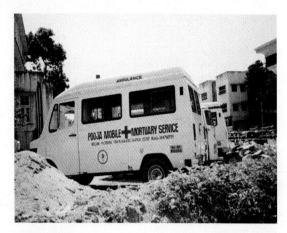

Mortuary vans may have the dual role of patient transport in India.

most injured people who make it to a hospital are transported by taxis and minibuses. In one study, ambulances brought in 3% of patients, all of whom were interhospital transfers.[14]

Where EMS is more organized and dedicated ambulances exist, rapid patient and hospital access can still be very difficult. High-density, traffic-congested cities, such as many in India, result in long transit times for traditional four-wheel vehicles. Different methods have been used to circumvent this problem. Auto-rickshaw drivers in parts of Kerala, India, have been supplied with first-aid boxes and basic training to encourage them to provide a basic but accessible EMS service when necessary. Along some busy highways in India, ambulance "cubicles" are stationed, staffed by a technician skilled in ALS (Figure 4-2). Having ambulances based on the highway reduces the response time

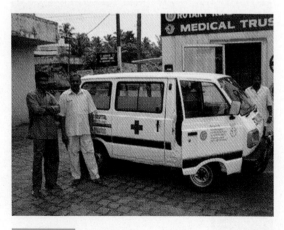

Ambulance and staffed station on highway in India.

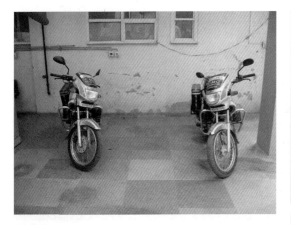

FIGURE 4–3

Ambulance motorcycles in the Punjab, India.

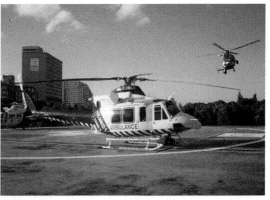

FIGURE 4–5

Ambulance helicopter.

to a motor-vehicle collision scene. One center in Ludhiana, Punjab, relies on motorcycle paramedics to bring ALS skills more rapidly to the patient in advance of the arrival of the conventional four-wheel EMS transport (Figure 4-3).

In developed EMS systems, the predominant medium of EMS transport is the road. Four-wheel vehicles are required to transport the patient; two-wheel vehicles may be used to facilitate the transport of skilled EMTs to the patient. Most mature EMS systems also have air transport capability. This includes rotary and/or fixed-wing aircraft.

The pattern of EMS transport used in developed EMS systems depends on a combination of terrain and population density. Four-wheeled vehicles are the predominant form of ambulance in almost all countries (Figure 4-4). For a single jurisdiction, as the region becomes larger and less densely populated, the

additional mode of EMS transport shifts along the spectrum from most flexible/least fuel and carriage capacity (i.e., motorcycle) to least flexible/greatest range (i.e., fixed-wing aircraft).

In countries, or regions within countries that are sparsely populated, with large distances to the closest *appropriate* hospital, an aircraft-based EMS is invaluable. Australia, Canada and Iceland, for example, rely on fixed-wing aircraft to provide nationwide EMS to remote areas.

While rotary wing aircraft are unable to cover great distances, they serve as a rapid and flexible form of EMS transport over medium distances, especially over terrain that cannot accommodate road vehicles (e.g., sea, ice, and snow). Rotary wing is a critical form of EMS transport in developed systems that bypass the closest hospital in order to deliver patients to the nearest appropriate urban center (Figure 4-5). In recent decades, such integrated systems have been created to provide optimal and timely emergency and trauma care.

In a number of developed nations, nonpatient transport vehicles may provide a first response service. Such vehicles, whether four- or two-wheel, are equipped with medical equipment for ALS. Sometimes the first responder may arrive in a police van or fire truck.

Some countries, because of specific characteristics, require unique forms of EMS transport. The terrain in sparsely populated Norway is particularly suited to rotary wing EMS transport, but there are also many high-speed marine ambulance boats. Israel has a number of armored ambulances (Figure 4-6).

Staffing

Human resources are considered in detail in **Chapter 10, Staffing of Ambulances.**

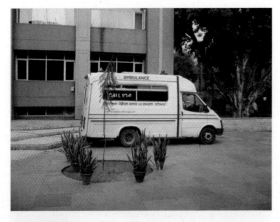

FIGURE 4–4

Road ambulance in the Punjab, India.

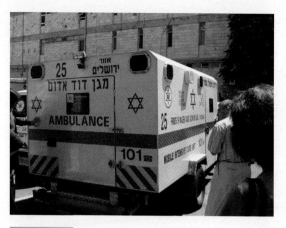

FIGURE 4–6

Armored ambulance in Jerusalem.

Processes

Operations

While there are various approaches to the actual operational delivery of EMS and the clinical governance linked to these operations, it has become useful to summarize the modus operandi of a national EMS under one of two headings: the Anglo-American and the Franco-German models.[15]

The features that separate the two models are provided in Table 4-3. This classification is a generalization; most developed nations have features taken from both models. The "stay and play" approach, for example, is not exclusive to the Franco-German model; as paramedics have developed more expertise under the Anglo-American model, scene times may be more prolonged. Notwithstanding the overlap, the model description provides a helpful taxonomy by which to describe a national EMS system.

In general, of the developed nations, those which follow the Franco-German model include France, Italy, Germany, Austria, Switzerland, and to some extent, Israel. The Anglo-American model is practiced by the UK, US, Canada, Hong Kong, Singapore, South Africa, Australia, and New Zealand.

Paramedics are the key feature of the Anglo-American model. In France, the role of the paramedic remains largely unknown. In Germany, paramedics do exist but operate under the direct supervision of a physician. That is, those in the paramedic role are only permitted to practice many of their advanced skills while assisting a physician who is physically present or if they are confronted by cases of immediately life-threatening emergencies.[16] Even in these countries, however, the model of care is changing.

In the Anglo-American model, paramedics normally function under the authority (medical direction) of one or more physicians charged with legally establishing the emergency medical directives for a particular region. Paramedics are credentialed and authorized by these physicians to use their own clinical judgment and diagnostic tools to identify medical emergencies and to administer appropriate treatment according to predetermined clinical protocols. In these cases, paramedics are regarded as a self-regulating health profession. The final common method of credentialing is through certification by a medical director and permission to practice as an extension of the medical director's license to practice medicine. The authority to practice in this semi-autonomous manner is granted in the form of standing order protocols (off-line medical control). Under this paradigm, paramedics effectively assume the role of out-of-hospital field agents to regional physicians, with independent clinical decision-making authority using standing orders or protocols.[17]

Triage

In most developing nations, in the absence of an organized EMS, there is no opportunity for effective triage. Even where there is a local EMS system functioning to deliver patients to a hospital, the prioritization is generally based on a "first call" basis.

Table 4–3	The Principal Features Separating the Two Operational Models of EMS	
Domain	**Anglo-American**	**Franco-German**
Approach	"Scoop and run"	"Stay and play"
Staff	Paramedic	Physician
Time at scene	Short-to-medium	Medium-long
Receiving hospital staff	Emergency physician	Other – no specialty of Emergency Medicine
Dispatch	Central	Hospital

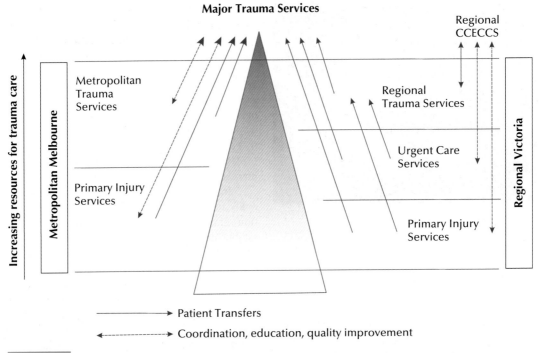

Major Trauma Services

Patient Transfers

Coordination, education, quality improvement

FIGURE 4–7

Structure of the integrated **Victoria state trauma system.** *Abbreviation*: CCECCS = Consultative Council on Emergency and Critical Care Services. Reprinted with permission of Atkin C, Freedman I, Jeffrey V, et al. The evolution of an integrated state trauma system in Victoria, Australia. *Injury* 36(11):1277; 2005.

Unfortunately, in both developing and developed nations, the ability of the patient's ambulance transport to be pre- or co-paid may contribute to the triage decision-making process.

The impetus for integrated trauma systems, and more recently, the approach to ST elevation myocardial infarction (STEMI) and stroke, is that the patient's best chance for survival is through rapid transfer to the place where the appropriate level of care can be provided (specifically the operating room for the trauma patient and the angioplasty [PCI] lab for the patient with a STEMI). EMS triage has been based upon immediate transport to the "closest *appropriate* hospital" rather than simply the "closest hospital" (Figure 4-7).[18]

For trauma care, the designation of centers with the capacity to provide varying levels of care have been linked with trauma triage guidelines predicting those patients who warrant such care (Table 4-4). More recently, similar hospital designations and triage guidelines have been developed to deal with the *nontrauma* presentations needing time-critical hospital-based interventions, including those with S-T elevation myocardial infarction and stroke.[5,19]

To ensure that a patient is delivered rapidly to a center that can provide all of the necessary lifesaving care, central dispatch is necessary. Those developed nations where EMS is *provided* centrally will usually coordinate EMS dispatch centrally.

In most developed nations, the EMS is summoned by members of the public (upon recognizing the need for EMS) via an emergency telephone number that puts them in contact with a control facility, which will then dispatch a suitable resource (EMS transport with EMT) to respond. The setting in which a call to EMS is made may be illness or injury in the home, in the workplace, on a street or road, or other site in the field.

The preferred initial link to a system of central dispatch is a common, easy-to-remember, ideally toll-free, publicly accessible phone number. The UK, most countries of Europe, the US, Australia, and New Zealand, have a national number. Across multiple European countries, the number is "112." This is also the number for emergency calls by mobile cellular phones, globally. In Italy, the EMS number is "118." In UK the number is "999" and in the US "911."

EMS transport used for dispatch is stationed in various locations, depending upon the national

Table 4-4	**Predictors of Life-Threatening Injury Appropriate for Use in Prehospital Trauma Triage**
Mechanism	Ejection from vehicle High-speed collision (>60 kph, 37 mph) Motorcycle/cyclist impact >30 kph (20 mph) Fall >5 meters (16 feet) Vehicle rollover Fatality in same vehicle Explosion Pedestrian impact >30 kph (20 mph) Extrication >30 minutes

Injuries (any of the following)	Serious or suspected serious penetrating injuries:
	    Head/neck/chest/abdomen/pelvis/axilla/groin
	All significant blunt injuries as assessed by ambulance
	All injuries involving
	    Evisceration
	    Explosion
	    Severe crush injury
	    Any amputation
	    Suspected spinal injury
	    Serious burns
	    Pelvic fracture

Vital signs	Respiratory rate <10 or >30 per min Systolic blood pressure <100 mm Hg (<75 mm Hg for child) GCS <15 Oxygen saturation <90%

Treatment
Patients who have undergone any
  of the following prehospital
  interventions
	Intubation
	Any airway maneuver at any time
	Assisted ventilation
	Chest decompression
	Failure to control external bleeding
	    >500 mL fluid
	Sedatives

Other criteria	All interhospital trauma transfers Significant comorbidity Pregnancy

GCS = Glasgow Coma Scale.

or regional approach and the type of ambulance. In most mature EMS systems, road ambulances are predominantly stationed at dedicated ambulance stations, while in less developed systems and some mature systems, road ambulances are located at hospitals (Figure 4-8). As mentioned previously, in parts of Kerala, India, small roadside ambulance points are positioned at places along the highway to maximize the ability to quickly access road trauma patients.

Dispatch technologies, including automated vehicle locating (AVL) and decision-making support software, are comparable across North America, Europe, Israel, and Australia. The logistic coordination of dispatch according to triage guidelines is relatively similar across different EMS systems, with some examples as follows:

In Australia, the emergency number (000) rings at the telephone company, where an operator determines the caller's needs and then directs the caller to the appropriate emergency service (police, fire, ambulance).

In France, the SMUR (Service Mobile d'Urgence et Reanimation) teams are typically hospital-based.

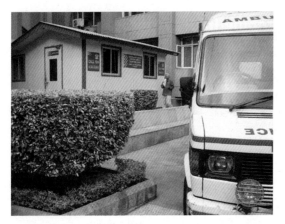

FIGURE 4-8

Hospital-based ambulance station in the Punjab, India.

All requests for emergency ambulance service are received and processed by the local SAMU (Service d'Aide Médicale Urgente). Calls are screened and patients interviewed by a physician, with a variety of possible outcomes. The French philosophy for medical emergencies allows the reanimation units to be dispatched only in life-threatening cases. Because of aggressive triage only about 65% of requests for ambulance service actually receive an ambulance response.[20]

In Israel, all EMS resources are dispatched from a single National Response Center (Figure 4-9). The national emergency number for an ambulance in Israel is "101." This number is answered by MDA around the clock. MDA claims rapid response times of less than six minutes for major emergencies the majority of the time. This is likely to be the result of extremely dense ambulance coverage and the high number of volunteer first responders.[12]

All 25 EMS regions in the Netherlands are self-dispatching. Some regions have more than one center, but all are interconnected. The EMS dispatch centers participate in the national emergency number scheme and EMS calls in the Netherlands are nurse-triaged. Most dispatch centers use computer-based decision-support systems, and in approximately 40% of cases, the call is triaged with the result that an ambulance response is avoided entirely.[3]

In South Africa, EMS dispatch operates from a variety of sources, and in many cases, especially for the private companies, has involved self-dispatch. The government is endeavoring to centralize dispatch.

All ambulances in Poland are dispatched from centralized regional dispatch centers. In Hong Kong, dispatch occurs through the Police Service. In Italy, there is centralized dispatch but a nonstandardized response given the variable mix of EMS agents and levels of training from one region to the next. In Sri Lanka, the four major cities now have the number "110" as a dedicated EMS number.

In the US, there are as many methods of dispatching EMS resources as there are approaches to providing EMS service. In some larger communities, EMS may be self-dispatching. Where EMS is operated as a division of the Police or Fire Departments, it will generally be dispatched by those organizations. Dispatching may occur through state-licensed EMS dispatch centers, which are operated by one service but provide dispatch to several counties.

SUMMARY

Most of the world's population does not have access to a formalized EMS system. In those countries *with* an EMS, the EMS system is built upon elements common to all: point(s) of administrative authority; agents of EMS provision; EMS transport, equipment, and human resources; and processes of dispatch. Across different nations and regions, however, there remain considerable variations in each of these domains of EMS structure. While both the operational models and the levels of authority and agency are broadly divided, EMS development is generally heading in the same direction, toward an "Anglo-American model," using paramedics as the primary EMS staff. Similarly, the natural progression of EMS development has been toward the increased "centralization" of authority and agency, allowing for a coordinated and integrated delivery and monitoring of EMS.

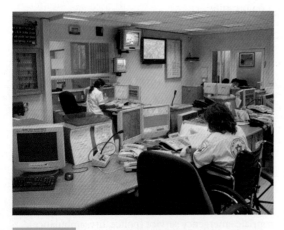

FIGURE 4-9

Ambulance dispatch center in Jerusalem.

References

1. UK NHS Ambulance Service Information. http://www.nhs.uk/NHSEngland/AboutNHSservices/Emergencyandurgentcareservices/Pages/Ambulanceservices.aspx accessed December 2009. (updated February 2010)

2. Hjaite L, Suserud B-O, Karlberg I. Initial emergency medical dispatching and prehospital needs assessment: a prospective study of the Swedish ambulance service. *Eur J Emerg Med* 4(3):134; 2007.

3. The CIA World Fact Book, https://www.cia.gov/library/publications/the-world-factbook/index.html accessed December 2009.(updated February 2010)

4. Consolidated Newfoundland and Labrador Regulation 999/96, www.assembly.nl.ca/legislation/sr/regulations/rc960999.htm, accessed December 2009.

5. Moyer P, Ornato J, Brady W, et al. Development of systems of care for ST-elevation myocardial infarction patients: the emergency medical services and emergency department perspective. *Circulation* 116(2):e42; 2007.

6. Trauma Secretariat, www.traumaseclanka.gov.lk/ems.html, accessed December 2009.

7. Mock C, ed. International approaches to trauma care. *Trauma Quart* 14(3):191; 1999.

8. Joshipura MK. Trauma care in India: current scenario. *World J Surg* 32:1613; 2008.

9. British Red Cross Voluntary Ambulance Service, www.redcross.org.uk/standard.asp, accessed December 2009.

10. St. John Ambulance First Aid Cover for Events, www.sja.org.uk/sja/what-we-do/event-first-aid-cover.aspx, accessed December 2009.

11. Metro EMS Western Cape, South Africa, www.metroems.org.za, accessed December 2009.

12. MDA Training website, www.mdais.org, accessed December 2009.

13. Pandian JD, Kalra G, Jaison A, et al. Factors delaying admission to a hospital-based stroke unit in India. *J Stroke Cerebrovasc Dis* 15:81-7; 2006.

14. Forjuoh S, Mock CN, Freidman D, Quansah R. Transport of the injured to hospitals in Ghana: the need to strengthen the practice of trauma care. *Prehospital Immed Care* 2:66; 1999.

15. Ghosh R, Pepe P. The critical care cascade: a systems approach. *Curr Opin Crit Care* 15(4):279; 2009.

16. Ummenhofer W, Scheidegger D. Role of the physician in prehospital management of trauma: European perspective. *Curr Opin Crit Care* 8:559; 2002.

17. Benitez FL, Pepe P. Role of the physician in prehospital management of trauma: North American perspective. *Curr Opin Crit Care* 8:551; 2002.

18. Harrington DT, Connolly M, Biffl WL, et al. Transfer times to definitive care facilities are too long. A consequence of an immature trauma system. *Ann Surg* 241(6):961; 2006.

19. Acker JE, Pancioli AM, Crocco T, et al. Implementation strategies for emergency medical services within stroke systems of care: a policy statement from the American Heart Association/American Stroke Association expert panel on emergency medical services systems and the Stroke Council. *Stroke* 38(11):3097; 2007.

20. Service d'Aide Médicale d'Urgence (SAMU) www.samu-de-france.fr/en, accessed December 2009.

CHAPTER 5

EMS Interactions with Governments

*Juliusz Jakubaszko, Shingo Hori,
Pairoj Khruekarnchana, Somchai Kanchanasut*

KEY LEARNING POINTS

- There is a great *intellectual barrier* between medicine and politics, resulting in difficulties in communication and understanding about emergency medicine.

- *Advocacy groups* can bridge the gap between medicine and politics.

- The *mass media* is a pivotal force for educating politicians, health system managers, and the public about quality emergency care.

- Change is often stimulated by an incident that causes instability in a stable system. Directional movement by *emergency physicians, public officials, fire departments, politicians,* and *public*

opinion is an important force to mold EMS system development.

- An EMS unit or system is typically confused and misunderstood as synonymous with emergency medicine, impeding full growth of the specialty.

- Factors important for the development and growth of EM and EMS are comprehensive improvement of health care, health insurance, economic growth of a country, and government leadership.

- National legislation is the common denominator of EMS development.

EMS AND THE POLISH EXPERIENCE

Health care organization is a critical issue facing developing societies. The need to create sensible structures of emergency medicine (EM) and EMS is the most prominent task. Systems need to be designed so every person with acute serious illness or injury has rapid access to emergency medicine (EM) specialists. An informed public will have sophisticated expectations and demand quality emergency care once exposed to information obtained from friends and neighbors, the mass media, and

the Internet. Communication and education are pivotal for providing our communities and nations with an understanding of the global model of contemporary emergency medicine—an integrated part of the health care system starting with prehospital care and continuing to a hospital's ED.

EMS and Emergency Medicine

EMS units and their functions are clearly identifiable to the public and to politicians. **In developing countries though, EMS units are often equated with the specialty of EM.** Such confusion results in a lack of understanding of the role of the emergency physician in EMS system development, organization, and function and considerably delays the development of the full scope of EM.

The factors that spur development of EM include urbanization, population density, an increase of cardiovascular diseases, injuries of more active workers, aging of society, and an increase of social expectations and awareness about health care. The prehospital medical procedures performed for life-threatening emergencies should be advanced and extremely timely —with time a pivotal factor. All these factors require an educated and organized EMS system to provide the first link of emergency care.

Politics, the Media, and EMS

The development of EM, including the establishment of EDs and EMS systems, requires the support of political and government decision-making circles.

The factors that speed up streamlining of EM structures and EMS are comprehensive nationwide improvement of health care, health insurance, and economic growth of a country. **International contacts and influence can help persuade national leadership about the importance of EM.**

Politicians and health care system managers responsible for the political and financial decisions of their health care systems need an understanding of the importance of EM and the EMS system. The proper understanding of EMS structures and their cross-references to EM is a hard task in countries that are just starting their organization of contemporary EM. **The intellectual barrier between the realms of medicine and politics is commonly underestimated and underappreciated.** In the minds of politicians and managers, most often the concept of EM is inappropriately simplified and equated with EMS units.

The mass media plays a pivotal role in health education. Relationships with journalists, newscasters, and other prominent media individuals should be cultivated. Mass media and journalism can shape consciousness and improve understanding of the problems of emergency care for health system managers and in political circles. The media should educate the public that prehospital care is a set of advanced medical procedures that must be performed by a qualified team that includes emergency physicians, nurses, and EMTs as the active participants.

Advocacy Groups

The need for creating strong advocacy groups for EMS and EM arises at the intersection of medical and political circles. The primary role of advocacy groups is to work out and skillfully convey the concepts of both EM and EMS to decision-makers so that an entire EM system can be introduced.

Such advocacy groups are formed within medical circles and leaders of EM-related disciplines who understand the function of advocacy. Advocates can popularize the specialty and provide sensible legislative lobbying for EM to facilitate building and maintenance of EM medicine structures. Services responsible for public safety and emergency rescue services can also be powerful advocates for the EMS system: firefighters, police, civil defense, and HAZMAT workers.

The Polish Experience

Poland is an example of a country that underwent a relatively quick process of contemporary EM medicine development.

Health Care Reform and Advocacy

In terms of reforming the health care system in Poland, the breakthrough moment was the political revolution of *Solidarnosc*[†] at the turn of the 1980s and 1990s. The new government that emerged in Poland after the Communist regime was overthrown in 1990 opened the country to international cooperation. Political change resulted in comprehensive reorganization of the health care system, the energizing of medical sciences, and the creation of emergency medicine. The concept chosen for EM was that of a complete, independent medical discipline.

Advocacy leader groups formed from the disciplines of anesthesiology, intensive care, surgery, internal medicine, and pediatrics. These specialties wanted to distinguish EM from other structures within the health care system in Poland and helped to develop a network of hospital-based EDs. The network conceived was composed of 250 EDs created within general

---

[†]Solidarity was the first non–Communist-controlled trade union in a Warsaw Pact country. In the 1980s it constituted a broad antibureaucratic social movement. The government attempted to destroy the union during the period of martial law in the early 1980s and several years of repression, but in the end it had to start negotiating with the union. The Round Table Talks between the government and the Solidarity-led opposition led to semi-free elections in 1989. By the end of August a Solidarity-led coalition government was formed and in December 1990 Lech Walesa was elected President of Poland. Since then Solidarity has become a more traditional trade union.

hospitals, which could secure sufficient health care for the 40 million citizens of Poland.

Improved Medical Education

Measures were taken to secure new vehicles and specialized medical equipment for ambulance teams working out-of-hospital. Raising the qualifications of the ambulance staff was secured by phasing in EM specialties for doctors, nurses, and paramedics.

This meant designing new education programs on undergraduate levels for EMTs and paramedics, and postgraduate specialist training for doctors and nurses. **A new medical profession came to life then—licensed paramedics, which required a new type of study and certification at Polish medical universities.** All medical universities have Departments of Public Health that are responsible for educating nurses and paramedics. Paramedic training consists of 3,500 hours of training over 3 years. After certification, paramedics can work on EMS units or in hospital EDs. Next, specialized Departments of Emergency Medicine within Polish Medical Universities were established. All medical universities now have such units.

Legislative Initiatives

Such thorough transformation required the introduction of new legislation and the establishment of a budget for the system. In order to realize such full-scale transformation, the Minister of Health, assisted by the leaders of EM, prepared an "Integrated Emergency Medicine System" program. The program gained popularity within the government, and initial funds were secured in the year 2000 budget plan. Thus, within the several successive years, a modern and nationally integrated EMS system was supposed to emerge, based on a network of affiliated EDs.

The Polish legislature enacted the ***Emergency Medical Services Act*** to develop the entire program. The Minister of Health organized an advisory group consisting of experts from EM–related disciplines and representatives of the state institutions involved in health care management. Legal professionals were selected to reframe existing and operating law.

Refining the ***Emergency Medical Services Act*** demanded a mobilization of the Parliamentary Health Commission within the Polish parliament to promote the act in forthcoming debates. The debates identified a scope of contradictions and irreconcilable expectations among some circles. The medical circle demanded a particular set of special arguments and additional justifications, even though the physicians were poorly oriented to the concepts and demands of the new discipline that EM was going to become.

Everyone Wanted a Voice

The first unforeseen experience was that the program, with all the budgetary investment required to bring it to life, spurred a great deal of local ambition and claims. Lobbyists from the tiniest segments were demanding a voice. Polish counties (Polish: *powiaty*) with their own hospitals illustrated the situation best. Nearly every local leader felt it was a point of honor to create an independent ED in his or her own hospital.

Every fire chief thought it was absolutely necessary to create his or her own emergency communications center. I believe the importance of this phenomenon was greatly underrated. The reactions had not been properly anticipated.

EM Resulted in Hospital System Change

Most hospital directors thought the EM program was an opportunity for extra funding to save their hospitals from utter deterioration. The directors full well understood the goals but tended to sign agreements with the Minister of Health that promised to open EDs in their hospitals. At the same time, new or additional equipment for the EM departments was requested. Sometimes resources were distributed among other hospital departments, not to the ED. Hospitals were so seriously underequipped to begin with that equipment needs became the weakest spot, an imperfection in the program itself. In spite of this, or maybe even thanks to it, the mere ambitions for budget money envisaged for the EM program resulted in a national understanding of the need to create a brand new, quality hospital structure. New hospitals emerged and started creating self-funded EDs. This was an extra positive and unforeseen effect of newly spurred interest in EM and EMS.

Unification of EMS and Emergency Medicine

Next, a better understanding of EMS integration arose. It was starting to be more widely recognized and it was stressed that the very shape, organization, and administration of EM as a health care service was a true comprehensive specialty. **There are not just two separate realms: EMS and in-hospital EM. The services are one and cannot be separated.** Whatever direction the changes take, the rule must be remembered. **EM is a system of care.** It is not a kind of knowledge to be taught separately and independently from EMS. It is an organization system defined as readiness of staff, resources, and facilities to be used immediately to take medical action in case of acute serious injuries and sudden, unexpected critical illness.

The Emergency Medicine Act

The development of the **National Emergency Medicine Act** in Poland took over 2 years. Over that time, several drafts of the act were proposed, many popular debates took place, and a great many state-level interdepartmental agreements were made. The final version was proposed to the Polish lower house (*Sejm*), and after further debate was finally passed in July 2001. This act constructed the emergency medical system in Poland with the following organizational units:

1. Hospital EDs.
2. Specialist EMS units (with EMTs, and with EM physicians on board).
3. Basic EMS units (with EMTs, and without a physician on board or with a nonemergency physician on board).

The Polish Society for Emergency Medicine and International Conferences

In the process of the promotion of EM as a new medical discipline and as a new part of the health care system, the role of the brand new "**Polish Society for Emergency Medicine**" cannot be underestimated. What also played an important role was "The First International Congress of Polish Society for Emergency Medicine," which took place in 2000 and hosted 700 participants and lecturers from all over the world. The congress was widely promoted in the media and medical and political circles and brought to life the importance and attractiveness of our newly created medical discipline.

The formation of the Society and its first congress was a milestone in the development of EM in Poland and encouraged its further development.

Politics Again

Unfortunately, the political scene in Poland resulted in the changing of political groups and decision-makers responsible for health care reform. A change in government in late 2001 resulted in the departure of a strong advocate for EM, the Minister of Health (a physician). His departure caused a significant slowing of the realization of the "Integrated Emergency Medical Services" program. The budget could not accommodate the costs of the newly created EMS system.

However, EM training programs had already begun, and a specialty board examination had been developed. The group of EM specialists was growing with strong motivation for system improvement. Three years after creation of the EM and EMS system, only 50% of the goals were completed. By 2004 about 100 departments were organized in selected hospitals. **As of the November 2009 certification examination, there are 645 board-certified emergency physicians in Poland. As of this writing, there are about 7,000 certified EMTs.** Finally, a new **Emergency Medical Services Act** was approved in September 2006 to correct the organizational and budgetary deficiencies of 2001.

A brand new phenomenon previously unnoticed was the exceptional and increasing social interest in the new medical discipline, EM. An appreciation of its role and importance in the scope of healthcare services was noticed in more and more circles. Society pressured improvements of the discipline. Public media became a strong and stimulating influence on politicians and healthcare system leaders.

In 2009, after ten years of EM in Poland, I can say that the task of development is really arduous, demands a great amount of time, and requires changes of some deeply-rooted habits of both those working in the system and those organizing health care.

EMS IN JAPAN

As society changes over time, the demands upon medicine change. Thus, EMS systems must change along with society. However, EMS in general is a gigantic organization and must meet government regulations, so the system is not always flexible enough to meet citizen demands rapidly.

In Japan, as EMS is organized by the government, all the ambulances are owned by the government, and all the EMS providers are employed by the government. In over 70 years of Japanese EMS history, the last 20 years have been most remarkable. This article examines the interaction between EMS and the government by reviewing key milestones of Japanese EMS history.

Definition

The Japanese name for a paramedic is an **Emergency Lifesaving Technician** (ELST). The term was legislated in Japan in 1991.

The Meiji Restoration

Japan is an island country with only one race and one language, with a unique culture over 1,500 years old. Until the Meiji Restoration 150 years ago, the only medicine was Chinese medicine. Patients were treated in clinics, or doctors came to the home. There were no hospitals. The Meiji Restoration began the process of westernization, and the Japanese government chose Germany as the standard. Japanese medicine was modeled after German medicine, and a medical licensure system was developed and regulated by the government. A system of medical education was established for doctors and nurses, and hospitals were constructed. Fire Defense organizations were developed by each city, town, or village under the Police Department.

The War Years

In 1935, a philanthropist donated six ambulances to the Tokyo metropolitan government (Figure 5-1). Traffic and workplace accidents had increased because of industrialization and the introduction of automobiles, and ambulances were needed to transport the injured to hospitals. The Fire Defense Organization obtained the command authority for ambulances, and 119, the universal emergency call number was established. Tokyo became the EMS managing center. In 1937, the start of the Sino-Japanese War made it impossible to expand the number of ambulances and rescue teams. Throughout the Second World War, because of heavy air raids and deaths (over 100,000 died in the Great Tokyo Air Raids on March 10, 1945), fire-fighting was prioritized over EMS.

World War Two ended on August 15, 1945, and the Allies occupied Japan for 6 years. During this period, the Japanese Constitution and the government were reorganized, and Fire Defense was separated from the National Police Organization. It is said that the manpower in Fire Defense was rather reduced by this revision because the number of existing houses in Tokyo dropped sharply due to the heavy air raids.

Industrialization Creates Need for Ambulances

As economic reconstruction progressed, Fire Defense expanded and more ambulances were added. Postwar economic reconstruction resulted in more than 10,000 traffic accidents annually. Newspapers called this the "*Traffic War.*" In 1957, when the author was 7 years old, a middle-aged man died from a motorbike accident in a Tokyo neighborhood. Many people gathered at the scene, but no one performed CPR or called an ambulance. At that time there were few ambulances and the concept of calling for an ambulance was unknown.

The Firefighting Organization Act

In 1963, the **Firefighting Organization Act** legislated Japanese EMS. Until this time the rescue teams carried vitacampher and wines to the rescue scene for the victims. Vitacampher (1,7-dimethyl-2-oxo-bicyclo[2.2.1] heptane-7-carbaldehyde)[1] was used as a cardiotonic drug, and wines seemed to be used as analeptics. The Japanese understanding of emergency transport had long been "transport of victims of severe trauma" but not "calling an ambulance for sick patients." There were only about 300,000 ambulance calls/year.

In 1975 the ex-prime minister of Japan and the 1974 Nobel Peace Prize laureate, Mr. Eisaku Sato, fell into a coma at a restaurant in Tokyo. Ambulances still were not commonly called for illnesses. Doctors treated him at the restaurant for 4 days before transferring him to the hospital.

However, as citizens began to appreciate the utility of ambulances, the number of ambulance calls has increased to about 5 million a year (Figure 5-2 and Figure 5-3). The Japanese concept of ambulance use has changed dramatically (Figure 5-4, Figure 5-5, Figure 5-6).

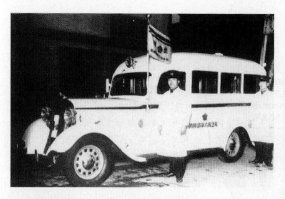

FIGURE 5–1

An ambulance donated to Tokyo City in 1935. Six ambulances started to transport victims in central Tokyo. A white coat was put on over the uniform of fireman. Photo courtesy of Tokyo Fire Department.

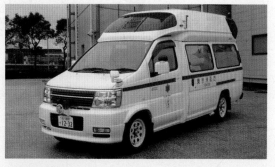

FIGURE 5–2

A typical Japanese ambulance in 2009. Photo courtesy of Tokyo Fire Department.

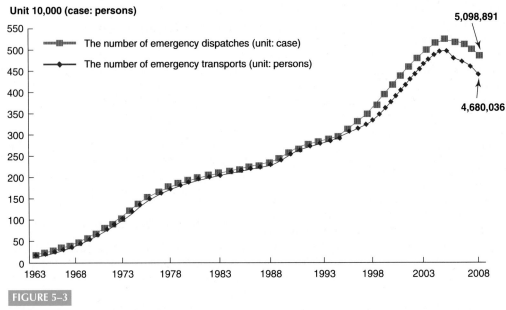

FIGURE 5–3

Numbers of emergency dispatches and transportation of victims in Japan (1961–2008). Numbers transported were less than 0.3 million when EMS was first legislated. They then increased to 5 million.[2]

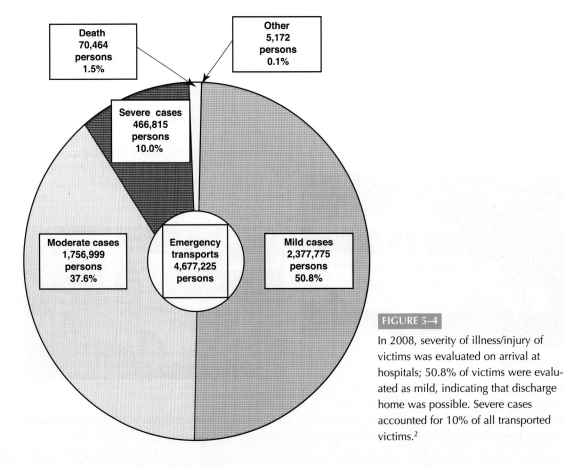

FIGURE 5–4

In 2008, severity of illness/injury of victims was evaluated on arrival at hospitals; 50.8% of victims were evaluated as mild, indicating that discharge home was possible. Severe cases accounted for 10% of all transported victims.[2]

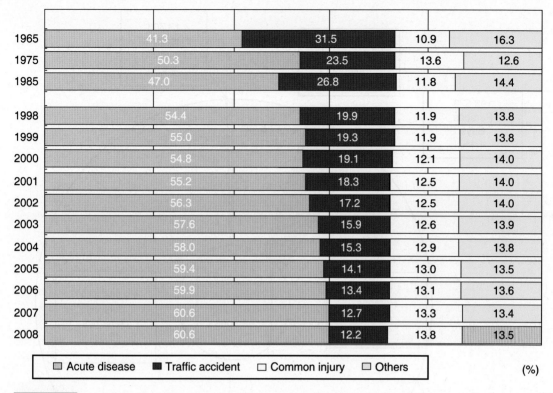

	Acute disease	Traffic accident	Common injury	Others
1965	41.3	31.5	10.9	16.3
1975	50.3	23.5	13.6	12.6
1985	47.0	26.8	11.8	14.4
1998	54.4	19.9	11.9	13.8
1999	55.0	19.3	11.9	13.8
2000	54.8	19.1	12.1	14.0
2001	55.2	18.3	12.5	14.0
2002	56.3	17.2	12.5	14.0
2003	57.6	15.9	12.6	13.9
2004	58.0	15.3	12.9	13.8
2005	59.4	14.1	13.0	13.5
2006	59.9	13.4	13.1	13.6
2007	60.6	12.7	13.3	13.4
2008	60.6	12.2	13.8	13.5

☐ Acute disease ■ Traffic accident ☐ Common injury ☐ Others   (%)

FIGURE 5–5

Categories of illness/injury of transported victims (1965–2008). In 1965, numbers of illnesses and injuries were equal. Because of the decrease in traffic accidents, trauma decreased to 25.8% and illnesses accounted for 60% of all victims.[2]

The Japanese Association for Acute Medicine was established in 1973 as the first association for EM in Japan. Around this period, a close relationship developed between Fire Defense government bureaucrats and emergency physicians. The Fire and Disaster Management Agency controls 803 Fire Headquarters that handle emergency transport (Figure 5-7, Table 5-1). The Tokyo Fire Department is the largest in scale, has the largest information-gathering capacity, and handles all emergency transportation in the Tokyo Metropolitan District. The Fire and Disaster Management Agency in the Ministry of Internal Affairs and Communication has the authority and the Tokyo Fire Department has the actual rescue units.

The Tokyo Fire Department is proud of its role in leading the Japanese EMS. It sponsors many EMS meetings and works closely with emergency physicians. As most Japanese emergency physicians in Japan live in Tokyo, and since most major meetings are held in Tokyo, the Tokyo Fire Department has adopted the opinions of those emergency physicians, who have learned EMS administration and practice from other

countries. The Tokyo Fire Department has become the center of movements to modernize the Japanese EMS system, and it has acquired more power than the Fire and Disaster Management Agency to drive EMS measures and policies.

The Birth of the ELST (Emergency Lifesaving Technician or Paramedic) and the Role of the Media

By the 1980s, it became common practice to transport patients to the hospital while doing CPR. However, Japanese ambulance crews were not yet legally allowed to perform defibrillation, tracheal intubation, or administer any medication, despite the fact that such paramedic procedures were standard practice in Europe and the United States.

In the late 1980s, the US TV drama "ER" was broadcast in Japan, and it became very popular. This drama taught citizens about the emergency medical

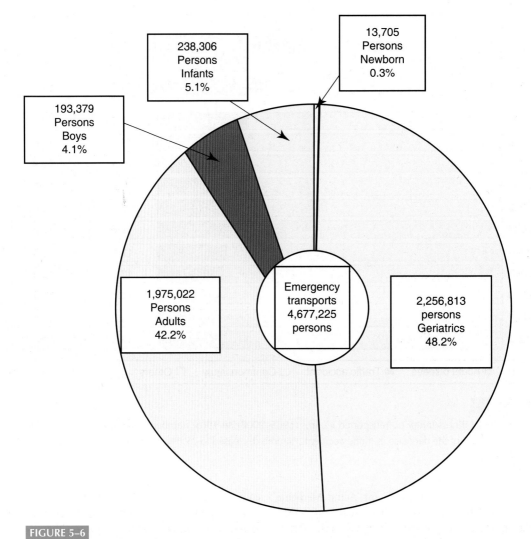

FIGURE 5–6

Age distribution of transported victims in 2008. Geriatric population accounts for 48.2%.[2]

services of foreign countries. Also in 1989, Mr. Yuji Kuroiwa, a newscaster of **Fuji TV** (a Japanese TV company) began a campaign to enable ambulance crews to perform defibrillation. Mr. Eikichi Nakajo, the chief of the EMS Division of the Tokyo Fire Department, took advantage of this campaign. Lawmaking proposed by a local public entity is uncommon in Japan, but the idea was signed into a national law in 1991—the **Emergency Lifesaving Technician (ELST) Law**. It is believed that the passage of this law would have been much later if not for the political activity of the Tokyo Fire Department.

Japanese paramedics, or Emergency Lifesaving Technicians (ELSTs), began training in 1992. They were allowed to perform defibrillation, provide venti-

latory support with specific devices, and provide intravenous fluid infusion. However, a physician's order was needed prior to defibrillation. Ventilatory

Table 5–1	Summary of Japanese EMS
Number of fire headquarters	803
Number of cities, towns, and villages adopting EMS	1,742
Number of ambulance units	4,920
Number of ELSTs	20,000+
Number of ambulances	5,933

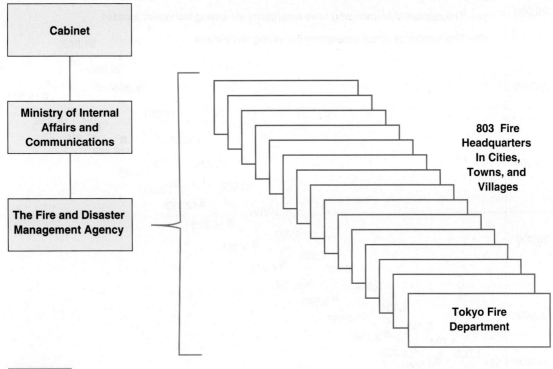

Organization of EMS in Japan. The Fire and Disaster Management Agency in the Ministry of Internal Affairs and Communications controls 803 Fire Headquarters distributed throughout the country. The Tokyo Fire Department is the largest.

support allowed only the use of the laryngeal airway or Combitube™. Administration of any medication was prohibited. These practice limitations severely limited our ability to demonstrate the benefits of prehospital care, and cardiac arrest survival rates did not improve.

Today there are more than 20,000 ELSTs working in Japan (Figure 5-8). The introduction of Japanese paramedics has changed not only the attitude of our citizens but also the attitude of ambulance crews. The focus of EMS care has moved from simple transportation to the actual provision of prehospital care.

However, this led to an unfortunate incident in Akita City.

The Incident in Akita City

Akita City was famous for the high survival rate of its cardiac arrest victims, and this fact attracted national attention. Then, a newspaper reported "*Illegal tracheal intubations by ELSTs for cardiac arrest victims in Akita City.*" Details of this report are included on the website of the Japanese Association for Acute Medicine: http://www.jaam.jp/html/report/index.htm.

Akita City is a city of 300,000 located in the northwest part of the Japanese islands. The city government had been budgeting 7,000,000 yen each year for public education for basic life support. No other regional government had ever made such an investment before, and that effort was nationally viewed as "extraordinary." As a result, bystander CPR was done by Akita citizens in up to 50% of cardiac arrest victims. Many doctors and health care workers applauded their efforts. Akita City also gave high priority to education of ambulance teams, including ELSTs. The high quality of prehospital care in Akita City was frequently reported in the media. However, Akita's ELSTs were routinely performing endotracheal intubation. The Akita City Fire Department tacitly approved the procedure, knowing it was illegal (see ELST Law above). The city had 200 cardiac arrest victims transported by ambulance a year, with intubation of 70% to 80% of victims. ELSTs were trained by the Department of Anesthesiology in Akita

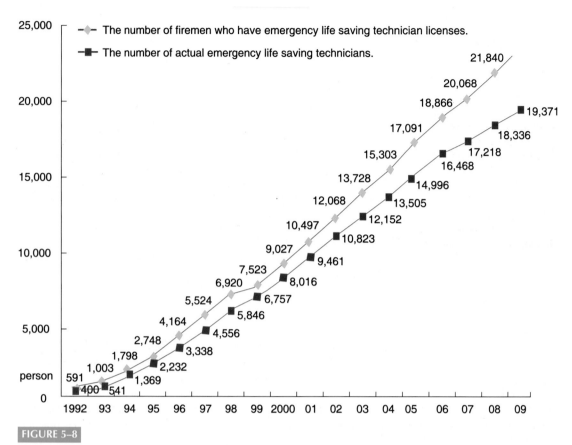

FIGURE 5–8

Number of ELSTs. Training and national board examinations have been ongoing since 1992. The number of ELSTs is over 20,000.[2]

University Hospital. The doctors felt that "airway control" implicitly included "tracheal intubation" and that the need for the procedure should be decided by ELSTs at the scene. Although the "why and how" of the start of prehospital tracheal intubation were obscure, it was performed routinely. At the same time, ELST documentation was silent about tracheal intubation.

The "illegal procedure" was first reported in local newspapers, then nationwide. In Akita City, paramedics became targets of criticism, and their children were ill-treated in schools. A national newspaper began a vindictive campaign. However, ultimately Akita citizens rose up to defend the ELSTs, and the Akita City council and the Akita prefectural assembly also defended them and refused to indict them.

This incident led to an expansion of the role of the ELSTs. Mr. Ryuichi Ishii, the chief of the Fire and Disaster Management Agency of Japan (2002–2004) allowed specially trained ELSTs to perform tracheal

intubation in 2002 and allowed the administration of intravenous epinephrine in 2004 (Figure 5–9).

The Sarin Attack in the Tokyo Subway System in 1995

At 8:10 AM on March 20, 1995, the Tokyo Fire Department announced a gas explosion in the Tokyo subway system and alerted all hospitals to be ready to receive emergency victims. In reality, this was the chemical terrorist incident by Aum Shinri Kyo cult members. The terrorists put bags filled with sarin liquid on five subway cars of three metro lines. They broke the bags with umbrella tips, and then ran away. These five subway cars were to arrive at Kasumigaseki station from 8:13 to 8:19. There are many government buildings around Kasumigaseki station, and the attack on the subway passengers meant an attack on the Japanese government. Cars immediately filled with sarin vapor. Twenty-six subway stations were

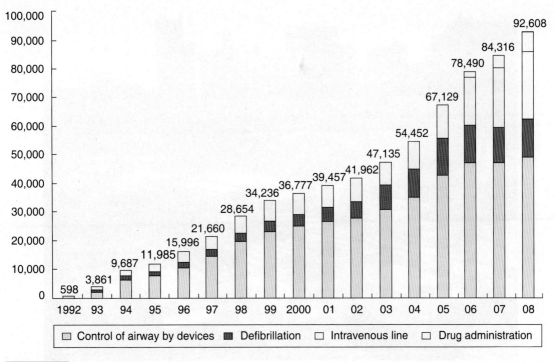

Number of lifesaving procedures performed by ELSTs. Airway control by device was performed in 48,939 cases, defibrillation in 13,718 cases, intravenous line in 24,057 cases, and epinephrine administered in 6,434 cases in 2008. The number of ELSTs who were able to do tracheal intubation was 6,477; the number of ELSTs who were able to administer epinephrine was 8,330; and number of ELSTs who were able to do both procedures was 4,468.[2]

closed, and two subway lines stopped their service. The Tokyo Fire Department directed all 200 ambulances to the site, for triage and hospital transport (Figure 5-10). The newspapers reported the effectiveness of the Tokyo Fire Department (Figure 5-11). In this attack, 5,513 victims were treated in EDs for sarin intoxication, and 12 of them died (Figure 5-12 and Figure 5-13). Victims included firefighters, police officers, and hospital workers with secondary sarin intoxication.[3]

In this chemical disaster not only the Tokyo Fire Department but police and self-defense forces were involved. The Tokyo Fire Department sent forth its chemical specialists to analyze the substance left at the site and announced at 11 AM that the chemical was methyl cyanide, which turned out to be wrong later.[4] The specialists did not have the reference sample of sarin and could only identify methyl cyanide, which was the solvent of sarin. The metropolitan police department made the correct announcement that the

toxin was sarin by noon, one hour later. Because the causative agent was not known at first, many hospitals did not give the correct treatment, that is Pralidoxime (2-PAM), atropine, and diazepam. After this attack, special fire department teams (600 personnel and 10 chemical teams) were developed to counter biological, chemical, and nuclear disasters (Figure 5-14). The public media reports and their comparisons with police, self-defense forces, and the fire department actions in the sarin gas attack facilitated the leadership of the Fire Department and EMS in disaster management.

A Sudden Death in the Imperial Family

The automated external defibrillator (AED) was imported to Japan from the United States in 1988, but at first the Ministry of Health, Labor, and Welfare only allowed physicians to use it. As a result, AEDs were not widely available or used.

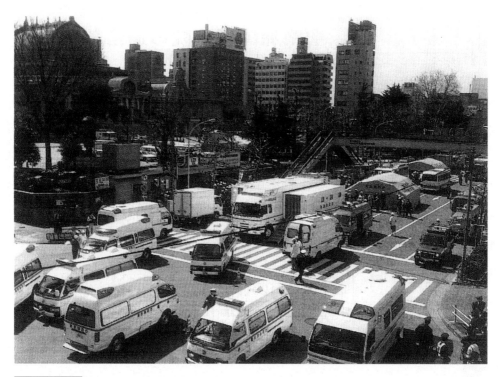

FIGURE 5–10

One of exits of Kasumigaseki subway station on the day of the sarin attack. More than 200 ambulance units were called together by the Tokyo Fire Department. A large-scale ambulance, called a super-ambulance, is seen in the center of the figure. Photo courtesy of Tokyo Fire Department.

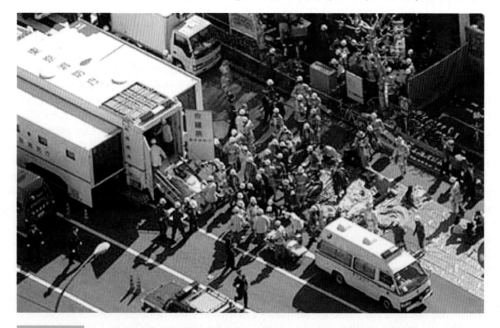

FIGURE 5–11

Super-ambulance. A king-size ambulance that seats eight victims for prehospital care. Its presence was reported as a symbol of prehospital care by the Tokyo Fire Department. Photo courtesy of Tokyo Fire Department.

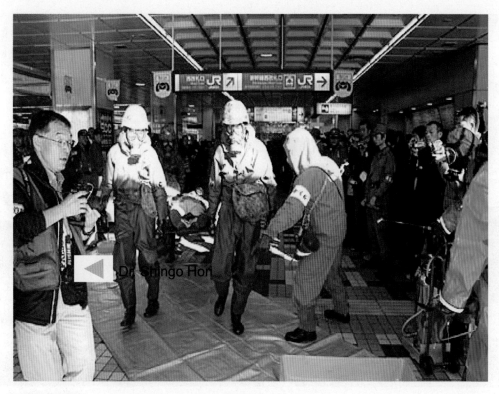

FIGURE 5–12
Scene of the sarin attack. Photo courtesy of Tokyo Fire Department.

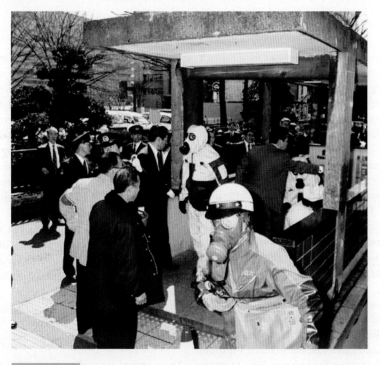

FIGURE 5–13
Sarin victims brought to the ED. Photo courtesy of Tokyo Fire Department.

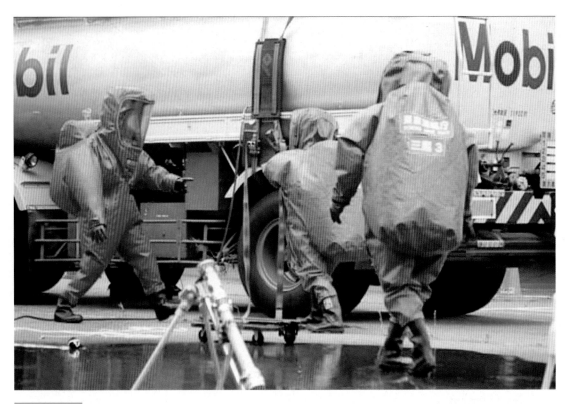

FIGURE 5–14
Training of chemical disaster teams in the Tokyo Fire Department. Photo courtesy of Tokyo Fire Department.

Prince Takamado was a nephew of the Emperor and one of the most popular and respected members of the imperial family. He was also the honorary president of the Japanese Football Association. On November 21, 2002, he suffered cardiac arrest while playing squash near the Canadian Embassy in central Tokyo. An ambulance crew arrived and started CPR. The crew identified ventricular fibrillation, but the law required a phone call and explicit permission from the doctor on call at the Tokyo Fire Department before defibrillating with an AED. The physician ordered defibrillation, but by then, asystole had developed. The paramedics restarted CPR, and Prince Takamado was brought to Keio University Hospital. Despite aggressive measures, including extracorporeal circulation, he could not be resuscitated.

The newspapers reported his sudden cardiac death widely, and this was the first time the words "ventricular fibrillation" were used in a Japanese newspaper. The death of Prince Takamado made ventricular fibrillation into a household phrase. The Ministry of Health, Labor, and Welfare and the Ministry of Internal Affairs and Communications then approved "defibrillation without a doctor's suggestion" and "AED usage by citizens" in 2004. As of 2008, the one-month survival rate for out-of-hospital cardiac arrest is 10.5%, and the rate of full recovery is 6.4% nationwide (Figure 5-15). The rate of bystander CPR and of AED use by citizens is also increasing (Figure 5-16). In 2008, about 800 citizens performed defibrillation by using an AED. One month survival rate for this patient series was 43.7%, and the rate of full recovery was as high as 38.8% (Figure 5-17).[4]

The sarin gas attack and the sudden death of Prince Takamado were examples of events that resulted in strong positive effects for EMS. Both cases were widely publicized, and the press encouraged further upgrading of the EMS system.

Making a Difference

These stories show that emergency physicians, public officials, the Fire Department, politicians, media, and

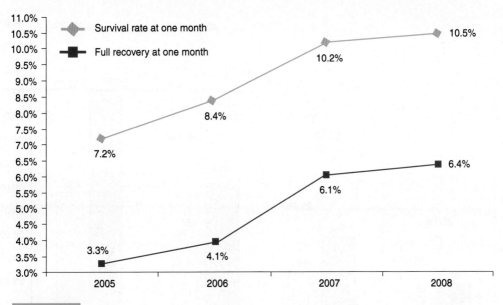

Nationwide survival and full recovery rates of witnessed cardiogenic cardiac arrest victims in Japan (2005–2008).[2]

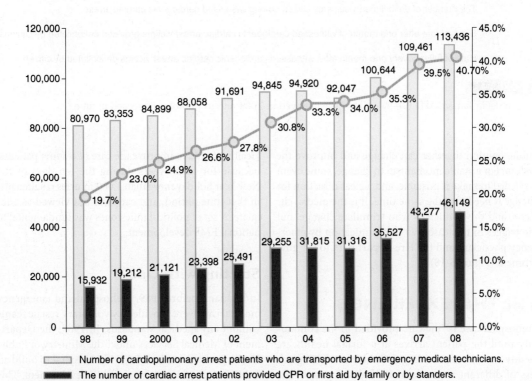

CPR and first aid by family or other bystanders (1998–2008). The number of cardiac arrest victims has increased, indicating the aging of society.[2]

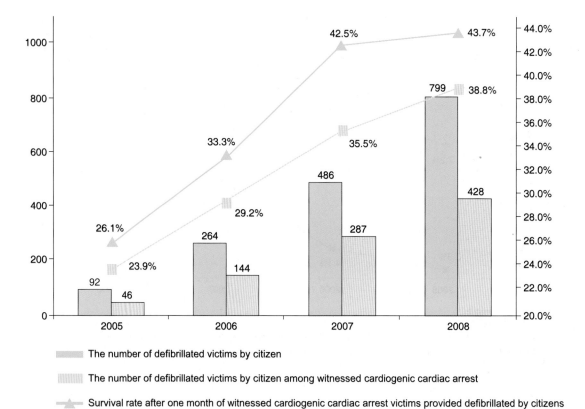

The number of defibrillated victims by citizen

The number of defibrillated victims by citizen among witnessed cardiogenic cardiac arrest

Survival rate after one month of witnessed cardiogenic cardiac arrest victims provided defibrillated by citizens

Rate of full recovery one month after witnessed cardiogenic cardiac arrest victims defibrillated by citizen

FIGURE 5–17

Citizen defibrillation. AED use by citizens was allowed in 2004 and its numbers increased in time.[2]

public opinion together can change and improve the system. For a stable mechanism to change, some event is needed to make it unstable, and a clear direction for change is needed at the same time. It is the media, citizens, and the politicians who stimulate change, but the trigger in this case was communication by emergency physicians and the Fire Department to the government (Figure 5-18).

THE THAI EXPERIENCE

Prehospital care is "the care provided in the community until the patient arrives at a formal healthcare facility capable of providing definitive care."[5] Regardless of different methods of EMS development, the final objective of an EMS system is shortening the time to deliver the patient to an appropriate hospital with adequate emergency medical care. In Thailand, EMS developed because of a close relationship with the Thai Ministry of Public Health. The Ministry of Public

Health wanted to improve the care of trauma patients, because for many years during the ten days of the New Year holiday more than 1,000 injuries resulted just in that time period, and care was not viewed as adequate. A set of political milestones was fundamental to national EMS development.

Starting with One

In Thailand before 1989, prehospital and emergency medical care were provided by voluntary rescue teams without any medical standards. In 1989, the Department of Medical Services under the Ministry of Public Health granted funds to Rajavithi Hospital to build an "EMS Building" as a center of EMS development. This was the first use of the term "EMS" in Thailand. International support was very important in this early period. The World Health Organization supported a project to set up an EMS unit. The Franco-Asian Medical Association (AMFA) supported a project to gain

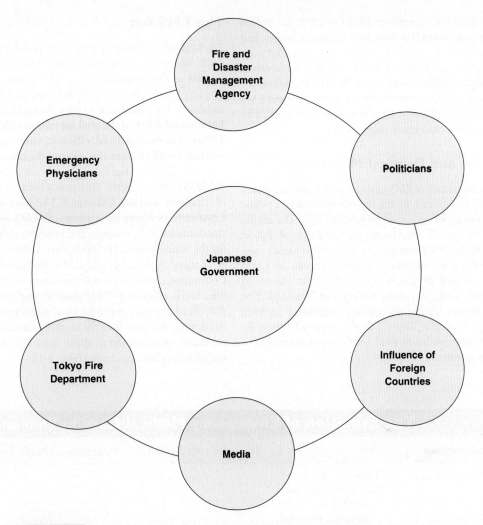

Figure 5–18 — circles labeled: Fire and Disaster Management Agency; Politicians; Emergency Physicians; Japanese Government; Influence of Foreign Countries; Tokyo Fire Department; Media

Factors impacting the role of government on the EMS system. Communications between emergency physicians, the fire department, government bureaucrats, the media, and politicians are the key factors that influence the government.

EMS experience at SAMU of France for Thai EMS personnel. The state of New South Wales in Australia helped to set up the Basic-EMT training course at Rajavithi Hospital. The George Washington University in Washington, D.C. provided EMS education to the administrative team of the Ministry of Public Health. However, no strategic plan for the system existed until 1995, when a prototype prehospital care unit was established at Rajavithi Hospital in Bangkok.

Leading up to 1995, the Ministry of Public Health formed a group whose members were all committed to providing better care for the injured during the New Year holiday. The group consisted of active members from the Department of Epidemiology, the Department of Permanent Secretary, and the Department of Medical Services. The Department of Epidemiology set up a system of injury surveillance, the Department of Permanent Secretary set up a system of trauma care, and Dr. Somchai Kanchanasut of the Department of Medical Services negotiated the support of Rajavithi Hospital to set up the EMS Pilot Project and the Basic EMT training course. Dr. Somchai then assumed leadership of the EMS Building under the Department of Emergency Medicine.

The pilot EMS project was one EMS unit, with 24-7 capability, based in Rajavithi Hospital. The unit was called the Narenthorn EMS Center. It was staffed by one physician (Dr. Somchai), volunteer nurses, and basic EMTs. Based on the results from this pilot project, EMS units gradually developed in many hospitals without specific government funds earmarked for EMS. However, hospitals were eager to support EMS development because they were all overburdened by trauma and emergency care patients.

Media and Political Milestones

The importance of EMS units for each hospital became widely recognized. Media reports resulted in a public movement for increased prehospital care. The media and the public convinced the Ministry of Public Health that EMS was an essential part of health care. In 2002, the Narenthorn Center (Bureau of EMS) was founded by the Ministry of Public Health to develop an EMS system throughout Thailand. The Narenthorn Center successfully negotiated an EMS budget from the National Health Security Office. By 2005, hospital-based EMS services had expanded to every province.

The EMS Act

The Ministry of Public Health developed the EMS Act draft, and it was approved by the Thai parliament in 2008 as **The EMS Act.** The events of the previous 12 years and the success of each hospital's EMS units convinced the parliament to pass the legislation. **The EMS Act established the goal for nationwide EMS of Thailand as standardized, efficient, and timely EMS services for all citizens throughout the country.**

The EMS Act legislated three bodies: the National EMS Committee, the Emergency Medical Institute of Thailand, and the EMS fund. The *National EMS Committee* develops the nationwide EMS plan, sets standards for EMS systems, and provides supervision for the entire system. The *Emergency Medical Institute of Thailand* implements the plans of the National EMS Committee, coordinates education and research activities, and is a liaison for EMS agencies worldwide. The *EMS fund* provides grants to local municipalities for developing and managing the local EMS units and also provides compensation to those units that have met the national EMS standards (Table 5-2).

Table 5–2	The Evolution of Emergency Medical Care in Thailand		
National Plan	**EMS**	**Emergency Medicine**	**Ministry of Public Health**
1986–1991	1989 First initiating fund for EMS to Rajavithi Hospital		
1992–1996 Starting first EMS program	1995 EMS Pilot Project by Rajavithi Hospital	1995 Injury Surveillance and Trauma Audit	1995 Injury Prevention Program
1997–2001 Expanding EMS to all provinces	2001 EMS provided by main hospital	1999 Establishment of Thai Association for Emergency Medicine	2001 EMS development as one main policy
			2002 EMS funded by National Health Security Office
2002–2006 EMS by community participation	2005 Full establishment of countrywide provincial EMS	2003 Starting of emergency medicine training program	2008 EMS Act
		2007 First graduated Emergency Physician	

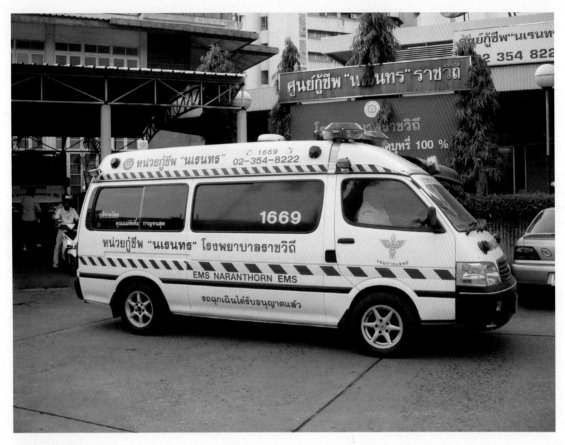

FIGURE 5–19

ALS ambulance, Narenthorn EMS Center. Rajavithi Hospital, Bangkok, Thailand. Photo courtesy of Barbara Steckler, EMT-P.

The objective of the EMS Act is to designate the individual municipality as the lead organization of EMS in own responsible area.[6] Any organization (such as a hospital, a voluntary foundation, or another agency related to emergency medical care) can be an EMS provider after applying to the individual municipality and being certified by the Emergency Medical Institute of Thailand. Penalties can be levied on those providers that do not meet standards or that do not demonstrate effective performance.

During the transition period to complete national EMS coverage, the Ministry of Public Health monitors local management while the municipalities are learning the process of leading each local EMS system. The national EMS hotline is the universal call number "1669." The 1669 Call and Dispatch Centers are located in every main provincial hospital and are supervised by physicians. The preference is, of course, for emergency physicians to be responsible for supervision, but this will not be possible until the number of certified emergency physicians increases.

There are three levels of ambulances providing the emergency medical services: the hospital-based Advanced Life Support Units (Figure 5-19), the volunteer-based Basic Life Support Units, and the community-based First Responder Units. The patients pay nothing for this ambulance service, as the National Health Security Fund reimburses directly based on cases serviced.

Emergency Physicians as EMS Leaders

The emergency physician has the lead role in both pre- and in-hospital emergency medical care. As of this writing, there are 200 board-certified emergency physicians in Thailand and 2000 EDs. The first certification was established by the Medical Council of Thailand in 2003.

The Ministry of Public Health is the main provider of all medical care in Thailand because more than 80% of the EDs belong to the Ministry. The EMS Act requires that every ED be staffed by emergency physicians. EMS development is possible because of government initiative and leadership, and the intense involvement of key individuals and stakeholders with the Ministry. The keys to the development of more emergency physicians for the Thai population of 64 million and the keys to quality control and improvement of emergency medical care are strong planning and cooperation between emergency physicians and the Thai Ministry of Public Health.

References

1. On the Treatment of Asphyxia Neonatorum with Vitacampher, with Special Reference to the Comparison of the Effects of Allo-p-oxocamphor and Trans-π-oxocamphor [in Japanese] (date unknown).
   • 安井 修平 Yasui Shuhei
   • 東京逓信病院産婦人科　Gynecological and Obstetrical Section of the Tokyo-Teishin Hospital
   • Acta Obstetrica et Gynaecologica Japonica [Journal Detail].
   • 日本産科婦人科學會雜誌　3(11) pp. 517–520 19511101 [Index].
   • Japan Society of Obstetrics and Gynecology (JSOG)
2. The Fire and Disaster Management Agency Present status of emergency and rescue (in Japanese); Annual Report, 2009.
3. Nozaki H, Hori S, Shinozawa Y, et al. Secondary exposure of medical staff to sarin vapor in the emergency room. *Intensive Care Med* 21(12):1032; 1995.
4. Nozaki H, Aikawa N, Shinozawa Y, et al. Sarin poisoning in Tokyo subway. *Lancet* 345(8955):980; 1995.
5. Kobusingye OC, Hyder AA, Bishai D, et al. Emergency medical systems in low-and middle-income countries: recommendations for action. Bull World Health Organ 83:8, 626; 2005.
6. Sinthavalai R, Memongkol N, Patthanaprechawong N, et al. A Study of Distinctive Models for Pre-Hospital EMS in Thailand: Knowledge Capture. World Acad Sci Engineering Technol 55:140; 2009.

EMS and Public Services: Lessons Learned in Lebanon

Amin Antoine Kazzi, Nabih Jabr

KEY LEARNING POINTS

- Key public services include the Ministry of Health, national, regional, and local authorities and legislative bodies, existing patient transportation services, hospitals, health care provider organizations, the media, police authorities, the fire department, and any other crisis response systems.

- EMS systems cannot operate in isolation. They are intimately linked to the level of education of the population and to key public services that should work closely with them.

- Stability of the government is an important prerequisite for a stable and advancing EMS system.

- One should ask not only how relationships are established between public services but also *if* they have been established, whether roles have been defined and accepted by all stakeholders, and whether or how they are maintained and sustained.

- Planners need to be familiar with the peculiarities of each agency and community and to understand the history and reasons behind the development of such complex organizations and the challenges they face.

- Public legislation is a core requirement to develop and deliver proper EMS services.

- A crucial key public service component of an effective EMS system is an available, capable, accessible ED that welcomes patients and provides basic screening, evaluation, and stabilization for every patient who comes through its doors.

- Committed and persistent emergency physicians and seasoned prehospital provider leadership provide momentum for improvement of the EMS system.

INTRODUCTION

It would be very challenging to determine the historical roots of EMS systems. Some people trace

them back to the parable of the Good Samaritan. Others argue that such systems originated in the carnage of battlefields. In this chapter, we shall describe the key public services that our experience in

Lebanon indicates should work closely with EMS. We shall also discuss how we believe such services relate to each other with regard to EMS. Our experience indicates that such key public services include the Ministry of Health, national, regional, and local authorities and legislative bodies, existing patient transportation services, hospitals and health care provider organizations, the media, police authorities, the fire department, and any other existing similar crisis response systems.

AN OVERVIEW OF EMS IN LEBANON

To better frame our discussion of key public services, we shall first provide an overview of the current status of EMS in Lebanon, while assuming that other developing nations face similar challenges with regard to their prehospital emergency services. In 1966, the National Academy of Sciences in the United States published a report called "Accidental Death and Disability: The Neglected Disease of Modern Society." This report concluded that both the public and the government were "insensitive to the magnitude of the problem of accidental death and injury" in the US; that the standards to which ambulance services were held were diverse and "often low"; and that "most ambulances used are unsuitable, have incomplete equipment, carry inadequate supplies, and are manned by untrained attendants."

More than 40 years later, EMS in Lebanon (and in many developing or underdeveloped nations) is in a somewhat better but fundamentally similar situation. The public's awareness of prehospital emergency care is low. Expectations are mostly focused on having any kind of ambulance with a siren and stretcher respond to an emergency, regardless of the personnel on board or their training and equipment. The government, with the support of local and international organizations and the Lebanese Red Cross, is attentive to this issue, but nothing concrete has been done yet to improve the system nationwide. There is no nationwide standardization of training for EMS personnel nor are ambulance specifications and equipment regulated in any way. Several EMS provider systems work in the country, with very little, if any, coordination.

As a result, the sick or injured in Lebanon or any country with similar challenges receive varying qualities of prehospital care, depending on where and when the emergency occurred, the identity of the injured, the type and severity of the injury, the number of casualties, who made the call for assistance if one was made, which emergency number was used, and which agency responded. This contradicts **the fundamental principle that access to good quality emergency prehospital care is a basic right that should be enjoyed by every sick or injured person throughout the country.**

To better frame interactions with key public services we listed above, we shall first briefly explore the essential components of a prehospital emergency care system and the priorities to improve a national system.

The 10 Main Elements of a Successful EMS System

An EMS system, as described by the World Health Organization, should be simple, sustainable, flexible, and efficient. As such, the country's existing capacity should be utilized and strengthened, and we should not fall into the temptation of importing an expensive European or North American EMS model before ensuring that we can provide rapid, high quality, *basic* prehospital emergency care to the population. This is especially important since "**there is scant evidence that more advanced approaches to prehospital care are inherently superior to less expensive but effective treatments.**"[†]

First responders represent the first and most basic tier of any EMS system. First responders can be ordinary citizens, police officers, taxi drivers, municipal employees, or other community members. The role of a first responder is to activate EMS and provide first aid until the arrival of formally trained personnel.

Basic prehospital emergency care should be the backbone of any EMS system. Basic care providers should have formal training in prehospital care, scene management, rescue, stabilization, and the transportation of injured or sick people. The Lebanese Red Cross is currently upgrading the training of its 2,600 volunteers and improving the ambulances and equipment used.

In advanced prehospital emergency care, in many countries, a physician or highly trained professional paramedics follow the first responders or basic providers to the scene and can provide advanced care before the patient reaches the hospital. **These systems are expensive and difficult to sustain and should be implemented only after the basic response has already proven its effectiveness and has been established nationwide.**

A system of medical oversight should be in place. Every EMS system should have a physician, preferably with extensive training and experience in out-of-hospital emergency care, assigned as medical

---

[†]Prehospital trauma care systems, World Health Organization, Geneva. 2005.

director. This is especially important in Lebanon, since EMS personnel are not independently licensed health care providers. The term **medical oversight** describes all of the prospective, concurrent, and retrospective activities conducted by the physicians who assume the ultimate responsibility and authority for the medical care provided by an EMS system. Medical oversight can also include providing on-line medical direction to EMS teams facing a difficult or exceptional situation in the field. In Lebanon, as EMS is still largely unregulated, this element is often missing. The Lebanon Red Cross EMS teams have, however, largely benefited from the medical direction provided by a team of emergency physicians since 1995.

Dispatch is a key element in the effectiveness of any EMS system. Dispatch is the mobilization of appropriate resources in response to a call for help made to a free designated telephone number. The "140" emergency number operated by the Lebanon Red Cross has been in service for more than 16 years, and the four 140 dispatch centers are currently being upgraded through better training of dispatchers and the introduction of computers, GPS navigation, and tracking systems. For the system to be effective nationwide, all calls related to prehospital medical emergencies should be routed through this single free emergency number. This measure would ensure that the closest, most appropriate unit is sent.

Training and protocols should be in place in order to raise the level of care. The most critical issue is to develop a minimum standard of care for patients in the out-of-hospital setting. When this standard of care is developed, training curricula can be implemented at all levels, and a national certification system can eventually be adopted. Currently the personnel of many ambulance services operating in Lebanon have no or little formal training in emergency care. The Red Cross has recognized the need to modernize and standardize the training of its EMS volunteers throughout the country and has started working since July 2008 on developing a new training curriculum, a rigorous certification and coaching process, and yearly mandatory continued education.

Documentation is needed in order to evaluate compliance and ensure medical accountability. All actions and interventions should be properly documented. A standardized patient care report would also provide essential data for assessing the system, taking corrective action, and implementing preventive measures.

Legislation and public policy also must be developed. Whereas the authority to operate a prehospital emergency system is usually derived from laws adopted by the country's governing bodies, the EMS systems in Lebanon currently operate in a legal vacuum. It is the role of EMS personnel and physicians to work together to ensure that appropriate legislation is put into place. Such legislation would address critical issues such as minimum standards of care, training and certification, and minimum requirements for ambulances and EMS equipment.

Financing the emergency response in Lebanon should not become a for-profit activity. Care should never be withheld because a person cannot afford it. However, a combination of funding from the government, insurance companies, and the community should be secured in order to be able to develop and maintain a high-quality system.

The issue of public awareness also needs to be addressed. The effectiveness of the best EMS system will never reach its full potential without a solid public education program. The public should be taught how and when to activate the system and what to do while waiting for the ambulance. It should also address the prevention of illnesses and injuries. Some good examples for Lebanon would be child safety seat education and motorcycle helmet use.

Relationships Between Key Public Services

EMS systems cannot operate in isolation. They are intimately linked to the level of education of the population and to key public services that should work closely with EMS. Therefore any effort to improve prehospital emergency care in the country should involve all concerned public service professionals and stakeholders. It must not be limited to health care providers.

Linkage between the EMS system and public services requires an understanding of the resources, strengths, and shortcomings of public services. Planning should therefore first identify what key public services are available. In undeveloped or under-developed nations, regions, or communities, services that developed nations consider "public" may not exist. Availability of services may vary from region to region or change from period to period. Some services that we assume are public in the world we know, including some that are essential to providing proper EMS care, may be private and some traditionally private services may be public in some nations. Peculiarities exist and healthcare planners should even expect to find additional public services that are unique to a specific community and have direct or indirect influence on EMS operations and development.

Such realism is therefore essential to understand an EMS system and public services in any international community. **One should ask not only how**

relationships are established between these public services but *if* they have been established, whether roles have been defined and accepted by all stakeholders, and whether or how they are maintained and sustained.

Following our discussion of the potential complexity in international EMS and its relationship with its key public services, we will describe our experience in Lebanon.

The Ministry of Health

The Ministry of Health is perhaps the most important of all public services and is a constant in all cabinets and governments of sovereign nations. The Ministry of Health provides structure, leadership, and services to its population(s). Of course, allocated resources and responsibilities vary from nation to nation and over time. A government and its Ministry of Health may choose to delegate varying degrees or all of its health care services to the private, nongovernmental or public sector. It may retain varying degrees of control or scrutiny over essential resources or health care agencies and providers, including medical personnel, nurses and physicians, patient transportation services, and health care facilities such as hospitals, clinics, and outpatient and diagnostic centers. Ministries of Health exert varying degrees of authority and effort in introducing, implementing, and/or regulating national or regional health care laws and policies, many of which have direct influence on the status, performance, type, composition, structure, and development of EMS services.

This highlights the importance of

1. The National Cabinet in how it supports, restricts, or controls its own Ministry of Health.
2. The functional and actual existence of a National Cabinet and Ministry of Health, considering that such entities may be totally or partially absent or ineffective in conflicted or war-ridden countries.
3. Local governments in nations with varying degrees of federal or regional authorities and their relationship with their Ministry of Health or central National Cabinet.

How can a sovereign Cabinet and Ministry of Health, in Lebanon or any other nation, require, introduce, and implement ambulance and prehospital certification, if or when the Cabinet or Ministry of Interior refuses to require such compliance from local municipality-based ambulance response and providers? Such ambulance response and its providers are financed and controlled by the Ministry of Interior, and it is common for such fragmentation or overlap to cause stalling of performance improvement initiatives.

How can the Ministry of Health require and enforce AED training or cervical spine immobilization by EMS providers in regions that are under the direct authority of militia? These are regions where EMS personnel are financed by, or are members of, armed groups, and where no one will bother responding to national decrees. How can national government require inspection of patient transport vehicles when local communities have their own ambulances and volunteers operating them, with no funds available to purchase equipment or pursue expensive training recommended by Ministry of Health planners? How can the Ministry of Health support the needs of EMS for laws and support to protect and empower them during their services when national government and/or the Cabinet has not agreed to convene for 18 months, or when the Cabinet cannot be formed for more than 6 months after its prior cabinet members have resigned?

Regional Authorities

In many countries, federated states, regions, counties, provinces, and municipalities have their own form of government authority, which may or may not overlap or contradict the national governance and entities. Their legislative process or structure may cause national initiatives to stall or fail. Opposition, which is sometimes armed or in conflict with central or other regional government, may intentionally or unintentionally refuse to comply or simply remain indifferent to national decrees or initiatives.

How can a national EMS authority require and enforce ACLS training or credentialing of ambulance personnel who fall under the authority of a dissenting governor or state cabinet? How can one select one emergency call number for the whole nation if the regional authority wants to use its own number because of local separatist parties and powers that want to declare their region independent from the rest of the country? How can the national EMS authority authorize female prehospital providers to ride on ambulances in regions where local official or unofficial authorities, parties, or powers insist on segregating workers of different sexes?

To what degree is a national initiative attentive to the special needs of a region or municipality where resources or challenges require special attention and exceptional measures? **Some regions may be remote, require different vehicles for transportation, different security support and measures, or special attention to ethnic, religious, tribal, or sociocultural considerations.** Calling off resuscitation in the field on non-resuscitatable patients may unnecessarily endanger rescuers, and while this could be done in a Beirut tertiary care center ED for a medical arrest in asystole, it certainly cannot be done and should not be mandated in the middle of the street of a refugee camp. Some municipalities may be rich enough to purchase an AED or to secure new C-spine collars for every trauma transport. However, others may not be able to afford the provision of single-use devices.

Legislative Bodies

Sovereign nations have their own structure and procedures to develop, define, and refine and to introduce the laws, rules, and regulations that directly impact the delivery of EMS and the practice of emergency medicine. Sovereign bodies can legislate, restrict, or approve the scope of practice, the logistic framework, the work force structure, the credentials, training, and qualifications, remuneration, and all forms of support for EMS providers and personnel.

Legislative bodies play a key role-in defining the authority to perform medical acts; in providing funding for and determining the capacity of the EMS system; for protecting EMS personnel and equipment; for helping retain experienced personnel; and for providing the structure and framework for EMS operations.

Public legislation is a core requirement to develop and deliver proper EMS services. How can EMS be supported with laws and budgeted allocations to protect and empower its personnel during their services when the national Parliament and its elected leader have refused to convene for more than 2 years?

This situation emphasizes a common challenge faced by EMS providers in developing nations and in conflict-ridden nations. What do EMS providers do when they find themselves forced to operate in a legal vacuum? They often just do it.

Media

In any nation, EMS providers and authorities should operate very carefully when interacting with the "media" because a double-edged sword can result when information is provided, received, or concealed. Indeed, first-line responders typically have the earliest and often perhaps the most accurate information about the circumstances, magnitude, and casualty profile of an incident.

While such information may be of great value to the ED in order to promptly prepare to receive serious or mass casualties, public information can have grave unintended consequences on the safety of the public, the victims, and the ED or EMS providers. Releasing inflated or inaccurate information can be as harmful as publicizing the count or identifying the victims or assailants, or those who may have been involved in causing or responding to an incident.

Certainly, **carefully worded information** may help reduce the risk of public or individual hysteria. It can guide the public and stakeholders, mobilize support, momentum, donations, and volunteers. It can guide and provide directions and directives that would reduce primary and secondary loss and injury, remove potential victims from harm, or facilitate relief efforts. It can also help reduce the chance for an unnecessary activation of mass casualty response by authorities, hospitals, and other public agencies or crisis response teams.

Should you tell the media who the victims are? Should you give them a count or identify who survived or was wounded? You will find vengeful assassins or distressed crowds barging into your ED to finish the victims off. Should EMS tell the media where the victims were transported, or their identity or count during a riot or civil strife? That will only add to the chaos and possibly guide assailants to the hospital. Distraught friends and families will also come searching for their relatives who may or may not be missing, disrupting ED operations for mass casualty incidents. Danger, distress, and the burden on EMS personnel and ED staff receiving victims should be minimized. **Destination hospitals, those potentially responsible or involved, and the casualty profile should be concealed. Information released should be carefully worded and limited to what is necessary.**

Accordingly, the role and responsibility for communication and dissemination of information should be delegated to those with the proper experience and training to properly assume that role. This assumes there is an incident command, or crisis response protocol, or a community or national plan defining who should speak to the media. Unfortunately, there are many nations where there is no plan, no proper training or experience, no predefined agency or responsible leadership. In others, the picture is more complicated: plans, authorities, and agencies overlap and many may believe they have the responsibility to release information to the media. This is a recipe for problematic errors – often compounded by poor, variable, or lack of training and experience, which often endangers patients, EMS and ED personnel or compromises relief and medical operations.

Patient Transport Services

Any national, regional, or community EMS system requires the existence of patient transportation services, typically those including ground transportation by ambulances. Developed nations with an established

EMS system have properly trained and supported staff (paramedics, nurses, physicians, inhalation therapists, and EMTs) providing prehospital emergency and non-emergency patient transportation through properly equipped land, air, sea, or train vehicles. Formal credentialing, certification, oversight, and audits ensure there is formal training and compliance for all prehospital staff and vehicles. Such systems include dispatch coordination and command centers, ambulance and personnel stations, medical control, logistic structures and networks, and treatment and transportation protocols.

Nations, regions, and communities *traditionally* have one agency primarily assigned to the provision of prehospital or patient transportation services. Such agencies may be publicly or privately owned and run or may be for profit, nonprofit, and nongovernmental or volunteer-based. This picture becomes more complex when prehospital patient transportation for a nation or specific regions or communities may be assigned to or in actuality delivered by more than one agency, with a variable degree of coordination, team play, compliance with expectations, credentialing, training, and operational standards and protocols. This heterogeneity among agencies is further complicated by variability and erratic and unreliable performance and the absence of protocols, standards, day-to-day implementation, oversight, and credentialing processes. Even if protocols and standards exist, they may not be disseminated to the providers or implemented in daily operations.

To illustrate this problem, we should indicate that in Lebanon, our prehospital response is primarily assigned to the Lebanese Red Cross, a nongovernmental volunteer-based not-for-profit organization, which receives direct support from the Ministry of Health. Throughout the Lebanese Civil War, it fell upon the Lebanese Red Cross to provide prehospital service to the population and the warring parties. After the end of that war, the Lebanese Red Cross was mandated by the Lebanese government to be the main provider of EMS services in the country. Today, the Lebanese Red Cross finds itself working with a multitude of partners and continuously seeking to modernize and improve its EMS service to better serve the population of Lebanon. Partners include key public and nonpublic, national and international, governmental and nongovernmental services and organizations such as the Lebanese Ministry of Health, the International Committee of the Red Cross, and a variety of official and unofficial stakeholders. After having established its reputation as a pioneering EMS provider in Lebanon, the Lebanese Red Cross is currently in the process of modernizing its services through a 5-year development plan (2008–2012).

Overlapping with the Lebanese Red Cross, the Lebanese Civil Defense is another EMS public service, which provides search and rescue and fire-fighting response as well as patient transportation. It is directly administered and supported by the Ministry of Interior and Municipalities. In some communities, municipalities, or regions, these two organizations may not consistently provide prehospital services 24/7. Volunteers may not be available around the clock, or municipalities may not have the proper budget to operate an effective service 24/7. In other Lebanese communities, both agencies may be mobilized and dispatched to the same incident by a caller or by the public. Both agencies can only provide basic life support and/or basic transportation.

To further complicate this situation, additional organizations provide prehospital and patient transportation services in certain regions and communities in this small country (10,452 square kilometers). They include:

1. Municipality-owned and run ambulances.
2. Nongovernmental organizations (NGOs) such as the "al-*Issaaf Shaaby*" (The People's Ambulance) and the Palestinian Red Crescent.
3. Militia-affiliated and/or militia-owned ambulances (e.g., parties such as Hezbollah and Amal).
4. Armed Forces (Lebanese Army).
5. Private for-profit ambulance services (PTS, PTC).
6. Hospital-owned/dispatched ambulances.

Understandably, any planning, coordination, oversight, or development of prehospital services becomes a daunting task. Planners need to be familiar with the peculiarities of each agency and region or community and to understand the history and reasons behind the development of such complex structures and the challenges faced by that community and agency. It is only then that one perhaps may have a chance to succeed at (1) introducing, requiring, and providing standards for operations, equipment, training, credentialing, and coordination for medical providers, dispatching center operators, and ambulances; (2) introducing structure for a national oversight, authority, or leadership for all prehospital agencies; (3) securing improved capacity and functionality of ambulances; (4) identifying and addressing change for communities with special challenges (e.g., geography, infrastructure, demography, sociocultural, ethnic, or religious considerations); (5) coordinating an effective and reliable 24/7 dispatch center or national number to call for emergencies; (6) ensuring stability of patients, the procurement of necessary records, and completion of proper calls between facilities and physicians before transfer; (7) dealing with special transportation requests and needs of patients and families and going to the closest appropriate hospital facility; (8) properly interfacing with national and local dispatch or hospital diversion requests (assuming such a national, regional, or community dispatch or interface even exists).

Simply stated, major problems can be identified in nations where patient transportation is administered by a wide variety of heterogeneous, overlapping, and sometimes conflicting agencies and organizations and where there is no national EMS authority or head. Accountability and available resources are limited or variable. There are conflicting or warring parties, militias, and warlords and therefore overlapping fluctuating resources, turfs, and territories. Therefore how can one define, establish, and implement change, process, and proper procedure? How can one introduce uniformity in standards, in training, equipment, and operations where it is needed?

In such nations, the patient transportation, dispatch, and medical control aspect of EMS — normally a public service — face everyday serious operational problems, challenges, and shortcomings. The negative impact of such heterogeneity, overlap, and difficulty with oversight is best illustrated by examples we experience in certain or all regions in Lebanon: ambulances drive with sirens on while they carry no patients; ambulances transport patients for dialysis or for convenience thereby becoming unavailable for rescue missions; or ambulances elect to transport unstable patients to hospitals that do not have the proper beds or resources for emergency care; or ambulances transfer patients without any attention to stability or completion of proper procedure or availability of equipment or personnel to deal with any en route deterioration. Ambulances carry victims with accompanying armed friends or militia into the EDs, or through checkpoints. Ambulances are misused to smuggle militia, weapons, or supplies during times of conflict. Some ambulance drivers and personnel may perform poorly, drive recklessly, or simply omit standard transport precautions (e.g., cervical or spine immobilization). One should note that such poor performance does not apply to all ambulance transport providers in Lebanon or in any nation.

Emergency Crisis Response Providers

In any nation, EMS does not operate in a vacuum. There are other stakeholders and teams involved in responding to all emergencies, including those that may or may not involve injuries or medical emergencies. We mentioned how Lebanon's Health and Interior Ministries support the Lebanese Red Cross and the Civil Defense, respectively. In addition, there are police, army forces, and other security agencies that may or may not respond or be called to the scene. In some regions, there is a fire department response that works with the Civil Defense.

Who calls the agencies and how do we ensure consistent and timely response? How do agencies interact or interfere with the staff of the ambulance or with the family or bystander request to take a victim by car to the nearest hospital? Will the responders hold an injured patient on the scene until the police arrive? Who makes such decisions at the scene? Who trains them? Who oversees responder performance and how are responders held accountable? How are calls routed and how does such routing ensure that all types of needed responders are promptly mobilized to the scene?

Problems do occur. Police will take the call from a crime scene or from the witnesses of an accident victim and may not alert any medical prehospital provider to respond. Prehospital providers may get a call and respond to a dangerous site, to a crime scene, or to a burning car or structure without alerting or mobilizing the police or fire department. Gunshot wound patients could (and have been) held on the scene until the police arrive to take pictures! Bystanders or ill-trained ambulance providers have transported victims to inadequately prepared hospitals (e.g., no ED physician or surgeon in house or no blood bank) 100 meters away from a tertiary care center for a variety of unacceptable reasons. Spinal cord injury patients have been carried manually over an untrained responder's shoulder to the doors of EDs. Local police may not have a transportation vehicle and have asked the ambulance provider to come by the police station to carry police to the scene. Another consideration is incident command and leadership on site during a mass casualty event: Who should be in charge early on and when other responders appear on site? Should it be the Red Cross, the Civil Defense, the police, the army, or the local militia leader or his party's own ambulance provider? How are such issues handled all over a nation with such heterogeneity and many variable providers?

Hospitals

A crucial key public service component of an effective EMS system is an available, capable, accessible ED that welcomes and provides basic screening, evaluation, and stabilization for every patient who comes through its doors. Hospitals play a key public service role in supporting prehospital response, namely through:

1. ED personnel response to ambulance arrivals and to requests for transfer.
2. ED, critical care, and hospital baseline and surge capacity.
3. Administration and admitting office/staff response and responsiveness to the ambulance provider and patient family who are seeking transport or transfer.
4. Available on-call specialty services and ambulatory services.

Again, a nation can have complex heterogeneity in its types of hospitals. There is wide variability in

1. Ownership (private, public, for-profit, nonprofit, religious, or political party affiliations).
2. Scope of practice: Is it a tertiary care or single-day hospital? Is it a teaching institution? Is it a specialty hospital where available services are limited to a single discipline (e.g., obstetrics, pediatrics, otolaryngology, ophthalmology, plastics, rehabilitation)?
3. Actual emergency and critical care capacity: Does the hospital have a properly equipped ED and properly qualified emergency physicians and nurses? Does it have an ICU and/or CCU capacity? Does it have a PICU or a polyvalent capacity?
4. Actual capacity to consistently deliver 24/7 specialty services (cardiac care, neurosurgery)?

Hospital variability can cause major problems and shortcomings for EMS providers and the patients they carry. Hospitals end up putting ramps obstructing ambulance entry or exit or refuse to accept or unload arriving ambulances because of alleged or actual lack of adequate resources or capacity (ICU, ED, floor, specialty service). Yet many hospitals refuse or resist any efforts at categorization based on emergency or critical care preparedness and capacity. Hospitals may have the sign "emergency" at the doors even if there is nothing more than a reception room with no staff, monitors, supplies, or equipment. The cause behind all of this is typically financial, driven by an institutional push to limit or divert unfunded or underfunded patient access into the institution through the ED. Such practices, including the lack of attention to prop-erly assessing and supporting basic medical screening and stabilization; nondisclosure of hospital capacity; the lack of public and EMS provider understanding of differences in hospital capacity; and duplication and fragmentation of hospital-based services are harmful to patients and result in significant distress and wasting of EMS resources.

The House of Organized Medicine

Under this title, we have lumped together various forms of professional groups, hospital and employee syndicates, and professional organizations that may or may not exist to represent public and private hospitals, physicians and their various specialties, nurses, and prehospital personnel. In Lebanon, we have a syndicate for private hospitals, a national Order of Nurses, two National Orders of Physicians (Lebanese Order of Physicians and the Order of Physicians of Tripoli and the North), and a number of specialty societies that currently function under the Lebanese Order of Physicians. This includes a Lebanese Society for Emergency Medicine. Public hospitals are not organized as an entity and are perhaps represented by the Ministry of Health. Prehospital personnel are not organized into any groups or syndicates.

Understandably, efforts led by these organizations have tried at various times to support and give momentum to the development and improvement of the national EMS system at all levels. By doing so, these entities constitute an additional form of public service with a key role with regard to EMS. Fragmentation, erratic communication, inadequate attention, and conflicts between these houses of organized medicine cause delays in the development and introduction of badly needed improvements. Solidarity and regular communication between them and with the Lebanese Red Cross and the Ministry of Health have led to major improvements in the last 10 years. Certainly, the emergence of committed emergency physicians and the persistence of experienced seasoned prehospital provider leadership over the last 10 years has provided EMS development with significant momentum and will further facilitate any improvement initiatives led by any stakeholders in any developing nation.

CHAPTER 7

EMS Role in Public Health and Public Education

Paul A. Jennings

KEY LEARNING POINTS

- EMS is being increasingly seen as part of an integrated health care sector.

- EMS is uniquely placed to contribute to public health activities and to provide effective public health education.

- Participation of EMS in primary prevention activities has the potential to significantly reduce healthcare costs and the burden of injury.

- There is a clear role for EMS in disease surveillance and reporting.

- Expanding the scope of practice of paramedics has the potential to reduce the burden on the healthcare system and the number of inappropriate ED admissions.

- EMS personnel are well placed to be an initial point of contact for the most needy cases within our communities.

Provision of acute health services is changing dramatically, with continued rationalization of services in spite of increasing demands. Hospital closures, difficulties accessing inpatient beds, nursing shortages, and an aging population all impact heavily on emergency health demands. Consideration of alternative models of health care delivery has never been more active. Roles such as the nurse practitioner, extended care paramedic, and physician assistant are emerging in response to healthcare demand and work force shortages. In some countries, the gap between high and low socioeconomic status is widening and having a direct impact on the number of people able to afford health insurance.

The inability to afford health insurance can significantly reduce the primary healthcare options available to people. There is a far greater reliance on EMS to extend or adjust roles and fill gaps in the health care system.[1]

Work force shortages at urgent care centers, general practitioner practices, or walk-in clinics have led to greater reliance on EMS for primary care, much of which ought to be managed within the community rather than the hospital system.

Currently EMS focuses on secondary and tertiary prevention, that is, identifying and treating people with established disease. Secondary prevention aims to detect serious disease early, while tertiary prevention aims to institute interventions to reduce mortality and morbidity and improve quality of life. While these are clearly important roles of EMS, more can and should be done in an effort to prevent injury or illness. Primary prevention focuses on inhibiting the development of disease before it occurs, and it is a prevention strategy that could be readily and effectively delivered by EMS.

One of the goals within the US Department of Health and Human Services' strategic plan is to "prevent and control disease, injury, illness, and disability across the life span and protect the public from infectious, occupational, environmental, and terrorist threats."[2] EMS professionals are uniquely placed to identify, document, and respond to such public health concerns from within the communities they serve. This could significantly reduce the number of inappropriate ED presentations.

BENEFITS OF EMS INVOLVEMENT IN PUBLIC HEALTH

1. Reduction in health care costs due to treatment in the field or direct referral for investigation/admission as appropriate.
2. EMS units are strategically placed and mobile within the community. Health care professionals are able to reach clients within the community who otherwise may be missed. Prehospital professionals can make timely referrals to appropriate agencies. Early detection and prompt action are crucial to effective prevention efforts.[3]
3. EMS systems collect a wealth of demographic, epidemiologic, and injury information that can be used to enhance surveillance and assist with the evaluation of various health intervention programs.
4. Increasing the scope of practice of paramedics to include injury prevention and health promotion is both possible and timely and has the potential of increasing job satisfaction through the accomplishment of wider-reaching health solutions.

There are numerous public health initiatives to which the EMS systems could provide significant contributions, some of which are listed in Table 7-1.

IMPORTANCE OF EMS INVOLVEMENT IN PRIMARY PREVENTION

The most common causes of death worldwide are cardiovascular disease, cancer, and injuries.[4] When all

Table 7–1	Potential EMS Public Health Initiatives

Road safety messaging
Risk assessment in homes of elderly (falls)
Risk modification
Chronic disease treatment
Needle exchange
Chronic wound care
Tuberculosis surveillance
Disposal of out-of-date patient medications
Referral to trauma counseling services

World Health Organization member states are aggregated, the median age standardized mortality rate (per 100,000 population) is 364, 129, and 68, respectively.[4] Injuries, whether intentional or unintentional, remain a significant public health problem (see Table 7-2).

EMS CONTRIBUTION TO PREVENTION OF INJURIES

Low- to middle-income countries are unfortunately overrepresented on global injury statistic tables, as are individuals of low socioeconomic status living in high-income countries.[5] Primary prevention is an effective way to reduce health care costs and the burden of injury. To reduce deaths from injury, prevention interventions must focus on the type of injury, such as drowning, falls, fire or burns, firearms, or motor vehicle accidents. Other agencies such as law enforcement and fire departments have been developing and delivering primary prevention programs for many years. Fire departments have been very successful in changing fire safety behavior and encouraging homeowners and landlords to install functioning smoke detectors. Law-enforcement agencies have been instrumental in reducing road traffic fatalities through their drunk-driving and seatbelt initiatives. Whereas EMS has always regarded primary prevention programs as desirable, the potential impact of EMS programs on reducing the burden of disease and injury needs to be revisited. A study in North America found that the majority of paramedics believe primary injury prevention should be a core mission of the EMS, and yet only about a third routinely educated their patients on how to modify injury risk behaviors.[6] An Australian EMS has recently developed an innovative secondary school program aimed at identifying the risks associated with drug and alcohol use and providing young people with skills in assessing and dealing with emergency

Table 7–2 | Cause-Specific Mortality in 2004[4]

WHO Member State	Age-Standardized Mortality Rates by Cause (per 100,000 Population)		
	Cardiovascular	Cancer	Injuries
Australia	136	126	32
Canada	131	135	33
China	279	143	73
France	123	154	45
Ireland	190	155	30
Japan	103	120	39
New Zealand	162	136	39
South Africa	389	151	159
United Kingdom	175	147	26
United States	179	133	50

World Health Organization. The Top Ten Causes of Death. Geneva; 2008. Available at http://www.who.int/mediacentre/factsheets/fs310/en/index.html.

situations. ADAPT: Ambulance Drug & Alcohol Program for Teenagers — is delivered by paramedics to secondary school–aged students and encourages "safe partying and going out" practices to prevent medical emergencies from occurring.[7] Despite the importance of primary prevention programs, they do tend to be resource-intensive. It is for this reason that programs should be routinely evaluated to ensure continued effectiveness. Regular reviews also provide the opportunity to update the content of the educational programs and materials and reassessment to ensure that the information is still relevant.

EMS CONTRIBUTION TO PREVENTION AND MANAGEMENT OF HEART DISEASE

Coronary heart disease (CHD) remains the leading cause of death worldwide, and in 2004 accounted for 12.2% of all deaths,[8] with the burden of CHD contributing substantially to the overall health cost.

EMS has much to contribute to integrated systems to reduce death and disability from myocardial infarct. As an integrated community primary health care provider, EMS is extremely well placed to contribute to all three phases of a patient's healthcare journey: pre-symptom, immediately following the onset of symptoms, and during rehabilitation following a heart attack.

The community health care focus of EMS provides opportunity for partnerships for the provision of primary prevention strategies. This may include support to the primary physician and other primary health service engagement, the delivery of appropriate messaging around early identification of heart attack symptoms, and accessing help early.

Apart from the prehospital management and transport of patients suffering from acute coronary syndrome, there are three key strategic areas where EMS can play a pivotal role in significantly reducing the burden of disease. These include

1. Primary prevention of heart disease.
2. Recognition of early heart attack symptoms.
3. Cardiac rehabilitation.

Primary Prevention of Heart Disease

EMS's participation in primary prevention of CHD activities provides an important public health function. EMS is ideally placed to provide sustainable and cost-effective primary prevention information campaigns. Opportunities for collaboration with various heart foundations and other primary prevention campaigners to promote consistent messaging around cardiac risk factor minimization strategies should be explored. Specifically, EMS could contribute through

1. Distribution of health and cardiac risk reduction strategy material consistent with national heart foundation programs. This may be achieved through information mailings with subscription accounts, billing material, or other health messaging methods.
2. Regular media releases reinforcing the importance of healthy living strategies.

3. Joint branding of important primary prevention messages.

4. Making healthy living information available on EMS public websites.

5. Provision of regular health checks, including blood pressure monitoring, random blood glucose analysis, cholesterol analysis, and acquisition of 12-lead ECGs.

Early Heart Attack Symptom Recognition

Knowing when to call an ambulance has been shown to be poorly understood by heart attack patients. "Patient delay" constitutes the majority of prehospital delays in the delivery of a heart attack patient to the hospital[9] for a condition we know to be time-critical. Failure of patients to recognize a heart attack is a source of considerable delay in treatment[9,10] and may result in worse outcomes.

Participation of EMS in early heart attack symptom recognition education provides an important public health function. People experiencing symptoms of Acute Coronary Syndrome (ACS) should activate their EMS as soon as possible.[11] It is likely that delays are contributed to by a lack of community awareness of early warning symptoms and the importance of early EMS activation.

While there have been several studies examining the effectiveness of mass media campaigns on reducing chest pain delay, the evidence is unconvincing.[9] Having said this, EMS still has an important part to play in community education regarding symptom recognition and the encouragement of people with chest pain to activate EMS as soon as possible.

International cardiac public health campaigns identify a range of common warning signs of heart attack, including pain in the chest, pain spreading away from the chest, discomfort in the upper body, and other symptoms such as nausea or vomiting, a cold sweat, or feeling dizzy or light-headed.[12] Guidelines usually advise if any of the above symptoms are severe, get worse quickly, or last longer than 10 minutes; these constitute a medical emergency and an ambulance should be contacted immediately.[12]

EMS is well placed to actively promote early symptom recognition messaging consistent with the recommendations from peak coronary heart disease organizations. Opportunities for collaboration with these groups and other primary prevention campaigners to promote consistent messaging around early symptom recognition should be explored. Again, EMS should be contributing by

1. Distribution of early symptom recognition material consistent with heart foundation messaging, perhaps through information mailings.

2. Regular media releases identifying symptoms related to coronary heart disease and the appropriate early actions to be taken.

3. Joint branding of early symptom recognition messages.

4. Making early recognition information available on EMS public websites.

Cardiac Rehabilitation

Partnership of EMS with cardiac rehabilitation providers would constitute an important public health function. EMS and the Coronary Heart Disease peak organizations recognize the importance of cardiac rehabilitation services for ongoing prevention following diagnosis of cardiac disease. The broad aims of cardiac rehabilitation include assisting patients to recover quickly, improving their overall physical, mental, and social functioning, and preventing the reoccurrence of cardiac events.[12] Unfortunately, participation rates for such programs are low and more effort is needed to encourage people to participate. One barrier to the lack of participation may be limited accessibility to such programs, particularly in the more remote areas.

EMS is well placed to assist in the provision of cardiac rehabilitation services in partnership with and under the guidance of various cardiac rehabilitation service providers. EMS should contribute through

1. Partnerships with cardiac rehabilitation service providers to assist with the provision of cardiac rehabilitation programs, particularly in more remote area.

2. Education, which is an important aspect of cardiac rehabilitation. EMS can create more awareness in the community through media and marketing and encourage patients to monitor their health more vigilantly. This includes heart rate and blood pressure monitoring.

EMS CONTRIBUTION TO PREVENTION OF OTHER DISEASE STATES

There are numerous other disease states in which EMS can play a role by participating in primary prevention intervention and screening programs. Health commentators have already suggested that EMS should focus pilot testing on disease clusters with existing strong public support for aggressive interventions, such as smoking-related cancers.[13]

EMS IDENTIFICATION OF THOSE AT RISK IN A COMMUNITY

EMS professionals are uniquely placed to identify those at risk for a range of vulnerabilities by virtue of their work environment. Very few health professionals find themselves consulting in the patient's home or workplace. It is the living and working environment of a patient that provides the most valuable information regarding his or her social circumstances. Risk can be manifest in a number of forms: risk of fall, spousal or child abuse, suicide or self-harm, drug and alcohol abuse, or an inability to care for oneself. With appropriate education and collaboration with the wide network of relevant support agencies, paramedics can readily provide education to mitigate risk and initiate appropriate referrals. Historically, EMS professionals achieved this role by proxy; patients deemed to be at risk were transported to the local ED irrespective of clinical need. The expectation of EMS was that the EDs would be sufficiently networked to refer the patient to appropriate support services.

Identification of the elderly at risk of falls is an important and achievable EMS objective. Falls are a major concern to the elderly, resulting in injury and psychological impact, and risk profiles effectively identify those at risk. A history of a fall is a strong risk factor for future falls.[14] EMS professionals frequently attend elderly patients who have had a minor slip or fall caused by tripping and have not sustained an injury, often to assist them to a chair or back to bed. It is these patients who would benefit from direct referral to community and health services that could assist with physical therapy and fall risk assessments of their homes. There are a range of other risk factors that may

Table 7–3	Risk Factors for Falls in the Elderly Residing in Supported Homes or Apartment Houses[10]

- Immobility
- Poor mental state
- Orthostatic hypotension
- Dizziness
- Stroke
- Polypharmacy

predict recurrent falls in the elderly, and these are illustrated in Table 7-3.[10]

Suicide and self-harm are serious and complex public health problems that are frequently encountered by EMS. Suicide is among the top three causes of death among young people aged 15 to 35 years and the psychological, social, and financial impact on the family and community is devastating.[15] Depression is strongly associated with suicide and about a third of cases of suicide have been related to alcohol abuse. The risk of suicide can be assessed by considering three factors:[15]

1. The person's current mental state and thoughts about death and suicide.
2. The person's current suicide plan — how prepared the person is, and how soon the act is to be committed.
3. The person's support system, including family and friends.

When a person is assessed as being at risk of suicide, he or she should be referred to a mental health professional or a doctor. Those with psychiatric illness, history of a previous suicide attempt, a family history of suicide, alcoholism, or mental illness, physical ill-health, or no social support must be referred for further assessment.[15]

EMS ASSISTANCE WITH SURVEILLANCE AND DISEASE REPORTING

Surveillance is "the ongoing, systematic collection, analysis, interpretation, and dissemination of data regarding a health-related event for use in public health action to reduce morbidity and mortality and to improve health."[16] Often routine disease surveillance, known as "baseline operations", collects data on the incidence of communicable diseases and alerts the appropriate authorities. It aims to identify outbreaks of communicable diseases[17] (Figure 7-1).

EMS has the ability to provide disease and injury surveillance data effortlessly by data already collected in patient care records. This data, when collected electronically, can be reported and analyzed in real time. Public health surveillance is an ongoing process monitoring acute and chronic health issues or symptoms. Historically, notification of reportable indicators or conditions was limited to those mandated by legislation. There are now more reportable conditions that are notified voluntarily. Public health authorities use surveillance to identify and track disease outbreaks. Monitoring and reporting of infectious diseases such as *meningococcal meningitis* have particular relevance

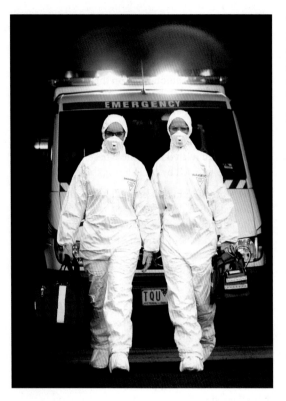

to EMS. First, they allow identification of *who* was infected, *when* the disease occurred, and *where* the case arose. Second, they allow opportunity for public health authorities to notify EMS providers that clinicians were in contact with a confirmed case, permitting prophylaxis where appropriate. Despite rates of meningococcal disease being the lowest they have been in the US (Figure 7-2) and other industrialized countries, the disease continues to cause substantial morbidity and mortality in all age groups.[18]

EMS data such as location of frequent traffic crashes could be used to identify significant traffic hazards, allowing the relevant authorities to make changes. After giving due consideration to issues surrounding patient confidentiality, the locations of assaults, violent behavior, or illicit drug use, such information could also be provided to law enforcement agencies, allowing the implementation of focused remedial intervention. Ultimately these data can be used to evaluate the effectiveness of specific countermeasures or interventions.

Surveillance systems must have two-way communication, allowing surveillance data to flow to the data repository and supporting safety data/epidemiologic information feedback to the EMS.[17]

FIGURE 7–1

EMS professionals prepare for H1N1 outbreak. Photo courtesy of The Herald and Weekly Times Photographic Collection. (Australia)

EMS ROLE IN EDUCATION CAMPAIGNS

Educational campaigns can be targeted at the community or patient level. Sometimes a combination of the

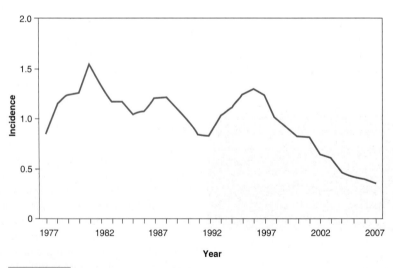

FIGURE 7–2

Meningococcal disease. Incidence (per 100,000 population) by year – United States, 1977 to 2007.[18] Centers for Disease Control and Prevention: Summary of notifiable diseases, United States: 2007. MMWR 56:53, 2009.

Table 7–4	**Potential EMS Public Education Initiatives**

Responsible use of alcohol and drugs
Safety around water – drowning prevention
Cardiopulmonary resuscitation training
Warning signs for stroke and heart attack
Safety around bushfires
Safety in extremes of temperature
Reducing the likelihood of falls in the elderly
What is a medical emergency?
Reducing the risk of sudden infant death syndrome (SIDS)
Mental health programs
Reducing road trauma
Instruction and supervision of parents undertaking emergency medical skills (PR diazepam/EpiPen™ administration)

two provides the greatest success. As described previously, EMS has been integral in community education programs, historically focused on first aid, resuscitation, and emergency care training. More recently the role of EMS in broader primary health care education has been embraced, and there are many successful examples of such programs. Table 7-4 lists some examples of public education initiatives in which EMS would be an ideal contributor.

When planning an educational program, the following (IDEA) tenets may be useful.

1. **I**dentify target audience and focus efforts (and resources) here.
2. **D**evelop audience-specific education packages. A general rule of thumb is to design educational materials to a level no higher than the sixth grade. Plan for culturally and linguistically different (CALD) groups.
3. **E**nsure an educational setting appropriate to the audience.
4. **A**llow opportunity for regular refreshing of information. The educational message often needs to be delivered in a recurrent, ongoing fashion to have lasting results.

EMS-driven education is potentially available in every community. Due to the nature of EMS work and education, EMS professionals are skilled communicators, able to rapidly disseminate pertinent health information in an understandable format to patients with a range of educational and cultural backgrounds. Paramedics are generally considered trustworthy and enjoy a high level of credibility within the community.

Although many paramedics may not be aware of it, they constantly deliver patient education through their contact with the patient. This may be as simple as informing patients of appropriate healthcare options other than ambulance transport to an ED or correct administration of prescribed medications. Paramedics have a unique "window of opportunity" within which to identify health education needs and to deliver information when it would be of most relevance — at a time of need. A recent North American study strategically placed stroke education media by EMS personnel in one county over a two-year period to increase public stroke awareness. EMS education interventions demonstrated a positive effect on the stroke knowledge of residents, with a significant increase in awareness observed in the proportion of respondents who named two stroke risk factors and three symptoms in comparison to those in the control counties.[19]

EMS professionals are often called upon to provide advice regarding health conditions or emergency prehospital care outside of the normal patient–paramedic setting. Such informal health education occurs in a range of forums. Career expositions, standby at sporting events, and picking up a meal from the local takeaway store provide opportunities for incidental primary prevention education.

The provision of pre-arrival health care instructions to patients and bystanders is now commonplace across EMS. Often scripted, emergency call takers provide lifesaving first-aid advice (such as CPR instruction or first-aid management of the choking or bleeding patient), which has the potential to buy precious minutes prior to EMS arrival. Some systems provide health advice for patients who are deemed not to require EMS attendance. Other systems arrange referral to services that can provide such advice.

As with all health education, it is important that the information provided is accurate, contemporary, and delivered in a standardized form supported by effective educational practice. Availability of brief patient information brochures for a range of commonly encountered problems is a useful way of providing patients and their families with information they can take away with them or refer to later. A disadvantage of information brochures is that they can take up space, which unfortunately in the EMS environment is at a premium. Also, in this age of the "online information superhighway," printed material is at far greater risk of losing currency, whereas online material can be quickly updated as required. Of course health information made available on the Internet relies on the patient and his or her family's having ready access to a computer that can connect with the Internet. The electronic clinical information systems that are becoming commonplace across EMS systems worldwide could potentially provide a solution to the provision of hard copy health information to leave with a patient. Up-to-date patient information brochures could readily be printed at the point of care, the patient and significant others familiarized with the information it contains, and brochures left with the patient to refer to later. Other pertinent information such as the contact details of the closest primary health care provider or health facility could also be left with the patient as appropriate.

EMS professionals must be aware of local public health initiatives, programs, and procedures to ensure timely referral. A large proportion of patients are not transported to EDs for various reasons, including patient refusal, condition not warranting assessment or management at an ED, or resolution of symptoms. It is this group in particular that is at greatest risk of being neglected when the EMS is not integrated into the local network of programs.

APPROPRIATE USE OF HEALTH SERVICES

As primary health services, general practitioner practices, walk-in clinics, and EDs struggle to keep up with an ever-increasing demand, EMS are relied upon to fill the gap. Hospital overcrowding, bypass, and ambulance diversion are becoming common language. This creates problems where EMS is resourced purely to respond to health emergencies and not for the assessment, management, and referral of day-to-day minor health ailments. The EMS is a significant driver of ED and hospital demand. Appropriate application of EMS public health care can potentially alleviate some of the ED overcrowding by assessing and managing the high proportion of patients seeking primary health care for the range of minor ailments that can be effectively managed in the community. Like most health services, EMS reports increasing demand annually. Without interventions targeted at ensuring that EMS resources are allocated to those in most need, some are either sure to miss out or receive a delayed response. This delayed response may impact a patient's recovery. Several studies[20-23] have identified inappropriate transport by EMS and suggested that education of care providers in the use of EMS and utilizing alternate means of transport would make the system more efficient and productive. Other studies highlight circumstances in which the EMS should have been involved in the management and transport of patients when other forms of transport were selected instead. [24,25]

There are four key ways of dealing with increased EMS demand.

First, educating the community regarding when to call an ambulance. All EMS members advise the community to call for an ambulance when somebody is seriously ill or injured or a life is at risk. Many EMS organizations provide examples of situations when an ambulance should be requested and often advise people to consider other options (apart from an emergency ambulance) when immediate medical attention is not required (Figure 7-3).

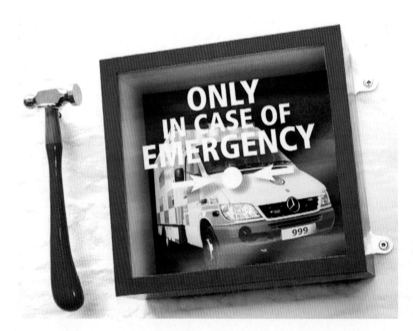

FIGURE 7–3

London Ambulance Service "use us wisely" campaign. Photo courtesy of London Ambulance Service NHS Trust.

Second, requests for ambulance attendance can be screened to identify cases not appropriate for ambulance care. These callers can be referred to alternative healthcare providers (general practitioners, walk-in clinics, or EDs) or to telephone services to provide over-the-phone triage, health advice, or referral. Some states within Australia offer a phone service known as nurse-on-call that provides immediate health advice from a registered nurse 24 hours a day, 7 days a week. England has a similar system known as NHS Direct. It provides health advice, out-of-hours support for general practitioners, and pre- and postoperative support for patients and remote clinics via the telephone. Likewise, telephone-consulting nurse programs are utilized in some parts of North America and Canada. Several studies have shown that it is possible to safely triage EMS calls to alternative resources when valid decision rules are accurately employed.[26,27]

Third, provide a range of alternative transport options for patients requiring transport to a health facility but not requiring acute prehospital management such as that provided by an emergency ambulance. These alternative options may include a nonemergency ambulance with stretcher-carrying capacity, outsourced transport agencies, or volunteer groups that provide nonemergency transportation.

Finally, systems need to be in place that support treat-and-release programs, whereby EMS professionals are supported to assess, treat, and refer patients with low acuity presentations to alternative primary health care options rather than transporting patients inappropriately to EDs. Interestingly, only a small proportion of EMS formally sanctions paramedic-initiated refusal of transport, and even fewer have formal alternatives to emergency ambulance transport.[28] While this final option does not reduce the EMS demand, it does increase the time the ambulance resource is available to attend more critical emergencies and make more efficient use of the health system.

ACCESS TO HEALTH SERVICES FOR THE NEEDY

Despite the inappropriate use of EMS, it is the ease of access to a health service that is of benefit to those who either avoid health care when it is required or have difficulty in gaining access. Some of those who are most at risk are the socially disadvantaged, the homeless, and those with psychiatric disorders or addiction to drugs and alcohol. A number of countries have identified a widening gap between socioeconomic deprived and nondeprived communities. With retrenchment, low employment, and financial hardship comes a reduction in those who can afford health insurance, which significantly limits the range of health options available to those people. International consensus is that access to community health resources is worse in deprived communities. EMS offers a readily available, integrated health service that may be considered less threatening than some of the acute services and traditional models of care. Furthermore, EMS is generally equally accessible in deprived and nondeprived neighborhoods. Programs that could be particularly effective in these settings are opportunistic immunization and safe needle exchange. Immunization currently prevents 2.5 million deaths every year from diphtheria, tetanus, pertussis (also known as whooping cough), and measles.[29] Rates of immunization vary among countries, with most achieving acceptable (greater than 90%) public health targets. Still, 23.5 million children under the age of 1 year missed out on the diphtheria toxoid, tetanus toxoid, and pertussis vaccine.[29] Missed opportunities are significant contributors to this shortfall, particularly in the disadvantaged cohort and could be further reduced through immunization by EMS professionals. There are also opportunities to assist in the reduction of bloodborne infectious disease transmission through the provision of needle exchange programs. Needle exchange programs have been shown to reduce the incidence of HIV among injection drug users and can reduce ED utilization among high-risk injection drug users.[30] Prehospital care providers are well acquainted with the various local health and community services available within their catchment areas. This local knowledge allows for timely and seamless referral of patients to appropriate community services for a segment of society that might otherwise be missed.

SUMMARY

As a community integrated primary health care provider, EMS is extremely well placed to contribute to public health and community education. EMS's community healthcare focus and strategic spread of paramedic resources throughout metropolitan, rural, and regional localities provide opportunity for healthcare partnerships.

EMS globally needs to actively embrace opportunities to contribute to public health initiatives. This can be achieved through partnership and collaboration with other health and community public health agencies. EMS is uniquely placed to provide a significant contribution to community health education and primary prevention promotion, supporting chronic disease management programs, disease surveillance, and reporting, provision of definitive primary health care, and identification of those at risk in our communities. Although some or all of these initiatives have started in some EMS jurisdictions, it is incumbent upon all of us to promote these important public health initiatives in each and every EMS throughout the world.

DEFINITIONS

Public Health

An organized activity of society to promote, protect, improve, and, when necessary, restore the health of individuals, specified groups, or the entire population. This sector is a combination of sciences, skills, and values that function through collective societal activities and involve programs, services, and institutions aimed at protecting and improving the health of all the people.[31]

Primary Health Care

Health care, or medical care, begins at the time of the first contact between a physician or other health professional and a person seeking advice or treatment for an illness or injury. It may be provided by non-specialized physicians and other health workers.[30]

Primary Prevention

Strategies, tactics, and procedures that prevent the occurrence of disease.[31]

Secondary Prevention

This includes the use of screening tests or other suitable procedures to detect serious disease as early as possible so that its progress can be arrested and, if possible, the disease eradicated.[31]

Surveillance

Surveillance is the ongoing, systematic collection, analysis, interpretation, and dissemination of data regarding a health-related event for use in public health action to reduce morbidity and mortality and to improve health.[16]

Tertiary Prevention

Such prevention includes interventions aimed at arresting the progress of established disease.[31]

Web Resources

1. World Health Organization http://www.who.int/en/. (accessed Sept 2009)
2. Centers for Disease Control and Prevention http://www.cdc.gov/. (accessed Sept 2009)
3. Healthy People (Developing Healthy People 2020) http://www.healthypeople.gov/. (accessed Oct 2009)
4. US Dept. of Health & Human Services, Office of the Surgeon General: Public Health Priorities http://www.surgeongeneral.gov/priorities/index.html. (accessed Oct 2009)

References

1. Bissell RA, Seaman KG, Bass RR, et al. Change the scope of practice of paramedics? An EMS/public health policy perspective. *Prehosp Emerg Care* 3:140, 1999.
2. US Department of Health and Human Services. US Department of Health and Human Services Strategic Plan - FY 2007– 012. Washington, D.C.; 2007 Available at http://aspe.hhs.gov/hhsplan/(accessed 20 October 2009).
3. Mann NC, Hedges JR. The role of prehospital care providers in the advancement of public health. *Prehosp Emerg Care* 6: S63–S7, 2002.
4. World Health Organization. World Health Statistics 2009. In Geneva; 2009. Available at http://www.who.int/whosis/whostat/2009/en/index.html (accessed 20 October 2009).
5. Razzak JA, Sasser SM, Kellermann AL. Injury prevention and other international public health initiatives. *Emerg Med Clin North Am* 23: 85, 2005.
6. Jaslow D, Ufberg J, Marsh R. Primary injury prevention in an urban EMS system. *J Emerg Med* 25: 167, 2003.
7. Neely H, Kropp J. ADAPT: It's Your Call. Melbourne: Ambulance Victoria; 2009.
8. World Health Organization. The top ten causes of death. Geneva; 2008 Available at http://www.who.int/mediacentre/factsheets/fs310/en/index.html (accessed 20 October 2009).
9. Finn JC, Bett JH, Shilton TR, et al. Patient delay in responding to symptoms of possible heart attack: can we reduce time to care? *Med Journal of Australia* 187: 293, 2007.
10. Tanner H, Larsen P, Lever N, Galletly D. Early recognition and early access for acute coronary syndromes in New Zealand: key links in the chain of survival. N Z Med J. 2006; 119(1232). http://www.nzma.org.nz/journal/119-1232/1927.
11. Aroney CN, Aylward P, Kelley A-M, et al. Guidelines for the management of acute coronary syndromes *Med Journal of Australia* 184: S1, 2006.
12. Heart Foundation - Recommended Framework for Cardiac Rehabilitation. 2008. (accessed 20 October 2009, at http://www.heartfoundation.org.au/SiteCollectionDocuments/cr%2004%20rec.pdf).
13. Maclean GC. The future role of emergency medical services systems in prevention. *Ann Emerg Med* 22: 11, 1743, 1993.

14. Graafmans WC, Ooms ME, Hofstee HM, et al. Falls in the elderly: a prospective study of risk factors and risk profiles. *Am J Epidemiol* 143: 1129, 1996.

15. World Health Organization. Preventing Suicide a Resource for Primary Health Care Workers. Geneva; 2000 Available at http://www.who.int/mental_ health/media/en/59.pdf (accessed 20 October 2009).

16. CDC. Guidelines for evaluating surveillance systems. *MMWR* (No. S-5), 1988.

17. O'Connor RE, Lerner EB, Allswede M, et al. Linkages of acute care and emergency medical services to state and local public health programs: the role of interactive information systems for responding to events resulting in mass injury. *Prehosp Emerg Care* 8: 237, 2004.

18. CDC. Summary of Notifiable Diseases–United States, 2007. *MMWR* 56(53); 1, 2009.

19. Tardos A, Crocco T, Davis S, et al. Emergency Medical Services–based community stroke education pilot results from a novel approach. *Stroke* 40: 2134, 2009.

20. Rosenberg N, Knazik S, Cohen S, et al. Use of Emergency Medical Service transport system in medical patients up to 36 months of age. *Pediatr Emerg Care* 14: 191, 1998.

21. Vardy J, Mansbridge C, Ireland A. Are emergency department staffs' perceptions about the inappropriate use of ambulances, alcohol intoxication, verbal abuse and violence accurate? *Emerg Med J* 26: 164, 2009.

22. Little GF, Barton D. Inappropriate use of the ambulance service. *Eur J Emerg Med* 5: 307, 1998.

23. Richards JR, Ferrall SJ. Inappropriate use of emergency medical services transport: comparison of provider and patient perspectives [comment]. *Acad Emerg Med* 6: 14, 1999.

24. Davis C, Rodewald L. Use of EMS for seriously ill children in the office: a survey of primary care physicians. *Prehosp Emerg Care* 3: 102, 1999.

25. Poltavski D, Muus K. Factors associated with incidence of "inappropriate" ambulance transport in rural areas in cases of moderate to severe head injury in children. *J Rural Health* 21: 272, 2005.

26. Schmidt T, Neely KW, Adams AL, et al. Is it possible to safely triage callers to EMS dispatch centers to alternative resources? *Prehosp Emerg Care* 7: 368, 2003.

27. Smith WR, Culley L, Plorde M, et al. Emergency medical services telephone referral program: an alternative approach to nonurgent 911 calls. *Prehosp Emerg Care* 5: 174, 2001.

28. Jaslow D, Barbera JA, Johnson E, Moore W. EMS-initiated refusal and alternative methods of transport. *Prehosp Emerg Care* 2: 18, 1998.

29. World Health Organization. Global Immunization Data. Geneva; October 2009. Available at http://www.who.int/immunization/newsroom/GID_englis h.pdf (accessed 20 October 2009).

30. Pollack HA, Khoshnood K, Blankenship KM, et al. The impact of needle exchange-based health services on emergency department use. *J Gen Intern Med* 17: 341, 2002.

31. Last JM. A Dictionary of Public Health. New York: Oxford University Press; 2007.

CHAPTER 8

EMS Research

Jane H. Brice, Lawrence H. Brown, Helen Snooks

KEY LEARNING POINTS

- Resources needed for EMS research are
  1. Skilled researchers.
  2. Adequate funding.
  3. Appreciation for and demand by EMS professionals for evidence-based practice.
  4. Integrated information systems, including links to patient outcomes, and
  5. An environment and processes that support ethical research, including ethics review and approval.

- EMS is uniquely positioned for research at the intersection of medical care, emergency services, and public health. Much EMS research is oriented toward population health.

- Finding methodologically sound avenues to integrate medical care and research is essential to understanding how to deliver the safest and most effective EMS care.

- Much work has been undertaken in the areas of cardiac arrest, trauma, and pediatrics. Emerging areas of investigation include stroke, public health, and field triage on medical necessity whether that be performed at the scene or via telephone.

- The future will see an emphasis on multicenter and multinational EMS research.

INTRODUCTION

Much of the medical care provided in the EMS environment has been derived from hospital practice with improvisations and adjustments to accommodate the drastically different demands of providing care in the field. In the past 40 years, however, medical science has begun to examine the EMS arena as a distinct practice area with its own unique demands on medical care and medical providers. It is now well recognized that medical care provided in hospital does not always translate into effective EMS care. EMS care must be based on research evidence taken from studies performed in the field with EMS providers and EMS patients.

The EMS environment is difficult to study because EMS entails the provision of unscheduled care to persons with acute emergencies. Time is often of the essence and, as in other medical disciplines, performing research takes a back seat to clinical care. **Finding methodologically sound avenues to integrate medical care and research is essential to understanding how to deliver the safest and most effective EMS care.**

HISTORY OF EMS RESEARCH

For centuries, people have fashioned litters to carry injured or sick persons to medical care. The birth of modern EMS systems is attributed to the research of visionaries such as J.F.Pantridge from Northern Ireland, who in the early 1960s studied the possibility of delivering cardiac care directly to patients in their homes.[1] In the US, the publication of *Accidental Death and Disability: The Neglected Disease of Modern Society* by the National Academy of Sciences in 1966 led to the development of EMS systems of care throughout the country.[2] The pioneering work of Pantridge and others led to the development of modern prehospital care.[3,4]

As EMS systems began to develop, so did the demand for improving those systems. With that demand for improvement came a cry for field research to better understand the nuances and particularities of the EMS environment. As researchers began to look at EMS medical care, they soon found that what works in a hospital often does not often work in EMS.[5-8]

EMS research has suffered the typical growing pains of a new field of investigation. The methodology for conducting EMS research has developed along a typical path. The first studies were case series and observational studies only. Before 1980, few randomized trials were conducted.[9-11] Investigators were slow to recognize that interventions must be linked to patient outcome in order to demonstrate effectiveness.[12]

In the last decade, EMS has benefited from research-trained investigators who are applying creative and scientifically sound methodology to efficiently answer the most pressing questions facing EMS. These investigators are utilizing large data sets, multicenter and international research groups, and randomized clinical trials. Investing in training young and talented scientists interested in pursuing careers in research will be critical to the continued development of EMS research.

CURRENT STATE OF EMS RESEARCH

Research in emergency care and particularly in EMS is in its infancy. The lack of evidence underpinning current clinical, educational, operational, and managerial practices has been highlighted and practices vary widely both within and across countries.[13] The effectiveness of historically accepted models of care, such as widespread introduction of paramedics and implementation of helicopter emergency ambulance services, is being subjected to scientific evaluation[14-17,19], although once introduced, models of care are extremely difficult to evaluate with robust study designs, thereby limiting the strength of evidence that can be gathered.

In recent years, there has been an expansion and shift in EMS research, from small-scale studies with weaker study designs to a greater number of multicenter randomized controlled trials. Research funding and infrastructure to support these efforts are now in place. EMS research is beginning to mature.

NECESSARY SKILLS AND TOOLS

The National EMS Research Agenda from the US identified five general impediments to EMS research. While the Agenda was specific to EMS research in the US, the identified impediments correspond well with the resources and attributes required of successful EMS research initiatives anywhere. **Essentially, these resources and attributes are 1. skilled researchers; 2. adequate funding; 3. appreciation for and a demand by EMS professionals for evidence-based practice; 4. integrated information systems, including links to patient outcomes; and 5. an environment and processes that support ethical research, including ethics review and approval.**[18,20]

Skilled Researchers

As with any clinical discipline, many EMS researchers might not be traditional scientists; they will often be clinician-researchers—health professionals who have an interest in the expansion of the evidence base for EMS. These clinician scientists could be medical doctors, nurses, paramedics, or other health care workers. However, the pool of EMS investigators should not be limited to clinician-researchers—traditional scientists with pure research backgrounds make valuable contributions to EMS research. More than vocation or formal education, what truly defines a researcher is inquisitiveness and healthy skepticism.

Specific knowledge and skills are necessary, however, and these can be obtained in numerous ways. Non-clinicians with traditional scientific backgrounds can learn about the intricacies of EMS by working with clinicians, riding along on ambulances, or undertaking some EMS-related training. Clinicians can acquire and refine their research skills by undertaking professional development courses or postgraduate education in epidemiology and/or biostatistics. As a less common path, a scientist might choose to pursue formal education and licensure or certification as a healthcare worker, and some clinicians might choose to pursue formal doctoral (PhD) research training.

Research Funding

Funding is a challenge for researchers in all disciplines. Just as many clinicians would prefer not to be burdened with the business aspects of health care, likewise many researchers prefer not to be saddled with the business aspects of research. Yet, both delivery of health care and the conduct of research require resources. The financial issues are unavoidable. Sometimes existing resources can be diverted to support research endeavors. Investigator time, administrative support, computer equipment and software, office supplies, and research-related travel are often supported by clinical and academic organizations as part of their core business operations. Research conducted with such internal support should not be viewed as "free." There is a cost to the organization even if it is not directly accounted for.

While meaningful EMS studies have been conducted using existing internal resources, larger, more sophisticated studies with wider impact—particularly multicenter trials—usually require significant external funding. It is possible to obtain funding for prehospital care research, although traditional funding streams are rarely focused on this area. Funding may come from government organizations (e.g., the Ministry of Health), charitable and nongovernmental organizations (e.g., the Gates Foundation), or even private for-profit corporations seeking to have a product evaluated. Here, there is a distinct relationship between researcher background and funding: researchers with more formal credentials and greater experience are typically more successful at attracting funding.

Networking and collaboration are valuable skills relevant to both research expertise and funding. Almost every EMS research effort requires an interdisciplinary team of investigators, so typically it isn't necessary for a single investigator to possess all of the required knowledge, skills, credentials, and experience.[19] The ability to assemble (and manage) a diverse, productive research team may be the most important skill of all.

Demand and Appreciation

Beyond the interests of individual researchers, the EMS professionals in an organization must appreciate the importance of—and in fact demand—evidence-based practice. As with all health disciplines, it is not necessary for every EMS professional to be a researcher, but researchers and systems administrators must foster an environment that supports and values research. Without the support of in-field EMS providers, most EMS research is doomed to failure: access to data (or patients) will be obstructed, research protocol violations will be common, and/or research data collection will be shoddy. Even if an investigator is successful in completing a research study, a system

in which research is not valued is unlikely to implement any changes suggested by the study. Fortunately, this is not the challenge it once was. Current EMS texts nearly ubiquitously include information on the importance of research.[20,21]

The remaining two necessary resources and attributes, information systems and research ethics, are discussed separately below.

APPROACHES TO EMS RESEARCH

Study Design

It is important that EMS research follows the same guidelines and reaches the same standards as clinical research in other disciplines where the scientific paradigm and evidence-based culture are more established. A range of research study designs can be utilized in EMS research, as appropriate to the question being posed. Research can be carried out on a small, local scale or on a large, multicenter and/or international scale—or anywhere in between. However, it is important to recognize that carrying out research in EMS carries particular challenges. These challenges must be met effectively so that clinical, operational, and management questions are answered rigorously and reliably.

In EMS, research interventions are likely to be complex—for example, implementing a new intervention incorporates aspects of additional training, skills acquisition, patient assessment issues, and administration of that intervention. EMS researchers may find the recent guidance from the UK's Medical Research Council on evaluating complex interventions helpful.[22]

Primary and secondary research, observational, qualitative studies, and quantitative modeling approaches all have their place, as do single-center as well as multicenter studies. When selecting the most appropriate research design to use in a study, there are several considerations that need to be taken into account, including:

- What is the question that the research needs to answer?
- What is possible in the real-world setting of EMS research?
- What level and type of funding are available?

Experimental and Observational Designs

It is important that the study design selected matches the research aim and objectives. In addition, the feasibility of implementing and successfully completing research needs to be considered at the research design stage.

The strongest study design for evaluation of clinical and cost effectiveness is the randomized controlled trial across multiple sites. However, the number of randomized controlled trials in EMS is low.[23-25] In a well-conducted randomized controlled trial, the outcomes are compared between groups of patients who are similar in terms of demographics and clinical condition, so that any differences found are likely to be due to the intervention being tested rather than any intrinsic differences between the patients themselves. By contrast, an observational design that relies on taking measurements and making comparisons between groups as they arise in real life is open to criticism, as results may always be confounded by known or unknown differences between groups. For instance, many helicopter evaluations—where it is extremely difficult to introduce any element of random selection—have been criticized for the inability of statisticians to adjust for all factors that may differ between groups. In addition to injury severity there are often differences between helicopter- and ground ambulance-attended patients related to location, age, and mechanism of injury.[26] However, there are many practical difficulties in undertaking studies with randomized designs. Persuading ambulance services to randomly dispatch advance life-support paramedics or BLS-trained EMTs to emergency calls for serious trauma proved to be almost impossible in a trial undertaken in the UK in the early 1990s, even though earlier observational study results indicated that patients attended by EMTs had better outcomes than those attended by paramedics.[27]

Randomization at the cluster level can overcome some of these difficulties. In cluster randomization, patients still have an equal chance of being allocated to the intervention or control arm of the trial, but at a group rather than individual level. The North American "Public Access Defibrillation Trial" is one example of an EMS study that used cluster randomization.[28] Randomization can also be by paramedic,[29] ambulance station,[30] or time.[31-34]

Quantitative and Qualitative Designs

Studies in prehospital care may utilize quantitative (numbers or data that can be measured) or qualitative (descriptions or observations) data collection methods and may indeed use a mix of both. Again, the choice of design is dependent on the research question(s) to be

answered through the study. Questions of effectiveness can only be answered through quantitative methods, although related questions about compliance with protocols and factors that encourage or impede the use of new interventions may be suitable for exploration through qualitative methods such as semi-structured interviews or focus groups with practitioners or managers. Quantitative and qualitative methods may be used for both experimental and observational study designs, but they do vary in terms of the evidence generated.

Quantitative data collection methods are used in order to produce evidence that is generalizable beyond the sample, so that conclusions can be drawn about a wider population than those included in the research. For this reason, multicenter studies are stronger than single-system projects. Attention is paid to the importance of achieving high response rates and minimizing dropouts—or attrition. It is seen as vital to document numbers of participants, including those eligible, consented, enrolled, and followed up, usually following accepted standards for reporting.[35-38] By contrast, qualitative research methods emphasize the depth and richness of data gathered from relatively small numbers of participants. Qualitative methods can be particularly suitable for gaining insight alongside quantitative data collection about how an intervention is implemented and received, both by practitioners in the EMS system and partner services as well as by patients and caregivers. Qualitative methods have been relatively underused as an approach within EMS research, with notable exceptions.[39,40]

INFORMATION SYSTEMS FOR EMS RESEARCH

Utilizing Databases

Both existing and purpose-built databases can be used for EMS research. A number of registries exist for various conditions for which a prehospital component is a key phase of care, including major trauma and myocardial infarction.[41-44] These databases can provide an extremely rich source of data for use in quality improvement and research projects, and a significant proportion of published EMS research is generated from such databases.[45-47] There are also many databases in other medical disciplines as well as public health databases and local or regional socioeconomic databases. However, the uniqueness and peculiarities of individual databases often limit their usefulness in cross-agency or multicenter research. A recent European-wide project evaluated databases to determine if they were suitable for implementation of studies across regional boundaries, finding few that could potentially be expanded in this way.[48,49]

Routinely Collected Health and Operational Data

Routinely collected patient care and operational data are another source of information for EMS research. The quality of routinely collected data, however, can be problematic. Common issues in routinely collected data (in all disciplines) include accuracy, completeness, timeliness, and appropriateness. The quality of clinical documentation can be variable and may depend on local information management and audit procedures.[50] Operational data produced for performance management may be of higher quality, but these data also have limitations. One particular example is artificial effects produced by established performance targets. For example, time-based performance standards in the UK have been shown to produce a large blip of responses in the last few seconds before 8 minutes and again at 14 minutes.[51]

Nevertheless, routinely collected data can provide an invaluable and cost-effective source of information related to patient demographics, clinical condition, care received, and early outcomes for research. The advantages of using routinely gathered data over purpose-built data sets for health-related research have been documented.[51] These advantages may be especially relevant to EMS research, where the addition of new data collection forms or tools is particularly difficult due to the nature of emergency care, and completion of additional documentation is likely to be low.[53]

Where routinely collected sources are used, researchers need to be aware of the limitations of this type of data and quality checks are needed for completeness and accuracy. Timeliness of retrieval also needs to be considered in the emergency field situation. If patients need to be contacted for consent in the aftermath of an emergency incident, then clinical documentation may need to be intercepted on station or along the route between completion and inputting or scanning/storage. This will be highly dependent on local systems for clinical and management information and may be hugely improved where electronic patient records are in use.

Linking Data

A particular challenge for prehospital research is the need to link data between different parts of the patient pathway and often across service providers. With identifiers such as name, age, and address often missing from (or inaccurate on) EMS reports, especially for the sickest patients, it is not a simple matter to link data. Even within a service the linkage of data between the dispatch center and records completed on scene can prove to be a challenge, especially with multiple calls, multiple patients, and multiple responders all being frequent occurrences per incident. But the challenge increases enormously when it comes to tracking patient information across different agencies (e.g., hospital, rehabilitation, law enforcement)—in practical and logistical terms as well as in relation to consent, confidentiality, and information governance. The linkage of clinical and operational data across systems is difficult, but in the case of EMS research it is vital in order to understand outcomes beyond the initial field phase of care.[54]

Even when data can be linked, identifiable data often cannot be shared for research purposes without explicit patient consent. Anonymous data linkage systems are now being developed and tested that may overcome many of these problems,[55] but anonymous data give rise to other issues in the context of clinical trials, such as the reporting and investigation of serious adverse events.

Quality Improvement Data

Another source of routinely collected or existing data is the quality improvement activities of EMS systems. Both the scope and accessibility of such data will depend on the sophistication of the EMS agency and its quality improvement initiative, but typical quality improvement databases (or files) can be expected to contain both clinical and operational data. Quality improvement data have been used in a large number of EMS studies, including (for example) studies of cardiac arrest,[56,57] intubation success rates,[58] and nontransport decisions.[59]

Importantly, studies utilizing quality improvement data suffer the same limitations of all retrospective studies and other studies utilizing routinely collected data. Specifically, the data are recorded for some purpose other than the specific study being undertaken, potentially threatening both the validity and reliability of the data. Investigators who make use of quality improvement data must take extra efforts to ensure that the data definitions used in the quality improvement process are consistent with those of the research protocol, that the data are complete, and that the data are representative of those from the broader target population.

Investigators must also understand the distinct differentiation between quality improvement and research. Different guidelines exist for distinguishing between the two activities,[60-63] but the key differences are:[64]

1. Quality improvement is part of the clinical enterprise; it generates organization-specific data for the purpose of improving that organization's operational and/or clinical performance, and

2. Research is part of learning and knowledge development; it generates data that are intended for generalization to other organizations, for the purpose of improving the performance of similar organizations or improving the care of similar patients.

Whenever an investigator undertakes research, even when using existing quality improvement data, that investigator must ensure that the research is conducted in accordance with the principles of ethical research, often including external review by an independent ethics board.[65] Instituting a new (or altering an existing) quality improvement activity for the explicit purpose of collecting research data is a research activity; that, too, must be subjected to appropriate ethics review. Utilizing quality improvement as a guise to avoid research ethics oversight is not ethical.

FOCUSED AREAS OF EMS RESEARCH

Cardiac Arrest

Alongside motor-vehicle crashes, cardiac arrest has been one of the driving forces behind the development of modern EMS systems. The epicenter of EMS cardiac arrest research has long been Seattle, Washington, in the US, where 25 years ago investigators began to report the positive influence of aggressive prehospital intervention—including bystander CPR on survival from out-of-hospital cardiac arrest.[66] In collaboration with other researchers, those investigators have pursued studies into the quality of prehospital CPR,[67] the effectiveness of telephone CPR instruction,[68] the use of automatic defibrillators,[69] intercity differences in survival rates and their associations with EMS system design,[70] and the effectiveness of antiarrhythmic agents.[71]

In the last decade, investigators from Ontario, Canada, have further advanced EMS cardiac arrest research through the Ontario Prehospital Advanced Life Support (OPALS) trials. They have demonstrated that optimization of the EMS system—specifically, reducing response intervals, increasing bystander CPR rates, utilizing police- or fire-based first responders, and providing rapid defibrillation—improves survival,[72,73] whereas adding other advanced life support interventions does not.[74]

EMS cardiac arrest researchers are a close-knit community, and a number of multicenter trials have been conducted. The "Public Access Defibrillation Trial," conducted at 24 different sites,[75] and the "ASPIRE" trial of an automated CPR device, conducted in 5 communities[76] are just two examples. A new multicenter research group, the Resuscitation Outcomes Consortium (ROC), includes 10 communities and is currently investigating early versus delayed rhythm analysis and defibrillation as well as the use of impedance threshold devices in cardiac arrest.[77,78]

Despite the vast amount of research completed already, and the ongoing efforts of multicenter groups, much remains to be investigated about the prehospital management of cardiac arrest. For example, the rate of bystander CPR continues to be poor,[79] and the best strategies for increasing the rate remain to be determined. Indeed, most of what we know about the societal issues surrounding cardiac arrest—bystander CPR rates; delays in seeking care; and gender, racial, and ethnic differences in survival rates—is based on research from western nations. As EMS research expands into more countries and different cultures, much of what we "know" may not be accurate.

Stroke

Stroke is one of the leading causes of death worldwide; however, in comparison to cardiac arrest or trauma, there have been few EMS studies of stroke. With the advent of the use of thrombolytics for acute intervention in stroke,[80] EMS has begun to embrace the urgency associated with stroke.

EMS researchers are in the early stages of studying ways to improve EMS recognition and care of stroke.[81] Emphasis has been placed on early recognition of stroke by EMS dispatchers and the delivery of the most appropriate resources to the patient in a timely fashion.[82-85] The development of stroke education tools to improve EMS recognition during patient assessment has resulted in several creative systems of EMS stroke education.[86,87] Other priority areas for research are the development of assessment tools or scoring systems to aid EMS personnel in stroke recognition.[88-90] Further, efforts are under way to determine the most efficient means to deliver the patient with acute stroke to stroke centers of care capable of intervening and mitigating the effects of ischemic stroke.[91,92]

Trauma

Trauma, particularly from motor vehicle crashes, was one of the driving forces behind the establishment of EMS in the US[93] and remains a primary focus of both EMS care and EMS research around the world. Yet, despite more than 40 years of research, many questions about the optimal prehospital care of injured patients remain. For example, the need for spinal immobilization following a motor vehicle crash, the ability of EMS personnel to adequately assess individual patients for spinal injury, and the best methods of effecting spinal immobilization have not been conclusively determined.[94-97] Questions also persist about the optimal approach to resuscitating hypovolemic trauma patients with regard to both the volumes and types of intravenous fluids that should be administered.[98-100]

Additional areas of EMS trauma-related research include interpersonal violence,[101] occupational injury, penetrating trauma,[102] poisonings, and drowning. One of the most successful EMS-based trauma-related action research initiatives used EMS system data to drive a community education campaign and legislative efforts to reduce childhood drownings in San Diego, California.[103]

Much of the research into EMS trauma care has been conducted by investigators associated with "trauma centers" using data from local, regional, and national trauma databases. These studies have contributed greatly to our understanding of EMS trauma care, but they are potentially affected by selection bias. Berkson's fallacy, for example, is a well-known example of selection bias that occurs when case-control studies are restricted to hospital (or, similarly, trauma center) populations.[104] Certainly, the most severely injured people in countries with well-developed trauma systems are typically transported to and treated at trauma centers, but many gaps remain in our understanding of EMS care for patients with mild to moderate injuries and for those in areas with developing health systems.

Pediatrics

Children present unique challenges in EMS: many providers are uncomfortable caring for children,[105] and the epidemiology of childhood emergencies differs from that of adults.[106,107] Care for children also requires unique interventions and therefore unique equipment, supplies, and skill sets. The adage is true: "Children are not just small adults."

In 1999, a consensus committee of the National EMS for Children (EMSC) Resource Alliance in the US published a 15-item list of research priorities relevant to the emergency care of pediatric patients.[108,109] Many of the items addressed epidemiologic, organizational, educational, and public health–related issues. A number of clinical entities were also identified, including:

- Shock
- Asthma
- Multiple organ trauma
- Poisoning
- Burns
- Pain
- Respiratory distress
- Brain injury
- Seizures
- Behavioral disorders
- Fever
- Resuscitation

These are not the only areas in need of pediatric-related EMS research, and in other nations and societies the priorities might differ—for example, dehydration from diarrheal disease would likely be a priority in some developing countries. The more important issue is to recognize that the foci of pediatric EMS research will often be different from those of adult EMS research, and sufficient resources need to be allocated to those efforts.

It is also important to recognize that true pediatric emergencies are relatively rare, and large multi-center studies are typically required for substantial investigations. To this end, the Pediatric Emergency Care Applied Research Network (PECARN) was developed to support pediatric research in North America.[110] Funded by the US Maternal and Child Health Bureau's EMSC program, the network incorporates four research nodes, a data-coordinating center, and more than 20 hospital emergency departments.[111] PECARN is not exclusive to prehospital care, and much of its work has focused on emergency care in EDs. Still, the infrastructure is now in place, and similar networks would be of great value to EMS researchers in other parts of the world.

Public Health

Health, from a public health perspective, "…is a state of complete physical, mental and social well-being and not merely the absence of disease or infirmity."[112] Further, health is a basic right of all people, and it is necessary for both the economic and social development of societies.[113] On the surface, this holistic view of health may seem nearly antithetical to the typically immediate, episodic, patient-based perspective of EMS; **in fact, EMS is uniquely positioned at the intersection of medical care, emergency services,**

and public health. According to Brown and Devine,[114] "EMS professionals see firsthand—in people's bedrooms and living rooms, in their cars and in their workplaces, in neighborhoods and communities—the interactions between individuals, their health, economic and social circumstances, community structure and resources, and environmental factors."

Ultimately, EMS is part of the public health infrastructure,[115] and much EMS research is oriented toward population health rather than individual illness and injury. Many of these EMS and public health research efforts overlap with the focus areas described above: efforts to improve the rate of bystander CPR in cardiac arrest[116-118] or to implement and evaluate injury prevention strategies[119,120] are examples of EMS and public health research. Disaster and mass-casualty research is simultaneously public health and EMS research.[121] Additionally, elder issues have fairly recently been identified as an area where the synergies of EMS and public health can have positive impacts.[122,123] The potential role of EMS in injury and illness surveillance is also well-recognized.[124-126]

Interestingly, as of December 2009, if one searches the National Library of Medicine index of published research using the intersection of the MeSH terms "emergency medical services" and "public health," only 48 citations are returned. This is a shortcoming of the indexing system, however, and not an accurate representation of the overlap between EMS and public health research. Whenever EMS research addresses health system infrastructure or population health (rather than the care of individual patients) it is undeniably public health research.

Outcome Measurements and Performance Indicators

Identifying the most appropriate outcome measure can be a challenge for any researcher, as often a balance must be achieved between the effort and costs required to obtain the optimal measure versus available measures. In any event, the outcome measure must appropriately represent the desired or anticipated result of the intervention under investigation. For operational research questions, these will likely be operational measures, such as time measures, costs, or patient satisfaction. For educational studies, the outcomes will likely be educational measures, such as performance on examinations or demonstrated skill success rates. For clinical studies, the outcomes will necessarily be clinical indicators.

By far, the greatest amount of work in developing and validating outcome measures for EMS research has centered on clinical studies and clinical outcomes.

The most well-developed and widely accepted of these is probably the "Utstein Style" (http://circ.ahajournals.org/cgi/content/full/110/21/3385) for reporting studies of out-of-hospital cardiac arrests, which is endorsed by the American Heart Association, the European Resuscitation Council, the Heart and Stroke Foundation of Canada, and the Australian Resuscitation Council.[127] Developed and reported in the early 1990s, the Utstein template for reporting out-of-hospital cardiac arrest includes information about the number of arrests, the number of attempted resuscitations, and the epidemiology of the arrests—that is, ventricular arrhythmias versus other causes. The recommended outcome measures are 1. any return of spontaneous circulation; 2. admission to hospital ward or intensive care unit; 3. discharge from the hospital alive; and 4. alive at one year.

A broader effort to establish outcome measures for EMS research was the EMS Outcomes Project (EMSOP) funded by the US National Highway Traffic Safety Administration.[128] This project looked at the broader scope of prehospital care and considered outcome measures for all types of emergencies, including those unlikely to result in mortality. Indeed, the process identified that survival (or mortality) is an inappropriate outcome measure for the great majority of EMS cases. The authors provide a matrix of conditions and appropriate outcome measures, including survival, physiologic improvement, limiting disability, alleviating discomfort, patient satisfaction, and cost-effectiveness. Alleviating discomfort was often identified as the most relevant outcome measure for EMS care, and in a subsequent iteration of the project, the authors proposed specific approaches to measuring pain in EMS research.[129]

The Utstein and EMSOP guidelines are essential approaches to outcome measurement in clinical EMS research; there is no reason to reinvent that wheel. Educational and operational outcome measures are less well defined, but investigators can look to the published literature for countless examples. One critical point in selecting an outcome measure, however, is to not misconstrue endpoints. The time required to place an intravenous catheter is an operational endpoint, not a clinical endpoint; likewise, skill performance in a classroom setting is an educational endpoint. While either may be a worthwhile outcome measure, **investigators must be careful not to presume that outcome measures translate into clinical outcomes.**

Transport Appropriateness and Nontransport of Patients

What constitutes an "emergency" is a continuing point of contention in EMS, with widespread reports of "unnecessary" ambulance use from countries around the world including the US,[130-133] the UK,[134-138] Australia[139], Canada,[140] and South Africa.[141] Medical necessity, however, is not easy to define. Physicians themselves often do not agree on what constitutes an emergency or medical necessity.[142-144] Some authors use hospital admission, including intensive care unit admission, as an indication of medical necessity for ambulance transport.[145-149] Hospitalization, however, might be a misleading reference standard, as Snooks and colleagues explain: "[A]ssessing appropriateness of use based on information only available after the patient has been assessed in a hospital setting . . . will tend to overestimate inappropriate use."[134]

Two systematic reviews have addressed this issue. A 2004 review of the UK and international literature concerning outcomes of patients not transported by ambulance, and the ability of ambulance crews to triage patients to nontransport, alternative transport means, or transport to alternative destinations concluded there is "...a lack of evidence to indicate that there is a clinically safe approach to identifying patients who call for an emergency ambulance but do not need conveyance to ED."[150] A more recent systematic review and meta-analysis of the US literature also found insufficient evidence to support paramedic determinations of medical necessity for ambulance transport, finding a negative predictive value (NPV) for paramedic determinations of medical necessity for ambulance transport of 0.91, with a lower confidence limit of 0.71.[151]

Still, the evidence examining this issue is weak, and additional studies—particularly in other health care and medical-legal environments—are needed.

Telephone Triage

The importance of providing appropriate care at the right time and in the right place to people who seek emergency medical aid is widely recognized, so that those who can benefit from an immediate response and treatment at the highest level of care are identified and those who can wait can receive advice or be directed to an appropriate service for further care with less urgency. National policy documents in the UK have portrayed a vision in which the spectrum of providers, such as EDs, general practitioners, the ambulance service, nurse-led telephone "help lines," and local authorities, should come together in networks to provide appropriate care to the patient.[152] However, the whole system hinges on one critical factor—efficient and effective triage. Triage (French: to sort) needs to be carried out—often remotely—quickly and accurately. The traditional response to this imper-

ative has been to err on the side of caution and tolerate a high rate of "over triage." However, increasing call volumes have put EMS systems under strain, and there has been an increasing impetus to provide more effective triage. Usually telephone triage is accomplished with the use of computer-assisted decision support software, but the research evidence is equivocal about the effectiveness of such systems.[153,154] Despite this, ambulance services are increasingly implementing a range of control room and field-based initiatives, reflecting a gap between service development and research in this area.[155,156]

Future Focus Areas

There are several emerging focus areas for EMS research that can generally be characterized as addressing clinical, operational, or educational issues.

Respiratory distress is a common prehospital complaint that encompasses many potential disease processes. Differentiating between those diseases and choosing the appropriate management continues to be a challenge of the prehospital environment.[157-160] Recently, investigations have evaluated the prehospital use of noninvasive positive-pressure ventilation,[161,162] and the intervention appears to be efficacious and cost-effective,[163] but this requires further evaluation. With the increasing prevalence of respiratory disease, particularly asthma, the prehospital management of respiratory distress will likely continue to be an emerging focus of EMS research. Another emerging area of clinical EMS research is medical errors.[164,165]

In addition to clinical issues, a number of operational issues are emerging as foci of EMS research. Currently, offload delays—or "ramping"—are gaining great attention. These delays not only cause congestion in the EMS system but they potentially threaten the patients waiting in ambulance bays or ED vestibules.[166] Other emerging operational issues include the sustainability of EMS services,[167] the hazards associated with providing care in ambulances,[168] and growing concerns about the safety of air-medical services.

While education of prehospital providers has long been an area of EMS research, greater emphasis is beginning to be placed on the empirical basis for education design. The rapid development of high-fidelity simulation equipment presents an opportunity to dramatically change the educational experience of EMS providers, and many educational programs now use such equipment and are beginning to report their experiences in both simulation-based teaching and evaluation.[169,170] However, the true effectiveness of simulation and the best way to incorporate it into education programs remain to be determined.

Ultimately, the future focus areas of EMS research will be driven by need. As existing EMS systems evolve, and as new systems develop in settings with diverse populations, different endemic diseases, and unique environments, the science of EMS will need to respond to address the new challenges presented by those evolutions and developments. In nations that have yet to undergo the epidemiologic transition, the predominant emergencies encountered by EMS will differ from those in developed nations, and thus the foci of EMS research will necessarily be different. Similarly, as the most industrially and economically developed nations continue to transition into postindustrial societies, they may well experience a new epidemiologic transition after which EMS systems will face new demands and different challenges. EMS systems and EMS researchers should not constrain their thinking to only current models of EMS.

ETHICS OF EMS RESEARCH

Research ethics stand on three firm principles— autonomy, beneficence, and justice. EMS research is no different. First the research subject must have the autonomy to decide whether or not to participate in research. The subject should be provided with a full description of the purpose and methodology of the research. The subject should understand the risks and benefits of participating and be allowed to make an informed decision about whether or not to participate. The research should preferably benefit the subject in some way or at the very least, not harm the subject. There must be equitable distribution of the study's risks among the population. This last principle is sometimes difficult to fully appreciate. The research will benefit a larger number of persons (i.e., society) than are enrolled in the study and only those subjects participating in the study will bear the burden of potential risk or harm. There should be an even distribution of research risk among populations. In the past, certain groups, such as prisoners, minorities, or developmentally delayed persons, were enrolled in studies in much higher percentages than other populations. The principle of justice demands that there be equitable distribution of risk when enrolling subjects in research.

These three principles form the core of The Belmont Report.[171] The Belmont Report is derived from the work of ethicists who developed the Nuremberg Code after the atrocities of the Second World War.[172] Today, the principles of the Nuremberg Code and The Belmont Report are the foundation of research ethics worldwide. Each country applies these principles in a fashion appropriate and acceptable to the population they serve. There is no universal checklist for an investigator to follow. When conducting research within an investigator's home country, the investigator must adhere to the standards of that country. When conducting multinational research, it is imperative to include co-investigators from each country who understand and are fluent in the research ethics of their country.

EMS research perhaps requires more effort and thought in the development of ethical methodology and protocols than other research areas. The research conducted in the EMS environment concerns subjects who are experiencing an emergency and who are physically, intellectually, and emotionally invested in their health and not invested in participating in research.

THE FUTURE OF EMS RESEARCH

When one looks at EMS systems today compared with those of 20 or even just 10 years ago, the changes have been dramatic. Similarly, when one looks at where EMS research is today compared with 20 or even just 10 years ago, it is clear that much progress has been made. There are established investigators who identify themselves specifically as EMS researchers; there are multicenter collaborations that focus on EMS issues; there are scientific journals specific to EMS; and there is an expanding evidence base for prehospital care. Still, much of EMS practice has not been subjected to rigorous scientific evaluation—more work is needed.

EMS is anything but static, and prehospital clinical care, EMS systems, and paramedic education will continue to evolve, particularly as EMS systems emerge and expand in developing nations. What EMS is today is not what EMS will be in 10 years; what EMS research is today is not what EMS research will be in 10 years. More researchers will enter the field, new interventions will require evaluation, and disease and injury patterns will evolve. As John F. Kennedy said, "The one unchangeable certainty is that nothing is unchangeable or certain."

While uncertainty and change are difficult for many people, they are realities of EMS and EMS research. Fortunately, most people attracted to EMS thrive on its dynamic nature; hopefully, most people attracted to EMS research share that characteristic. If so, then the future of EMS research—the uncertainties and the changes—presents an exhilarating opportunity rather than a daunting challenge.

References

History of EMS Research

1. Pantridge JF, Geddes JS. A mobile intensive-care unit in the management of myocardial infarction. *Lancet* 2(7510): 271, 1967.
2. Accidental Death and Disability: The Neglected Disease of Modern Society. National Academy of Sciences, National Research Council; Prepared by the Committee on Trauma and the Committee on Shock. 1966.
3. Nagel EL, Hirschman JC, Mayer PW, Dennis F. Telemetry of physiologic data: an aid to fire-rescue personnel in a metropolitan area. *South Med J* 61(6): 598, 1968.
4. Baum RS, Alvarez H, III, Cobb LA. Survival after resuscitation from out-of-hospital ventricular fibrillation. *Circulation* 50(6): 1231, 1974.
5. Ambulances and the injured. *Br Med J* 5489: 691, 1966.
6. Hazards of ambulance journeys. *Br Med J* 4(516): 373, 1967.
7. Committee on Public Health. Ambulance service in New York City. Report by the Committee on Public Health; the New York Academy of Medicine. *Bull N Y Acad Med* 43(4): 336, 1967.
8. Committee on Acute Medicine. Community-wide emergency medical services. Recommendations by the Committee on Acute Medicine of the American Society of Anesthesiologists. *JAMA* 204(7): 595, 1968.
9. Valentine PA, Frew JL, Mashford ML, Sloman JG. Lidocaine in the prevention of sudden death in the pre-hospital phase of acute infarction. A double-blind study. *N Engl J Med* 291(25): 1327, 1974.
10. Hampton JR, Nicholas C. Randomised trial of a mobile coronary care unit for emergency calls. *Br Med J* 1(6120): 1118, 1978.
11. Diederich KW, Fassl H, Djonlagic H, et al. [Lidocaine prophylaxis in the pre-hospital phase of acute myocardial infarction] (author's transl). *Dtsch Med Wochenschr* 104(28): 1006; 1979.

Current State of EMS Research

12. Sayre MR, White LJ, Brown LH, McHenry SD; National EMS Agenda Writing Team. National EMS Research Agenda. *Prehosp Emerg Care* 6(3 Suppl): S1–43, 2002.
13. Edstrom M, Waks C, Winblad-Spangberg U. States, Regions, and EMS: Levels of decision, funding and evaluation. The Hesculaep Project. www.hesculaep.org. Accessed December 27, 2009.
14. Stiell IG, Wells GA, Field B, et al. Ontario Prehospital Advanced Life Support Study Group. Advanced cardiac life support in out-of-hospital cardiac arrest. *N Engl J Med* 351(7): 647, 2004.
15. Nichol G, Stiell IG, Laupacis A, et al. A cumulative meta-analysis of the effectiveness of defibrillator-capable emergency medical services for victims of out-of-hospital cardiac arrest. *Ann Emerg Med* 34 (4 Pt 1): 517, 1999.

16. Joyce SM, Davidson LW, Manning KW, et al. Outcomes of sudden cardiac arrest treated with defibrillation by emergency medical technicians (EMT-Ds) or paramedics in a two-tiered urban EMS system. *Prehosp Emerg Care* 12(1): 3, 1998.
17. McVey J, Petrie DA, Tallon JM. Air versus ground transport of the major trauma patient: a natural experiment. *Prehosp Emerg Care* 14(1): 45, 2010.

Necessary Skills and Tools

18. Sayre MR, White LJ, Brown LH, McHenry SD, The National EMS Research Agenda Executive Summary: Emergency Medical Services, for the National EMS Research Agenda Writing Team. *Ann Emerg Med* 40: 636, 2002.
19. Gebbie KM, Meier BM, Bakken S, et al. Training for interdisciplinary health research: defining the required competencies. *J Allied Health* 37(2): 65, 2008.
20. Bledsoe BE, Porter RS, Cherry RA. Paramedic Care: Principles and Practice, 3rd ed, (5-volume set). Upper Saddle River, NJ: Prentice Hall, 2009.
21. Evans BE, Dyer JT. Management of EMS. Upper Saddle River, NJ: Brady Publishing, 2010.

Approaches to EMS Research

22. Craig P, Dieppe P, Macintyre S, et al. Developing and evaluating complex interventions: the new Medical Research Council guidance. *Br Med J* 337: a1655, 2008.
23. Callaham M. Quantifying the scanty science of pre-hospital emergency care. *Ann Emerg Med* 30(6): 785, 1997.
24. Osterwalder JJ. Insufficient quality of research on prehospital medical emergency care—where are the major problems and solutions? *Swiss Med Wkly* 134(27–28): 389, 2004.
25. Sayre MR, White LJ, Brown LH, McHenry SD; National EMS Agenda Writing Team. National EMS Research Agenda. *Prehosp Emerg Care* 6(3 Suppl): S1, 2002.
26. Karanicolas PJ, Bhatia P, Williamson J, et al. The fastest route between two points is not always a straight line: An analysis of air and land transfer of nonpenetrating trauma patients. *J Trauma* 61(2): 396, 2006.
27. Nicholl J, Hughes S, Dixon S, et al. The costs and benefits of paramedic skills in pre-hospital trauma care. *Health Technol Assess* 2(17), 1998.
28. Ornato JP, McBurnie MA, Nichol G, et al. PAD Trial Investigators. The Public Access Defibrillation (PAD) trial: study design and rationale. *Resuscitation* 56(2): 135, 2003.
29. Dale J, Higgins J, Williams S, et al. Computer assisted assessment and advice for "non-serious" 999 ambulance service callers: the potential impact on ambulance dispatch. *Emerg Med J* 20(2): 178, 2003.
30. Snooks H, Kearsley N, Dale J, et al. Towards primary care for non-serious 999 callers: results of a controlled study of "Treat and Refer" protocols for ambulance crews. *Qual Saf Health Care* 13(6): 435, 2004.

31. Mason S, Knowles E, Colwell B, et al. Effectiveness of paramedic practitioners in attending 999 calls from elderly people in the community: cluster randomised controlled trial. *Br Med J* 335(7626): 919, 2007.

32. Dixon S, Mason S, Knowles E, et al. Is it cost effective to introduce paramedic practitioners for older people to the ambulance service? Results of a cluster randomised controlled trial *Emerg Med J* 26(6): 446, 2009.

33. Snooks H, Foster T, Nicholl J. Results of an evaluation of the effectiveness of triage and direct transportation to minor injuries units by ambulance crews. *Emerg Med J* 21(1): 105, 2004.

34. Dale J, Williams S, Foster T, et al. Safety of telephone consultation for "non-serious" emergency ambulance service patients. *Qual Saf Health Care* 13(5): 363, 2004.

35. Moher D, Schulz KF, Altman DG. The CONSORT statement: revised recommendations for improving the quality of reports of parallel-group randomised trials. *Lancet* 357(9263):1191,2001.

36. Altman DG, Schulz KF, Moher D, et al. The revised CONSORT statement for reporting randomized trials: explanation and elaboration. *Ann Intern Med* 134(8): 663, 2001.

37. Zwarenstein M, Treweek S, Gagnier JJ, et al. Improving the reporting of pragmatic trials: an extension of the CONSORT statement. *Br Med J* 337: 1223, 2008.

38. von Elm E, Altman D, Egger M, et al. The Strengthening the Reporting of Observational Studies in Epidemiology (STROBE) statement: guidelines for reporting observational studies. *The Lancet* 370(9596): 1453, 2007.

39. Bruce K, Suserud BO. The handover process and triage of ambulance-borne patients: the experiences of emergency nurses. *Nurs Crit Care* 10(4): 201, 2005.

40. Porter A, Snooks H, Whitfield R, et al. 'Covering our backs: ambulance crews' attitudes towards clinical documentation when 999 patients are not conveyed to hospital.' *Emerg Med J* 25: 292, 2008.

Information Systems for EMS Research

41. Boyle MJ. The experience of linking Victorian emergency medical service trauma data. *BMC Med Inform Decis Mak* Nov 17;8: 52, 2008.

42. Gabbe BJ, Cameron PA, Hannaford AP, et al. Routine follow up of major trauma patients from trauma registries: What are the outcomes? *J Trauma* (6): 1393, 2006.

43. B. Roudsari, A. Nathens, C. Arreola-Risa, P. Cameron, I. Civil, G. Grigoriou, R. Gruen, T. Koepsell, F. Lecky, R. Lefering, Emergency Medical Service (EMS) systems in developed and developing countries *Injury*, Vol 38:9, pg 1001–1013.

44. Horne S, Weston C, Quinn T, et al. The impact of pre-hospital thrombolytic treatment on re-infarction rates: analysis of the Myocardial Infarction National Audit Project (MINAP). *Heart* 95(7): 559, 2009.

45. Roudsari BS, Nathens AB, Cameron P, et al. International comparison of prehospital trauma care systems. *Injury* 38(9): 993, 2007.

46. Newgard CD, Sears GK, Rea TD, et al. ROC Investigators. The Resuscitation Outcomes Consortium Epistry-Trauma: design, development, and implementation of a North American epidemiologic prehospital trauma registry. *Resuscitation* 78(2):170, 2008.

47. Mulholland SA, Gabbe BJ, Cameron P. Victorian State Trauma Outcomes Registry and Monitoring Group (VSTORM). Is paramedic judgement useful in prehospital trauma triage? *Injury* 36(11): 1298, 2005.

48. Rebollo Garcia NE, Muhedini GK, Perea-Milla E. Public funding for research: a way into investigation in urgency and emergency medicine. *Emergencias* 20: 335, 2008.

49. Fairhurst R. Prehospital care in Europe *Emerg Med J* 22: 760, 2005.

50. Porter A, Snooks H, Whitfield R, et al. 'Covering our backs: ambulance crews' attitudes towards clinical documentation when 999 patients are not conveyed to hospital.' *Emerg Med J* 25: 292, 2008.

51. Turner J, Nicholl J. Changing ambulance service response time targets – Do patients benefit? World Congress on Disaster & Emergency Medicine, Edinburgh; May 2003.

52. Williams A. "Is the QALY a Technical Solution to a Political Problem? Of Course Not." *Int J Health Services* 21;2: 365, 1991.

53. Close JC, Halter M, Elrick A, et al. Falls in the older population: a pilot study to assess those attended by London ambulance service but not taken to A&E. *Age Ageing* 31(6):488, 2002.

54. Mears GD, Pratt D, Glickman SW, et al. The North Carolina EMS Data System: A Comprehensive Integrated Emergency Medical Services Quality Improvement Program. *Prehosp Emerg Care* 14(1): 85, 2010.

55. Lyons RA, Jones KH, John G, et al. The SAIL databank: linking multiple health and social care datasets. *BMC Med Inform Decis Mak* 9: 3, 2009.

Quality Improvement

56. Scliopou J, Mader TJ, Durkin L, Stevens M. Paramedic compliance with ACLS epinephrine guidelines in out-of hospital cardiac arrest. *Prehosp Emerg Care* 2006;10:394, 2006.

57. Lerner EB, Billittier AJ, Shah MN, et al. A comparison of first-responder automated external defibrillator (AED) application rates and characteristics of AED training. *Prehosp Emerg Care* 7: 453, 2003.

58. Allen TL, Delbridge TR, Stevens MH, Nicholas D: Intubation success rates by air ambulance personnel during 12- versus 24-hour shifts: does fatigue make a difference? *Prehosp Emerg Care* 5: 340, 2001.

59. Persse DE, Key CB, Baldwin JB. The effect of a quality improvement feedback loop on paramedic-initiated nontransport of elderly patients. *Prehosp Emerg Care* 6: 31, 2002.

60. Lynn J. When does quality improvement count as research? Human subject protection and theories of knowledge. *Qual Saf Health Care* 13: 67, 2004.

61. Doyal L. Preserving moral quality in research, audit and quality improvement. *Qual Saf Health Care* 13: 11, 2004.

62. Kofke WA, Rie MA. Research ethics and law of healthcare system quality improvement: the conflict of cost and quality. *Crit Care Med* 31(suppl.): S143, 2003.

63. Baily MA, Bottrell M, Lynn J, Jennings B. The ethics of using QI methods to improve health care quality. *Hastings Cent Rep* 36: S40, 2006.

64. Department of Health & Human Services: protection of human subjects. 45 CFR 46, 1991.

65. Brown LH, Shah MN, Menegazzi JJ. Research and quality improvement: drawing lines in the grey zone. *Prehosp Emerg Care* 11: 350, 2007.

Cardiac Arrest

66. Cummins RO, Eisenberg MS, Hallstrom AP, Litwin PE. Survival of out-of-hospital cardiac arrest with early initiation of cardiopulmonary resuscitation. *Am J Emerg Med* 3(2):114,1985.

67. Cummins RO, Eisenberg MS. Prehospital cardiopulmonary resuscitation. Is it effective? *JAMA* 253(16): 2408, 1985.

68. Eisenberg MS, Hallstrom AP, Carter WB, et al. Emergency CPR instruction via telephone. *Am J Public Health* 75(1): 47, 1985.

69. Cummins RO, Eisenberg MS, Litwin PE, et al. Automatic external defibrillators used by emergency medical technicians. A controlled clinical trial. *JAMA* 257(12): 1605, 1987.

70. Eisenberg MS, Horwood BT, Cummins RO, et al. Cardiac arrest and resuscitation: a tale of 29 cities. *Ann Emerg Med* 19(2): 179, 1990.

71. Kudenchuk PJ, Cobb LA, Copass MK, et al. Amiodarone for resuscitation after out-of-hospital cardiac arrest due to ventricular fibrillation. *N Engl J Med* 341(12): 871, 1999.

72. Stiell IG, Wells GA, DeMaio JV, et al. Modifiable factors associated with improved cardiac arrest survival in a multicenter basic life support/defibrillation system: OPALS study phase I results. Ontario prehospital advanced life support. *Ann Emerg Med* 33(1): 44, 1999.

73. Stiell IG, Wells GA, Field BJ, et al. Improved out-of-hospital cardiac arrest survival through the inexpensive optimization of an existing defibrillation program: OPALS study phase II. Ontario prehospital advanced life support. *JAMA* 281(13):1175, 1999.

74. Stiell IG, Wells GA, Field BJ, et al. Ontario Prehospital Advance Life Support Study Group. *N Engl J Med* 351(7): 647, 2004.

75. The Public Access Defibrillation Trial Investigators: Public-Access Defibrillation and Survival after Out-of-Hospital Cardiac Arrest. *N Engl J Med* 351: 637, 2004.

76. Hallstrom A, Rea TD, Sayre MR, et al. Manual chest compression vs use of an automated chest compression device during resuscitation following out-of-hospital cardiac arrest: a randomized trial. *JAMA* 295(22): 2620, 2006.

77. Stiell IG, Callaway C, Davis D, et al. ROC Investigators. Resuscitation outcomes consortium (ROC) PRIMED cardiac arrest trial methods part 2: rationale and methodology for "analyze later vs analyze early" protocol. *Resuscitation* 78(2): 186, 2008.

78. Aufderheide TP, Kudenchuk PJ, Hedges JR, et al. ROC Investigators. Resuscitation outcomes consortium (ROC) PRIMED cardiac arrest trial methods part 1: rationale and methodology for the impedance threshold device (ITD) protocol. *Resuscitation* 78(2): 179, 2008.

79. Lerner EB, Sayre MR, Brice JH, et al. Cardiac arrest patients rarely receive chest compressions before ambulance arrival despite the availability of pre-arrival CPR instructions. *Resuscitation* 77(1): 51, 2008.

Stroke

80. Tissue plasminogen activator for acute ischemic stroke. The National Institute of Neurological Disorders and Stroke tPA Stroke Study Group. *N Engl J Med* 333(24): 1581, 1995.

81. Brice JH, Griswell JK, Delbridge TR, Key CB. Stroke: from recognition by the public to management by emergency medical services. *Prehosp Emerg Care* 6(1): 99, 2002.

82. Reginella RL, Crocco T, Tadros A, et al. Predictors of stroke during 9-1-1 calls: opportunities for improving EMS response. *Prehosp Emerg Care* 10(3): 369, 2006.

83. Evenson KR, Brice JH, Rosamond WD, et al. Statewide survey of 911 communication centers on acute stroke and myocardial infarction. *Prehosp Emerg Care* 11(2): 186, 2007.

84. Buck BH, Starkman S, Eckstein M, et al. Dispatcher recognition of stroke using the National Academy Medical Priority Dispatch System. *Stroke* 40(6): 2027, 2009.

85. Deakin CD, Alasaad M, King P, Thompson F. Is ambulance telephone triage using advanced medical priority dispatch protocols able to identify patients with acute stroke correctly? *Emerg Med J* 26(6): 442, 2009.

86. Lellis JC, Brice JH, Evenson KR, et al. Launching online education for 911 telecommunicators and EMS personnel: experiences from the North Carolina Rapid Response to Stroke Project. *Prehosp Emerg Care* 11(3): 298, 2007.

87. Tadros A, Crocco T, Davis SM, et al. Emergency medical services-based community stroke education: pilot results from a novel approach. *Stroke* 40(6): 2134, 2009.

88. Kidwell CS, Starkman S, Eckstein M, et al. Identifying stroke in the field. Prospective validation of the Los Angeles prehospital stroke screen (LAPSS). *Stroke* 31(1): 71, 2000.

89. Bergs J, Sabbe M, Moons P. Prehospital stroke scales in a Belgian prehospital setting: a pilot study. *Eur J Emerg Med* 17(1): 2, 2010.

90. Kothari RU, Pancioli A, Liu T, et al. Cincinnati Prehospital Stroke Scale: reproducibility and validity. *Ann Emerg Med* 33(4): 373, 1999.

91. Konstantopoulos WM, Pliakas J, Hong C, et al. Helicopter emergency medical services and stroke care regionalization: measuring performance in a maturing system. *Am J Emerg Med* 25(2): 158, 2007.

92. Mechem CC, Goodloe JM, Richmond NJ,et al. Resuscitation Center Designation: Recommendations for Emergency Medical Services Practices. *Prehosp Emerg Care* 14(1):51,2010.

Trauma

93. Accidental Death and Disability: The Neglected Disease of Modern Society. Washington D.C.: National Academy of Sciences National Research Council, 1966.

94. Hauswald M, Ong G, Tandberg D, Omar Z. Out-of-hospital spinal immobilization: its effect on neurologic injury. *Acad Emerg Med* 5: 214, 1998.

95. Hauswald M, Hsu M, Stockoff C. Maximizing comfort and minimizing ischemia: a comparison of four methods of spinal immobilization. *Prehosp Emerg Care* 4(3): 250, 2000.

96. Domeier RM, Frederiksen SM, Welch K. Prospective performance assessment of an out-of-hospital protocol for selective spine immobilization using clinical spine clearance criteria. *Ann Emerg Med* 46(2): 123, 2005.

97. Domeier RM, Swor RA, Evans RW, et al. Multicenter prospective validation of prehospital clinical spinal clearance criteria. *J Trauma* 53(4): 744, 2002.

98. Bickell WH, Stern S. Fluid replacement for hypotensive injury victims: how, when and what risks? *Curr Opin Anaesthesiol* 11(2): 177, 1998.

99. Bickell WH, Wall MJ Jr, Pepe PE, et al. Immediate versus delayed fluid resuscitation for hypotensive patients with penetrating torso injuries. *N Engl J Med* 331(17): 1105, 1994.

100. Brasel KJ, Bulger E, Cook AJ, et al. Resuscitation Outcomes Consortium Investigators. Hypertonic resuscitation: design and implementation of a prehospital intervention trial. *J Am Coll Surg* 206(2): 220, 2008.

101. Ernst AA, Weiss SJ, Cham E, et al. Detecting ongoing intimate partner violence in the emergency department using a simple 4-question screen: the OVAT. *Violence Vict* 19(3):375,2004.

102. Mackay B. Gunshot wounds: the new public health issue. *CMAJ* 170: 80, 2004.

103. Griffiths K. Best practices in injury prevention: national award highlights programs across the nation. *J Emerg Med Serv* 27(8): 60, 2002.

104. Buettner PG, Mueller R, Joyce C. Epidemiology for Public Health, 3rd ed. Townsville, QLD: James Cook University, 2006.

Pediatrics

105. Warren L, Sapien R. Your most feared calls: assessing and treating pediatric patients with undiagnosed pre-existing conditions. *J Emerg Med Services* 34(1): 48, 2009.

106. Gerein RB, Osmond MH, Stiell IG, et al. OPALS Study Group. What are the etiology and epidemiology of out-of-hospital pediatric cardiopulmonary arrest in Ontario, Canada? *Acad Emerg Med* 13(6): 653, 2006.

107. Kannikeswaran N, Mahajan PV, Dunne RB, et al. Epidemiology of pediatric transports and non-transports in an urban Emergency Medical Services system. *Prehosp Emerg Care* 11(4): 403, 2007.

108. Seidel JS, Henderson D, Tittle S, et al. Priorities for research in Emergency Medical Services for Children: results of a consensus conference. EMSC Research Agenda Committee, National EMSC Resource Alliance. *J Emerg Nursing* 25(1): 12, 2009.

109. Seidel JS, Henderson D, Tittle S, et al. Priorities for research in Emergency Medical Services for Children: results of a consensus conference. *Pediatr Emerg Care* 9;15(1): 55, 2009.

110. Zuspan SJ. The pediatric emergency care applied research network. *J Emerg Nursing* 31(4): 299, 2006.

111. Pediatric Emergency Care Applied Research Network. www.pecarn.org. Accessed 27 Dec 2009.

Public Health

112. Grad FP. The preamble of the World Health Organization. *Bull World Health Organ* 80: 981, 2002.

113. Declaration of Alma Ata. Geneva: World Health Organization, 1978.

114. Brown LH, Devine S. EMS and health promotion. *Emerg Med Serv* 37(10): 109, 2008.

115. Delbridge TR, Baily B, Chew JL, et al. EMS agenda for the future: where we are … where we want to be. *Ann Emerg Med* 31: 251,1998.

116. Swor RA, Jackson RE, Walters BL, et al. Impact of lay responder actions on out-of-hospital cardiac arrest outcome. *Prehosp Emerg Care* 4(1): 38, 2000.

117. Swor RA, Jackson RE, Compton S, et al. Cardiac arrest in private locations: different strategies are needed to improve outcome. *Resuscitation* 58(2): 171, 2003.

118. Mitchell MJ, Stubbs BA, Eisenberg MS. Socioeconomic status is associated with provision of bystander cardiopulmonary resuscitation. *Prehosp Emerg Care* 13(4): 478, 2009.

119. Garrison HG, Foltin GL, Becker LR, et al. The role of emergency medical services in primary injury prevention. *Ann Emerg Med* 30: 84, 1997.

120. Mackay B. Gunshot wounds: the new public health issue. *CMAJ* 170: 780, 2004.

121. Savoia E, Massin-Short SB, Rodday AM, et al. Public health systems research in emergency preparedness: a review of the literature. *Am J Prev Med* 37: 150, 2009.

122. Shah MN, Lerner EB, Chiumento S, Davis EA. An evaluation of paramedics' ability to screen older adults during emergency response. *Prehosp Emerg Care* 8: 298, 2004.

123. Weiss SJ, Ernst AA, Miller P, Russell S. Repeat EMS transports among elderly emergency department patients. *Prehosp Emerg Care* 6: 6, 2002.

124. Hinman AR, Davidson AJ. Linking children's health information systems: clinical care, public health, emergency medical systems, and schools. *Pediatrics* 123(Suppl. 2): S67, 2009.

125. Aldana-Espinal JM, Garcia-Leon FJ. [Opportunities for the 112 emergency service to collaborate in public health surveillance.] (Spanish) *Gac Sanit* 19: 172, 2005.

126. Chretien JP, Tomich NE, Gaydos JC, Kelley PW. Real-time public health surveillance for emergency preparedness. *Am J Public Health* 99: 1360, 2009.

Outcome Measurements and Performance Indicators

127. Cummins RO, Chamberlain DA, Abramson NS, et al. Recommended guidelines for uniform reporting of data from out-of-hospital cardiac arrest: the Utstein Style. *Circulation* 84(2):960, 1991.

128. Maio RF, Garrison HG, Spaite DW, et al. Emergency medical services outcomes project I (EMSOP I): prioritizing conditions for outcomes research. *Ann Emerg Med* 33(4): 423, 1999.

129. Maio RF, Garrison HG, Spaite DW, et al. Emergency medical services outcomes project (EMSOP) IV: pain measurement in out-of-hospital outcomes research. *Ann Emerg Med* 40(2): 172, 2002.

Transport Appropriateness and Ntransport of Patients

130. Heilicser B, Stocking C, Siegler M. Ethical dilemmas in emergency medical services: The perspective of the emergency medical technician. *Ann Emerg Med* 27(2): 239, 1996.

131. Billittier AJ, Moscati R, Janicke D, et al. A multisite survey of factors contributing to medically unnecessary ambulance transports. *Acad Emerg Med* 3(11): 1046, 1996.

132. Gibson G. Measures of emergency ambulance effectiveness: Unmet need and inappropriate use. *Journ AmerCollEmergPhys.* 6(9): 389, 1977.

133. Kamper M, Mahoney BD, Nelson S, Peterson J. Feasibility of paramedic treatment and referral of minor illnesses and injuries. *Prehosp Emerg Care* 5(4): 371, 2001.

134. Snooks H, Wrigley H, George S, et al. Appropriateness of use of emergency ambulances. *J Accid Emerg Med* 15(4): 212, 1998.

135. Mann C, Guly H. Is the emergency (999) service being misused? Retrospective analysis. *Br Med J* 316(7129): 437, 1998.

136. Gardner GJ. The use and abuse of the emergency ambulance service: Some of the factors affecting the decision whether to call an emergency ambulance. *Arch Emerg Med* 7(2): 81, 1990.

137. Morris DL, Cross AB. Is the emergency ambulance service abused? *Br Med J* 281(6233): 121, 1980.

138. Volans AP. Use and abuse of the ambulance service. *Pre-hosp Immediate Care* 2:190,1998.

139. Sosnin M, Young D, Dunt DR. A study of emergency ambulance utilisation. *Aust Fam Physician* 18(3): 233, 1989.

140. Rademaker AW, Powell DG, Read JH. Inappropriate use and unmet need in paramedic and nonparamedic ambulance systems. *Ann Emerg Med* 16(5): 553, 1987.

141. Frank SA, de Villiers PJ. An analysis of the appropriate use of the Caledon ambulance service in the Overberg. A short report. *S Afr Med J* 85(11): 1185, 1995.

142. Foldes SS, Fischer LR, Kaminsky K. What is an emergency? The judgments of two physicians. *Ann Emerg Med* 23(4): 833, 1994.

143. Patterson PD, Moore CG. Inter-rater agreement using one component of the Neely conference criteria for determining medical necessity of EMS transports [abstract]. *Prehosp Emerg Care* 10(1): 121, 2006.

144. Patterson PD, Moore CG, Brice JH, Baxley EG. Use of ED diagnosis to determine medical necessity of EMS transports. *Prehosp Emerg Care* 10(4): 488, 2006.

145. Haines CJ, Lutes RE, Blaser M, Christopher NC. Paramedic initiated non-transport of pediatric patients. *Prehosp Emerg Care* 10(2): 213, 2006.

146. Zachariah BS, Bryan D, Pepe PE, Griffin M. Follow-up and outcome of patients who decline or are denied transport by EMS. *Prehosp Disaster Med* 7(4): 359, 1992.

147. Levine SD, Colwell CB, Pons PT, et al. How well do paramedics predict admission to the hospital? A prospective study. *J Emerg Med* 31(1): 1, 2006.

148. Price TG, Hooker EA, Neubauer J. Prehospital provider prediction of emergency department disposition: implications for selective diversion. *Care Prehosp Emerg* 9(3): 322, 2005.

149. Richards JR, Ferrall SJ. Triage ability of emergency medical services providers and patient disposition: a prospective study. *Prehosp Disaster Med* 14(3): 174, 1999.

150. Snooks HA, Dale J, Hartley-Sharpe C, Halter M. On-scene alternatives for emergency ambulance crews attending patients who do not need to travel to the accident and emergency department: a review of the literature. *Emerg Med J* 21(2): 212, 2004.

151. Brown LH, Hubble MW, Cone DC, et al. Paramedic determinations of medical necessity: a meta analysis. *Prehosp Emerg Care* 13: 516, 2009.

Telephone Triage

152. Snooks H, Nicholl J. Sorting patients: the weakest link in the emergency care system. *Emerg Med J* 24:74, 2007.

153. Dale J, Williams S, Foster T, et al. Safety of telephone consultation for "non-serious" emergency ambulance service patients. *Qual Saf Health Care* 13(5): 363, 2004.

154. Dale J, Higgins J, Williams S, et al. Computer assisted assessment and advice for "non-serious" 999 ambulance service callers: the potential impact

on ambulance dispatch. *Emerg Med J* 20(2): 178, 2003.

155. Cone DC, Benson R, Schmidt TA, Mann NC. Field triage systems: methodologies from the literature. *Prehosp Emerg Care* 8(2): 130, 2004.

156. Brown LH, Hubble MW, Cone DC, et al. Paramedic determinations of medical necessity: a meta-analysis. *Prehosp Emerg Care* 13(4): 516, 2009.

Future Focus Areas

157. Brown LH, Gough JE, Seim RH. Can quantitative capnometry differentiate between cardiac and obstructive causes of respiratory distress? *Chest* 113: 323, 1998.

158. Snooks H, Halter M, Palmer Y, et al. Hearing half the message? A re-audit of the care of patients with acute asthma by emergency ambulance crews in London. *Qual Saf Healthcare* 14: 455, 2005.

159. Eckstein M, Suyehara D. Ability of paramedics to treat patients with congestive heart failure via standing field treatment protocols. *Am J Emerg Med* 20: 23, 2002.

160. Cathomas RR, Rade DU, Reinhart WH, Kuhn M. [Ambulance transport of patients with respiratory problems: a prospective observational study.] (German) *Praxi* 91: 4441, 2002.

161. Kallio T, Kuisma M, Alaspaa A, Rosenberg PH. The use of prehospital continuous positive airway pressure treatment in presumed acute severe pulmonary edema. *Prehosp Emerg Care* 7:209, 2003.

162. Hubble MW, Richards ME, Jarvis R, et al. Effectiveness of prehospital continuous positive airway pressure in the management of acute pulmonary edema. *Prehosp Emerg Care* 10: 430, 2006.

163. Hubble MW, Richards ME, Wilfong DA. Estimates of cost-effectiveness of prehospital continuous positive airway pressure in the management of acute pulmonary edema. *Prehosp Emerg Care* 12: 277, 2008.

164. Hobgood C, Bowen JB, Brice JH, et al. Do EMS personnel identify, report, and disclose medical errors? *Prehosp Emerg Care* 10(1): 21, 2006.

165. Fairbanks RJ, Crittenden CN, O'Gara KG, et al. Emergency medical services provider perceptions of the nature of adverse events and near-misses in out-of-hospital care: an ethnographic view. *Acad Emerg Med* 15(7): 633, 2008.

166. Ting JY. The potential adverse patient effects of ambulance ramping, a relatively new problem at the interface between prehospital and ED care. *J Emerg Trauma Shock* 1: 129, 2008.

167. Blanchard IE, Brown LH. Carbon footprinting of EMS systems: a proof of concept study. *Prehosp Emerg Care* 13: 546, 2009.

168. Slattery DE, Silver A. The hazards of providing care in emergency vehicles: an opportunity for reform. *Prehosp Emerg Care* 13: 388, 2009.

169. Hall RE, Plant JR, Bands CJ, et al. Human patient simulation is effective for teaching paramedic students endotracheal intubation. *Acad Emerg Med* 12:850, 2005.

170. Lammers RL, Byrwa MJ, Fales WD, Hale RA. Simulation-based assessment of paramedic pediatric resuscitation skills. *Prehosp Emerg Care* 13:345, 2009.

Ethics of EMS Research

171. National Commission for Protection of Human Subjects of Biomedical and Behavioral research. The Belmont Report: Ethical principles and guidelines for the protection of human subjects of research, OPRR Publication 887–806. Washington, D.C., 1979.

172. Trial of war criminals before the Nuremberg Military Tribunals under Control Council law 10. Vol 2. Washington, D.C.: US Government Printing Office; 181, 1949.

Part 2

Basics of Organization

First Responders and Bystanders

Rick Bissell, Christoph Redelsteiner

KEY LEARNING POINTS

■ The percentage of the population (bystanders) trained in first aid in different countries varies from over 30% to near zero.

■ First-aid training norms vary considerably from country to country and even within countries.

■ Wealthy countries are more likely to have first-aid trained bystanders and first responders, but the countries of the European Union have shown that comparative wealth is only one of the determinants.

■ It is unwise to assume that nonmedical first responders have first-aid training.

■ In most countries the Red Cross/Red Crescent is the single most important provider of first-aid training and related services.

Although there are specific definitions for first responders and bystanders in some countries, usually related to the kinds of or depth of training received, these definitions are of limited value when comparing and describing first responders and bystanders across the broad spectrum of nations. For this reason, we have chosen to provide a brief description for each country we are able to highlight in this chapter. In general, although organized differently, the more advanced countries (in socioeconomic terms) are more likely to have a higher percentage of first responders who have first-aid training, and among the general public (potential bystanders) there is also likely to be a broader distribution of first-aid training. "First-aid training" does not mean the same thing across countries, hence limiting even further the ability of interna-

tional response personnel to predict the capacity of first-aid assistance that might be provided by local citizens and their first response personnel.

In disasters the vast majority of first aid and rescue/extrication is performed by bystanders or local first responders. International disaster responders hope to augment the care and services that are first available through local personnel. Hence, the importance of dedicating this chapter to the kinds of training and organization bystanders and first responders may have in various spots around the world.

This book defines "first responders" in terms of specific training received by fire, rescue, and law enforcement personnel. The definition, as described in Chapter 1, is based on training programs designed and based in the United States with somewhere around 40 hours of formal training, including such topics as hemorrhage control, airway management, splinting and positioning, hyper-/hypothermia management, and transport. In researching information for this chapter, we found that first responders, defined as people who belong to an organized team (career or volunteer) that takes responsibility for responding to various kinds of emergencies (commonly encompassed in fire, police and rescue services), have radically different standards for first-aid training in different countries. These range from no training at all in a huge number of countries to more than 200 hours of first-aid training for fire fighters in Japan.

First-aid training for the general population of a country is training that will be available when they become bystanders in emergencies and disasters. Experience in places like Seattle, Washington, have demonstrated that well-trained bystanders can make a substantial difference in patient outcomes in certain kinds of emergencies.[1] However, the kinds of first-aid training provided and the percentage of citizens trained in first aid can be expected to have a substantial impact on the probability that bystanders will be able to provide useful assistance to those who need immediate help. We hope that this chapter will help illuminate some of what international responders can expect to find. However, it is important to note that direct comparisons between one country and another are of limited value because of differences in vocabulary, training standards, and data keeping. This chapter is not intended as a definitive comparison study.

The world is too big and its countries too numerous to allow for a description of first responder and bystander training in each country. Additionally, a large number of countries simply have no published reporting system describing the variables we focus on in this chapter. Therefore, we have organized this chapter by continent. Obviously, some continents, such as Asia, offer such vast extremes of socioeconomic and government systems development that any broad continent-wide stereotyping would be both foolish and useless. Therefore, we provide a brief overview of what we have found in each continent and then more specific descriptions of several countries within each continent in an attempt to demonstrate some of the variance that exists. The continents/regions appear in the following order: Europe, North America, Central America and the Caribbean, South America, Africa, Asia, the Middle East, and Oceania. At the beginning of each continental section we identify which countries are included. Some countries such as the Soviet Republic span more than one continent but are included only in a single continent in our descriptions. Antarctica is not included.

DEFINITIONS

As mentioned previously, there are few consistencies in definitions regarding first aid and some of the trained response groups. For the purposes of this chapter, we provide the following broad definitions.

First aid: Actions taken to assist an individual in an emergency in such a manner that it helps the individual (or group) escape further harm or stabilizes the person such that he or she can be transported to a place for definitive health care. There are two subsets of first aid:

1. Untrained first aid, provided by people who are doing the best they can without formal training.
2. Trained first aid, provided by people who have completed a formal course in the provision of first aid. In this chapter we concentrate on those who have received some kind of formal first-aid training.

Bystander: person who is in the vicinity when an emergency event occurs and is not part of a pre-organized response group.

First responder: person who has a recognized responsibility to respond to people who need emergency assistance. It is unimportant whether this person is part of a volunteer group or a career or professional group, but first responders must be members of some locally recognized group with preassigned roles for emergency assistance. Some examples of first response groups commonly found in many countries are fire fighters, police, and rescue personnel. EMS personnel are included among first responders, but they are covered in other chapters of this book and are omitted here.

EUROPE

Countries covered include Albania, Andorra, Armenia, Austria, Azerbaijan, Belarus, Belgium, Bosnia and Herzegovina, Bulgaria, Croatia, Cyprus, Czech Republic, Denmark, Estonia, Finland, France, Georgia, Germany, Greece, Hungary, Iceland, Ireland, Italy, Kazakhstan, Kosovo (not acknowledged by all nations), Latvia, Liechtenstein, Lithuania, Luxembourg, Macedonia, Malta, Moldova, Monaco, Montenegro, Netherlands, Norway, Poland, Portugal, Romania, Russia, San Marino, Serbia, Slovakia, Slovenia, Spain, Sweden, Switzerland, Turkey, Ukraine, United Kingdom, and Vatican City.

Europe consists of 47 nations, some of which also stretch into Asia. More than 700 million inhabitants live in Europe. The over 50 different languages are an indicator of the high degree of cultural variety in

Europe. European healthcare systems also are very different and represent every possible type of care delivery and finance system. This also influences the first responder and bystander situations. The range varies from only basic health care systems with three hours of daily access similar to that found in some "developing" countries to high-level medical care that can be reached within 20 minutes in more densely populated and wealthy nations. The health care may be high quality and free, or expensive enough to bankrupt a person, or of low quality and too costly for financial and personal well-being. The European Reference Center for First Aid Education, part of the International Federation of Red Cross and Red Crescent Societies, estimates that there are 100 million medical emergencies annually within Europe.

The European Union (EU) encompasses 27 nations with more than 500 million inhabitants. Twenty-three languages are official EU languages. The EU member nations leave the operational part of healthcare delivery to the individual nations; hence there is no EU-based regulation on first responders or bystanders. However, the EU provides overall public health policy, which all member nations have to follow. A major directive is to provide the right of everyone to the same high standards of public health and equity in access to quality health care, and free mutual health care for citizens of the EU during travel. Prevention is also a major strategic goal of European Union health care; hence there are special national laws in most nations that require:

1. First-aid training for every person obtaining a drivers license.
2. On-site presence of first-aid trained people, EMTs, paramedics, registered nurses, or medical doctors in special work or school settings, depending on the type of industry and number of employees. Even small enterprises with fewer than 10 employees usually have to have at least one person trained in a basic first-aid course of around 20 hours.
3. Specific professions to have a mandatory first-aid training session of at least 4 hours, including policemen, firefighters, soldiers, teachers, childcare-takers, railroad workers, public traffic employees, and staff of sport or recreational resorts.

Some nations such as **Austria** and **Germany** still have mandatory military service, resulting in every single male who is healthy enough for military duty receiving some first-aid training during his service time. The young men may choose alternative duties instead of the military and are frequently assigned to institutions involved in emergency medical service

such as St. John Ambulance or the Red Cross, where they receive a Basic-EMT registration. For example, Austria trains more than 1,500 young men per year to become Basic EMTs for 9 months. Over the course of the years many former EMTs have become part of the Austrian Society and still have basic first-aid skills and can act as trained bystanders. European Red Cross societies train 3.5 million people per year in basic first aid, and St. John's Order trains more than 500,000 lay people annually within the **United Kingdom**.[2,3] The Order of Malta and SAINT, an Association of Samaritan Ambulance Service along with ("Boy") Scouts also is very active in the training of the general public. It is estimated that 6.2 million Europeans get first-aid training per year.[4]

Every motor vehicle must carry a first-aid kit, described for example in the Austrian "*ÖNORM V 5101 First Aid Equipment for Multi-Track Motor Vehicles.*"

Within the European Union, every nation has to have "**112**," the single European emergency phone number. Most nations still have additional, older numbers for their ambulance services or a central emergency number such as "999" in the **United Kingdom**. However, when one dials 112 within the EU he or she will be able to access the EMS system. Any citizen or visitor in the EU should be able to reach emergency services when dialing 112 from their fixed line or mobile phones or from public pay phones. "People calling 112 — whether from a fixed line or a mobile phone — are connected to an operator. Depending on the national organization of emergency services, the operator will either deal with the request directly or transfer it to one of the emergency services (such as ambulance, fire brigade, or police). Six countries (**Denmark, Finland, the Netherlands, Portugal, Sweden,** and most recently **Romania**) have established 112 as their main national emergency number and have been promoting it as the single number for all emergency services. The EU executive body, the European Commission, also takes legal action against countries that fail to comply with EU rules. To ensure the effective implementation of 112, the Commission has so far launched 17 infringement proceedings against 15 countries because of the lack of availability of 112, of caller location, or of appropriate handling of 112 calls. Thirteen of these have been closed following "corrective measures."[5]

Bystander first aid in Europe is greatly enhanced in those nations where callers get advice from telephone communications. The whole **United Kingdom** uses caller instructions. Some of the **Austrian, French, German, Serbian, Czech, Swiss,** and **Slovak** EMS answering centers also provide over-the-phone first-aid instructions to callers who can assist victims of an emergency.

It is almost unknown in Europe for police and fire departments to serve as a permanent medical first tier among first-response providers for specific emergencies such as cardiac arrest. Some fire departments that also run ambulance services would use a fire engine if the expected response time of the ambulance would be too long or if the district ambulance is unavailable. Police departments engage themselves in rural areas, often on an informal basis due to personal commitment of the officers to better serve the community. Some parts of the **United Kingdom** use community first responders, private people with basic first-aid training as the first level of help. Parts of **Germany** and **Austria** use off-duty EMS personnel or local volunteers of the Red Cross or Samaritan Ambulance Services who live in close proximity to the caller as first responders. The information is usually provided via Short Message Service (SMS) to mobile phones. The first responders will drive to the scene in their private cars without emergency lights and may use BLS and AEDs to treat the patients. Public access defibrillation is fairly widespread in the **United Kingdom** and **Austria**. AEDs can be found in some Austrian bank chains next to the ATM machines.

Relatives of patients with a history of cardiac problems get the option of first-aid training during the rehabilitation treatment of their significant others. This is currently available in **France, Spain, Norway, Sweden,** and **Finland**. Some nations also provide an AED for the relatives of cardiac risk patients as a "leased medical subscription device."

The city of Amsterdam, the **Netherlands,** has Europe's most progressive first-responder project. Trained citizens from the general public, public safety, and health care institutions are encouraged to register themselves and ideally their AEDs with the emergency dispatch center. In the case of a cardiac arrest, the dispatch service will send them an SMS if they are in close proximity to the patient.

In summary, Europe covers about 700 million inhabitants with a wide range of economies, languages, cultures, and ways of resolving policy. However, through the work of the European Union, certain common rules and expectations govern the provision of first response and first-aid services in most European countries. Because there are so many countries involved, it is impossible to obtain a count of the number of citizens who are first-aid trained across the continent. However, we estimate that some countries, such as **Germany, Austria, Switzerland,** and others would reach *at least* the 30% mark, given the requirement that

all drivers must be first-aid trained, many industries and businesses must have first-aid trained employees, and all military personnel have been trained in first aid. This greatly enhances the probability that a number of bystanders at emergencies or disasters will have first-aid training. Volunteer first response organizations such as St. John's Order contribute to the availability of first-aid trained bystanders. To add to the uniformity of first-aid provision in Europe, there is a movement in the EU to pass a uniform basic curriculum for first-aid training.

NORTH AMERICA

North American countries include Canada, the US, and Mexico.

There are many similarities between the **US** and **Canada** that cannot be extended to Mexico. Canada and the US are generally characterized by

1. Citizens who have easy access to first-aid training, but with vastly different percentages actually participating in such training when comparing jurisdictions or regions within each country.
2. Volunteer citizen first-response groups for local emergencies (i.e., CERT, Red Cross, Boy Scouts), all of whom train at least a part of their members in first aid.
3. Many fire fighters (volunteer and career), who have at least basic first-aid training.
4. Police and sheriff services that require basic first-aid training. Rural law enforcement may actually be more likely to assist with first aid.
5. Disaster response that is usually managed at the scene by fire departments.
6. National Guard personnel, some of whom are first-aid or EMT trained, some of whom are also physicians and nurses.
7. Civil protection/emergency management groups that typically do more coordinating than on-scene hands-on care of victims.

Military participation in domestic disaster response is rare in both the US and Canada.

One should expect to find first-aid trained first responders throughout both countries, many with at least a 40-hour first responder first-aid training course. In **Canada**, first responder first-aid training follows a 40-hour schedule and is provided by a variety of organizations, including the Red Cross, St. John Ambulance, and the Canadian Department of National Defense. St. John Ambulance also offers a shorter 24-hour course. Trainees serve in a broad variety of organizations, including law enforcement, parks service, local and regional rescue squads, fire departments, campus safety teams, and a variety of commercial organizations that require such training (including large event organizers and telephone companies). St. John Ambulance squads are local voluntary organizations that provide primary first response service in some rural areas of Canada and often back up or supplement career EMS in some of the more urban/suburban areas.

Both countries offer an adequate quantity of high-quality first-aid courses for the public. National heart associations provide widespread CPR courses, and national Red Cross organizations provide a full range of first-aid courses, including even several courses on first aid for pets. Numerous commercial companies require first-aid training for personnel, including telephone companies and power suppliers. The American Red Cross has a growing nationwide program to combine first aid and disaster preparedness courses for home and businesses into the same package (Ready Rating Program).

First-aid training is also part of several local citizen-based response organizations. In the **US,** The **Federal Emergency Management Agency (FEMA)**-sponsored Citizen Emergency Response Team (CERT) program trains local people how to train for and respond to emergencies within their own neighborhoods, to cover the first few precious hours before outside help can arrive. Some of the CERT members are first responder and first-aid trained. In some places in California and other states, local governments have helped organize neighborhood block-by-block disaster committees, which include a certain proportion of participants who take it upon themselves to become trained in first aid and be available to assist neighbors in an emergency.

It is difficult to estimate what percentage of a country's population is first-aid trained. The American Red Cross provides the following numbers for people who are Red Cross- or American Heart Association-trained and who annually recertify.[6] (Table 9-1).

As we mentioned earlier, there are other providers of first-aid courses who are not captured in this information, but we do not have reliable figures for them. If you consider the total number above, divided by a total estimated US population of about 304 million, we find a rough estimate of a minimum of about 6% of the US population having current first-aid training, loosely defined. If you restrict the number to only those who are currently certified in a Red Cross first-aid course, you have a figure of less than 2%. Of course, this does not count those who have their training from other sources or who have first-aid training but who are not in the annual recertification database. Nor does it fig-

Table 9–1	American Red Cross and American Heart Association Numbers Trained[6]
Type of Training	**Numbers Trained and Recertified**
Lay rescuer CPR	7,000,000
Professional CPR	6,000,000
Full first-aid course	5,000,000
Total	18,000,000

Source: Thomas C. Heneghan, Senior Associate, Business Planning, American Red Cross National Headquarters. Personal communication, December 28, 2009.

ure in the fact that American Red Cross (ARC) first-aid trainees are required to recertify only every third year, and basic CPR every second year. We would conjecture that somewhere between 6% and 10% of the US population has some kind of first-aid training.

The **Canadian** Red Cross reports training about 500,000 persons per year, and the St. John Ambulance about 700,000.[7] There is no registry reporting the number of first response personnel trained in first aid in Canada, nor is there a national reporting requirement for civilian first-aid trainees, and therefore there is no confirmable record of the number of Canadian first-aid trainees. If one takes a conservative approach and counts only the 1,200,000 annual recipients of civilian training, approximately 4% of the Canadian public is currently trained in first aid. Actual numbers are likely significantly higher, perhaps more than double that figure, given that recertification is, in many cases, only every second or third year.

Both the **US** and **Canada** share the same nationwide emergency phone number: "911."

In **Mexico,** as compared to the US and Canada, there are fewer first-aid trained personnel at all levels, including trained first responders and the general citizenry. Many ambulance service providers lack EMT-B level training; full paramedic level (US standards) is unusual but can be available in some jurisdictions. Red Cross/Green Cross volunteer teams make first-aid services available in disasters and other emergencies. One particular agency (National Center for Prehospital Evaluation—CENEVAP) has been training first responders, EMS providers, and law enforcement agencies on trauma care (e.g., PHTLS, Advanced Medical Life Support [AMLS]) but has not extended its programs to the general population.[8]

- Some fire services require basic first-aid training; many do not. There is a high level of difference from jurisdiction to jurisdiction regarding first-aid training among the fire services, including among adjacent jurisdictions in the same urban/periurban region. In general, wealthier urban jurisdictions are more likely to have fire fighters who also have at least some basic first-aid training.
- Police generally have no formal first-aid training.
- Civil Protection coordinates disaster response using local and external resources. Military personnel are also used in disaster response; it is unknown how many military personnel outside of the medical corps have any first-aid training.
- Volunteer organizations are sanctioned in the national General Law of Civil Protection, but no mention is made of first-aid standards. In practice, the level of training and first-aid competency of these organizations varies considerably, even within the same jurisdiction.

The Mexican Red Cross offers first-aid courses to the public that are, in general, on par with similar courses offered by Red Cross agencies in the US and Europe. It is unknown what percentage of the general population has any formal first-aid training, but it is expected to be low.

Mexico has three universal emergency phone numbers ("060," "066," and "080," depending on the jurisdiction), which are not yet universally available.

CENTRAL AMERICA AND THE CARIBBEAN

Countries include Guatemala, Nicaragua, El Salvador, Honduras, Belize, Costa Rica, Panama, Jamaica, Cuba, Haiti, Dominican Republic, Puerto Rico (US Protectorate), British Virgin Islands, US Virgin Islands, Bahamas, and more than a dozen small Caribbean island states.

Although resource constrained, in general, **Costa Rica, Cuba, Puerto Rico**, the **Virgin Islands** and the **Bahamas** have well-organized and reasonably well-trained emergency response forces available to most of their territory. The other countries may have clusters of first-aid trained emergency personnel in some urban areas but fail to extend those services broadly. Voluntary groups such as the Red Cross and Green Cross may make up the majority of available disaster responders in many countries of this region, working alongside Civil Protection and local fire service personnel.

- The US, British, and Dutch protectorates or colonies benefit from the standard training available in the "home" countries, although resource constraints may limit their extension.
- The Pan American Health Organization (PAHO) offers the Caribbean Course on Emergency Care and Treatment (ECAT) region-wide, which is available through health ministries and emergency preparedness/response organizations. Available in English, Spanish, and French, the course covers basic first aid, patient packaging, and light extrication. The American Red Cross also partners with several Caribbean national Red Cross organizations to offer Red Cross first aid and preparedness courses in both English and Spanish.
- In these same countries, fire service personnel can be counted upon to have basic first-aid training, as is also the case in **Costa Rica** and **Cuba**. In the rest of the region's countries, fire service personnel are unlikely to have useful first-aid training.
- Throughout this region, it will be rare to find police personnel with substantial first-aid training.
- Civil Protection/Defense coordinates disaster response in most of these countries, working through local fire departments, police, military, and voluntary groups. For the most part, first-aid training is limited to a minority of the personnel of these first response groups in this region.
- In most Central American and Caribbean countries the level of first-aid training among the general population is quite low. **Cuba, Costa Rica,** and **Puerto Rico** all have programs designed to bring first-aid training to the general public via courses designed for adolescents and young adults. The percentage of coverage is unknown.
- **Cuba** has a high level of well-trained primary care medical and nursing personnel who are well distributed throughout the country.
- Regional countries that have universal emergency phone numbers are listed in Table 9-2.

Puerto Rico, as part of the US, uses "911" to reach all emergency services, with operators who are generally bilingual. Regional countries not shown in Table 9-2 are not known to have country-wide emergency phone numbers.

SOUTH AMERICA

Countries include Colombia, Venezuela, Guyana, Surinam, French Guiana, Brazil, Ecuador, Peru, Bolivia, Uruguay, Paraguay, Chile, and Argentina. Excluded from this description are various small, low-population

Table 9–2	**Central America and the Caribbean Emergency Phone Numbers**			
Country	Police	Medical	Fire	Notes
Guatemala	110	120	123	**Note:** The number 911 exists but this is only for private services like medical insurance
El Salvador		911		
Costa Rica		911		
Panama		911		
Barbados	211	511	311	
Cayman Islands		911		
Dominican Republic		911 or 112		
Jamaica	119		110	
Trinidad and Tobago	999		990	
Nicaragua		118		
Honduras		199		

Source: Original by Rick Bissell and Christoph Redelsteiner.

island countries or protectorates: Ascension Island, Tristan da Cunha Group, St. Helena, Fernando de Noronha, Trinidad, and the Falkland Islands.

Almost all of these countries are characterized by a well-developed urban core in one or more cities, with considerably less resource availability and organization outside of those cores. This description is somewhat less apt for **Chile, Argentina**, and **Uruguay**, all of which have well-educated populations with resources distributed throughout their territories. **Brazil** has great wealth in huge urban centers and extreme resource-poor rural and periurban environments. In general, first-aid trained first responders can be expected mostly in the urban cores of the wealthier countries (**Argentina, Brazil, Chile, Colombia, Uruguay, Venezuela**), but rarely in the periurban or rural areas or in the rest of the countries of this region.

- Fire service personnel are likely to have first-aid training in the core centers of the wealthier countries, and, to some extent, in the outlying areas of those same countries. In the poorer countries, fire service personal are less likely to have any useful first-aid training.
- First-aid training for police personnel can be found in some areas of **Chile, Argentina**, and **Uruguay**. For the most part, police in South America lack formal first-aid training.
- Civil Protection/Defense coordinates disaster response in most of these countries, working through local first response personnel, voluntary organiza-

tions, and the national military. The militaries in the wealthier countries are likely to have deployable medical detachments; this is much less predictable in the less developed nations of this region.

Volunteer organizations vary considerably in this region, with the Red Cross being the primary voluntary response organization throughout the region. The reach of the Red Cross and other volunteer organizations that have deployable first aid–trained personnel is wider in the group of wealthier countries and quite limited elsewhere.

Population-level first-aid training is emphasized most in **Cuba, Chile, Argentina**, and **Uruguay** but lags behind the levels of training found in Europe and North America. A study was recently completed in Cuba proposing to offer first aid and health training for students between the fourth and ninth grades, and it found that knowledge of first aid in that age group was lacking. The extent to which this proposal has been enacted could not be confirmed at the time of this publication.[9] Currently, active Cuban public first-aid training focuses on the Pioneers and Boy Scouts groups. In **Chile** and **Argentina** the *Fundación Escuela de Socorrismo y Primeros* (EASPA Foundation) provides to the general public and outdoor sports enthusiasts several North American-structured courses in first aid, wilderness first aid, and basic search and rescue techniques. The extent of distribution of these courses could not be confirmed. The existence of trained civilian bystanders in the rest of the region is quite limited, particularly outside of the urban centers of South American countries.

In the majority of South American countries the primary source of population level first-aid training is provided by the national Red Cross, using curricula that are relatively standardized throughout the Red Cross movement. The strength and successful activity levels of the national Red Cross organizations vary considerably from country to country and even within countries. Again, the economically stronger countries tend to have the stronger Red Cross organizations. Chapter coauthor Bissell has had very successful collaborative disaster response and research interactions with local and regional Red Cross organizations in the **Dominican Republic, Costa Rica,** and **Bolivia** and would suggest that international responders to a Latin American country make it a priority to establish contact with the local and national Red Cross officials in their destination country for further information on means of coordinating the provision of assistance. In the poorer countries, these organizations may have limited resources but have long experience with getting their available resources to the places that may do the most good in a short timeframe.

The universal emergency access numbers for South America are shown in Table 9-3.

Table 9–3	**Emergency Numbers in South America**			
Country	**Police**	**Medical**	**Fire**	**Notes**
Argentina	101	107	100	Emergency dispatcher for Buenos Aires (city), Santa Fe (city), Rosario (city), Salta and Buenos Aires (provinces) **911**
Bolivia	110	118	119	
Brazil	190	192	193	Federal highway police **191**; federal police **194**; civil police **197**; state highway police **198**; civil defense **199**; human rights **100**; emergency number for Mercosul area **128**; **112** will be redirected to 190 when dialed from mobile phones and **911** will also be redirected to the police number (**190**)
Chile	133	131	132	
Colombia	112 or 123 (land lines and mobile phones)			Traffic accidents **127**, GAULA (anti-kidnapping) **165**. More specialized three-digit numbers are available
	156	132	119	
Ecuador	911 (land lines and mobile phones)			All types of emergencies in Guayaquil (**112** land lines, ***112** mobile phones), traffic accidents in Guayaquil **103**, Red Cross **131**
	101	911	102	
French Guyana	17	15	18	
Guyana	911	913	912	
Paraguay		911		
Peru	105		116	
Suriname		115		
Uruguay		911		
Venezuela		171		

Source: Original by Rick Bissell and Christoph Redelsteiner

ASIA

Countries include Uzbekistan, Turkmenistan, Afghanistan, Tajikistan, Kyrgyzstan, Kazakhstan, Pakistan, India, Sri Lanka, Nepal, Bangladesh, Bhutan, Myanmar, Thailand, Laos, Cambodia, Vietnam, Malaysia, Singapore, Philippines, China, Mongolia, South Korea, North Korea, and Japan. Country excluded: Russia (included in Europe).

Asia incorporates such extremes of socioeconomic development and cultures that it is unproductive to lump these countries together in anything but a geographic unit. Japan and Singapore are high-income, high-productivity, tightly organized societies with excellent educational systems and broad social safety nets. Uzbekistan, Kazakhstan, Bhutan, Mongolia, and Nepal all represent countries with poor levels of income, education, and social services. India and China are huge in size and population and are in a very dynamic time of emerging from being resource-constrained countries with largely agricultural underpinnings into the hypercompetitive world of industrial production and high-stakes economic investment. However, both countries still have large areas of population with poor resource availability and few options. As is the general rule in the other continents examined in this chapter, the wealthier countries tend to have better first-aid training available, more first-aid trained first responders. and more expectation that bystanders will have some first-aid training. Japan, for example, has one of the world's most rigorous first-aid training requirements for fire fighters, which is over 200 hours of training. In the poorer countries of this region one can expect to find few first responders with usable first-aid training, and first-aid training in the general public would be highly unusual.

Japan requires that all recently graduated fire fighters take a 250-hour first-aid course, which includes the standard basic life support topics typical of an EMT-Basic in the US Japan also has a number of volunteer fire fighters, all of whom reportedly also have first-aid training, although not of the same intensity as that of the career fire fighters.[10] Thus, every fire fighter in the country is first-aid trained. Because Japan's Fire and Disaster Management Agency (emergency management/civil protection) depends largely on local fire fighters to make up the majority of the personnel engaged in disaster response, a huge percentage of Japan's official disaster responders are first-aid trained. These trained fire fighters are also part of the personnel make-up of the Japanese Disaster Medical Assistance Teams, who do not have civilian EMS-trained personnel like their American NDMS/DMAT counterparts.

Japan has recently further enhanced its percentage of citizens who are first-aid trained by requiring that all licensed drivers complete a first-aid course, similar to the requirement in Germany. It is unknown what that percentage is, but it would be likely to exceed 10%. Japan's universal emergency access numbers are "110" for police and "119" for fire and medical.

India lacks quality EMS services in many parts of the country but has been building an interesting variety of citizen-based and first responder–based programs to deal with emergencies and disasters. Many Indian police personnel (quantity unknown) receive first-aid training as part of their basic police academy education.[11] Although the quantity is unknown, many Indian fire fighters and civil defense workers also receive first-aid training as part of their basic training.[12,13]

Often the largest provider of first-aid training in many countries, the Red Cross in India has decided to place its focus on disaster response and preparedness. Within this, first aid plays a relatively minor role. The response and preparedness programs, which are receiving significant nationwide attention, focus on community skills related to light rescue, shelter set-up and management, clean water provision, food preparation, and reestablishment of community health services. It is unclear from the literature how many Indians have been trained in these areas. Interestingly, the Indian Red Cross Society has recently developed a rapid-deployment emergency water and sanitation team for deployment to disaster sites.

The government of India has recently required the establishment and provision of disaster preparedness education in all public schools in grades 8, 9, and 10, with topics covering hazard management, mitigation, survival skills, and some components of basic first aid.[14,15] This should greatly augment the number of citizens who have basic familiarity with first aid, although it will not reach some of the most vulnerable populations for which secondary school education may not be available. No numbers of trainees are yet available.

Formed under the Ministry of Youth Affairs, the National Services Scheme (NSS) trains high school, college, and university students to respond to disasters and other emergencies in which basic first aid is one of the components. NSS participants can be involved in[16]

1. Assisting the authorities in distribution of rations, medicine, and clothes.
2. Assisting the health authorities in inoculation and immunization and medicine supplies.
3. Working with the local population in reconstruction of their homes, cleaning of wells, and building roads.

4. Assisting and working with local authorities in relief and rescue operations, and
5. Collection of clothes and other materials to be sent to the affected areas.

There is no information available on the number of students who have been trained or how immediately deployable these assets are.

As is the case in a number of other former British colonies, St. John Ambulance plays an important role in India. St. John Ambulance India is made up of 23 State centers, 9 railway centers, 3 Union centers, and over 670 regional, district, and local centers of the Association. There are 29 districts comprising over 2,400 divisions and corps where over 50,000 St. John volunteers are trained to deliver first aid.[17] As such, St. John volunteers represent a well-distributed source of first-aid volunteers, reaching into all major regions of the country.

Finally, India has National Disaster Response Force battalions. These eight multidisciplinary, multi-skilled, well-equipped battalions, stationed at different locations, have 1,185 members in each of them.[18]

In summary, although we have scant numbers, and recognizing the fact that the number of Indians who are trained in first aid is surely miniscule compared to the country's population of over one billion inhabitants, India has taken a strong multifaceted approach to meeting the need for trained first-aid responders to everyday emergencies and disasters.

China: There is extremely little information available on the web about Chinese first response force training, and we have been unable to find anything about civilian training in first aid in the country. There are hundreds of Chinese web sites promoting their sales of Chinese-made first-aid materials and kits.

MIDDLE EAST

Countries include Syria, Israel, Palestine, Jordan, Saudi Arabia, Yemen, Oman, United Arab Emirates, Qatar, Bahrain, Kuwait, Iraq, and Iran.

Middle Eastern countries are among the most difficult from which to gather reliable information. In most of these countries, civil protection is run by the national government (instead of states/provinces/local jurisdictions) with close administrative coordination between civil protection and routine law enforcement and fire protection. In **Jordan**, the Civil Defense agency manages routine emergency response agencies, with assistance from the Jordanian Red Crescent Society (Red Cross affiliates in Muslim countries). The

Red Crescent Society offers first-aid courses to the public, but it is unknown how many people have taken such courses. Some other public institutions, such as the Jordanian University of Science and Technology (JUST), offer first-aid and preparedness courses, but they are usually targeted to the university community or other special groups. Jordanian Civil Defense offers workshops to the public and members of targeted organizations on first aid and preparedness, but with limited dissemination. The agency also sponsors public television announcements on seasonally apropos first-aid advice, but it is unknown what kind of effect these efforts have. As is the case in all Middle Eastern countries, disaster response quickly incorporates and is dependent upon resources from the military. We have been unable to ascertain what percentage of civilian first response personnel or military disaster responders have first-aid training.

Israel provides an example of a Middle East country that has a strong program that combines national-level civil defense with a Red Cross affiliate (Magen David Adom in the case of Israel).

Magen David Adom (MDA) serves many roles, including providing routine ambulance service, training of civilian first responders, provision of disaster services ranging from on-scene first-aid assistance to shelter management, and management of the nation's blood supply. MDA claims to have over 10,000 first-aid trained volunteers on its roster who are ready for response at any given time. All volunteers complete a 60-hour course on first aid, self-protection at emergency sites, and disaster scene logistics.[19] Much of the training available to citizens focuses on management of trauma in multi-casualty incidents, such as bombings or other terrorist attacks. MDA reports training over 50,000 first-aid responders per year in Israel but does not have public reports on how many MDA-trained civilians and first responders the country has at any given time. Given the country's experience with terrorist attacks and earthquakes, motivation for civilian first-aid training is quite high.

Israeli police have a combination of regular duty officers and an auxiliary police force (Civil Guard), which may number 70,000 volunteer officers.[20] Israeli police report that a significant portion (no exact numbers) of the Civil Guard have first-aid training, with focus on transportation- and terrorism-related trauma. Israel has a very small career fire-fighting force, estimated to be about 1,800 career fire fighters for a national population of over 7 million. All career fire fighters have a basic first-aid course, although they do not consider the provision of first aid to be among the agency's top priorities. Fire personnel work closely with MDA ambulance and rescue workers, who focus on first aid and medical assistance.

Israel's universal emergency phone numbers are "100" (police), "101" (medical), and "102" (fire).

AFRICA

Countries include Algeria, Angola, Benin, Botswana, Burkina Faso, Burundi, Cameroon, Canary Islands (Spain), Cape Verde, Central African Republic, Ceuta (Spain), Chad, Comoros, Congo, Côte d'Ivoire, Democratic Republic of the Congo, Djibouti, Egypt, Equatorial Guinea, Eritrea, Ethiopia, Gabon, Gambia, Ghana, Guinea, Guinea-Bissau, Kenya, Lesotho, Liberia, Libya, Madagascar, Madeira Islands (Portugal), Malawi, Mali, Mauritania, Mauritius, Mayotte (France), Melilla (Spain), Morocco, Mozambique, Namibia, Niger, Nigeria, Réunion (France), Rwanda, Saint Helena, Ascension and Tristan da Cunha (UK), São Tomé and Príncipe, Senegal, Seychelles, Sierra Leone, Somalia, South Africa, Sudan, Swaziland, Tanzania, Togo, Tunisia, Uganda, Western Sahara, Zambia, and Zimbabwe.

There are more than one billion people living in the 55 African nations and six territories belonging formally to European nations. Languages spoken include Arabic, English, French, Spanish, Portuguese, Swahili, and around 50 other local languages.

Health care in Africa in general is a huge challenge. Large areas of territory with few people alternate with very high-density cities, making it difficult to provide care in both settings. Civil wars, flooding, and long periods of drought impact the people of many African nations and decrease needed resources for medical care. Virtually all humanitarian and religious institutions such as the Red Cross, St. John, Doctors Without Borders, Caritas, and Catholic, Protestant, and all other major churches are engaged in relief work. Priorities are frequently to assist the local communities with water purification, sanitation, and infrastructure for policlinics and hospitals. Basic first aid and informal first response for the people in the vicinity of the relief or missionary centers is part of the daily work of humanitarian workers and religious organizations.

Major multinational industries, international institutions, or embassies frequently contract with private air and ground ambulance providers to provide first aid and air evacuation for their staff, to ensure access to a modern level of care. Capital cities typically have private health-care facilities designed for this target group that perform on a "western" medical level.

International military peacekeeping operations provide their own local first-aid units and independent medical units at central points, the latter being usually on a tertiary care level with full surgical capabilities. It is not uncommon for staff members of private and military hospitals to be interested in providing first aid and medical care to the general public, although this is frequently against the stated policy of their institutions. Limited resources force many such institutions to limit their service offerings so as not to threaten the viability of the medical missions to their target groups.

The parts of Africa that still belong to European nations, such as the Canary Islands, have health, first aid, and ambulance structures very close to and similar to the respective "mainland" nations. These islands commonly host high-level tourist resorts, having most medical amenities accessible in close proximity to resorts and in different languages.

Ambulance services in many African nations are influenced by the structures of their former colonial nations and have shared know-how and donated equipment from their former "motherland."

Egypt, Libya, Morocco, and the Seychelles usually have reliable health care systems, particularly in the tourist and urban regions.

South Africa is using a structure of province-based ambulance services, as is now operative in the UK, supplemented by private ambulance services. In rural areas, volunteers of the province ambulance service "Metro," South African Red Cross, and St. John are engaged in providing first response and first-aid training in their communities. In preparation for the world soccer games in 2010 Johannesburg has started initiatives in the healthcare sector such as Community Emergency Response Teams to provide basic first aid in the immediate neighborhood or township and trained 1,000 policemen in first aid. The plan is also to train teachers in every high school to become first-aid teachers for their students.[21] First Aiders of the South African Red Cross are also active as stand-by teams at large public events, such as the 2009 elections, in which volunteers were present at polling stations.[22]

Basic first-aid courses in South Africa have to be delivered under minimum requirements set by the Department of Labor; the three basic levels take 18, 32, and 42 hours to attend.[23]

Ambulances, Missionary Stations, and Hospitals

A situation typical for many African nations is found in **Cameroon** in central Africa, at the eastern border of Nigeria. For purposes of illustration, we will provide a brief discussion of Cameroon's reality, keeping in mind that each country is different although there are many similarities between Cameroon and many other African nations regarding first aid. Cameroon has a population of almost 19 million people[24,25] and occupies a surface area of 279,100 square miles. The country does not have the local equivalent of the 911 number for emergency medical services. However, some private hospitals and provincial and military hospitals may possess ambulance services. These services are limited to the wealthy in most cases. In some small towns and villages ambulances are mainly used for commercial purposes to transport the deceased to the mortuary from hospitals. They are not used in the true sense of an emergency. Any person who needs an ambulance has to call the hospital and negotiate a price before the ambulance can leave the hospital premises. Other ambulances are attached to private mortuaries and also function in the transportation of bodies either during a funeral ceremony or from one town to the other. In fact, talking about ambulances to some local residents is often linked to the notion that there is a corpse to be transported. Some people are unaware of the importance of emergency ambulance services.

In this community, critically sick people are transported to the hospital by their loved ones or neighbors. They may either hire a private car or a taxi for the transportation. This is the case when an emergency happens at home. Citizens of this community use their basic knowledge and judgment to identify physical signs of an emergency (signs of impending death). These signs may include severe bleeding from any part of the body, difficulties in breathing, vomiting of blood, loss of consciousness, and abrupt falls. Their main objective is to make sure the patient reaches the nearest health center or hospital to seek medical help. There is no treatment given en route to the hospital.

On the other hand, emergencies that occur in an organized gathering may be responded to by the Red Cross or Boy Scouts. These include mountain races, public demonstrations, tournaments, and national day celebrations where provisions are made in preparation for any emergency. The Red Cross members and Boy Scouts are volunteers who have basic training to identify an emergency, but very few offer response to daily emergencies. Therefore, they only offer their services on demand and for organized occasions. Their typical configuration would be to have one ambulance to help transport an emergency patient to the hospital.

Cameroon has considerable cultural diversity which influences many aspects of life, but there is an almost uniform way that people respond to motor vehicle accidents or other emergencies. Bystanders or the first person at the scene of the accident has the obligation to do something to help the victim(s). If this person(s) cannot completely help the victim to the hospital, they either shout and seek help or quickly rush to where there are people to help, since there is no local universal emergency phone number. Depending on the nature of the accident and the location, as people gather around, they start developing ideas in a cooperative manner on how best to transport the victim to the hospital. If the accident is in the forest where there is no passable road, people will devise a method of taking the victims to the road for transportation. The victim can either be carried on the rescuers' backs, on the shoulders, or by holding the legs and hands, depending on how many persons are available and how strong they are. Very often the first vehicle driver who comes in contact with the victim involved in an accident opts to transport him or her to the hospital. If there are passengers in the vehicle they will volunteer to drop off and let the victim be transported to the nearest health center or hospital. In case of a big passenger bus, space might be created for the victims to be transported to the hospital. Most drivers already know that in the event of an accident they have to stop in order to give a helping hand.

Various occupational groups have specific means of identifying accidents within their field. For example, drivers of a particular transport company know each other, including the various vehicles they drive. A driver cannot bypass the first loaded vehicle on the way without finding out if there is a problem. If a vehicle loads after another and arrives first, then the whereabouts of the first loaded car will be questioned and searched for. Another example can be given with tree cutters. If a tree falls and the sound of the chain saw engine is not increased, a colleague will immediately rush in that direction to see if help is needed. In this field there is a rule that one must increase the sound of one's chain saw engine when the tree finally falls down. If this is not done, it is a sign that the falling tree has hurt the cutter.

Police officers play a very limited role as first responders in an emergency as compared to the 911 emergency services in more economically developed countries. At present each district has a phone number to the local police station. Even if this number is called, depending on the location, it often takes at least 30 minutes for police to arrive at the scene of an incident. This is often because of the lack of resources and staff. Even when they reach the scene of an accident, immediate help may have been provided by nearby witnesses. The only job left will be to investigate the circumstances of the incident and write a report, identify the victims of the accident, and communicate to the family members of the victims, directing them to the identified hospitals.

In the final analysis Cameroon does not specifically have any central emergency medical services system to compare to the 911 Emergency Medical Services system in the United States. There are some discussions under way to create EMS systems in Cameroon and some other African nations.[26] There are some trained first aiders who participate in covering organized events, but it is unknown how these individuals or their organizations would respond in a disaster: as individual bystanders or as an organized response force? Given the culture of bystander participation in helping in emergencies, we expect that disasters in many parts of Africa would see many bystanders stepping in to provide assistance, but that very few of these individuals would have any formal first-aid training.

Most African nations share issues as described above and common topics in health care policy, planning, and delivery:

- lack of data to monitor healthcare problems.
- no common emergency access numbers such as 911 or common numbers for emergency medical services.
- no awareness about the importance of bystander first-aid training and mobile ambulance services.
- problems in regard to coordination of existing institutions from local, national, and international resources.
- a high prevalence of motor vehicle crashes.
- diseases like HIV, TB, hepatitis, and malaria, which are still major health problems.
- lack of local first aiders and people skilled in basic birth attendance.
- access to medium and higher levels of health care is difficult.
- cultures of medical care and local healing paradigms may collide with traditional "western" medicine.
- religious and cultural paradigms of help, fate, and death, combined with historical experience that "help" from western nations has not always been altruistic and second thoughts about such help (monetary, religious) show us the need to think about our intentions to provide assistance and to find alternative approaches to support and empower local people.

For those interested in learning more about specific African countries, refer to the Country Briefs and overviews of the nations' health systems found at http://www.usaid.gov/ and http://www.who.int/countries/en/.

OCEANIA

Countries include Indonesia, Papua New Guinea, Timor, Australia, New Zealand. Countries excluded: the numerous small island states of the South Pacific.

Australia and **New Zealand** are relatively well-organized wealthy countries with a long tradition of providing effective professional first response services to all citizens. As is the case in all countries that have a large expanse of rural land, the quality and quantity of first response available is much higher in urban/periurban areas and decreases in the rural and wilderness regions.

Indonesia is a large country with a large population, spread out over a number of islands with considerable distance between some of them. While it has several highly urbanized cores, much of the population lives in relatively rural areas with a limited infrastructure.

Papua New Guinea, Timor, and the numerous small island nations are characterized by relatively low levels of economic productivity and resource availability, with exceptions in limited urban areas. For the most part, in Indonesia and the poorer countries the availability of first aid among bystanders and first responders can be expected to be quite low.

Australia has an interesting overlay of 81 field medical response teams that deploy to large incidents in addition to the local first response organizations. These field response teams (physicians, nurses, paramedics) are not covered in this chapter but can constitute an important part of the medical/first-aid assistance provided at large events. Because of its large land mass and low population density, Australia has many volunteer first response agencies, the largest of which is St. John Ambulance, which provides primary ambulance service to some jurisdictions and secondary or back-up service in others. More importantly for the concerns of this chapter, St. John Ambulance is Australia's largest provider of first-aid training, averaging about 400,000 trainees per year.[27] Its trainees include the general public as well as members of first response organizations such as volunteer fire departments, rescue squads, and government agencies. The Australian Red Cross is the country's second most important provider of first-aid courses, although we do not have numbers of those trained. Its most popular first-aid courses are one, two, and three-day courses, with the last being designed for occupational sites.

The first-aid roles of Australian fire departments differ from state to state. For example, in the state of Victoria, the state's fire department has no first-aid responsibilities,[28] while in Western Australia first aid is an integral part of the fire service.[29] Likewise, some of Australia's police departments require first-aid training (i.e., Victoria) while others do not. We have been unable to obtain a reliable estimate of what percentage of Australia's police and fire-fighting community are first-aid trained.

While **New Zealand**'s first-aid and first response services are not exactly identical to those in Australia, the similarities are too frequent to merit separate discussion in the limited space of this chapter.

SUMMARY

First aid is the core focus of this chapter, whether provided by organized first responders or by individual bystanders. Unfortunately, the very definitions of first aid, what it contains, how it is used, and by whom, differ dramatically from country to country and even within countries, making it possible only to discuss relative differences rather than absolutes that can be counted on by international responders. The International Red Cross and Red Crescent movement are the most stabilizing forces and providers of training in a world of some 200 countries, but even its standards and practices vary considerably from one place to the next. In general, wealthier countries are likely to have more first-aid trained first responders and bystanders than will economically more disadvantaged countries. However, the example of the European Union, with its standards and first aid–friendly laws, demonstrates that countries with fewer economic advantages than those found in the US and Canada can have a significantly stronger first-aid presence within their borders.

An equally important finding in this chapter is that many countries have an adequate or even good presence of first-aid providers in their urban cores but may have virtually no trained providers in poverty-stricken periurban and rural environments. While it is not highlighted in the text of this chapter, another important finding is that there are many countries for which there is very little information available from common sources about their first response forces or first-aid training. Some of these countries are quite large, like China.

In short, we must be very careful about any stereotyping as to the probable availability and quality of first-aid resources at any given response site. Local Red Cross/Red Crescent–affiliated organizations may be the best rapidly available sources of information about local first-aid availability.

Acknowledgments

The authors extend thanks to the following people for helping us collect information where it was frequently missing from public documents: Buba Soweh, MD; Sako Narita, M.P.H.; Cornelius Chebo; Rick Caissee, MD; Luis Pinet, Ph.D. (cand); David Prakash, MD; Ala'a Oteir; and John Lindsay, M.P.A.

References

1. Eisenberg MS, Horwood BT, Cummins RO, et al. Cardiac arrest and resuscitation: a tale of 29 cities. *Ann Emerg Med* 19(2): 179, 1990.
2. St. John Ambulance http://www.sja.org.uk/sja/; accessed 12/30/2009.
3. European Reference Centre for First Aid Education, http://www.firstaidinaction.net/First-aid-in-Europe; accessed 12/30/2009.
4. United Nations Radio, http://www.unmultimedia.org/radio/english/detail/81138.html, Dominique Praplan, Head of the IFRC's Health and Care Department, accessed 12/30/2009.
5. Europa: Press Releases, http://europa.eu/rapid/press ReleasesAction.do?reference=MEMO/09/60&format= HTML&aged=0&language=EN&guiLanguage=en, accessed 12/30/10.
6. Thomas C. Heneghan, Senior Associate, Business Planning, American Red Cross National Headquarters, personal communication, 28 December 2009.
7. Rick Caissie, MD, Canadian Red Cross, communicated 30 December 2009.
8. Luis Pinet, Ph.D., personal communication, 15 December 2009.
9. Irayma Cazull Imbert, Aida Rodriguez Cabrera, Gisela Sanabria Ramos,Raul Hernandez Heredia. Enseñanza de primeros auxilios a escolares de cuatro a noveno grados. *Revista Cubana de Salud Pública* 33 (2), 2007.
   Raul Hernandez Heredia First aid teaching of a nursery school to ninth grade *Cuban Journal of Public Health,* April-June, 2007/ vol. number 002 Cuban Society of Health Administration Havana, Cuba Network of Scientific Journals of Latin America and the Caribbean, Spain and Portugal (Autonomous University of Mexico State)
10. Sako Narita, M.P.H., NREMT-P, personal communication, 22 December 2009.
11. Commonwealth Human Rights Initiative: Police Organisation in India http://www.humanrights initiative.org/publications/police/police_organisatio ns.pdf; accessed 30 December 2009.
12. Government of India, Ministry of Home Affairs: National Fire Service College, Nagpur http://nfscnag pur.nic.in/; accessed 30 December 2009.

13. Director General Civil Defence Ministry of Home Affairs Government of India (Training) http://dgcd.nic.in/training1.htm; accessed 30 December 2009.

14. Secondary Board of Secondary Education; towards a safer India: http://www.ndmindia.nic.in/WCDR DOCS/Towards%20A%20Safer%20India-CBSE.pdf; accessed 30 December 2009.

15. Together Towards a Safer India, part III, http://www.cbse.nic.in/DM%20ENGLISH.pdf; accessed 30 December 2009.

16. National Service Scheme (NSS) Special Camping Programme, http://nss.nic.in/speccamp.asp; accessed 30 December 2009.

17. St. John Association of India, http://www.orderofst john.org/india; accessed 30 December 2009.

18. Newsletter of the National Disaster Response Force, India Vol 1, April 2008, http://ndma.gov.in/ndma/newsletters/Final%20NDRF.pdf; accessed 30 Dec 2009.

19. Mogen David Adom in Israel, Volunteers layout, http://www.mdais.com/235/; retrieved 30 December 2009.

20. The Israel Police & the Community: Volunteers http://www.police.gov.il/english/Volunteers/Pages/default.aspx; accessed 30 December 2009.

21. The City of Johannesburg Alex community volunteers for EMS, E. Visser 15 Sept 2008 http://www.joburg.org.za/content/view/2964/200/; accessed 03 January 2010.

22. The South African Red Cross Society, http://www.redcross.org.za/; accessed 03 January 2010.

23. St. John, Johannesburg, South Africa, first aid courses http://www.stjohn.org.za/copy/courses/docc.asp accessed 03 January 2010.

24. Cameroon people (2009) CIA World Factbook. http://www.theodora.com/wfbcurrent/cameroon/cameroon_people.html. Accessed December 20, 2009.

25. NationMaster.com, Surface Area of Cameroon (2005). http://www.nationmaster.com/time.php?stat=geo_sur_are_sq_km&country=cm. accessed December 20, 2009.

26. Buba, Soweh and Chebo, Cornilius (2009). Personal communication December 21, 2009.

27. St. John Ambulance Australia, first-aid training, http://www.stjohn.org.au/index.php?option=com_content&task=view&id=14&Itemid=24; accessed 30 December 2009.

28. Country Fire Authority (CFA) State of Victoria, Australia http://www.cfa.vic.gov.au/about/whatwedo.htm.

29. The Fire and Rescue Service of Western Australia, History Fire & Rescue Service, http://www.fesa.wa.gov.au/internet/?MenuID=216&ContentID=376.

CHAPTER 10

Staffing of Ambulances

Silvio Aguilera, Jose G. Cabañas, Alberto Machado

KEY LEARNING POINTS

- No perfect ambulance staffing model exists, and EMS models are constructed around the needs of the community and according to the available economic resources.

- An EMS system can be a mixed model of private and public services with paid and/or volunteer providers. Even if providers are from different service agencies, they should be seen as part of *one* EMS delivery system.

- In general, the levels of ambulance service staffing fall into one of two categories: Care

given by EMTs as BLS (basic life support); and by paramedics, nurses, or physicians as ALS (advanced life support).

- Paramedics have great experience and are well adapted to the prehospital environment. They can provide care with minimal resources and in a difficult environment. In some settings, physicians can expand the scope of prehospital care and decrease the need for transport from the scene to the ED.

INTRODUCTION

Every other second, a request for emergency medical assistance is received at emergency dispatch centers around the world. Public expectations are largely based on prehospital response time. EMS has evolved considerably from its origins and is a branch of the specialty of emergency medicine that provides prehospital acute emergency care to a particular community. Depending on the country, an EMS unit may also be known as a first-aid squad, emergency squad, rescue squad, ambulance service, ambulance or life squad.

The goal of EMS systems around the world is to provide high-quality care to those in need of

urgent medical attention. Care includes recognition, treatment, and transport of the ill and injured to a point of definitive care. To meet this goal, EMS systems rely on competent healthcare providers who are trained to work in the prehospital arena. In this chapter we discuss the most common EMS staffing models utilized around the world.

EMS SERVICE CONFIGURATION MODELS

Prehospital care configuration models vary around the world. Every country has policy makers who determine EMS system delivery models, how prehospital care should be provided, and by whom. In general, the levels of service available fall into one of three categories: care provided by emergency medical technicians as BLS, care by paramedics as ALS, or care by nurses and physicians. There are regions in Europe where legislation mandates that ALS services must be physician-led, while other systems allow specially trained nurses to deliver care and have no traditional paramedics at all. Elsewhere, as in North America, the UK, and Australia, paramedics deliver ALS care. In paramedic-centered systems, the direct physician-led models are rare. **No perfect model exists, and most jurisdictions will construct their EMS model based upon the needs of the community and the available economic resources.**

Most systems rely on trained individuals who are certified as providers by a local government entity. Training and qualification levels for members and employees of EMS systems are different throughout the world. Some providers serve as volunteers, while others are employed by an agency. Some jurisdictions depend solely on volunteer providers due to a lack of economic resources. In other systems, besides patient care, EMS units are tasked to handle technical rescue operations such as extrication, water rescue, and search and rescue.

Basic Life Support

BLS providers have a specific skill set that includes basic airway management (bag-mask ventilation), adult and pediatric CPR, bleeding control, spine immobilization, and splinting techniques. The use of an automated external defibrillator (AED) along with CPR is the most critical skill BLS providers possess, and many EMS systems around the word use BLS providers as first responders during cardiac emergencies.

There are two classifications of BLS levels: medical first responder (MFRs) and EMT-Basic (EMT-B).

First responders are usually the first to arrive on the scene of an emergency incident. They can be part of the regular EMS response or part of the social fabric within a community group. They are capable of performing a primary patient assessment along with CPR, basic airway support, and hemorrhage control. In the US, MFRs receive 40 hours of classroom instruction, and depending on local regulations, 16 to 36 hours of refresher training.

The EMT-B certification is the minimum required to staff a basic ambulance. Most private non-emergency transport services utilize EMT-Bs as their sole providers. In the public model, it is common to have EMT-Bs and paramedics responding to emergencies. Public safety agencies like the fire department commonly train their personnel to serve as BLS providers during the emergencies they attend. This organization is particularly common in multitiered EMS models. The EMT-B has the skills of the first responder and can also perform scene triage, patient assessment, and patient monitoring during transportation. Depending on the country's regulatory agency, the hourly requirements to become an EMT-B will vary. In the US, the National Highway Transportation Safety Administration (NHTSA) mandates a standardized curriculum for EMT-Bs. The initial course requires approximately 110 hours of instruction and includes specific educational objectives and clinical experiences for mastery of skills.

Under special circumstances, some jurisdictions have expanded the training and scope of EMT-Bs under the supervision of a local medical director to include the use of epinephrine autoinjectors (e.g., EpiPen™), glucose administration, and albuterol administration by a metered-dose inhaler. Some jurisdictions have expanded the scope of practice of the EMT-B. For instance, prehospital care in Tehran is provided by Tehran's basic EMS system. EMTs are trained to provide BLS to trauma patients but can also administer intravenous fluid therapy.[1]

Advanced Life Support

Modern EMS has incorporated higher levels of prehospital providers to perform ALS. ALS system models provide a more comprehensive level of service by highly trained personnel usually certified at the paramedic level (EMT-P) or an equivalent level, depending on the country's certification levels. In some jurisdictions healthcare professionals like nurses or physicians serve as ALS providers for the system. The main distinction of an ALS provider is the knowledge and skills to perform invasive therapeutic procedures during a medical emergency.

Some systems may utilize intermediate certification levels between a basic and a paramedic provider for economic reasons or because the paramedic supply may be limited. This is particularly common in small cities or rural regions. EMT-Intermediates are considered ALS providers as well. However, their scope of practice is more limited compared to the paramedic level. In general, ALS providers function under the license and supervision of a system medical director.

Most EMS systems in major cities around the world operate at the ALS level of care. Traditionally, EMS care has evolved by bringing more care from the ED to the field.

Paramedic

The EMT-P is the most advanced prehospital provider. Paramedics have the capability to manage most life-threatening emergencies in the prehospital setting. These highly trained professionals are able to perform advanced airway interventions, IV or intraosseous (IO) line placement, medication administration, recognition and treatment of dysrhythmias, cardiac monitoring, chest decompression of a tension pneumothorax, needle or surgical cricothyrotomy for a failed airway, and transcutaneous cardiac pacing.

There are different models for paramedic education and certification. This will depend on the countries' regulatory and credentialing process. In the US, there is a National Standard Curriculum for paramedic training that consists of 1,200 educational hours including didactic, clinical, and a field practicum. As EMS management career options have expanded, many paramedic educational programs have evolved from a 12-month certificate to an associate or baccalaureate degree.

A large number of studies have evaluated the ability of paramedics to obtain a medical history, perform a physical examination, and provide a clinical assessment. There is good inter-rater reliability with emergency physicians in conditions such as chest pain and respiratory distress.[2,3] Depending on training and experience, paramedics can demonstrate excellent sensitivity and positive predictive value in the prehospital identification of ST-segment acute myocardial infarction.[4-6] Paramedics work in the prehospital environment, are familiar with trauma and violence, make decisions quickly, and can provide care with minimal resources. They work in a variety of physical and environmental conditions, tolerate noisy and chaotic situations, and make decisions when faced with uncertainty.[7]

Registered Nurse

The use of registered nurses in the prehospital environment is more common in countries that have a limited number of traditional EMS providers. Some EMS systems in Europe allow nurses to work independently, and some require supervision by a physician. Some jurisdictions have implemented nurses into their standard EMS staffing model, as they feel nurses bring unique skills to some clinical situations. In contrast, other jurisdictions, most notably in the US, use nurses mostly as critical care interfacility transport providers. Nurses may be part of a team with a respiratory therapist, a paramedic, or an emergency physician. Critical care teams are ground or air medical crews that transport critical patients to a facility with a higher level of care. Nurses on such teams are generally required to seek additional certification beyond basic nursing certification.

In Sweden, all emergency ambulances are staffed with a registered nurse with specialization in prehospital care, anesthesia, or intensive care. The second person in the ambulance is a nurse with additional specific prehospital training. In Stockholm County (population two million) this is complemented by a physician in the dispatch center who can respond by car or helicopter to very selected cases. There is a medical director within the county who supervises EMS services in the region.[8]

Physicians

There are many places in Europe where paramedics do not exist and most advanced prehospital care is performed by physicians. EMS systems in France, Italy, and Germany are well known for having specialized physicians take a more hands-on approach during high-acuity emergency calls. In fact, some countries legally require that a physician must be physically present for paramedics to perform ALS interventions.

The utilization of physicians as primary field providers is less common in the US. In the US, EMS medical directors may respond to an emergency call as part of medical quality assurance. Some critical care transport programs utilize the services of emergency physicians on a case-by-case basis. This may occur when a critical patient requires special monitoring or advanced therapeutic interventions during transport that are beyond the skills of a paramedic or a transport nurse.

PRIVATE VERSUS PUBLIC EMS STAFFING

Historically, public EMS systems of care developed from volunteer hospital-based initiatives to manage local emergency situations. But, as years passed, volunteers became older and resources started to become scarce as communities and service demand grew. Such factors pressed local governments to develop public and private EMS service models to help mitigate the increasing demand.

Public EMS models are subject to public policies established by government decision-makers and are regulated by available economic resources. Most private models do not possess these drawbacks. Most private EMS services work with a specific set of goals and objectives in return for payment. In addition, private

EMS agencies commonly respond to nonemergency transports. However, in some jurisdictions the government may contract private agencies to be the sole providers in the community. This decision depends mostly on the personnel and economic resources available to serve the region.

The model that serves the community (i.e., private or public) can affect the ambulance-staffing model. For instance, in the city of Buenos Aires, Argentina, (population eight million), the EMS system is a hospital-based public system staffed by physicians from municipal hospitals. In this EMS service, all bases are localized in municipal hospitals and emergency physicians from these institutions staff ambulances regularly. However, having physicians in ambulances does not guarantee a superior and consistent prehospital care because on occasion nonemergency physicians staff ambulances as well. Interestingly, despite having emergency physicians responding to prehospital emergencies with great acceptance in the public domain, emergency medicine as a formal specialty is still not recognized in Argentina.

It is common for public models to have specific government mandates that may create parallels between providers that staff private and public EMS services. Take for example the city of Buenos Aires, where law mandates that the public EMS system must respond to all incidents on public roads within the city. In addition, the law also states that the patient should then be transported to a public hospital, thus overloading the public system. Such a situation can create significant competency challenges for private-system providers because it becomes more difficult for private-system personnel to maintain trauma skills, a proficient knowledge base, and exposure to reasonable call volumes.

No Perfect Model

There is no perfect EMS delivery model, and models vary around the world. For instance, some Latin American countries have only paramedics and doctors in ambulances (Mexico), whereas in others the public services have paramedics. Other countries (Panama, Venezuela, Peru, and Ecuador) have private ambulances providing services with a general physician on the vehicle. In still other countries (Argentina, Brasil, Uruguay), all ambulances have physicians, and nurses and EMTs cannot provide medical care without direct medical supervision. As of 2010, Ecuador is obligated to have a physician on all ambulances.[9-14]

In South Africa, the EMS system is based on paramedics. Some public and private systems occasionally have a physician who comes to the scene in an automobile. Medical direction is frequently assumed by a paramedic.[15]

In China, the EMS team consists of physicians, nurses, and drivers with four different EMS models (Beijing, Shanghai, Chongqing, and Guangzhou). There are no ambulances using only paramedics or nurses.[16]

Among the different systems, the most convenient for the population are those that are properly managed and administered and meet the community needs. There may be instances where EMS provision to a region will be a mixed model of private and public services with paid and/or volunteer providers. In this case a good interaction between all services is essential to maintain healthy and quality service. **Ideally, even if all providers are from a different service agency, they should be seen as part of *one* EMS delivery system.** Volunteerism can create operational issues within the system due to lack of dependability if volunteers are not available and if there are performance issues with training and review. This deficiency is corrected by instituting a public paid service model.

PHYSICIANS IN EMS

EMS physicians need competencies in the clinical and administrative aspects of EMS. We can summarize them in two major categories: physician as medical director and physician as prehospital care provider.[17]

Physician as Medical Director

There are two main functions for an EMS medical director: direct medical oversight of clinical operations and continued education of system providers. An EMS medical director must be available immediately by telephone or radio communication as needed for consultation. Medical director functions are supplemented by other important tasks as well. These include direct supervision, quality improvement, development and revision of protocols, determining the scope of local EMS practice, and designing educational content and research.[18]

The presence of an active EMS system medical director is a key element of modern EMS. The training of emergency medicine physicians to become medical directors is not always complete. Even though residency graduates provide medical supervision and work as consultants to local EMS systems early in their careers, most still gain their experience and knowledge at work.

The training required to work in EMS varies greatly across Europe. Most countries require that EMS physicians be experts in at least one or more areas of medicine.

A very important aspect to consider is the status of the specialty of emergency medicine within a country's medical community, because this could drive support for a certified subspecialty in EMS. In the US, there is a proposal to consider EMS as a certified subspecialty within emergency medicine. This would allow the accreditation and standardization of EMS fellowship programs.

The concept of an EMS medical director varies widely around the world. In a recent review of prehospital EMS in 12 Caribbean countries, the Pan American Health Organization (PAHO) reported that in most countries there was no legal requirement for the position of a medical director. In fact, some countries had services in which there was no direct involvement of a physician.[19]

In contrast, a US survey including seven states in the mid-Atlantic region and the District of Columbia identified 273 EMS systems and a large majority of respondents (96%) indicated that a medical director was involved.[20]

The pilot implementation of medical director in 2007 in an EMS program in Qatar resulted in an overall improvement in clinical quality indicators for that system.[21]

The Physician as Prehospital Care Provider

There are two well-known philosophical models of EMS: the Anglo-American model, in which paramedics are the primary prehospital providers, and the Franco-German model, in which physicians have a more hands-on approach. Both models have a medical director who oversees clinical practice in the system. Countries that adhere to the Anglo-American model include Canada, the US, the UK, Ireland, Israel, Japan, the Philippines, South Korea, Australia and New Zealand. This system is based upon strict supervision and control by a qualified medical director. This model tends to exist where the specialty of emergency medicine is recognized, and medical direction is limited to emergency physicians.

In contrast, France, Germany, Switzerland, Norway, Austria, Belgium, Poland, Portugal, Spain, and many Latin American countries utilize a Franco-German model. This model has many variations in different countries. In some countries the specialty of emergency medicine still does not exist and in others physicians who work on ambulances are trained in specialties such as anesthesiology, critical care, internal medicine, or cardiology.

In other countries there is great degree of variability of experience and training of ambulance physicians. The usual reason is because career prospects as an ambulance doctor are poor, and most talented physicians choose other specialties.

It is difficult to determine if one of the two systems is superior to the other. A country must develop an EMS system based on economic opportunities, the health plan structure, cultural issues, and availability of personnel.

The European Union (EU) convened an expert group (project Hesculaep) to describe and evaluate EMS delivery models across Europe.[22,23] The survey reviewed the situation in 27 EU member states. Most of the member countries used physicians as prehospital care providers. EMS activity was often an assignment as part of training in another specialty. In some countries the mere title "physician" was considered sufficient to work as a prehospital provider.

In most European countries, medical control is provided by a medical director. Training required in order to work in EMS varies widely across Europe. Most countries require that EMS physicians become specialists in at least one or two areas. Table 10-1 summarizes different specialties required by country.

In the French EMS system, physicians perform telephone triage and decide what type of ambulance should be sent to the scene. The options are a BLS fire-department ambulance or a hospital-based ambulance with a physician. BLS fire ambulances are usually sent to less urgent cases or situations requiring extrication. Law prohibits fire-department ambulances from performing medical care. The hospital-based ambulances have a driver and an anesthesiologist and sometimes are accompanied by a resident physician.[24]

In the Netherlands there are two types of ambulances. The first has a team consisting of a driver and a nurse. The nurse decides if the patient requires transport to a trauma center or other hospital, or if a unit with a physician is needed to treat the patient on the scene without hospital transport. The physician unit has a nurse and a trauma surgeon or anesthesiologist. This unit is requested for multiple or entrapped victims. Physicians can perform tube thoracostomy, rapid sequence intubation, and amputations.[25]

In Sweden, since February 2008, emergency ambulances are staffed with a nurse with specialty training or experience in prehospital care, anesthesia, or intensive care; and a nonregistered nurse with specific prehospital training. Physicians may be called to the scene for selected cases. In Stockholm County (population two million), EMS care in four of five local districts is provided by private companies.[26]

Table 10–1 | Required specializations for EMS Physicians[9]

COUNTRY	Emergency Medicine	Internal Medicine	Anesthesia	Surgery	Cardiology	Other	No required
Austria	X	X					
Belgium	X	X					
Bulgaria							X
Cyprus	X						X
Czech Rep.	X						
Denmark							X
Estonia	X		X				
Finland							X
France	X		X				
Germany					X		
Greece	X		X	X			
Hungary	X		X				
Ireland							X
Italy							X
Latvia	X						
Lithuania							X
Luxembourg			X				
Malta						X	X
Nethrlands						X	X
Poland	X		X	X			
Portugal							X
Romania	X		X				
Solvakia	X		X				
Slovenia		X					
Spain							X
Sweden						X	
Total	11	3	8	2	1	2	11

In Spain, neither public nor private systems have paramedics. Técnicos en Emergencias Sanitarias (TES, Emergency Health Technicians) provide support for physicians and nurses on ambulances. There are two types of ambulances, basic and advanced life support. Basic ambulances have two emergency health technicians, and advanced units have a physician and nurse. There are about twice as many basic ambulances as advanced ambulances in Spain, but they are not evenly distributed. If needed, basic units can be transformed into advanced units. Most EMS service is public, although some areas have private services.[27]

In Argentina, where 100% of the ambulances are staffed by physicians, the proportion of patients transported to the hospital is only 23% (when the call is categorized as an emergency response). The proportion transported is greater for severe or moderate trauma. Experienced physicians can evaluate and treat patients at the scene without transport to the hospital.[28]

The presence of physicians in ambulances at events with large numbers of attendees may reduce the number of ambulances transporting patients. In a prospective observational study conducted during a major motor sport event at a California Speedway, the presence of physicians at the scene reduced ambulance transportation of patients to the local hospital by 89%. The scope of medical practice at this event, which exceeded paramedic capability, included care of lacerations, renal colic, pharyngitis, and need for medical prescriptions.[29]

The presence of physicians in ambulances at large sporting or mass gathering events may decrease the need for transport to the ED for evaluation and treatment. One study of football game attendees reported that while 206 people who were evaluated met the criteria for ALS care at the scene, 155 of these (75.2%) were treated by physicians on site without ED referral.[30]

Physicians as prehospital care providers can establish a primary diagnosis, provide treatment at the scene without necessarily transporting the patient to the ED, determine if hospitalization is necessary, and admit the patient directly to the appropriate inpatient unit. In Germany, physicians as prehospital care providers can provide palliative care in the prehospital setting to patients with advanced stage neoplastic disease, keeping the patient at home instead of transporting him or her to the hospital.[31]

The use of physicians as prehospital care providers can expand the scope of EMS care. Many countries around the world have embraced this staffing model with great success.

References

1. Modaghegh MH, Roudsari BS, Sajadehchi A. Prehospital trauma care in Tehran: potential areas for improvement. *Prehosp Emerg Care* 6: 218, 2002.
2. Ackerman R, Waldron R. Difficulty breathing: agreement of paramedic and emergency physician diagnoses. *Prehosp Emerg Care* 10, 1: 77, 2006.
3. Schaider JJ, Riccio JC, Rydman RJ, et al. Paramedic diagnostic accuracy for patients complaining of chest pain or shortness of breath. *Prehosp Emerg Care* 10: 245, 1995.
4. Le May MR, Dionne R, Maloney J, et al. Diagnostic performance and potential clinical impact of advanced care paramedic interpretation of ST-segment elevation myocardial infarction in the field. *CJEM* 8(6): 401, 2006.
5. Williams B, Boyle M, Lord B. Paramedic identification of electrocardiograph J-point and ST-segments. *Prehosp Disaster Med* 23(6): 526, 2008.
6. Davis DP, Graydon C, Stein R, et al. The positive predictive value of paramedic versus emergency physician interpretation of the prehospital 12-lead electrocardiogram. *Prehosp Emerg Care* 11(4):399, 2007.
7. Ummenhofer W, Scheidegger D. Role of the physician in the prehospital management of trauma: European perspective. *Curr Opin Anaesthesiol* 8(6):559, 2002.
8. Gunnar Ohlen, President European Society for Emergency Medicine, personal communication. January 2010
9. Victor Rodriguez. Past President, Sociedad Venezolana de Emergencias y Desastres, personal communication. January 2010
10. Guillermo Perez, Ecuador, personal communication. January 2010
11. Olga del Carmen Alonso, Mexico, personal communication. January 2010
12. Luciano Guerra, Marta Sandoya, Panamá, personal communication. January 2010
13. Abel Garcia, Past President Sociedad Peruana de Emergencias y Desastres, Past President ALACED, personal communication. January 2010
14. Agustin Blanco, Brasil, personal communication. January 2010
15. Lee Wallis, South Africa, personal communication. January 2010
16. Shao JF, Shen HY, Shi XY. Current state of emergency medicine education in China. *Emerg Med J* 26: 573, 2009.
17. Cone DC, Krohmer JR. EMS physicians certification: just one piece of the puzzle. *Prehosp Emerg Care* 9,3: 371, 2005.
18. Peterson T. The role of state medical direction in the comprehensive EMS system. *Prehosp Emerg Care* 8: 98, 2004;
19. Barnett AT, Segree W, Mattthews A. The roles and responsibilities of physicians in pre-hospital emer-

gency medical services: A Caribbean perspective. *West Indian Med J* 55(1):52, 2006.

20. National Highway Traffic Safety Administration. Configurations of EMS systems: a pilot study. *Ann Emerg Med* 52:453, 2008.

21. Munk MD, White SD, Perry ML, et al. Physicians medical direction and clinical performance at an established emergency medical system. *Prehosp Emerg Care* 13 (2): 185, 2009.

22. Fairhurst R. Prehospital care in Europe. *Emerg Med J* 22: 760, 2005.

23. Emergency Medical Services Systems in the European Union. Report of an assessment project co-ordinated by the World Health Organization, 2009. http://www.euro.who.int/document/e92038. pdf.

24. Nikkanen HE, Pouges C, Jacobs LM. Emergency medicine in France. *Ann Emerg Med* 31:116, 1998.

25. de Vries GMJ, Luitse JSK. Emergency medicine in The Netherlands *Ann Emerg Med* 38: 583, 2001.

26. Gunnar Öhlén, President European Society for Emergency Medicine, EuSEM Stockholm, Sweden, personal communication. January 2010

27. Tomás Toranzo. President, Sociedad Española de Medicina de Emergencia, personal communication. January 2010

28. Aguilera S. Prehospital Emergency Medicine in Argentina. Fifth Annual Mediterranean Emergency Medicine Congress. 14-17 September, 2009. Valencia, Spain.

29. Grange J, Baumann G, Vaezazizi M. On-site physicians reduce ambulance transports at mass gatherings. *Prehosp Emerg Care* 7,3:322,2003.

30. Pozner CN, Levine M, Listwa T, et al. Does the presence of physicians at professional football games reduce the number of patient transports? *Ann Emerg Med* 48: S55,2006.

31. Wiese CHR, Bartels UE, Ruppert D, et al. Treatment of palliative care emergencies by prehospital emergency physicians in Germany: an interview based investigation. *Palliat Med* 23:369,2009.

CHAPTER 11

EMS Medical Directors

Garry Wilkes

KEY LEARNING POINTS

- The medical director provides medical leadership and medical authority for the EMS.

- The medical director authorizes medical procedures and medication use by paramedics and other nonphysicians via Clinical Practice Guidelines (CPGs) or Protocols.

- A key role of the medical director is to ensure that EMS practice is consistent with current evidence and is formulated in conjunction with the local medical community.

- A rigorous clinical governance system, including incident review, monitoring of performance indicators, and complaint/incident management is essential for every EMS. The medical director is responsible for oversight of these processes either directly in small services or by delegation in larger services.

- The medical director is usually the spokesperson and liaison with local physicians and the media for EMS-related matters.

THE MEDICAL DIRECTOR

As a service industry, the principal deliverables of an EMS are medical care and transport. The medical director is primarily concerned with the former.

Medication administration and medical procedures are governed by statutes that require medical licensing. While some EMSs have physicians as part of the responding crew (most commonly seen in European countries), the majority of North American and other western EMSs have responding crews composed of paramedics, emergency medical technicians, nurses, or first-aid officers with varying degrees of training. The EMS practitioners within the service generally have delegated authority to provide medical care and administer

medications at the direction of and under the licensure of the medical director. This authority to practice is discussed further below.

Role

The role of the medical director varies considerably among jurisdictions. The position may be full time or part time and may be closely associated with conjoint practice in a local medical facility. In the majority of cases, the medical director is an acute care physician who works both in EMS in an advisory capacity and in a hospital-based practice in a clinical capacity in a specialty area.

In those services where physicians are part of the responding team, the medical director's role is more managerial. In other services there is no individual medical director; instead a panel or committee assumes the various roles of a medical director. This chapter will assume the viewpoint of a nominated medical director for the sake of simplicity while recognizing the variations that may occur. The roles, however, remain the same in general terms regardless of how the position is filled.

The medical director, as the name implies, is responsible for directing medical care provided by the organization, ensuring care delivered by the service is contemporary, appropriate, in keeping with accepted best practice, and delivered in a cost-effective manner.

The medical director has the principal responsibility for the content of the Clinical Practice Guidelines (CPGs) or Protocols. The CPGs specify the practices EMS providers within the service are authorized to perform and provide specific details regarding indications, contraindications, and dose of medications. Traditionally, protocols have been more commonly used than guidelines to ensure care delivered is in keeping with the delegated authority.

The CPGs are effectively the documentation of the service's medical policy. Practice outside of these guidelines by EMS personnel must therefore be authorized beforehand or within a reasonable timeframe after the event by a delegated authority. Without this authority, the individual EMS provider becomes directly liable for those actions and any consequences.

The principal responsibilities of the medical director are shown in Table 11-1.

Table 11–1	Medical Director's Role

- Remain current in medical practice
- Keep abreast of developments in practice, including research in related areas
- Ensure practice is in keeping with local medical expectations
- Monitor clinical activity within the service, including clinical indicators
- Provide direction for future developments in medical practice
- Oversee investigation of clinical incidents
- Oversee the organization's CPGs to ensure
  - Currency
  - Completeness
  - Compliance
  - Clinical efficacy
- Clinical governance
  - Clinical audit
  - Risk management

As the person responsible for determining the service's medical practice, the medical director will also typically be the spokesperson and primary respondent to inquiries from within and from outside the service regarding medical care, ensuring these are addressed appropriately.

REPORTING/RELATIONSHIPS

Management structure varies considerably with the size and function of the EMS. Smaller services may have a few vehicles and a very small number of EMS personnel operating within a relatively small geographical area. Larger services can have more than a thousand vehicles with tens of thousands of operational personnel providing services to vast geographic areas. For example, St John Ambulance Service in Western Australia has approximately 4,500 personnel providing services out of 200 locations in an area of 1 million square miles.

Whereas smaller services can be effectively managed by a few individuals, larger services will have a CEO, board of directors, and the typical management levels that accompany large businesses. What will be described below is the structure of a larger organization, recognizing that although many of the named roles will not exist in smaller services, the general principles still apply.

The medical director liaises closely with all directors, particularly the operational director, and should report directly to the CEO.

If present, the manager of clinical governance (see below) reports to the medical director for matters related to medical practice and policy such as CPG reviews, clinical audits, clinical issues, and suggested new practices. The manager of clinical governance usually also oversees audits and complaints regarding operational issues. For these matters, the reporting is via the operational director.

The medical director should oversee and guide clinical research within the service. Where resources permit, there may be a separate research capacity within the service or close links with external research bodies (see Chapter 8, EMS Research). Research conducted within the organization related to clinical care is evaluated by the medical director and action is taken accordingly.

AUTHORITY TO PRACTICE

Different services employ different degrees of medical oversight. In some services authority to practice for many procedures and/or medication administration requires direct communication with an authorizing medical officer from the scene. This can be achieved by telephone, radio, or by other means. Once authority is obtained, patient care continues with authority documented. This is referred to as "direct medical oversight."

In other services, the majority of procedural skills and medication administration are detailed in the CPGs and skills manuals, the officers are specifically trained and current in those practices, and authority to practice is provided within that framework without the need for direct communication at the time. Communication is only required in uncommon situations where existing guidelines do not cover the situation at hand. This is referred to as "indirect medical oversight."

Whichever system is in place, those practices that do not require authorization at the time are contained in the services' CPGs.

The CPGs have an important governance role because they limit clinical practice. Delegated authority exists for the contents of the CPG only. Therefore if individual EMS personnel practice outside those guidelines (by practice, dose, or indication), that practice will be deemed noncompliant and hence not authorized. As CPGs are specifically developed to reflect best practice and to cover the vast majority of circumstances likely to be encountered, practicing outside of these guidelines is likely to reflect practice that does not comply with accepted best practice. Not only does this increase the risk of adverse outcomes, but in the event of an adverse outcome the individual concerned may be placed at risk of legal action.

It is recognized that there are times when situations arise when CPGs are not sufficient for the particular circumstances encountered, and the practitioner on the scene believes practice outside of the guidelines is essential to ensure a good patient outcome. In these circumstances, there is the capacity to gain authority for out-of-authority practice. Typically this can be obtained by telephone/radio consultation using a predetermined process. Different services vary regarding the frequency with which this occurs.

In the exceedingly rare circumstance where out-of-practice authority is not able to be obtained and the practitioner at the scene is certain the intervention is vital for good patient outcome, the interests of the patient should always take precedence. However, the event must be reported and authority requested as soon as is practical and the individual practitioner still remains liable for any outcomes.

CLINICAL PRACTICE GUIDELINES

Purpose

The CPGs are a key document for the service. They may be printed, electronic, or both. Abbreviated versions may be produced as pocket guides. The CPGs specify in detail which procedures and medications are authorized for use by individual EMS personnel at various levels of training and expertise. CPGs are updated regularly, and some are available on line for public viewing (see Web resources).

As the medical director assumes responsibility for medical care delivered by EMS personnel who have been delegated authority, the CPG becomes the reference and manual for that practice. It is obviously impractical to expect all personnel to recall all the details of authorized practice, particularly so for less commonly employed agents or practices. In those circumstances the CPGs also act as a guide and aid document.

Development/Maintenance

CPGs are developed from a variety of inputs (Figure 11-1) and triggers (Table 11-2).

Table 11–2	Clinical Practice Guideline Review Triggers

Routine
- 5-year minimum

Responsive
- Incidents
- Complaints

New Evidence
- **Internal**
  - Audit
  - Research
  - Clinical group
- **External**
  - Research
  - Medical advisory panel
  - Other services
  - Other experts

Staff Input
- Staff forum
- Via on-road senior staff/clinical group
- Via medical director

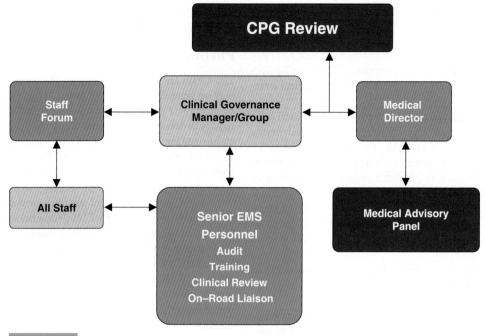

FIGURE 11–1

Clinical practice guideline review.

For new services, CPGs are designed to cover as many conditions as are likely to be encountered in clinical practice. Obviously it is not feasible to cover all possibilities, as the list of what may be encountered is enormous. However, it is expected that all common conditions and all rare but potentially deadly conditions should be included. For practical procedures, a separate skills manual may be developed (diagrams and images of equipment and step-wise procedures are highly recommended).

With time, CPGs are revised, new ones added as practices evolve, and others are removed when they are no longer necessary.

As a principle all should be reviewed at least every five years. The documentation should include inception, review, and revision dates along with time of next scheduled review. Not only does this provide clarity regarding currency but it also may act as a prompt for interested individuals to suggest changes for upcoming revisions.

Important sources of information that help refine practice are research, expert reviews, staff suggestions, and the results of investigations of complaints, incidents, and audit results.

CPGs should be based on the best available evidence and, wherever possible, provide an indication of the evidence evaluated in the form of a worksheet in accordance with standard evaluation practices. Locally collected data are the most relevant to local practice and are preferred where available. Research and evaluation of the literature are specialized skills that may need to be outsourced. If resources allow, a project officer with research training and skills is a valuable addition to the service (see Chapter 8, EMS Research).

Process

The following is an outline of the development/review process.

- Identify CPG for development:
  - Planned—as part of regular review process
  - Responsive
    - Outcome from analysis/review of incidents or complaints
    - New evidence
      - Internal—audit, research
      - External—publication, via medical advisory panel
  - Staff input
    - Staff forum
    - On-road discussion with senior staff
    - Suggestions ratified via the clinical governance operational group
- *Obtain relevant literature/existing clinical guidelines from other services

- *Prepare evidence evaluation worksheet assessing
  - Levels of evidence
  - Quality of evidence
  - Included/excluded studies
- Draft CPG developed by clinical governance group
  - Forward to relevant medical advisory panel member(s) for comment
  - Draft CPG posted for wider comment
- Final CPG developed by clinical governance group
- Medical director endorsement
- Revised/new CPG incorporated in CPGs
  - Dates, including next review recorded
- Implementation/training organized as required

It would be useful to have a project officer trained in these areas to assist where available.

STAFF FORUMS

Input from on-the-road and other staff is important for inclusion, ownership, and to provide a mechanism whereby the "end users" can provide direct input into their own practices.

Input can be achieved in a number of ways. Direct contact can be made with on-road senior staff or members of the clinical governance group (see below) or the medical director.

Staff forums are useful mechanisms to present, discuss, debate, and suggest changes to various practices. These may be conducted as formal or informal events but are most productive with a clearly defined structure for the process. Many services find a debate style most useful, with a number of senior clinicians presenting arguments for and against a particular practice. The evidence can be discussed in this fashion and the final decision determined shortly after the event and communicated back to staff.

Alternative methods of gaining wider staff input include "questions on notice" and open discussion forums, each of which can also be adapted to electronic formats such as notice boards and blogs.

A variety of in-person and electronic modes for staff input maximize staff engagement. Timely feedback of the discussion points and outcomes decided from meetings is important to encourage further input.

MEDICAL ADVISORY PANEL

Engagement of the local medical community is essential. The creation of a medical advisory panel is the most common method to facilitate this. Representation is from the various clinical specialties most relevant to EMS practice—emergency medicine, trauma, cardiology, neurology, pediatrics, obstetrics, and retrieval specialists will cover the vast majority of cases. Others can be consulted as required.

The engagement with local medical experts is a two-way process. Most hospital-based practitioners are not familiar with the prehospital environment and will assume hospital and prehospital practices are the same and therefore expect the same outcomes for practices in the two different environments provided by different practitioners. However, there is considerable research to indicate this is not the case. By engagement of the various specialty groups via the medical advisory panel, EMS providers can benefit from the specialty knowledge of those practitioners and the hospital-based practitioners can gain a greater understanding of prehospital practice and outcomes.

Members of the medical advisory panel assist in the development and revision of CPGs and may assist in investigation of incidents and complaints in their areas of expertise. As experts in their fields, members of the medical advisory panel will be aware of the latest practice developments and may suggest EMS practice changes in advance of this information's becoming available via other sources. Maximum currency in practice is therefore obtained.

The medical director is the chair of the medical advisory panel and ensures that liaison with the members is a continuous process.

TRAINING

Training is essential to ensure that all staff are provided with the skills necessary to perform the role for which they are employed. Once skills have been learned, they must then be practiced on a regular basis in order to maintain proficiency. As a rough guide, a skill must be completed successfully more than 20 times before proficiency reaches 85%, and the skill must be repeated at least every 6 months to maintain that proficiency.

For many skills, practices and courses have been established to teach and assess these skills, for example, BLS, ACLS, and ATLS. Other skills and procedures may be less commonly used and/or require specific circumstances that make observation of the skill in clinical practice impractical for educational purposes, such as surgical airway intervention. In these circumstances, training manikins or simulation provides an alternate learning platform.

Training may be provided internally within the service or by external agencies. Regardless of how the training is obtained, the medical director is responsible for ensuring that processes are in place to confirm that the standards required for practice are met by

EMS personnel prior to commencement of employment and at regular intervals thereafter.

Regular training updates can be achieved in a variety of ways. Modular learning including eLearning minimizes direct contact time, provides staff with flexible learning opportunities, and ensures consistency of information provided. Alternatively the training can be provided by appropriately skilled staff either in the field individually or in small groups or in a classroom-type setting. Regardless of the process employed for teaching the particular skill, a formative assessment is required to confirm that the skill has been learned correctly and this assessment must be in person.

A combination of in-field and block teaching in classroom-type settings enables new skills to be introduced more rapidly to all staff while also providing a forum where staff can also give feedback via the instructors on the various aspects of the teaching or, indeed, any other aspect of the service. An example of this was the change in International Liaison Committee on Resuscitation (ILCOR) recommendations regarding CPR. Following release of the revised guidelines in 2005, most EMS agencies modified their practice to align with the new guidelines. Initial information was circulated widely in the medical literature and internally within most EMS groups. Individual skills improvement was then achieved via classroom-type teaching for new staff and for scheduled refresher training, modular learning with self-directed learning followed by practical assessments, individual in-field training by senior personnel, or combinations of these activities. In small- to moderate-sized services, this process can be accomplished in 3 to 6 months. For larger services, 12 months may be required to complete the introduction of a new protocol of this type.

CLINICAL GOVERNANCE

Clinical governance is a framework or process by which EMS providers examine, review, and refine clinical practice. The intention is to ensure clinical practice is enshrined in the process of continuous quality improvement.

The medical director is responsible for ensuring the clinical governance structure is robust and maintaining the service quality and medical policy direction that has been established. Depending on the size of the service, the various components of clinical governance may be delegated to clinical managers and/or senior operational staff.

It is also important that all staff are aware of and have input into the service's clinical governance process. Ultimately, every individual who is part of the organization shares the outcome of the service provided to patients and should therefore be actively engaged in the processes that ensure that high quality and safe care are maintained.

Process

In order to maintain high-quality care, the components of service delivery must be assessed and monitored. This includes setting the standards, ensuring adherence to practice, and analyzing clinical outcomes to determine if the overall practice is achieving the intended targets. The persons responsible for each of these components must be clearly identified, and the results of the process readily available for review by all concerned. By this process, engagement of all stakeholders is achieved in an open and transparent way.

The key components of a clinical governance structure are

- Education/awareness of all staff of the process.
- Clearly defined reporting structures.
- Mechanisms to provide input from internal and external sources.
- Regular review of quality indicators.
- Structured audit processes.
- Complaint/incident/issue management processes.
- Timely resolution of identified risks/performance issues.

Structure

Clinical governance may be solely the responsibility of the medical director. However, in larger services, a number of the facets will be delegated to senior EMS personnel and/or a manager of clinical governance. Where a number of individuals are involved, a clinical governance group will be formed. The medical director determines the activity that will be undertaken by the members of the group. The group may then collectively manage the various tasks involved, reporting to the medical director at regular intervals as determined by the individual service. The medical director in turn reports to the CEO. In some services, senior EMS personnel lead the majority of the clinical governance activity with guidance and assistance, not direct line management, from the medical director.

Input from internal and external sources is vital for effective practice. This is achieved by the same processes as outlined in CPG review. Important sources of information guiding change are quality indicators, audit results, complaints, incidents, and expert review (formal or informal).

Activity

The clinical governance process includes collecting information on clinical practices employed, their frequency, compliance with CPGs, and complications and outcomes including adverse events. Further information is obtained from audits and reviews, quality indicators, incidents, complaints, and other sources of input from external sources.

The clinical governance group, led by the medical director, analyzes the information available from these various sources and decides if and how practice improvements may be made. Where necessary these include revision of the relevant CPGs. (Refer to Figure 11-1).

CLINICAL INDICATORS

Quality indicators are utilized in all modern businesses. EMS quality indicators should be developed to reflect the desired outcomes from the perspective of providers (clinicians), purchasers (funding agencies), or consumers (patients).

To be effective indicators, the parameter chosen should be easily measured, consistent in outcome, reflect EMS practice, and not be influenced by practices from other providers, including in-hospital practices. Very few indicators in use fulfill these criteria, and hence caution should be taken when examining the result of indicators that are influenced by factors external to EMS practices.

Indicators reflecting efficiency of resource use include number of vehicles operational at a given time, percentage of time crews are actively engaged (standby capacity), and response times. Although of interest to the medical director, these indicators are typically managed by the operational director. There will always be some overlap of operational and clinical indicators. An example is reattendance within 24 or 48 hours. Services that monitor and investigate these cases often find incidents where clinical practices can be improved.

Indicators reflecting EMS practices and patient outcomes are generally classified as clinical indicators, although this term is more applicable to those indicators that directly or indirectly reflect actual patient outcomes.

Indicators reflecting provider issues include performance of technical procedures such as advanced airway interventions or various other ALS procedures. The success rate of these procedures can then be compared to established standards to determine if skills are being maintained at the appropriate level. These

Table 11–3	Quality Indicators
Operational	Vehicles available
	Stand-by capacity
	Response times
	Complaints (rate/resolution)
	Satisfaction surveys
	Compliance with CPGs
	Reattendances
Clinical	Survival from cardiac arrest
	Survival from major trauma
	ASA administration in ischemic chest pain
	Scene time for major trauma
	Scene time for ischemic chest pain

ASA = Aspirin or acetylsalicylic acid; CPG = clinical practice guidelines.

indicators reflect training and continuous practice improvement and are therefore important to monitor. However, their relevance to patient outcomes is not always clear.

The indicators of most relevance to EMS medical directors are listed in Table 11-3. Further information on clinical indicators and other aspects of clinical quality assurance can be found in **Chapter 16, EMS Quality Improvement Programs.**

COMPLAINTS/INCIDENTS

A mature management system includes the ability to proactively identify areas of practice deficiency and areas where practice can be improved. In addition to the information obtained from quality assurance practices, complaints and adverse incidents are valuable sources of information that can help guide EMS practice. Investigation of complaints and analysis of adverse incidences in a systematic fashion, particularly over long periods of time, enable early detection of areas where practice can be improved.

The medical director is ultimately responsible for the management of complaints and incidents that involve clinical practice. However, complaints and incidents regarding operational issues often have clinical components. As such, both operational and medical directors are usually involved in management of all complaints and adverse incidents. Some, or all, of this role may be delegated to senior clinical personnel or other staff, depending on the particular structure of the EMS.

Complaints

Complaints indicate an unsatisfactory interaction between client (patient or accompanying person) and provider. Complaints most commonly arise out of adverse personal interaction but can also arise from deficiencies in patient care secondary to deficiencies in practice guidelines or incorrect application of or adherence to these guidelines. Complaints are therefore a valuable tool to provide direction for reviewing guidelines, compliance, interpersonal skills, and attitude.

Even when no error can be found in practice, a complaint indicates expectations have not been met and further interaction will be required with the complainant to determine why this is the case (Table 11-4).

All complaints must be followed up as quickly as possible. The complainant needs acknowledgment that the complaint has been received, especially if provided indirectly and not in person or verbally via telephone. This acknowledgment should include an indication of the likely timeframe for investigation to be undertaken and when feedback will occur. Acknowledgment of complaint should occur within 48 hours of receipt and most uncomplicated cases should be resolved within a month.

All customer complaints must be recorded, preferably in a log that tracks progress and flags unresolved cases. Complaints can also be generated by staff and are managed by the same process.

Table 11–4	Complaint Management
I Minor: no practice or clinical deficiencies	Manager clinical governance (Delegated officer)
II Moderate: some deficiencies in practice or clinical management	Manager clinical governance Delegated officer (Medical/operational director)
III Severe: major practice deficiencies and/or adverse outcome	Manager clinical governance Delegated officer Medical/operational director (CEO)
IV Sentinel event	Root cause analysis investigation

CEO = chief executive officer.

Complaints can be classified as minor, moderate, and severe. These will be addressed below.

Incident Reporting

A variety of incident reporting systems are used around the world in hospital, prehospital, and other areas of practice. The airline industry in particular has demonstrated major benefits from this process over decades.

It is recognized that prehospital practice is relatively unpredictable for individual practitioners and occurs in a less controlled environment with less staff available compared with hospital practice; it is therefore inherently prone to significant risk of adverse events.

The purpose of incident reporting systems is to collect information over time for a large number of adverse events or situations recognized as having a high risk of adverse outcomes ("near misses"). Greater amounts of information can be obtained in a shorter time frame when multiple providers use the same database. Information can be reported anonymously to increase reporting. Collated data can identify high-risk situations and the various factors contributing to them with a higher degree of reliability than evaluation of isolated incidents. Once risk factors are identified, the intention of incident reporting systems is to facilitate processes that mitigate those risk factors and therefore avoid or at least reduce future incidences.

Serious Adverse Events (SAEs) and Sentinel Events

More significant adverse outcomes can be classified as SAEs or sentinel events.

Sentinel events are predefined events that mandate immediate and high-level investigation. These events and the processes to follow are usually clearly defined within the incident-monitoring framework. Examples of sentinel events include unexpected patient deaths or permanent incapacitation as a result of incorrect procedure or medication error.

SAEs are defined as the following:

- Any medication error leading to harm of the patient.
- Any unexpected injury sustained by the patient during EMS care.
- Any action or omission during the delivery of prehospital care adversely compromising the patient's condition or causing death.
- Any staff injury associated with delivery of medical care.

Complaint/Incident Investigation

All complaints and incidents are logged in a register and the complaint acknowledged. The clinical governance manager (or medical director) rapidly assesses each complaint or incident and determines:

- If the issue is clinical, operational, or both.
- The level of severity (see below).

Level I-Minor: No Practice or Clinical Deficiencies

Minor incidents when no practice deficiency or adverse clinical event is identified are dealt with either by the manager of clinical governance or a delegated senior clinical officer.

In most cases, the matter is resolved by direct discussion with the complainant, and this is confirmed in writing. The medical and/or operational director reviews the updated log at regular intervals to ensure resolution of complaints and incidents.

Where further action is required, a level II response is commenced.

Level II-Moderate: Some Deficiencies in Practice or Clinical Management

After initial assessment by the manager of clinical governance, the medical and/or operational director is briefed and a senior clinical officer is delegated to commence an investigation. Typically, initial steps will involve reviewing the Patient Care Report or Patient Clinical Record (PCR) and interviewing staff concerned.

After collating the initial information, the delegated officer prepares a report for the manager of clinical governance. The report and other factors are reviewed by the clinical governance group and recommendations made to address identified deficiencies and avoid or minimize future occurrences.

Feedback to the complainant is provided by the investigating officer, the manager of clinical governance, or relevant director, depending on the individual circumstances. This is confirmed in writing and noted on the log.

Where corrective actions are undertaken, these are implemented and then reviewed after an appropriate interval (usually 3 months) to ensure the intended effect was achieved.

Level III-Severe: Major Practice Deficiencies and/or Adverse Outcome

Level III incidents are managed along the same principles as level II incidents with the inclusion of a briefing

for the CEO. Feedback to the complainant is more appropriate from the manager or director level.

Level IV-Sentinel Event

Sentinel events are investigated along predetermined processes and may have additional statutory reporting requirements that must be followed. Typically this will include a root cause analysis (RCA) investigation. Inclusion of external experts, representation from governing bodies, and consumer representation may individually, or all, be included in this process. In an RCA investigation, the incident is analyzed in detail to determine the precise issues that predisposed and precipitated the event. The presence or absence of risk mitigation strategies is evaluated, and recommendations are made on causality and methods to reduce further incidents.

The outcomes and recommendations of the RCA are communicated back to the complainant and implemented and routinely reviewed after an appropriate interval (usually 3 months) to ensure implementation is complete and the intended effect has been achieved.

EFFECTING CHANGES TO PRACTICE

Information collected from the various audits, investigations, and reviews should be collated for analysis by the clinical governance group to identify trends where practice review is required. Where a deficiency is identified in the CPGs or the performance of skills, recommendations are made to the medical and/or operational director so that corrective action can be undertaken. This may involve changes in training, CPGs, or some other areas.

Where the changes required involve a specific individual, directed training and/or provision of a clinical mentor are typically all that is required to effect change. For system issues such as an identified need to change a CPG, more detailed action is required.

In keeping with the quality assurance cycle described in **Chapter 16, EMS Quality Improvement Programs**, re-evaluation is important at an interval after a change has occurred to ensure the intended change has been effected, the underlying issue has been adequately addressed, and no other issues have arisen as a result of the change.

For the review process outlined in Figure 11-2 to be most effective, active engagement of clinical personnel is needed so that change is supported. Most clinicians support change once the positive benefits are apparent. It is therefore vital that the medical director

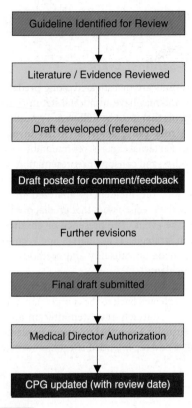

Guideline Identified for Review

↓

Literature / Evidence Reviewed

↓

Draft developed (referenced)

↓

Draft posted for comment/feedback

↓

Further revisions

↓

Final draft submitted

↓

Medical Director Authorization

↓

CPG updated (with review date)

FIGURE 11–2

Clinical practice guideline update process.

and/or other personnel involved in clinical management ensure the positive outcomes of change, and that clinical audits are communicated to on-road staff directly and on a regular basis.

Media and Other Relationships

From time to time, clinical issues will become topics for media discussion and/or legal proceedings. In these circumstances, the medical director is usually the spokesperson for the service regarding medical practices in general and any issues regarding practice guidelines specifically. A well-established relationship with local medical experts via the medical advisory panel will be of great support during these times.

For issues relating to outcomes of clinical practice, the results of audits, reviews, and research within the organization will be of significant assistance for clarification of specific details.

SUMMARY

Medical leadership and direction are vital to the successful function of an EMS. This can be accompanied by an individual or a panel of experts, depending on the organizational size and structure. The most common model throughout the world is a single medical director working part time in an EMS in an advisory capacity while engaged clinically in hospital practice in an acute care area.

The medical director provides delegated medical authority for nonphysicians to administer medications and perform procedures that would normally require authority for independent practice. This is usually achieved with proscriptive guidelines/protocols that are regularly reviewed and modified in response to new evidence and information derived from quality assurance, complaints, and incident investigations conducted at the direction of or with the assistance of the medical director.

In addition to determining and authorizing medical practices within the EMS, the medical director is the usual spokesperson for the media and other external purposes.

Web Resources

EMS Clinical Practice Guidelines Online
Australia
Ambulance Victoria http://www.ambulance.vic.gov.au/Paramedics/Qualified-Paramedic-Training/Clinical-Practice-Guidelines.html.

England
Joint Royal Colleges Ambulance Committee: UK Ambulance Service Clinical Practice Guidelines (2006) http://www2.warwick.ac.uk/fac/med/research/hsri/emergencycare/prehospitalcare/jrcalcstakeholderwebsite/guidelines/.

New Zealand
Wellington Free Ambulance: http://www.wellingtonfreeambulance.org.nz/ClinicalPractices.htm.

Ireland
The Pre-Hospital Emergency Care Council (PHECC) 2009 http://www.phecit.ie/Documents/Clinical%20Practice%20Guidelines/EMT%203rd%20Edition%20CPGs/EMT%20Introduction.pdf.

CHAPTER 12

Training Programs and Standardized Curricula

Tim Rainer, Colin Graham, Giles Cattermole

KEY POINTS SUMMARY

- A global EMS curriculum must include graded, detailed contents and standards that may be applied to different contexts, depending upon their resources, aims, and stages of EMS development.

- A global EMS curriculum will help those who plan to develop an EMS program. It will provide guidance on the important curriculum principles that need to be addressed.

- A global EMS curriculum will provide a standard against which EMS systems can evaluate their past, present, and future development.

- A standardized global EMS curriculum will ensure that a newly developed EMS program is robust and meets professional standards.

- Ultimately a standardized EMS program and curriculum are likely to improve patient care.

SETTING THE SCENE

You have been involved in leading the development of emergency medical services (EMS) in your country. Your leaders have asked you to extensively evaluate the current state of your EMS with a view to moving the whole process "to a higher level." You are not entirely sure of how your current EMS compares with those in other countries. You use the same words but know that in this big world, there are many different contexts and countries and these words may have very different meanings. Some sort of training is essential. Resources and equipment are essential. Some sort of training program is necessary. How can you assess the current level of your EMS? Is there an international standard against which you can benchmark your service? If you are to introduce or develop your training program, what should you do next? What are the next steps? What training and resources are needed? How much time do others give to training in order to reach a certain level of competency and provision of care?

This chapter will aid anyone who is looking to evaluate the past, present, and future of their EMS against a global standard. It will outline training programs that could form the basis of basic, interme-diate, and advanced levels of practice for EMS and emergency medical technicians (EMTs) globally. The basis of all teaching programs is the curriculum, which should not only describe the topics to be learned in detail but should also describe the manner in which they will be learned and the resources required to sup-port those learning activities.

We will present standardized curricula that may be applied internationally to different levels of EMS. Ultimately though, the exact teaching delivered will depend on the needs of the local community, the clini-cal and logistic resources available to them, and the cur-rent level of skills of any EMS personnel and students.

CHALLENGES

Across the globe, there are variations in language, culture, religion, resources, priorities, health care training, and expectations. Although the terms "basic," "intermediate," and "advanced" are somewhat subjec-tive, it is important to provide and appropriately apply some form of unified terminology. It will then be pos-sible to operate and evaluate within a defined frame-work of standardized skills and levels of clinical care. The terms basic, intermediate, and advanced are not intended to imply differential quality but rather a cer-tain standard of care based on available resources and training. The aim is to provide the highest possible quality of care at all times irrespective of whether it is at the basic, intermediate, or advanced level.

The primary purpose of the chapter is to lay out broad general principles, but there will always be "spe-cial populations" and "special circumstances" that will need to be addressed. Before embarking on a new pro-gram, it will be important to conduct a needs analysis, paying particular attention to general and special cir-cumstances. Some regions will be faced with the spe-cial challenges of AIDS, emerging infectious diseases, war and terrorism, limited infrastructure, or different languages, making communication difficult. In an area with many children or in areas where there are many schools, it may be necessary to have a curriculum and training program that emphasizes pediatric care and pediatric multi-casualty incidents. In areas where peo-ple gravitate to for retirement, there may be a need for geriatric programs, with emphasis on elderly care and nursing homes. Areas that are popular for tourists need different planning, as there will be language bar-riers to the provision of emergency health care. Those countries that are close to areas prone to natural disas-ters (China, Turkey, and Indonesia, for example) will also need special planning and preparation.

DEFINITIONS

It is important to understand the difference between a syllabus and a curriculum if a standardized training program is to be set up.

- What is a training program?
- What is a standardized curriculum?
- How do these differ from a syllabus?

The term **training** refers to the delivery by a teacher and the acquisition by a student of the knowl-edge, skills, and competencies relevant to a particular discipline. As a result of the teaching of specific practi-cal skills and knowledge, the student should become competent in certain areas. People within many pro-fessions and occupations refer to this sort of training as professional development.

Knowledge for the purpose of this chapter con-sists of the theory, facts, and information relevant to a specific discipline such as prehospital care. It is the theoretical aspect of the subject. **Skills** are the practi-cal abilities acquired by a person through experience or education. It is the practical understanding of a sub-ject in which there is a very strong emphasis on expe-riential learning. **Competency** is achieved when an individual can perform a specific task with the appro-priate knowledge and skills to a specified minimum verifiable standard. This includes an appropriate com-bination of knowledge, skills, and behavior for that task to be completely performed safely.

A **syllabus** is a general outline, list, or summary of topics to be covered in an education or training course. It describes the general content and quality of a course and will guide assessment and examination. Syllabi are used to ensure consistency among educa-tional institutions so that all teachers and assessors know what should and what should not be taught. Examinations should only contain assessments that are based on information included in the syllabus.

A **curriculum** (derived from the Latin word for race course) is a specific, precise, and detailed sum-mary of the actions and experiences in a course through which students grow to competence and maturity. A curriculum should set out the intended aims and objectives, content, experiences, outcomes, and processes of the educational program. In the con-text of this chapter, the curriculum should provide healthcare professionals with the skills, knowledge, and competence to provide state-of-the-art EMS.

The curriculum should be laid out logically and sequentially to meet international standards. A cur-riculum should be visionary, forward-looking, aspira-tional, and inspirational and should be centered on

EMS as the principal learning environment for students. The curriculum should direct and integrate the development of a training program.

For the purpose of this chapter it is not possible to lay out a full curriculum for reasons of space. However, we list a reasonably comprehensive syllabus and give an example of part of a curriculum.

A training program is a well-organized, practical summary of what will be taught, where, and when. It will closely match and reflect the curriculum.

A STANDARDIZED TRAINING PROGRAM

Elements of a Training Program

Outline training programs can be defined and implemented for each level of EMT training. The application of these training programs must be adapted to local circumstances. In particular, an assessment should be made of the needs of the community to be served, and training should be aimed at an appropriate level. For example, a rural Asian community 30 miles from the nearest basic medical facility might be best served by emergency care providers trained to recognize acutely ill patients, perform basic hemorrhage control, and identify obstetric patients with obstructed labor and postpartum bleeding and sepsis. It would be inappropriate to train care providers in oxygen therapy, defibrillation, and advanced airway care in this setting. However, in a high-income country with a highly developed healthcare system, such as Australia, this may be an entirely appropriate step.

A further part of this assessment must be the resources available to train the health care providers: training must be in keeping with the resources available in day-to-day practice, as lack of ongoing experience will rapidly lead to loss of skills and the need for retraining in that skill.

How are we to differentiate between basic, intermediate, and advanced? These terms apply primarily to certification at the end of the program and not to entry criteria into the program. This could be done based on duration of training, range of competency, and educational level attained or certification achieved. A suggested classification for entry into an EMS program taking into account competency, graduate level, and time is shown in Table 12-1.

Programs will lie in a spectrum from the least resourced to the most resourced contexts in the world. Depending upon resources and depth of training, practitioners may be classified into

1. Very Basic.
2. Basic.
3. Intermediate.
4. Advanced.
5. Very Advanced.

Very Basic implies the provision of emergency care in very limited resource areas at a level less than an emergency medical assistant (EMA I). Basic, intermediate, and advanced levels loosely match EMA I (non-paramedic), II (partial paramedic), and III (full paramedic) status. In some areas in the world, a full paramedic certification is an undergraduate qualification (e.g., the US), while in others it is a graduate qualification (e.g., Australia). Very Advanced is a term used for doctors or highly trained nonphysicians trained to specialist levels and working in the field of prehospital care (for example Germany, France, or China). Although these classifications are hard to apply rigidly, as there will always be some overlap in skills and training, a classification of this nature allows some uniform understanding of different systems.

There is debate as to whether competency or duration of training should drive the service. For example, one individual may achieve full competency in six months while another may take two years. Although competency is the primary goal, experience is also very

Table 12–1	An IFEM Global Classification of EMS Training and Curriculum				
	A	**B**	**C**	**D**	**E**
	Very Basic	**Basic**	**Intermediate**	**Advanced**	**Very Advanced (Medical)**
EMA equivalent	Pre-EMA	EMA I	EMA II	EMA III	EMA – M
Training hours	<300	300–1,000	1,000–3,000	3,000–5,000	>5,000
Level of Education	Primary	Primary	Secondary	Ug or Pg	Pg

EMA = Emergency medical assistant; Ug/Pg = undergraduate/postgraduate.

valuable and that can only come with time on the job. Also some programs may be full time and others part time, and the time requirements must recognize that fact.

Very Basic to Basic Levels of Care

Basic training programs should emphasize the priorities for emergency health care in that community. For most western countries and many developing countries, this will mean an emphasis on the immediate management of cardiovascular disease and trauma. A traditional approach to emergency care should be adopted in these regions, with an emphasis on airway care, breathing assessment and care, and circulation care, including advisory defibrillation where this is available and appropriate. Basic trauma care including external hemorrhage control and knowledge of local trauma resources (to allow trauma bypass to trauma centers) should be taught in all areas where transport is available and where trauma is common.

In many impoverished countries, including the majority of those in Africa and Asia, the priorities will be different. Training should focus on the main lethal medical problems in the community, and due consideration should be given to local culture and values. In many countries, the priority will be effective obstetric care and the establishment of basic referral pathways to ensure that women in labor and those with postpartum bleeding or sepsis can reach appropriate timely care. Early recognition of patients who are bleeding may improve outcome, as will improved transport facilities and referral options. Trauma is also increasing in these countries and basic trauma care, including hemorrhage control, can make a major difference to patient outcome.

Medical diseases such as tuberculosis, HIV infection, malaria, and childhood pneumonia may be the major medical burden in poor countries, and the challenge is to teach care providers to recognize the signs of severe medical disease before patients have deteriorated beyond salvage. Again, the major determinant of whether or not to train care providers in the general or specific recognition of these medical disorders will depend on the resources available to make a diagnosis and treat patients; there is little point in transporting a child with pneumonia far away from home to a hospital that has no antibiotics available. Basic care should consist of recognition of severe illness and rapid transport to an appropriate facility where possible. Oxygen therapy, while desirable, is unlikely to be available and therefore should not be taught to care providers.

Basic to Intermediate Levels of Care

Intermediate levels of training could usefully extend the basic training already described. For developed countries, the emphasis on cardiovascular disease and trauma could be extended to include the identification of acute stroke and care of diabetic emergencies such as hypoglycemia. The emphasis on airway care, breathing assessment and care, and circulation should continue, with advisory external defibrillation being more universally available. Trauma care can be extended to include spinal immobilization and oxygen therapy, and the emphasis again should be on knowledge of local trauma resources (to allow trauma patients to be bypassed to appropriate centers).

The priorities in Africa and Asia remain different. Training should focus on the main lethal medical problems in the community, and due consideration should be given to local culture and values. Effective obstetric care should be a priority and basic referral pathways to ensure that women in labor and those with postpartum bleeding or sepsis can reach appropriate timely care are mandatory. Clearly this relies on the availability of midwives and obstetricians or at least physicians and surgeons who are capable of emergency obstetric care. Early recognition of patients who are bleeding may improve outcome as long as that can be accompanied by rapid transport facilities to definitive care. Trauma care could also be increased to include basic airway management incorporating cervical spine control. Recognition and management of hemorrhage remain a priority.

Basic care of medical diseases should continue to emphasize the recognition of severe illness and rapid transport to a medical facility. Oxygen therapy is desirable and should be taught to care providers whenever it is available. Few other interventions have been demonstrated to make any difference in this setting and therefore little else should be taught.

Advanced to Very Advanced Levels of Care

Advanced training should extend beyond the intermediate level toward that expected of a full paramedic or a physician trained in prehospital care. It will involve greater depth, breadth, and quantity of training, often at the postgraduate level, and generally in resource-rich contexts. For developed countries, the emphasis on cardiovascular disease and trauma could be extended to include the identification and triage of acute stroke to specialist centers. The emphasis on airway care, breathing assessment and care, and circulation care should continue and be extended. Tracheal intubation and supraglottic airway device care can be introduced, and very advanced care could include prehospital drug-assisted airway care. Trauma care can be extended to include fluid resuscitation, chest decompression, pelvic binders, and specialist trauma triage and diversion to trauma centers.

Advanced care of medical diseases should emphasize the recognition and treatment of severe illness, including advanced care and triage of acute coronary syndrome, and where appropriate, prehospital thrombolysis. Rapid triage and transport of myocardial infarction patients to a facility capable of primary coronary angioplasty is desirable. Fluid resuscitation and the administration of selected drugs, including antibiotics for sepsis, should be considered at this level of care.

A Training Program for EMS Personnel

A training program for EMS should build on the existing foundation and experience of healthcare workers who already work in prehospital care. It should be generally understood by all and be relevant for medical doctors, ambulance personnel, nurses, police, fire service personnel, or other relevant voluntary agencies such as the St. John Ambulance, the Red Cross, and the military. It should also include aspects of communication, command, control, driving skills and other forms of transport, physical fitness, administration, ethics, teamwork, and leadership.

General Background and Description

It is important to understand why a course of instruction is needed and why it should be introduced into a community or country. Why do we need a training program in EMS? There is no community in the world that does not face medical emergencies and crises. EMS systems improve the delivery of emergency care, and the provision of high-quality coordinated, integrated emergency care in the community is a global challenge. The speed of response and quality of decision-making have been shown to affect outcomes. There is heterogeneity in the professional groups that provides emergency care, and there is no universally accepted common pool of knowledge. Care is enhanced when agencies work together to provide emergency care for the community, and globally when only a small number of care providers are university or college graduates.

An EMS training program can harness and enhance the enthusiasm and existing skills of healthcare providers to improve standards that benefit the community by improving the quality of care delivered

in the prehospital phase and the emergency department (ED).

Every training program should have a core set of values that may include:

- excellence in prehospital care
- patient-centered care
- professional approach to practice
- promotion of integrity, honesty, and academic rigor
- communication, teamwork, leadership, transport and driving skills
- promotion of a cohesive, integrated healthcare system.

Each of these values needs definition. For example, what does "professional" mean in the context of health care and particularly EMS? A detailed discussion of these concepts is beyond the scope of this book.

Objectives of a Training Program

The objectives of the training program are to improve the emergency care delivered to patients in the prehospital environment by enhancing the professional knowledge and skills of a group with interest in the field in order to help them become expert practitioners.

Each program should have clear general and specific objectives (Box 12-1).

Admission Requirements

It is important to decide what level of education is appropriate for each course, whether it is degree-based

BOX 12–1	Example of Course Objectives

On completion of this training course, EMS students should:

- Understand the scientific basis for common emergency problems
- Be able to assess common emergency problems in the prehospital environment
- Be able to manage common emergency problems in the prehospital environment
- Understand the importance of communication and coordination among the various service providing prehospital emergency care to the public
- Understand the principles of command and control for the emergency services and their importance during the management of mass casualty incidents

or not, the medium and language of teaching, or what level of experience is required.

Assessment

The training program should include a variety of methods of assessment that confirm that the student is competent across a broad and balanced range of the curriculum. They may include multiple choice questions (MCQs), objective structured clinical examinations (OSCEs), and clinical data interpretation. The assessment may involve a logbook or portfolio to facilitate reflective practice development. Practical clinical assessments are particularly important to ensure that clinical skills have been mastered to an adequate degree.

Supervision, Feedback, and Evaluation

All courses should have a clearly defined course director, preferably a tutor-student (mentoring) system and regular (for example, every 6 months) developmental appraisal meetings by trainers skilled in effective feedback. The purpose of the evaluation is to refine the learning materials and delivery, the appropriateness of content, the appropriateness of teaching style, the organization of the course, and how the course meets the needs of the healthcare community and the community it is serving.

Managing Curriculum Implementation

A course executive committee should conduct annual operational reviews that cover timing, venues, module/unit allocation, evaluations, communication processes, and faculty development requirements.

Curriculum Review and Updating

There should be a process of reviewing each course with records of when it was last reviewed and when next it should be reviewed (e.g., every 2 to 3 years). There should be an analysis of feedback, meetings with tutors, and also an external examiner assessment.

Program Organizers and Purpose

There should be a clear statement of who the program organizers are, their qualifications to direct this type of course, and the purpose of the course. Any bodies or organizations that approve, accredit, or endorse the course should be stated as well.

Program Structure and Duration

The training program should be clearly described, for example, part time or full time, modular courses, over two terms offered each year. The training program should ensure that everyone is competent in a full range of skills if they are to practice in the community. Therefore there should be no elective modules for a basic or intermediate course, but at advanced levels there may be scope for elective courses or some degree of selection, for example, in the performance of an operational audit or a research project. Students should undertake attachments to EDs, ambulance services, or other prehospital and emergency environments as arranged between the course directors and individual students, depending on the location and resources available to the organizers.

A STANDARDIZED CURRICULUM

The Curriculum

The curriculum will include a syllabus, or list of topics, such as is detailed in Appendix 12-1, but it will be far more than that. Each curriculum should have general and specific standards, as shown in Box 12-2.

General Curriculum Standards

Here are examples of general standards for a curriculum.

Standard 1: Rationale

The purpose of the curriculum is to describe the knowledge, skills, and expertise together with the

---

BOX 12–2   Essential Elements of a Curriculum

- A syllabus (i.e., a list of topics to be taught)
- General standards (i.e., relevant to most curricula but not specific to EMS)
- Special standards relevant to the work of EMS
- Context-specific standards relevant to EMS facing special circumstances
- Methods of teaching and learning
- Methods of formative and summative assessment
- Matching between the curriculum and the program (i.e., where in the program is a curriculum item to be taught?)
- Detailed objectives
- Categorization into areas of knowledge, skills, and attitudes

learning, teaching, feedback, and supervision that will be provided by an educational training program. In this context it is designed to provide safe, expert health care workers functioning as part of a team in a prehospital environment.

The curriculum should be developed and validated. For example, the content of the curriculum should been derived with the help of a specific academic body (e.g., International Federation for Emergency Medicine, [IFEM]), together with other expert comments. Expert advice should be sought from existing experts and ambulance personnel, as it is believed that the principles and practice will broadly apply throughout the globe.

The curriculum should have its foundation in the specialty of emergency medicine as practiced in the prehospital environment, and this should be reflected both in the generic and specific aspects of the curriculum. Throughout the curriculum, different stages of learning should be identified, e.g., basic, intermediate, and advanced levels of care.

Standard 2: Content of Learning

The content of learning should be clearly defined. Although many ambulance personnel may not have had a higher education in one of the professions, nevertheless a professional model may help to define the content or learning (see Box 12-3).

The curriculum sets out the general professional and specialist content to be mastered. The knowledge, skills, and expertise should be clearly and explicitly specified. The content of the curriculum is presented in a way that identifies what the health care professional will need to know about, understand, describe, and be able to do at the end of the educational program. For each of the content areas, there is a recommendation for the type of learning experiences.

Standard 3: Model of Learning

The training program, while building on the students' existing knowledge, skills, and attitudes, should allow opportunities for work-based experience, independent self-directed learning, and classroom-based teaching. The latter should include lectures, tutorials, and constructive feedback, and it should also allow time for discussion and reflection.

Wherever possible the curriculum should describe the appropriate model of learning, whether it is work-based experiential learning, independent self-directed learning, or appropriate off-the-job education. The method of learning for knowledge, competence, performance, and independent action needs to be specified.

BOX 12-3	Professional Model

Students should be able:

- to manage themselves
  - EMS personnel should be able to ask and answer questions, address personal safety, manage their time, have good communication skills, understand professional and ethical qualities, understand the different roles of leadership and teamwork.
- to manage patients
  - EMS personnel should have good clinical skills in safety and patient protection, general resuscitation skills, medical emergencies, traumatic emergencies, pediatric emergencies, obstetrics and gynecology, advanced prehospital care techniques, and triage.
- to manage their environment
  - students should have an understanding of safety, communication, transport, escort medicine, major incident and disaster management, heat and cold, hazardous materials, wilderness medicine, tactical medicine and management of terrorist incidents, violence, and threats; and aviation, diving, and altitude medicine.

Standard 4: Learning Experiences

Recommended learning experiences are specified. These are predominantly self-directed and work-based learning. The following methods will be used: learning from practice; learning from trainers either by working alongside or in specified one-to-one teaching; learning from formal situations such as group teaching within the department, and regional teaching programs. Focused personal study outside of contracted hours is essential. Educational strategies that are suitable for work-based experiential learning include the use of log books and personal audit.

Learning experiences can be summarized, simplified, or abbreviated as in Box 12-4.

Standard 5: Supervision and Feedback

The mechanisms for ensuring feedback on learning recommended and required are specified. These include one-to-one teaching, clinical evaluation exercises, multi-professional feedback appraisal, and mock clinical examinations.

The supervision of practice and the safety of healthcare professionals and patients is provided by means of direct supervision of students by course

BOX 12–4	Learning Experiences

- Learning from Practice
- Learning from Trainers
- Group Teaching (including lectures and tutorials)
- Personal Study
- Life Support Courses
- Skills Laboratory
- Emergency Department Training
- Out-of-Department Training in Ambulance
- Out-of-Department Training in Other Settings (e.g., ICU, anesthesia)

BOX 12–5	Assessment Options

Clinical
- Observed care
- Case-based discussion
- *Examination*
- Multiple choice questions
- Objective structured practical examination
- Clinical skills
- Slide assessment
- Written assignment
- Thesis

trainers, with a specialist always being available for advice, and by clinical governance mechanisms, including audit and risk management.

Standard 6: Managing Curriculum Implementation

It is intended that the curriculum identify the knowledge, skills, and expertise required of trainers and guide how they should deliver their training. It also identifies the means by which feedback should be given and assessment undertaken.

The curriculum should have an independent external expert to give feedback and appraisal of the course on a regular and ongoing basis. Alternatively, a national examination or system of professional registration allows for regular adherence to established standards of care or adherence to a stated curriculum for learning.

Standard 7: Curriculum Review and Updating

The executive committee is responsible for continuous review of the curriculum and receives feedback from external experts, national standards certifying bodies, trainers, and those specialists allocated segments of the curriculum.

Evaluation of the curriculum should be influenced by informal feedback from trainers and trainees and feedback from the executive committee.

The curriculum should be updated regularly (e.g., every two years).

Standard 8: Probity and Ethical Behavior

The curriculum should be in accord with local standards of professionalism, ethics, and personal integrity. Appropriate account should be taken of local laws and culture. Plagiarism should not be tolerated.

Standard 9: Assessment

The assessment methods must be clearly defined (see Box 12-5). They may be formative or summative and may be clinical and nonclinical. Formative assessment occurs when students are assessed and assess themselves while going through a course. Formative assessments help form the student's knowledge and skills. Success or failure does not usually contribute to final marks. Summative assessment is the final assessment at a given point in time, and it should be a reflection of the sum of all the training. Marks usually contribute to the final grade, typically a pass or fail. A combination of formative and summative assessments should be used.

Generic Skills Curriculum Contents

The important clinical skills are history and examination; documentation; diagnosis; decision-making; time management; safe prescribing; continuity of care; and therapeutic interventions.

The important communication skills are with colleagues; referrals; with patients and care-givers; in breaking bad news; and in exhibiting team work.

The important practice review and maintenance skills are life-long learning; audit and clinical outcomes; critical appraisal; information management; assessment and appraisal; and risk management.

The important professionalism issues are professional attributes and career and professional development.

The important ethics and legal issues are informed consent; patients without full capacity; "do-not-resuscitate" orders and advance directives;

Table 12–2	An Example of How EMS Curriculum Standards for Airway Management Could Be Adapted Across a Spectrum of Global Health-Care Situations				
	Pre-EMA	EMA I	EMA II	EMA III	EMA – M
Simple airway anatomy	E	E	E	E	E
Difficult airway anatomy and assessment	N	N	D	E	E
Basic airway care – the triple maneuver	E	E	E	E	E
Suction	D	E	E	E	E
Airway adjuncts	D	E	E	E	E
Oxygen	D	E	E	E	E
Endotracheal intubation without drugs	N	N	D	E	E
Endotracheal intubation with drugs	N	N	N	E	E
Laryngeal mask airway	N	N	D	E	E
Cricothyrotomy	N	N	N	D	E
Mouth-to-mouth ventilation	E	E	E	E	E
BVM ventilation	D	E	E	E	E
Mechanical ventilation	N	N	N	D	E
Universal airway algorithm	N	N	D	E	E
Crash airway algorithm	N	N	N	D	E
Difficult airway algorithm	N	N	D	E	E
Failed airway algorithm	N	N	N	D	E

BVM = Bag-Valve Mask, N, Not expected; D, Desirable; E, Expected.

withholding and withdrawing treatment; privacy and confidentiality; allocation of limited resources; and other medicolegal issues.

An EMS-Specific Syllabus

It should be recognized that the syllabus is a list of broad topics included in a teaching program and does not describe or relate the details of each skill and knowledge point to be taught or its method and place of assessment. Further, as programs range from the most limited to the highest of resource areas, it is necessary to map areas that are from the most simple and basic to the most complex and advanced. A syllabus can be part of a curriculum but a curriculum is not part of a syllabus. An example of an EMS-specific syllabus is shown in Appendix 12-1 at end of this chapter.

An EMS-Specific Curriculum

An EMS-specific curriculum will integrate aspects of the syllabus, objectives, teaching method, assessment, and modular position. An example of a portion of a curriculum for the History and Examination section of a core module is shown in Appendix 12-2 at the end of the chapter. A more comprehensive list of possible topics in a core module along with suggested hours of teaching taken from the Masters of Science in Pre-hospital and Emergency Care Course of the Chinese University of Hong Kong is shown in Appendix 12-3 at the end of the chapter.

An EMS-Specific Program

Programs will clearly vary depending upon the resources and intended competency level. An example of how EMS curriculum standards for airway management could be adapted across a spectrum of global healthcare situations is shown in Table 12-2. The time given to different aspects of teaching across a spectrum is shown in Table 12-3.

SUMMARY

In conclusion, an EMS curriculum needs to be differentiated from a syllabus. No single-sized EMS curriculum can fit all programs. However, there is a need for a standardized global framework against which programs can be compared, developed, and evaluated. This chapter is not intended to be didactic but illustrates many of the issues that need to be faced in developing and implementing EMS curricula.

Table 12–3	An Example of the Time for Teaching and Experience Expected in an EMS Program (Hours)				
	Pre-EMA	EMA I	EMA II	EMA III	EMA–M
Core Skills Module					
Introduction to prehospital and emergency care	½	½	½	½	½
BLS for babies	0	0	½	½	½
BLS for children	0	0	½	½	½
BLS for adults	½	½	½	½	½
Web access	0	0	0	2	2
Teamwork and leadership	0	1	1	1	1
Scene assessment and safety	½	½	½	1	1
General approach to the emergency patient	½	½	1	1	1
Command, control, and communication	0	1	1	1	1
Triage and transport	0	1	1	1	2
Airway assessment and management	½	2	4	6	8
Defibrillation and arrhythmias	0	1	3	5	6
Initial assessment and management of shock	½	1	2	3	4
Assessment and management of the unconscious patient	½	1	2	3	4
Pain assessment and management	½	1	1	1	2
Basic wound care	½	1	1	1	1
Assessment (MCQ)	0	½	1	1	1
Assessment (clinical slides)	0	0	½	½	½
Assessment (clinical examination)	½	½	½	½	½

MCQ = multiple choice questions.

Web Resources

1. National EMS Management Curriculum Committee, http://home.gwu.edu/~mikeward/FESHE_EMS.html.

References

1. Jackson WP. Conceptions of curriculum and curriculum specialists. In Jackson Philip W, ed. Handbook of Research on Curriculum: A Project of the American Educational Research Association, pp 3-40. New York: Macmillan Publishing Co., 1992.
2. Pinar WF, Reynolds WM, Slattery P, Taubman PM. Understanding Curriculum: An Introduction to the Study of Historical and Contemporary Curriculum Discourses. New York: Peter Lang, 1995.

An EMS-Specific Syllabus

These items cover the broad area of EMS. Some should be touched upon in all curricula, although the level of depth will vary among basic, intermediate, and advanced levels. Others may receive special emphasis relevant to local context. In general, the core skills should exist in all EMS curricula and training programs.

CORE SKILLS

Introduction to EMS systems and to the course
General learning for students
BLS
Basic airway management
Cardiac arrest/peri-arrest
Recognition and basic treatment of hemorrhage and shock
Recognition and basic treatment of pain
Recognition and basic treatment of coma
Recognition and basic treatment of wound care
Focused history, examination, and diagnosis
Triage
Multi-casualty incidents

MEDICAL EMERGENCIES

Respiratory emergencies
Cardiologic emergencies
Abdominal emergencies: undifferentiated abdominal pain
Abdominal emergencies: gastrointestinal hemorrhage
Neurologic emergencies, including stroke
Hepatic emergencies
Toxicologic emergencies
Diabetic and endocrinologic emergencies

Sepsis and severe sepsis
Infectious diseases
Dermatologic emergencies
Oncologic emergencies

TRAUMATIC EMERGENCIES

Integrated trauma care
Trauma airway care
Head injury
Chest trauma
Shock due to trauma
Pelvic injury
Abdominal trauma
Spinal injury
Limb injuries
Trauma in women
Trauma in the elderly
Burns
Thermal injury: burns and cold
Miscellaneous aspects of trauma care

PEDIATRIC EMERGENCIES

Introduction to pediatric anatomy and physiology
Principles and practice of managing the acutely ill child
Principles and practice of managing the acutely injured child

OBSTETRIC AND GYNECOLOGIC EMERGENCIES

Gynecologic emergencies
Obstetric emergencies
Neonatology

ADVANCED MANAGEMENT OF PREHOSPITAL SITUATIONS

Transport medicine
Major incident management
Disaster medicine
Advanced airway protection
Rescue in difficult circumstances
Tactical medicine and management of terrorist incidents
Aviation emergencies

ETHICAL AND LEGAL ASPECTS OF PREHOSPITAL AND EMERGENCY CARE

Legal aspects of emergency medicine
Ethical aspects of emergency medicine
Professionalism

RESEARCH METHODS AND STATISTICS

Research for prehospital and emergency care
Statistics for prehospital and emergency care

OTHERS

Administrative management
Training the trainers
Urologic emergencies
Ocular emergencies
ENT emergencies
Dental emergencies
Environmental emergencies
Psychiatric emergencies
Geriatric care

Example of History and Examination Section Taken from an EMS-Specific Curriculum

The general content of a curriculum falls into one of three parameters: knowledge, i.e., the candidate will know_____; skills, i.e., the candidate will be able to _____; and attitudes and values, i.e. the candidate will value/encourage/_____.

Detailed objectives are stated clearly and can be matched to course module, learning and teaching methods, and types of assessments. The detailed nature of this method, although cumbersome and sometimes tedious, ensures that the course teaches what it says it will teach.

The learning and teaching method for each objective is stated clearly. There are different methods of teaching that may be abbreviated as follows: BT – bedside teaching; GT – group teaching; LT – learning from teachers; OC – observed care; LP – learning from practice.

Each objective needs to be a clear definition not only of how it is to be taught but also of how it is to be assessed. There are different methods of assess-ment, and these may also be abbreviated as follows: for example, CS – Clinical Skills; SA – Slides Assessment; MCQ – Multiple Choice Questions.

Finally, the module in the program is stated so that it can be clearly shown where in the program this part of the curriculum is covered, for example, EMS-1 – Emergency Medical System Module 1.

The following example illustrates detailed but key aspects of a curriculum.

CLINICAL SKILLS: HISTORY AND EXAMINATION

Objectives

At the conclusion of this EMS course, the candidate should

1. Be able to take a focused history from patients in all emergency circumstances.
2. Be able to clinically examine patients and detect and interpret relevant clinical signs.

Parameter	Detailed Objectives	Learning Method	Assessment	Module
Knowledge	Know how to recognize critical symptoms and symptom patterns	BT	MCQ/CS/SA	EMS1
	Know the difference between open and closed questioning and when to utilize each type	GT	MCQ/CS/SA	EMS1
	Know some of the cultural and language differences in the description of common symptoms	GT	MCQ/CS/SA	EMS1
	Know and be familiar with methods to elicit accurate histories	GT/BT	MCQ/CS/SA	EMS1
	Know how to recognize the relevance of clinical signs in a given clinical situation	GT/BT	MCQ/CS/SA	EMS1
	Know some of the considerable health inequalities that exist between different groups	GT	MCQ/CS/SA	EMS1
Skills	Be able to incorporate clinical, social, and psychological factors in the history	OC	MCQ/CS/SA	EMS1
	Be able to elicit a relevant, focused history and identify and synthesize problems	GT	MCQ/CS/SA	EMS1
	Be able to take a history in difficult circumstances, (e.g., busy, noisy department with competing demands, patients who are often abusive, aggressive, confused, or unable to co-operate)	BT	MCQ/CS/SA	EMS1
	Be able to apply knowledge of symptoms to determine the likely differential diagnosis	GT BT	MCQ/CS/SA	EMS1
	Be able to take a history from a third party	GT/BT/ LP	MCQ/CS/SA	EMS1
	Be able to examine a patient while maintaining his or her dignity and privacy	LP LT	MCQ/CS/SA	EMS1
	Be able to elicit clinical signs effectively	GT LP BT	MCQ/CS/SA	EMS1
Attitudes	Value and appreciate the diversity of cultural backgrounds	LP	MCQ/CS/SA	EMS1
	Encourage the difficult historian and actively encourage and explore alternative ways of communicating	LP	MCQ/CS/SA	EMS1
	Appreciate the importance of time and attention to detail in talking to patients	LP	MCQ/CS/SA	EMS1
	Be prepared to allow the patient to take his or her time	LP	MCQ/CS/SA	EMS1
	Be effective in eliciting facts while being empathic in approach	LP	MCQ/CS/SA	EMS1

BT = Bedside Teaching; CS = Clinical Skills; GT = Group Teaching; LP = Learning from Practice; LT = Learning from Teachers; MCQ = Multiple Choice Questions; OC = Observed Care; SA = Slides Assessment; EMS1 = Emergency Medical System Module 1.

Example of Core Module Taken from Chinese University of Hong Kong Masters of Science for Prehospital and Emergency Care*

CORE SKILLS

1. Introduction to prehospital and emergency care; BLS refresher for all ages; web access; teamwork and leadership; scene assessment and safety and approach to the emergency patient (4 hours).
2. Principles of communication, triage, and transport (4 hours).
3. Airway assessment and management (basic airway care; the use of suction, airway adjuncts, and oxygen; endotracheal intubation and use of the laryngeal mask airway; cricothyrotomy; artificial ventilation; pneumothorax and hemothorax, including needle thoracostomy) (8 hours).
4. Defibrillation and arrhythmias (6 hours).
5. Initial assessment, management of shock, intravenous cannulation and therapy (4 hours).
6. Assessment and management of the unconscious patient (including head injury) (4 hours).
7. Principles of pain assessment and management, and basic wound care (4 hours).
8. Special circumstances: children, the vulnerable, and mass casualty incidents (4 hours).

9. Assessment (MCQ, Clinical Examination, Clinical Slide Examination) (2 hours).

PEDIATRIC EMERGENCIES

1. Introduction to pediatric anatomy and physiology (7 hours).
2. Principles and practice of managing the acutely ill child (9 hours).
3. Principles and practice of managing the acutely injured child (9 hours).
4. Assessment (MCQ, Clinical Examination, Clinical Slide Examination) (2 hours).

TRAUMATIC EMERGENCIES

1. Trauma airway care: oxygen, suction, simple airway adjuncts, endotracheal intubation, rescue devices, surgical airway principles (6 hours).
2. Spinal immobilization: techniques, devices, indications, and when to remove (4 hours).
3. Thoracic trauma: needle and tube thoracostomy, chest x-ray. Predictors of major injury (4 hours).

*This is suitable for a country with a comprehensive health care setting. (*in title)

4. Abdominal trauma: mechanisms, injury patterns, emergency management (4 hours).
5. Pelvic fractures and their initial management (4 hours).
6. Head and spinal cord injury (4 hours).
7. Limb injuries and splintage techniques. Femoral nerve block (4 hours).
8. Burns: prehospital and emergency care (4 hours).
9. Trauma moulage scenarios (4 hours).
10. Assessment (MCQ, Clinical Examination, Clinical Slide Examination) (2 hours).

OBSTETRIC AND GYNECOLOGIC EMERGENCIES

1. Emergencies in obstetrics: emergency delivery, eclampsia, pre-eclampsia, PV (Blood loss *per vaginam)* bleeding (8 hours).
2. Emergency gynecology (4 hours).
3. Assessment (MCQ, Clinical Slide Examination) (1 hour).

ESCORT MEDICINE

1. Principles of emergency medical transport (5 hours).
2. Practical experience with ambulance service (10 hours).
3. Helicopter transport and safety (5 hours).
4. Helicopter practical session (5 hours).
5. Principles of interhospital transfer of the critically ill (10 hours).
6. Assessment (MCQ, Clinical Examination, Clinical Slide Examination) (2 hours).

MEDICAL EMERGENCIES

1. Acute cardiology I: acute coronary syndromes, ECG interpretation, diagnosis of acute myocardial infarction (4 hours).
2. Acute cardiology II: management of myocardial infarction, thrombolysis, and percutaneous coronary intervention (PCI), commonly known as coronary angioplasty; acute aortic disease (4 hours).
3. Acute respiratory disease: asthma, chronic obstructive pulmonary disease, pneumothorax, pulmonary embolism, pneumonia (4 hours).
4. Acute neurologic emergencies: stroke, epilepsy, decreased conscious level (4 hours).

5. Acute poisoning: paracetamol (acetaminophen), opioids, tricyclic antidepressants, benzodiazepines, others (4 hours).
6. Endocrine emergencies: hypoglycemia, diabetic ketoacidosis, addisonian crisis (4 hours).
7. Abdominal pain; differential diagnosis and emergency management (4 hours).
8. Acute gastrointestinal bleeding and acute liver disease. Alcohol and drug abuse. Bloodborne viruses and their importance in prehospital and emergency care (4 hours).
9. Advanced life support scenario session (6 hours).
10. Assessment (MCQ, Clinical Examination, Clinical Slide Examination) (2 hours).

MAJOR INCIDENTS AND DISASTER MANAGEMENT

1. Management of civilian disasters.
2. Chemical, biological, radiologic, road traffic, maritime and aircraft/airport disasters.
3. Uncompensated disasters (where infrastructure and basic services [e.g., water supplies], are also lost to the rescuers).
4. Major infectious diseases outbreak disaster.
5. Role of the police (including tactical issues) (3 hours).
6. Role of the Fire Department (including a practical session on extrication) (3 hours).
7. Role of the Ambulance Service and mobile medical team (3 hours).
8. Role of Government Flying Service (GFS), Air-Sea Rescue, and Coast Guard (3 hours).
9. Introduction to major incident management. Triage sort and sieve (3 hours).
10. Tabletop exercise I (3 hours).
11. Tabletop exercise II (3 hours).
12. Major incident practical exercise (3 hours).
13. Assessment (3 hours).

ETHICAL AND LEGAL ASPECTS OF PREHOSPITAL AND EMERGENCY CARE

This module will explore the ethical aspects of prehospital and emergency care and apply the legal principles of medicine to these ethical problems. Examples of new developments which may affect emergency care include advance directives, and the full impact of these has yet to be determined for the emergency care provider. The interface between the legal requirements for emergency care providers and the ethical problems they create (for example, taking blood for ethanol levels in suspected drink driving cases) will be explored on an international basis. Further ethical and practical difficulties, such as stopping a resuscitation attempt in the prehospital situation, will also be discussed. Candidates will be encouraged to bring their own examples into the course and will be required to write an account of an ethical dilemma with a fully referenced commentary for assessment purposes (28 hours).

CHAPTER 13

EMS Health, Safety, and Wellness Issues

Mazen J. El Sayed, Jon Mark Hirshon

KEY LEARNING POINTS

- EMS personnel are at relatively high risk for work-related injuries and illnesses.

- EMS agencies need to actively promote and operate injury and illness prevention and wellness programs for their personnel.

INTRODUCTION

Prehospital healthcare providers are health professionals trained in the initial care of injured and ill individuals. Their training may be very minimal, such as basic first aid, through to quite advanced knowledge and skills, including endotracheal intubation. Their roles and responsibilities cover a wide range of activities from responding to emergencies to assessing patients and initiating treatment at the response scene, through initial stabilization and transportation of the patient to an appropriate medical facility for definitive care. Within their work environment, EMS providers encounter physical and emotional challenges that may impact their health and safety. Injuries ranging from minor to life-threatening, mental stress, communicable diseases, and chemical exposures are some of the risks encountered by these prehospital providers.

Health, safety, and wellness are fundamental in order to help reduce the effects of hazards encountered by EMS personnel. Preemployment screening, adequate training, injury prevention and

health maintenance programs, postexposure counseling, and treatment are all essential components of EMS wellness, health, and safety and will be discussed in this chapter. Many challenges and barriers exist to implementing appropriate occupational health and safety measures. These include lack of adequate funding, deficiencies in data collection, the absence of centralized databases, and lack of consensus over standards and policies. These issues will be discussed in this chapter as well as potential solutions to overcoming these problems.

OCCUPATIONAL HAZARDS

Occupational Injuries and Fatalities

Higher rates of work-related injuries were reported by the US Department of Labor in 2000 for EMS workers when compared with the national average and with rates from other industries.[1] The diverse EMS work environments predispose the providers to exposure to a vast array of hazards that may inflict physical injuries, some of which may be disabling and result in extended periods off work or even permanent disability. Physically demanding activities, including frequent lifting and bending, are part of the daily duties of EMS workers. Depending on the type of EMS system, the prehospital providers may be required to physically participate in the extrication of the injured from the accident scene in addition to carrying heavy equipment and/or patients over long distances prior to transfer.

A number of studies and surveys of EMS workers have tried to elicit the most frequent types of injuries.[1,2,9] The most commonly cited ones are back injuries, lifting and musculoskeletal complaints, falls, motor vehicle collisions, being struck by an object, and assault injuries. Sprains, strains, and muscle tears were the leading category of injury and the back was the body part most injured[1,2] (Table 13-1). In a survey of a national sample of US EMS workers, injuries within the previous 12 months were reported in up to 30% of responders. In this study, the incidence of back injuries was also compared between paid and volunteer EMS providers, revealing that these injuries were more common in experienced or paid providers or paramedics than in volunteer workers.[2]

A review by Maguire and colleagues of the available databases of EMS workers' occupational fatalities estimated a rate of 12.7 per 100,000 EMS providers annually. This rate is higher than the national average for occupational deaths of 5.0 per 100,000 for the same period (1992–1997). The leading categories of EMS personnel fatalities were vehicle crashes, cardiovascular or cerebrovascular accidents, and homicide.[3]

Risk factors for EMS vehicle crashes, as identified by Levick and coworkers in a literature review of ambulance safety, were the use of light and siren warnings, lack of use of restraints by EMS personnel, drivers with a history of prior collision, and driving through red lights at intersections.[4] Hazards during an ambulance crash are higher for rear compartment occupants, since ambulances are exempt from federal standards for vehicle safety in the US and, in most cases, are not crash tested like other commercial vehicles.[5]

More recently, an increase in the fatalities related to air ambulance transport has instigated a debate about the safety of air ambulance transport and potential measures to improve safety. The number of fatalities reached a peak of 29 in 2008, the deadliest year to date in the industry's history, from a yearly average of 10 fatalities according to data from the US National Transportation Safety Board (NTSB).[6] The main factors related to crashes were pilot error, nighttime operation flight, flights to remote terrains, and adverse weather conditions.[7] The rapid growth of the air ambulance industry in the US within the past few years, along with increasing competition between services, may have led to potential unsafe practices such as "call jumping" (responding to a scene without being officially dispatched by the local or regional dispatch authority). However, lack of quality data on actual flight activity limits the ability to draw conclusions about true trends in the air ambulance crash rate. Several measures have been taken by the Association of Air Medical Services (AAMS) and the Federal Aviation Administration (FAA) to improve the safety of this industry, including increased government oversight, regular inspections, more frequent pilot continuing education programs, higher maintenance standards, and improved safety technologies (e.g., night vision goggles), which can serve as examples for air ambulance services in other countries.

Violence

EMS workers can be exposed to a number of violent and abusive situations in their practice. This violence can be within the environment and not directed at the EMS providers, such as at the scene of a domestic dispute, or can be directed toward the EMS workers. Violence in the prehospital setting takes various forms and is fairly common. In one survey of EMS personnel of the Albuquerque, New Mexico (US) Fire Department, 90% of respondents reported being the target of an assault or a violent action during their career. Feelings of anger and irritability commonly resulted from this. Violence was even perceived as "part of the job" by 71% of respondents.[8] The source of abuse was not limited to violent patients but included family members and bystanders. Types of abuse ranged from obscene language and verbal harassment to other

Table 13–1	**Most Frequent Injuries to EMS Personnel**

Back strains
Falls
Motor vehicle collisions
Struck by an object
Assaults
Musculoskeletal

Source: Original by Mazen J. El Sayed, Jon Mark Hirshon.

abusive actions including threats of harm, kicking, spitting, pulling hair, and threats with weapons. The most cited stressors related to violence in the EMS workplace were lack of training and absence of protocols addressing violent situations not related to an angry or agitated medical patient (abuse from relatives or bystanders); inadequate equipment to handle dangerous situations; and frequency of exposure to violence.[9]

Unfortunately, deficiencies in collecting data about the frequency of abusive actions, in defining and identifying intolerable behaviors, and problems with assessing the long-term impact of violence on prehospital providers are prevalent among most EMS agencies, which causes difficulties in obtaining good quality data to evaluate the magnitude of this problem. Clearly, cultural and social patterns of any given jurisdiction or country, as well as the societal stability and ongoing conflicts between groups, will significantly impact the potential for EMS workers to face violence. (See **Chapter 44, EMS Violence** for more information.)

Occupational Exposure to Infectious Diseases

EMS workers can encounter significant infectious hazards while caring for patients, including the risk of contracting certain bloodborne and airborne infectious diseases. Well-known examples of such infections include, but are not limited to, human immunodeficiency virus (HIV), viral hepatitis (especially hepatitis B and C), tuberculosis, and respiratory viruses such as H1N1 influenza (a.k.a. swine flu). Numerous potential opportunities for disease transmission exist in the prehospital care settings, including droplet exposure while securing the patient's airway or blood exposure while inserting an intravenous catheter for fluid resuscitation. Contact with other body fluids, contaminated sharp objects, and needle-stick injuries are other mechanisms of infection transmission.

A number of studies have investigated the risks related to infectious disease exposure and transmission among EMS providers. Occupational blood contact frequency in a sample of EMS workers from three US inner city areas with high AIDS incidence was estimated to be 12.3 blood contacts per prehospital worker per year, including 0.2 percutaneous exposures per year.[10] More specifically, needle-stick injury rates among full time EMS and fire fighter paramedics were found to be comparable to other healthcare workers' rates (87 to 370 needle-stick injuries per 1,000 employees per year).[11] Concerning hepatitis B virus (HBV)

transmission, one study found a strong correlation between HBV infection and years of work exposure in EMS regardless of job description (paramedic versus emergency medical technician),[12] which highlights the importance of preventive measures such as vaccinations. Airborne disease hazards such as tuberculosis have also been examined in the prehospital setting. The tuberculin skin test conversion rate among New York City EMS workers was estimated to be 0.5% annually (1993–1996).[13] This rate was found to be lower than what was commonly perceived, even during a period where the prevalence of tuberculosis cases in New York City was comparable to that in some developing countries. It was also lower than the reported conversion rates in New York City hospitals (10%) during the same period.

In general, communicable disease transmission to prehospital workers is a significant concern, even though it may be only an infrequent problem in some EMS systems. Most EMS agencies in the US have protocols and infection control policies as stipulated by the department of public health in each state or other governing jurisdiction. However, these policies and procedures are frequently absent in many volunteer services and EMS services in developing countries where infectious diseases could constitute a major threat.[14] The particularly high incidence of tuberculosis in some countries, such as in South Asia, constitutes an example of a significant health threat to EMS personnel in these countries. Even if appropriate protocols exist, implementation and enforcement may be poor or inconsistent.

Occupational Exposure to Chemical Hazards

EMS providers are frequently first responders to incidents where there is potential for hazardous materials (liquid, solids, or gaseous) exposure. Once the on-scene hazard assessment is done, the incident commander identifies the appropriate zones (labeled hot zone, warm zone, and cold zone; See **Chapter 47, Disasters and HazMat** for more information on this classification.) based on safety and degree of hazard. EMS workers are usually restricted to and positioned in the cold zone where the exposure risk is only from hazardous materials still present on the patients. Once the appropriate levels of personal protective equipment (PPE) are defined and in place, there is usually minimal further contamination and occupational exposure, since all the patients must pass through decontamination procedures in the process of being transported to the cold zone. The only significant hazardous materials exposure should potentially occur during the initial scene response time when the nature of the incident may still be unknown by the EMS personnel or the hazards are not completely identified. Unfortunately, this has not always been the case in some previous disasters. Long-term medical conditions such as respiratory illnesses have been reported among EMS workers and first responders in previous major incidents.[15] The EMS personnel of the Fire Department of New York City incurred substantial exposures to toxic substances while working at the World Trade Center (WTC) site during the 9/11 attacks in 2001. Three years after the attack, at the initial (2204) and follow-up examination (2207), 24.1% of the WTC responders were found to have persistent impairment in their lung functions.[16]

Mental Health

EMS workers face challenging situations on a daily basis, some of which may impact the provider's well being and mental health. Stressors vary in severity and frequency and can be categorized as acute or chronic. Acute stressors can be unfamiliar situations or events that have the potential to cause post-traumatic stress symptoms, such as an injury secondary to an assault on the EMS provider or an incident with a seriously ill or injured child. Chronic stressors are frequent events or work conditions that EMS workers experience regularly, such as physically demanding activities including lifting a patient, lack of support from coworkers, lack of public appreciation, and/or dealing with abusive patients and personal threats. Stressors in the EMS workplace can also be categorized as ambulance-specific stressors and administrative organizational stressors. The ambulance-related stressors (physical demands and serious operational activities) tend to be more severe and more frequent than the general organizational stressors. The size of the population served has a direct impact on the frequency of the stressors experienced by EMS workers.[17] Job satisfaction and psychological well being of EMS providers and their attitude toward their career are adversely affected by these different stress sources. Failure to cope with the physiologic distress is evident through a high prevalence (up to 15.2%) of post-traumatic stress disorder (PTSD) symptoms experienced by EMS providers.[18] Disasters are also notorious for causing PTSD and other mental health problems among first responders and EMS workers. Studies that resulted from the 9/11 WTC disaster in New York revealed elevated rates of PTSD symptoms (up to 12%) among exposed EMS workers up to 3 years after the attacks.[19]

CHALLENGES WITH HEALTH, SAFETY, AND WELLNESS FOR EMS

EMS agencies worldwide face numerous challenges in dealing with health, safety, and wellness issues of their providers. These agency challenges tend to vary, depending on many factors such as the complexity, size, and organization of the agency, the practice environment, and the service expectations and demands.

There are many different types of EMS agencies including private, hospital-based, Fire Department–based, and municipal-based. The EMS staffing is either career- (professional) or volunteer-based or a combination of both. This variety in the types of EMS systems and providers creates major organizational and research challenges, which translates into difficulties in collecting data related to wellness, safety, and providers' health. Research results drawn from a study in one country may not be applicable to EMS workers in another country or city because of the different types of providers or different types of agencies involved. Differences are even present within one agency between its paid and its volunteer providers: paid providers report more injuries and their risk of injuries correlates with their level of training.[20,21] The lack of a unified code or group that identifies the EMS workers raises another challenge to data collection. Multiple databases available in the US such as from the Bureau of Labor Statistics, the Fatality Analysis Reporting System (FARS), and the Census of Fatal Occupational Injuries (CFOI) collect data on occupational injuries and fatalities of EMS workers. However, data extraction from these databases is problematic in part because of the variations between these databases in the types of personnel they categorize and include as "EMS personnel."

Lack of funding for research and training programs that deal with injury prevention and EMS workers' health and wellness is another source of concern for many EMS agencies. Much of the available funding is frequently channeled to other priorities within an agency such as infrastructure development or quality improvement, leaving the wellness and health and safety programs with scant or no funding at all. Research in the prehospital setting relies mainly on individual EMS agencies' databases, which may be of variable quality. Results vary widely among agencies and are usually agency-specific. Multiple factors should be taken into account when trying to reproduce these results or apply recommendations that emerged from previous studies, especially those recommendations related to providers' health, wellness, and safety. Examples of such factors are the type of agency and its setting, the type of providers involved, the education programs in place, and the support system that is available.

Despite all of the above-cited challenges, general recommendations and strategies to minimize the risk of occupational hazards for EMS providers can be developed for a specific agency and some are illustrated in the following section of this chapter. One way for EMS agencies and providers to utilize these recommendations is to conduct an occupational hazards assessment in order to identify areas for potential improvement for the wellness and safety of employees. These organizations can also test solutions that have been successfully implemented by other agencies with similar structure and needs. For example, one study in New Castle County in the state of Delaware (US), showed that the use of a self-capping intravenous catheter by ALS providers, while controlling for all other variables such as use of protective gloves and availability of sharp disposal containers, was associated with a statistically significant reduction in the absolute number of needle sticks and the rate of needle-stick injuries.[22] Such a simple, feasible measure can be used by an EMS agency with ALS providers to decrease the rate of needle-stick injuries.

ACTION CONSIDERATIONS FOR EMS AGENCIES AND PROVIDERS

Preventing Injuries and Reducing Fatalities

Vehicle crashes constitute the highest risk for occupational fatalities for EMS personnel. Ensuring EMS vehicle safety is a basic requirement to reduce this risk. Until recently, only minimal safety standards and few crash safety guidelines were applied to ambulances in most countries. National safety standards in Australia and the US have been established for EMS vehicles.[23,24] These standards or guidelines are aimed at improving EMS vehicles' safety and at decreasing the vulnerability of rear compartment occupants. Safety measures extending beyond the design of EMS vehicles and pertaining to EMS agencies and providers include mandatory personnel use of restraints (seat belt use and making seat belts available in the back compartment of ambulance vehicles), mandatory driver training, and driver screening for sensory or coordination deficits.

Introduction of "black box" technology (meaning the use of high technology sensors to monitor vehicle

Table 13–2	Summary of EMS Vehicle Safety Measures

Mandatory use of seat belts by EMS personnel
Having seat belts available in the rear compartment
Mandatory driver training
Driver screening for sensory or coordination deficits
"Black box" vehicle monitoring sensors
Priority dispatching
Decreased use of "lights and siren"

Source: Original by Mazen J. El Sayed, Jon Mark Hirshon.

position, stability, distance to nearby vehicles or structures) to warn drivers of dangerous conditions, priority dispatching, and reevaluation of "light and sirens" policies are other measures with potential safety benefit to EMS agencies. (see Table 13-2). Although the use of warning "lights and sirens" in emergency medical vehicle response and patient transport has been shown to shorten transport times,[25,26] controversy exists regarding the clinical significance of the time saved. One study that looked at using medical criteria for "light and sirens" transport based on the patient's condition showed no increase in adverse outcomes related to transport without lights and sirens.[27] These findings are dependent on the geographic nature of the EMS system (urban or rural) and the proximity of hospitals. The relationship between use of different EMS vehicle warning devices and transport safety is not yet clearly established.

The air ambulance industry in the US is undergoing major changes in response to the increasing number of air medical services helicopter crashes and fatalities. Numerous agencies and associations, including the National Transportation Safety Board, the Federal Aviation Administration, and the Association of Air Medical Services, have together stepped in to focus efforts on improving safety.

This has resulted in increased research into causes of crashes and how to improve training. Measures taken by the aviation authorities include regular and expanded inspection of air ambulance fleets by dedicated teams of inspectors, enhanced oversight and technical support, launching crash mitigation programs, and revision of standards for operations during adverse weather and for safe cruising altitude. Additional recommended strategies include collecting

Table 13–3	Methods to Increase Safety in Air Medical Services

Regular and expanded inspections of air ambulances

Enhanced oversight and technical support

Launching crash mitigation programs

Revision of standards for operations in bad weather

Revision of standards for safe cruising altitudes

Collecting enhanced operational data

Use of safety technology and warning systems

Improving operational control

Revising policies for appropriate dispatch and usage

Clarifying the government's role in oversight and regulations

Source: Original by Mazen J. El Sayed, Jon Mark Hirshon.

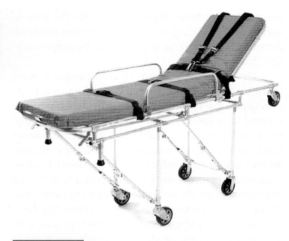

FIGURE 13–1

Type of ambulance stretcher which has self-deploying supports and wheels. From http://www.firesafety solutions.com.au/product_details.php?&556674866 1414874749426356297&pID=1120&rID=3&c Path=844.

accurate operational data on air ambulance flights (e.g., number of flight hours), encouraging use of safety technology such as terrain awareness and warning systems, improving operational control, revising policies for appropriate dispatch and usage of air ambulances, and clarifying government's role through oversight and regulations of air ambulance services[28,29] (Table 13-3). All of these measures require extensive collaboration among the various agencies to effectively reduce the number of air ambulance crashes and improve the industry's safety.

Preventing nontransportation-related occupational injuries is a complex process because of the diversity of injury types and mechanisms. Injury prevention programs for EMS providers have varied in efficacy. Effective components in back injury prevention programs are the use of mechanical lifts, zero lift policies, and the use of lift teams.[30-32] An example of a type of ambulance stretcher commonly used that has its support legs and wheels deploy to contact the ground before the stretcher is fully removed from the ambulance is shown in Figure 13-1. This type of stretcher enables the patient's weight to be fully supported before the stretcher exits the ambulance so the EMS personnel don't have to fully lift the patient to exit the ambulance.

A simple commonly used type of back brace is shown in Figure 13-2. Some EMS agencies have developed programs that start with preemployment screening and progress to physical strengthening while focusing on injury prevention training. Most of these

programs incorporate ergonomically improved equipment, patient extrication devices, and high-tech personal protective gear. Financial limitations and limited available numbers of EMS providers in some settings or areas (agencies relying on volunteers) may hinder the application of such programs.

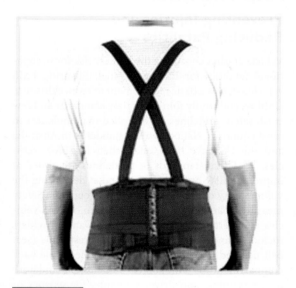

FIGURE 13–2

Commonly used type of back brace. From http://www. phc-online.com/Back_Support_p/safe-t-lift_dx.htm.

Preventing and Managing Communicable Diseases

Most programs for EMS providers designed to prevent occupationally related infectious diseases and promote health and wellness in the US are in accordance with the Centers for Disease Control and Prevention (CDC) and Occupational Health and Safety Administration (OSHA) standards. These programs include education related to bloodborne/airborne pathogens, immunizations, and occupational exposure management. Preemployment proof of completed immunizations and serologic tests for EMS workers are similar to those for other healthcare workers. These include requirements for tetanus and diphtheria, measles/mumps/rubella and varicella immunizations and current tuberculosis (TB) screening. Hepatitis B vaccination is also commonly provided to EMS workers after employment.

In addition to that, constant updates on emerging and prevalent diseases are made available to EMS workers through regular reports from the EMS agencies and public health departments. One excellent source for this information is the CDC web site http://www.cdc.gov/DiseasesConditions/. Finally, many EMS agencies have also established postexposure management protocols, based upon CDC and OSHA guidance, in collaboration with employee health departments and local institutions in order to provide assistance and treatment for employees exposed to communicable diseases.

Preventing Chemical and Hazardous Material (HAZMAT) Exposure

Education programs about chemical weapons, related chemicals such as pesticides, as well as other hazardous material are normally part of an EMS worker's training. Exposure of fire fighters and prehospital providers to toxins, especially from fires and industrial releases, is a major concern. Early detection and identification of chemical agents at the response scene in consultation with HAZMAT teams allows EMS workers to provide the necessary decontamination measures for victims while using the appropriate level of personal protective equipment (PPE).

Four Levels of PPE currently exist as defined by OSHA: these range from level A equipment (completely impervious suit with enclosed self-contained breathing apparatus), to level D equipment (least protective work uniform to be used for nuisance contamination only when there is no danger of chemical exposure)[33] (Table 13-4).

The development of protocols that deal with chemical exposure as well as early involvement of HAZMAT experts in suspicious scenes may prevent unnecessary exposure of unprotected individuals, including EMS providers. The HAZMAT experts can carry hand-held devices in order to detect chemical vapors on site within seconds, which can be important for response scene personnel safety.

Managing Stress and Maintaining EMS Workers' Mental Health

Maintaining a healthy lifestyle and having good social and familial support networks are some of the elements that alleviate the toll of chronic exposure to stress in the EMS workplace. Peer support groups in EMS have also been made available in some agencies to help colleagues deal with daily work problems and stressful events.[17] Some US agencies in approximately 16 states such as Virginia, Utah, and Nebraska have adopted the Critical Incident Stress Management (CISM) approach: a critical incident is any situation faced by personnel causing unusually strong emotional reactions that have the potential to interfere with their ability to function during or after the event.

Table 13–4	Personal Protective Equipment Levels	
PPE Level	**Contamination Risk Environment**	**Description and Components**
A	Highly contaminated	Vapor protective and chemically resistant suit, full face SCBA
B	Contaminated	Liquid splash protective suit, full face piece SCBA
C	Mildly Contaminated	Support function protective garment, face piece canister equipped respirator
D	Not Contaminated	Coveralls or gown, safety shoes, safety glasses

SCBA = self-contained breathing apparatus.
Source: Original by Mazen J. El Sayed, Jon Mark Hirshon.

Examples include a fellow EMS provider's suicide, serious injury or death of an emergency responder, and mass casualty events. CISM teams identify a critical incident and provide crisis support to EMS workers to lessen the impact of the incident and to accelerate the recovery process of stressed or injured EMS workers. These teams also provide pre-incident education and post-incident debriefings and defusing to EMS personnel. "Defusing" refers to the post-incident education of exposed individuals after the immediate impact of the event and the available resources to help with the physical and emotional recovery course. However, there is still a lot of controversy about the effectiveness of the CISM approach.[34] Some countries such as Australia have turned away from using only this model, especially the mandatory post-incident debriefing, and moved towards using selective postexposure counseling, depending on the affected EMS worker's preference and need.[35]

SUMMARY

It is clear that the health, wellness, and safety of EMS providers are the basis for a sound functioning EMS agency. Without adequate appropriately trained and motivated staff, an EMS agency will have difficulty providing needed services. The available literature has shown that there has been only sparse attention accorded to this topic.

Improving EMS providers' health, safety, and wellness starts by conducting research, providing education, developing and writing policies and procedures, and reviewing programs for efficiency and effectiveness. Appropriate budget allocation to the development of these programs is essential. Having well-prepared providers who can perform their duties in a safe manner within an agency that is concerned about their wellness and safety is what helps EMS personnel to enjoy their rewarding careers.

Web Resources

1. EMS Responder http://emsresponder.com/
2. JEMS magazine: http://www.jems.com.
3. US Dept. of Labor, Occupational Health & Safety Administration: http://www.osha.gov.
4. Centers for Disease Control: http://www.cdc.gov.
5. Dept. of Health & Ageing, Australia: http://www.health.gov.au.
6. Samu Emergencies de France http://www.samu-de-france.fr.
7. The Air Medical Physician Association http://www.ampa.org.
8. Association of Air Medical Services: http://www.aams.org.
9. National Association of EMS Physicians: http://www.naemsp.org.
10. Fire Rescue 1: http://www.firerescue1.com.
11. EMS.gov: http://www.ems.gov. (hosted by NHTSA)
12. National Highway Safety Traffic Administration (US) http://www.nhtsa.gov.

References

1. Maguire BJ, Hunting KL, Guidotti TL, Smith GS. Occupational injuries among emergency medical services personnel. *Prehosp Emerg Care* 9(4): 405, 2005.
2. Heick R, Young T, Peek-Asa C. Occupational injuries among emergency medical service providers in the United States. *J Occup Environ Med* 51(8): 963, 2009.
3. Maguire BJ, Hunting KL, Smith GS, Levick NR. Occupational fatalities in emergency medical services: A hidden crisis. *Ann Emerg Med* 40: 625, 2002.
4. Levick N, Mener D. "Searching for Ambulance Safety: Where is the Literature?" Paper presented at the annual meeting of the National Association of EMS Physicians, Registry Resort, *Naples, FL.* 2009-05-25 from http://www.allacademic.com/meta/p64904_index.html accessed on 8/24/09.
5. Becker LR, Zaloshnja E, Levick N, Miller TR. Relative risk of injury and death in ambulances and other emergency vehicles. *Accident Analysis Prev* 941, 2003.
6. "NTSB NEWS." Safety Board Issues. Additional Recommendations to the Helicopter Emergency Medical Services Industry. September 1, 2009. http://www.ntsb.gov/pressrel/2009/090901.html.
7. GAO, Aviation Safety: Potential Strategies to Address Air Ambulance Safety Concerns, GAO-09-627T (Washington, D.C.: April 22, 2009).
8. Pozzi C. Exposure of prehospital providers to violence and abuse. *J Emerg Nursing* 1998; 24(4): 320, 1998.
9. Fontanarosa P. Occupational considerations for the prehospital provider. *Emerg Med Clin North Am* 8: 119, 1990.
10. Marcus R, Srivastava P. Occupational blood contact among prehospital providers. *Ann Emerg Med* 25(6): 776, 1995.
11. Rischitelli G, Harris J. The risk of acquiring hepatitis B or C among public safety workers: A systematic review. *Am J Preventive Med* 20(4): 299, 2001.
12. Pepe PE, Hollinger FB, Troisi CL, Heiberg D. Viral hepatitis risk in urban emergency medical services personnel. *Ann Emerg Med* 15: 454, 1986.
13. Prezant D, Kelly K. Tuberculin skin test conversion rates in New York City emergency medical service health care workers. *Ann Emerg Med* 32(2): 208, 1998.
14. Mahomed OJ, Champaklal C, Taylor M, Yancey A. The preparedness of emergency medical services against occupationally acquired communicable diseases in the prehospital environment in South Africa. *Emerg Med J* 24(7): 497, 2007.
15. Banauch G, McLaughin M. Injuries and illnesses among New York City Fire Department rescue workers after responding to the World Trade Center attacks. *JAMA* 288(13): 1581, 2002.

16. Skloot GS, Schechter CB, Herbert R, et al. Longitudinal assessment of spirometry in the World Trade Center medical monitoring program. *Chest* 135(2): 492, 2009.

17. Sterud T, Hem E, Ekeberg O, Lau B. Occupational stressors and its organizational and individual correlates: A nationwide study of Norwegian ambulance personnel. *BMC Emerg Med* 2008; 8:16.

18. Jonsson A, Segesten K, Mattsson B. Post-traumatic stress among Swedish ambulance personnel. *Emerg Med J* 20: 79, 2003.

19. 9/11 HEALTH. Retrieved from http://nyc.gov/html/doh/wtc/html/know/know.shtml20. http://www.nyc.gov/html/doh/wtc/html/home/home.shtml.

20. Schwartz RJ, Benson L, Jacobs LM. The prevalence of occupational injuries in EMTs in New England. *Prehospital Disaster Med* 8: 45, 1993.

21. Hogya PT, Ellis L. Evaluation of the injury profile of personnel in a busy urban EMS system. *Am J Emerg Med* 8: 308, 1990.

22. O'Connor RE, Krall S, Megargel RE, et al. Reducing the rate of paramedic needlesticks in emergency medical services: the role of self-capping intravenous catheters. *Acad Emerg Med* 3: 668, 1996.

23. ANSI/ASSE Z15.1-2006 American Standard: Safe Practices for Motor Vehicle Operations, American National Standards Institute (ANSI)/American Society of Safety Engineers (ASSE) Accredited Standards Committee, Z.15, March 2006.

24. Joint Standards Australia/Standards New Zealand Committee ME/48 on Restraint Systems in Vehicles, Standards for Ambulance Restraint Systems, Joint Standards Australia/Standards New Zealand ASN/ZS 4535:1999.

25. Hunt RC, Brown LH, Cabinum ES, et al. Is ambulance transport time with lights and sirens faster than that without? *Ann Emerg Med* 25(4): 507, 1995.

26. Brown LH, Whitney CL, Hunt RC, et al. Do warning lights and sirens reduce ambulance response times? *Prehosp Emerg Care* 4(1): 70, 2000.

27. Kupas DF, Dula DJ, Pino BJ. Patient outcome using medical protocol to limit "lights and siren" transport. *Prehospital Disaster Med* 9(4): 226, 1994.

28. National transportation Safety Board Recommendations & Advocacy. Retrieved from http://www.ntsb.gov/Recs/index.htm.

29. (2009, June). FAA Regulations & Policies. Advisory Circulars. Emergency Medical Service/Airplane (EMS/A). Retrieved from http://www.faa.gov/regulations_policies/advisory_circulars/index.cfm/.

30. Collins JW, Wolf L, Bell J, Evanoff B. An evaluation of a best practices musculoskeletal injury prevention program in nursing homes. *Inj Prev* 10: 206, 2004.

31. Li J, Wolf L, Evanoff B. Use of mechanical patient lifts decreased musculoskeletal symptoms and injuries among health care workers. *Inj Prev* 10: 212, 2004.

32. Gatty CM, Turner M, Buitendorp DJ, Batman H. The effectiveness of back pain and injury prevention programs in the workplace. *Work* 20: 257, 2003.

33. (1994, August). OSHA Regulations (Standards - 29 CFR) General description and discussion of the levels of protection and protective gear. Retrieved from http://www.osha.gov/pls/oshaweb/owadisp.show_document?p_table=STANDARDS&p_id=9767.

34. Bledsoe BE. Critical incident stress management (CISM): benefit or risk for emergency services? *Prehosp Emerg Care* 7(2): 272, 2003.

35. Smith, Robin (2006, May 1). Australia: rethinking the strict CISM model. The Free Library. (2006). Retrieved August 30, 2009 from http://www.thefreelibrary.com/Australia: rethinking the strict CISM model-a0145473394.

CHAPTER 14

Dispatch and Communication Systems

Ian Patrick, Bill Barger, Conor Deasy

KEY LEARNING POINTS

- All EMS should have easy access through a single emergency number.
- Standardization of call taking and dispatch should reduce error and response times to critically ill patients.
- Communications and dispatch processes must be continually audited.

- Different communication methods are available such as radio/telephone/telemedicine, but certain principles apply to all.
- Standardized handovers should be used to avoid information loss.

INTRODUCTION

Coordination and communication are essential in the provision of EMS. An EMS system must be easy to access, have a prioritized dispatch system, be capable of communicating with and coordinating mobile resources in the community, and have a structured approach to patient handover between healthcare providers.

Figure 14-1 shows an illustration of a communications center.

A convenient access has evolved through the 911/112/999 emergency telephone system, allowing rapid access to emergency services: police, fire services, and emergency medical services. These emergency call services are operator-assisted and designed to connect callers to emergency service organizations in a life-threatening or time-critical situation.

Enhanced 911/112/999 allows the call taker to identify the caller's exact location when ringing from a land line. The call taker will confirm that the emergency is at the address from which the land line emergency call has been made, clarifying the exact location with the aid of a GPS coordinance map on which the caller location can be seen. This is the vital first step in emergency call-taking designed to ensure that no confusion exists as to the whereabouts of the emergency. If the caller disconnects or his or her condition deteriorates such that

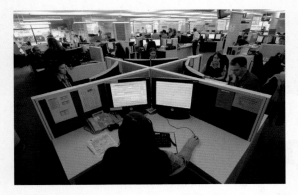

FIGURE 14–1

Communications center for ambulance, Victoria, Australia. Photo courtesy of Bill Barger.

developed to improve accuracy, efficiency, and professionalism of call takers. Some aim to create a "zero minute" response time to initiate lifesaving support such as initiation of bystander CPR through telephone instructions. The key function of any call-taking system is to prioritize the allocation of ambulance resources to calls for which the response time is crucial to the patient's outcome.

The systems of emergency call-taking can be divided into two broad groups: medical priority dispatch system (MPDS) and criteria-based dispatch systems (CBDS). The medical priority dispatch system (MPDS) differs from criteria-based dispatch systems by using algorithms rather than prompts.[4] There have been no comparative studies of the criteria-based dispatch with MPDS.

the phone call cannot be continued, the emergency can still be responded to.

Similar to land line calls, when a call is received from a mobile phone a set of coordinates is generated. In urban areas with a high density of phone masts, the Enhanced Information Service for Emergency Calls (EISEC) can locate a mobile phone position within a small radius, sometimes as little as 30 meters (m), although this can increase to over 3,000 m in rural areas with fewer masts. The EISEC system can also assist in identifying when the caller is not at the site of the incident being reported and in some cases this will also identify hoax calls. Since the introduction of the mobile phone locating system, the London Ambulance Service has seen a significant improvement in ambulance response times.[2]

Identification of a vehicle accident and the location of that event are possible without secondary callers with advanced technology. One such example is OnStar© tracking and monitoring equipment, which is present in some vehicles, both private and commercial. If that vehicle is involved in a collision, an automatic notification providing the exact location to a dispatch center is generated.[1]

The primary functions of emergency call-taking and dispatch are ascertaining and categorizing the caller's priority, providing first aid and scene safety instructions, and dispatching the most appropriate emergency response to that patient in a time-appropriate manner, all the while maintaining availability of appropriate medical resources for further callers. Emergency medical lights and siren responses may expose prehospital care providers and the public to increased risk of road traffic collisions. Systems have

EMERGENCY MEDICAL DISPATCH SYSTEMS (MPDS)

MPDS comprise a set of key questions, prearrival instructions, and dispatch priorities for medical emergencies that ambulance call takers provide over the telephone.[3] The advantage of MPDS is stated to be that it does not rely on the "exercise of good medical judgment" and is more amenable to quality assurance.[10] MPDS attempt to eliminate the potential for call-taker bias, errors, and omissions through the use of scripted questions and pre-arrival instructions that are structured and consistent. It is easy to audit and minimizes stress to the call taker/dispatcher.

MPDS call-taker training usually occurs over a 16- to 22-week period and includes basic clinical knowledge and specific call-taker techniques.

MPDS do not allow local customization of caller interrogation protocols or prearrival instructions. The National Academy of Emergency Medicine Dispatch controls MPDS and through its College of Fellows uses a systematic change process to ensure that changes to any protocol create the desired results relative to outcome. There are "cultural" versions that do reflect local terminology and situations: for example, adrenaline versus epinephrine or blue-ringed octopus which features in the Australian version and rattlesnake in the US version.

The automated version of the MPDS is ProQA™ (brand of dispatch software). It provides the caller interrogation script and on-line prearrival instructions. It time stamps protocol activation and provides response and referral recommendations. AQUA©

1. To identify the correct problem or situation and the proper response.
2. To determine the presence of conditions requiring the provision of prearrival instructions and special advice such as instructions on scene safety in the case of electrocution or on bystander CPR in the case of out-of-hospital cardiac arrest.
3. To provide necessary information to the responders so they can preplan their actions and collect appropriate equipment that will be needed while en route.
4. To provide for the safety of all those at the scene: patients, caller, bystanders, and responders.

(advanced quality assurance) software simplifies the process of case review, data collection, and analysis, facilitating quality control and improvement.

Quality review of the dispatch process should include assessment of the call-taking procedures, such as address verification, review of the taped conversations, the AQUA© data, the CAD data, and the subsequent event management.

Several studies have investigated the use of MPDS to triage emergency ambulance calls and assessed the subsequent resource allocation. In Delaware, US, inappropriate ALS responses were reduced by 19.9% using MPDS rather than a chief complaint–based system.[5] In the London Ambulance Service the detection of cardiac arrest increased by 200% by adapting MPDS as opposed to a criteria-based dispatch system. They also found an association between call-taker compliance and accurate cardiac arrest detection.[6]

The MPDS has been demonstrated to have a specificity of 99.2% for detecting cardiac arrest in an Australian study.[8] In this study, which examined 52,895 calls received, 403 responses were dispatched as priority 0, which subsequently did not turn out to be a cardiac arrest on assessment by the crew (403/52,895), while 172 cases were not dispatched as priority 0 and subsequently did turn out to be cardiac arrests (172/52,895).[8]

ProQA™ allows the option of overriding the recommended dispatch response-based code. Downgrading the code to a lower level may increase risk. Every override is captured in the ProQA™ system's coding records for review.[7]

CRITERIA-BASED DISPATCH

The Criteria-Based Dispatch (CBD) system was developed and is licensed by King County Emergency Medical Services in Seattle, Washington, US.[9] After asking a series of key questions, the call taker prioritizes the call and assigns the patient to a CBD category. The advantage of CBD is the freedom given to the person taking the call. For example, the initial information given by a caller may obviate the need for some questions; there is no need to ask about consciousness level if the caller is the patient. CBD allows the call taker to stop questioning as soon as a high-priority response is realized.

Each particular emergency service preassigns a response to each CBD or MPDS protocol endpoint or "determinant code." This code system allows an emergency service to best utilize the most appropriate response tailored to the likely needs of the particular situation. For example, some emergency services may have first responders, some BLS teams, some Advanced Life Support (ALS) teams, some physician response teams, or various combinations of these.

Not all patients who ring emergency services actually require an emergency unit response and may more appropriately and efficiently be dealt with by a general practitioner in the community, a nursing outreach service, or a community psychiatry service. Initial triage with MPDS or CBD is designed to rule out an emergency situation. Secondary triage requiring coordination between community and emergency services to meet the needs of the patient in a safe manner can then occur. An example here may be a nursing home patient whose urinary catheter falls out and needs to be replaced.

COMPUTER-AIDED DISPATCH (CAD)

CAD is a method of dispatching emergency services assisted by computer. The objective of CAD is to enable the dispatch center to easily view and understand the status of all units being dispatched. CAD provides displays so that the dispatcher has an opportunity to handle calls as efficiently and effectively as possible. A dispatcher may send call details to field units over a two-way radio or CAD systems may send text messages with call-for-service details to alphanumeric pagers or wireless telephone text services like SMS (short message service)

CAD systems have the following components: computer-aided dispatching software, mapping software, communications interface, radio system, alerting/

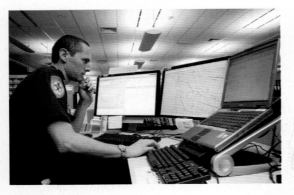

FIGURE 14-2

Dispatch screens for computerized dispatch.
Photo courtesy of Bill Barger.

paging systems, mobile data terminals in vehicles, automatic vehicle locating systems, and voice logging.

Computer technology has the advantage of being able to save at every step of data entry, allow for documentation in near-real time, allow sorting of information into categories, and permit quick on-line retrieval of data (see Figure 14-2).

In a CAD system, the caller's number and address are shown automatically at the call-taker's terminal in the communications center. The dispatcher makes an assignment based on the response preassigned to the MPDS dispatch code. GPS systems and the status of the unit (e.g., loaded, available, out of service) tell the dispatcher which unit is closest to the origin of the call and the appropriate unit is routed to the call.

CAD data and electronic patient care data provide information as to the performance of the emergency system as well as identifying opportunities for improvement both of a logistical and clinical care nature.

MOBILE DATA TERMINALS

Many emergency vehicles are fitted with GPS locators often built into their mobile data terminals, allowing the dispatcher to see the vehicle's location with respect to the call. A mobile data terminal (MDT) is a computerized device used in emergency vehicles to communicate with a central dispatch control. MDTs feature a screen on which to view information and a keyboard or keypad for entering information and may be connected to various peripheral devices. They are often used in conjunction with a "black box" that contains a GPS receiver, cell phone transceiver, or other radio devices. MDTs may be simple display and keypad units, where the keypad is activated to acknowledge response to call arrival at the scene, departure from the scene, arrival at

the hospital, and when free to take another call. Additionally, information such as hospital status, scene safety information, and messages related to previous attendances at the location or to that patient may be sent to the MDT to update the crew.

MDTs have the advantage of decreasing the amount of voice transmission over the airwaves. The use of visual data decreases the likelihood of error in communications that can occur with verbal communications. At the advanced end of the spectrum, MDTs may contain full, personal computing-equivalent hardware.

TELEMEDICINE AND ONLINE MEDICAL DIRECTION

Emergency response crews are increasingly utilizing telemedicine. Telemedicine is a rapidly developing application of clinical medicine in which medical information is transferred through the phone or the Internet and sometimes other networks for the purpose of consulting. On-line medical direction is available in many emergency systems. This may take the form of a Senior Clinician/Senior Advanced Paramedic based in the control room. Responsibilities may include clinical oversight, clinical advice, and recommendations on the appropriate clinical level of care and response needed for the particular situation. Many systems also allow for physicians to speak directly to the EMT involved in the patient's care by telephone or radio. These communications may involve communication of biotelemetric components such as transmission of an ECG to a specialist center or medical control facility.

RADIO

Key issues to consider for any communication system are guaranteed availability (the system will be working when you need it), guaranteed capacity (the system will be able to handle the amount of traffic you have when you need it), and guaranteed performance (the system will do what you need efficiently).

Two-way voice communication at fairly low band width remains the backbone of any telemedicine consultation and prehospital communications. Operation modes used for emergency medical services radio communications include simplex, multiplex, duplex, and trunked. The simplex mode means the transmitter and receiver operating on the same frequency transmit their message one at a time, obeying certain radio etiquette. The duplex mode uses two frequencies, allowing both parties to communicate at the same time. The multiplex mode has the advantage of transmitting telemetry and voice simultaneously from the field. A trunked radio system is a complex type of computer-controlled radio system. Trunked radio takes advantage of the probability that in any given number of user units, not everyone will need channel access at the same time. Therefore with a given number of users, fewer discrete radio channels are required.

In a trunk radio system, all users share a pool of frequencies from five up to a maximum of twenty-eight. Users are assigned a "group ID," and field radios are programmed to only pick up transmissions for that group. A computer, called the "site controller," automatically assigns a frequency for users belonging to the same group to communicate with each other. This is done over a data channel called the "control channel," which carries data that tell field radios what frequency they are on. Trunk radio systems may have one or more control channels and may rotate them every 24 hours.

For example, the ambulance emergency dispatcher is communicating on a frequency assigned by the controller. As soon as there is a break in the communications, the controller automatically moves all users in that talk group to the next available frequency. At the same time, the nonemergency transport is communicating on another assigned frequency, and as soon as there is a break in their communications, the controller moves them to the next available frequency.

Since communications on a trunked system never stay on one frequency, monitoring these communications with a conventional scanner is virtually impossible, especially in large metropolitan areas where a trunked system can have many users.

Digital radio systems allow for encryption of messaging as well as selectively alerting crew members when away from the vehicle.

The base station provides the hub for communications throughout the network. Base stations tend to be located at elevated positions to optimize transmission and reception. A base station will often be equipped with antennae to boost the signal. Communication between dispatch and the base station will often be through telephone lines. Vehicle-mounted transmitters usually operate at lower outputs than the base stations with a more limited range. They may be hampered by mountainous terrain or tall buildings. Portable transceivers are hand-held devices used by paramedics when away from the vehicle. These have a limited range. The signal may be boosted by a mobile or vehicular repeater. A repeater receives transmissions from a low-power portable at one frequency and at the same time retransmits them at a higher power on another frequency.

The "duress alarm" safety feature is a vital safety feature of a portable radio and vehicle radio system. These systems provide an alert back to the communication center and, in conjunction with Automatic Vehicle Location (AVL), allow the response of appropriate support.

CELLULAR PHONE

The cellular phone has more clarity, is a hands-free operation, allows simultaneous conversation, has an easier procedure to initiate communication, and has a low cost of system maintenance. However, cellular band width can be overwhelmed in the event of a major disaster. In such situations it is possible for the mobile network to only allow preassigned emergency mobile phones to operate. In addition, certain geographic areas continue to have inadequate network coverage.

Mobile phones may also be used by emergency services as part of a warning system designed to alert the community in the event of a life-threatening emergency, for example, bush fires or a toxic accident.

MAJOR/COMPLEX EVENTS

At times, planned and unplanned major or complex events occur; therefore a communications center needs to be able to manage this surge in demand while continuing to provide response to the "normal" day-to-day activity. Plans need to be in place and tested to deal with such occurrences. Such events require planning, communication, and coordination with other emergency services. Depending upon the complexity and anticipated duration of such events, the communication and coordination can be isolated from "normal" work and undertaken by those coordinating the event.

Surge capacity would be enhanced by a system that transparently captured the receiving hospital capacity and bed availability status in real time and coordinated this with the ambulance control room. Combining this information with ambulance distribution across the region would greatly enhance system capacity to respond.

Such a system would optimize coordination of ambulance availability with emergency department flow.

CLINICAL HANDOVER

The aim of effective clinical handover is seamless transfer of information and clinical responsibility between care providers. Handover between paramedics and the emergency receiving team provides challenges in ensuring that information loss does not occur. Handover is often time-pressured and paramedics' clinical notes are often delayed in reaching the trauma team. Documentation by emergency team members must be accurate.[11] Strategies that may be employed to decrease vulnerability to data loss are the use of cognitive aids such as acronyms ISBAR (Table 14-1)[12] or MIST (Table 14-2). These are standardized tools to increase the quality of information exchange. Electronic voice recognition technology incorporated into the electronic prehospital patient record and subsequent electronic transmission to the hospital record could offer great opportunity to improve patient handover safety and efficiency with further development.

Table 14–1	ISBAR[12]
I	Identify yourself and patient
S	Situation
B	Background
A	Assessment
R	Recommendation

From: Marshall S, Harrison J, Flanagan B. The teaching of a structured tool improves the clarity and content of interprofessional clinical communication. *Qual Saf Health Care* Apr;18(2): 137, 2009.

Table 14–2	MIST
M	Mechanism of injury, e.g., car versus pedestrian 60 kph (approximately 40 mph)
I	Injury, e.g., closed head injury, left femur fracture
S	Signs: Respiratory rate and effort, oxygen saturation on room air, heart rate and blood pressure, GCS
T	Treatment, e.g., 2 liters of IV fluids, 10 milligrams IV morphine, pelvic binder, Donway splint

GCS = Glasgow Coma Scale.
From: Ambulance Victoria Protocol Manual, Version 1, January 2009, available at: http://www.rav.vic.gov.au/Media/docs/CERT-Protocol-Manual-V1-January-2009-Final-7548caee-4beb-4716-b573-a3f6a0ed50a3.pdf.

SUMMARY

The communication system adopted by an EMS will determine the success of the EMS in accurate, timely dispatch of the appropriate resources to emergencies and the safe triage and handover of the patient to an appropriate healthcare facility. The communications architecture and protocols are fundamental building blocks for an EMS.

References

1. Ball WL. Telematics. *Prehosp Emerg Care* Jul-Sep; 10(3): 320, 2006.
2. Gossage JA, Frith DP, Carrell TW, et al. Mobile-phones, in combination with a computer locator system, improve the response times of emergency medical services in central London. *Ann R Coll Surg Engl* Mar;90(2): 113, 2008.
3. Larson RD. A conversation with Dr. Jeff Clawson. Emergency medical dispatch: looking back, looking ahead. 9-1-1 Magazine. Mar/Apr: 28, 1998.
4. Cocks RA, Glucksman E. What does London need from its ambulance service? *Br Med J* 306: 1428, 1993.
5. Bailey ED, O'Connor RE, Ross RW. The use of emergency medical dispatch protocols to reduce the number of inappropriate scene responses made by advanced life support personnel. *Prehosp Emerg Care* Apr–Jun;4(2): 186, 2000.
6. Heward A, Damiani M, Hartley-Sharpe C. Does the use of the Advanced Medical Priority Dispatch System affect cardiac arrest detection? *Emerg Med J* Jan;21(1): 115, 2004.
7. Clawson J, Olola CH, Heward A, et al. Accuracy of emergency medical dispatchers' subjective ability to identify when higher dispatch levels are warranted over a Medical Priority Dispatch System automated protocol's recommended coding based on paramedic outcome data. *Emerg Med J* Aug;24(8): 560, 2007.
8. Flynn J, Archer F, Morgans A. Sensitivity and specificity of the medical priority dispatch system in detecting cardiac arrest emergency calls in Melbourne. *Prehosp Disaster Med* Mar–Apr;21(2): 72, 2006.
9. Zachariah BS, Pepe PE. The development of emergency medical dispatch in the USA: A historical perspective. *Eur J Emerg Med* 2:109, 1995.
10. Clawson JJ, Martin RL, Hauert SA. Protocols vs. guidelines, choosing a medical-dispatch program. *Emerg Med Services* 23: 52, 1994.
11. Evans SM, Murray A, Patrick I, et al. Assessing clinical handover between paramedics and the trauma team. Injury. 2010 May;41(5):460-4. Epub 2009 Sep 6.
12. Marshall S, Harrison J, Flanagan B. The teaching of a structured tool improves the clarity and content of interprofessional clinical communication. *Qual Saf Health Care* Apr;18(2): 137, 2009.

CHAPTER 15

Patient Data Records and Patient Handover

Terrence Mulligan, Harm van de Pas, C. James Holliman

KEY LEARNING POINTS

- Patient care reports (PCRs) are an essential and required function of any prehospital/EMS system. PCRs should include pertinent data regarding the patient's complaint, history, physical and clinical condition, as well as documentation of any clinical changes, procedures done, or medications administered in the prehospital setting.

- PCRs should be automated and computerized whenever possible to aid in the collection, research, transfer, and dissemination of data as well as in quality improvement (QI).

- Handover procedures from prehospital personnel to the hospital medical staff should be performed with the utmost care and precision and should be a formal, official process involving strict adherence to protocol and regulation whenever possible.

- A QI system helps to provide ongoing improvement of the EMS system and education for personnel and can be used to maintain interest and morale. Physician involvement in QI for prehospital care is extremely important and should be included whenever possible.

While taking care of a patient, any health professional gathers data about the patient and the care given. This information has to be conveyed to the next person in the chain of care in a consistent, precise manner. In the case of EMS specifically, this transfer is often complicated and more difficult because it often involves time-sensitive information about critical, emergent, unstable patients as well.

It is no surprise that the transfer of information is prone to error. Like in the childhood game called "whispers," where the first person whispers a message into the ear of the next person, who then whispers the message to the next, information transfers will invariably be associated with some unavoidable degree of information omission, error, and noise. Sometimes handovers between different levels of ambulances occur as well, adding to the potential of information loss or distortion. It is the job of health care professionals to account for this information loss and to design information systems, patient data records, and patient handover procedures that limit this information loss and distortion to an absolute minimum wherever possible (Figure 15-1).

The Continuum of Care

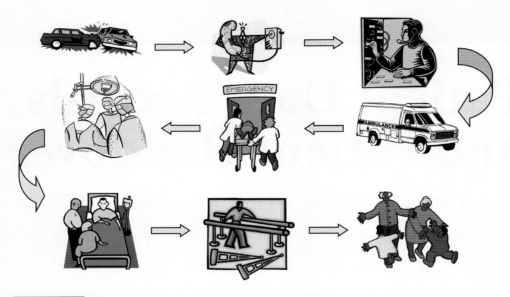

FIGURE 15–1

The continuum of care. Information relay in prehospital health care: accident → caller → dispatcher → ambulance personnel (who must also interact with patients, family, and others) → ED personnel → emergency physicians and acute care personnel → inpatient and outpatient services → rehabilitation and recovery services → reentry into home, family, and workforce.

PATIENT CARE RECORD – RUN REPORT/RUN SHEET

Also called the "patient data record," the "run sheet," and the "run report," the patient care record (PCR) is a collection of all the data of value to the hospital-based care providers that should be recorded to avoid information loss, decay, and omission.

Patient identifying information is recorded on the PCR. In some countries a unique numerical identifier is available. Laws may be applicable and even mandate recording of this person-specific number.

While taking care of the patient, a number of things are measured, done to, or communicated about the patient. Vital signs are recorded with the time they were obtained to get an overview of the vital signs as a function of time.

Application of cervical collars, splints, spine boards, and other immobilization methods are an essential part of the run report as they provide the necessary information for hospital care providers. Depending on the level of EMT, therapy is started according to protocol or after consulting with on-line medical direction. Time, dose, and route of all medication are all recorded. If therapy was started according to protocol, reference is made to this protocol by name and number.

In some countries, certain treatments can only be done by health care professionals of certain levels. These usually are treatments that if done without sufficient skill and training could harm patients. Examples of these are central IV cannulation, endotracheal intubation, and defibrillation. These should be recorded with extra care and the run report should contain enough information to show who provided this specific part of the care and why.

DISPATCH DATA

Historically since the beginning of ambulance care, dispatchers and EMTs alike have been recording data on tape (dispatch) or paper (ambulance). In the setting of increasing demand for information, for accountability and for quality improvement and liability claims, the need for data recording has only increased. In some systems this has led to a form of information overload with too much time spent gathering, transmitting, and transferring data. This may then lead to unnecessary delays and complications. This poses the question of what is the appropriate level of data provided by each link in the chain, such that no pertinent and important data are omitted and no unnecessary and superfluous data are included. The main initial data points must include the following:

Location

A major factor in timely delivery of ambulance care is the exact location of required care. Dispatch should provide the ambulance unit with a location as precisely as possible.

Safety

Safety of ambulance personnel is of paramount importance. Any concerns regarding safety should be apparent to the EMTs. If the dispatcher suspects an unsafe working environment for the ambulance crew, the ambulance should not proceed to the location itself but instead wait until the location has been made safe. This usually requires the presence of a police or fire department.

Reason for Dispatch

Depending on the information, EMTs will take different material to the scene from their ambulance. Although the information a caller provides at times necessitates the dispatcher to send an ambulance on nothing more than "unwell," usually the dispatcher will be able to provide more information. As this information can cause an EMT to make an incorrect diagnosis, the dispatcher should provide information that is as objective as possible: for example, "chest pain and shortness of breath" would be a better way to dispatch than "hyperventilation syndrome," as it keeps all possibilities open. This way of (mis)guiding the next person's thoughts is called a cognitive disposition to respond (CDR), specifically *Diagnostic Momentum*.[1]

We will use a sample template from the Maryland Ambulance Information System (MAIS), from the State of Maryland, US, which has a statewide, state-run prehospital/ambulance system, to discuss components of a PCR. This form was used throughout the entire state by all prehospital professionals from 2003–2007. This is a standardized computer form that is filled out by hand but that is then read into a computer to automatically capture the data. As of 2007, Maryland and many other EMS systems began the transition to fully computer-aided or computer-entry of PCRs and other prehospital/ambulance data. We will discuss these and other advances in prehospital information technology (IT) and electronic data sheets later in this chapter.

The Sample Patient Care Record of the State of Maryland EMS System, US, is available at http://www.nhtsa-tsis.net/ems/state/MD/Mais2003.pdf.

Sections marked are as follows:

1. Jurisdiction, Patient, and Provider Identification
2. Call Date/Case Number
3. Documentation of Response Times
4. Response Identification
5. Patient Demographics
6. Vital Signs, GCS, and other calculated trauma scores
7. Signs and Symptoms
8. Cardiac Arrest, CPR
9. Airway/Ventilation
10. Medications
11. Hospital Codes
12. Transportation and Communication
13. Provider Exposure
14. Documentation of Care Rendered
15. Narrative Information

We will discuss this Sample Patient Care Record in detail section by section as a description of some of the necessary and recommended data that need to be collected by the PCR. Each of the above sections will be discussed, with depictions whether certain sections or subsections should be **required, recommended, or optional**.

SECTION 1: Jurisdiction, Patient, and Provider Information

- Station Run Number, Jurisdiction Incident Number, Box Number, District: All data regarding selection of ambulance companies, jurisdiction, and other locally determined codes necessary for local record-keeping for private companies, legal requirements, and hospitals. OPTIONAL
- Receiving Facility: Record the name of the receiving facility to which you transported this patient. REQUIRED
- Other Units on Scene: Identify other emergency units responding to this call. RECOMMENDED

- Response Location: Record the location where your unit encountered the patient. Be as specific as possible. For example, record the exact street address to which you responded for a medical call, names of intersecting streets for vehicular accidents, or another geographic location description, such as Memorial Park, for a child with seizure. REQUIRED
- ZIP Code: Record the ZIP code/postal code for the location to which you responded. RECOMMENDED
- Incident Type, Occupancy type, Action, Disposition: Record the type of incident, the occupancy type, action and disposition required/encountered on this call. OPTIONAL
- Patient Name Print: The patient's last name, first name, middle initial. REQUIRED
- Parent/Guardian: In the case of a minor child, print the last name, first name of the child's parent or legal guardian. REQUIRED
- Patient Address: Print the patient's residential address. Note that the residence address may differ from the response location. REQUIRED
- Home Phone: Print the patient's home phone number. Include the area code. REQUIRED
- Provider 1 ID Number, Provider 1 Name: Record the unique numeric identifiers for the providers on this call. RECOMMENDED

SECTION 2: Call Date/ Case Number

- Call Date: Mark the month, day, and year responses for your call date in the fields provided. REQUIRED
- MAIS Number/Case Number: A preprinted unique ID/case number for each PCR, printed on original and carbon copies of this particular PCR. REQUIRED

SECTION 3: Documentation of Response Times

You should document each response time for your call in this section. Response time data allow standardized evaluation of time intervals within jurisdictions as well as statewide. Please darken the responses for all time intervals that apply to your current call.

- **911 CALL:** Time the 911/112/EMS dispatcher received the call for EMS intervention.
- **AMB CALL:** The time your station was notified of the call.
- **DPT STA:** The time your unit departed the station.

- **ARV LOC:** The time your unit arrived at the location of the incident.
- **DPT LOC:** The time your unit departed the location. The depart location time should be completed regardless of whether or not your unit transports a patient.
- **ARV HOS:** The time your unit arrived at the receiving facility. The arrive hospital time should be left blank if the call results in no patient transport.
- **RTN SERV:** The time your unit is available for the next request for EMS intervention. The return service time should be recorded each time you respond to a call.
- All of these time intervals should be REQUIRED or STRONGLY RECOMMENDED data points.

SECTION 4: Response Identification

CTY: (County, City code) Mark the responses that correspond to your unit's base county or city (CTY). This code should always reflect your unit's base jurisdiction number even though you may respond to another jurisdiction. REQUIRED

- Unit: Record your unit's identification number. REQUIRED
- Highest Staff: Indicate the highest certification level among the providers on your unit. RECOMMENDED
- Dispatch: Mark the **ALS** or **BLS** or other tiered-response based on the life support level assigned to this call at dispatch. Mark only one dispatch level.
- First Due: Mark **Yes** if your unit was considered the first due/first assigned unit for this call. If your unit was not the first assigned, mark the **No** response. OPTIONAL
- No Care Rendered: If you were dispatched to a call that resulted in no patient care by your unit, you should indicate the reason no care was required. Mark only one response. RECOMMENDED
  - PDOA: Patient was presumed dead on the arrival of your unit at the scene.
  - Cancel: Your response was cancelled while your unit was en route or upon the arrival of your unit at the scene.
  - False: The call was determined to be false; EMS was not required.
  - No Pt: The potential need for patient care existed but was not required.
  - Refuse: Patient refused all care and transportation.

- Unit 2: Your unit was not required to provide care because other unit(s) at the scene were managing the patient(s).
- Priority: Record the triage priority for your patient based on your local EMS guidelines. RECOMMENDED
  - One: Critically ill or injured. Requires immediate attention. A delay in treatment may be harmful to patient.
  - Two: Less serious condition. Requires emergency medical attention.
  - Three: Nonemergent condition. Requires medical attention but not on an emergency basis.
  - Four: Does not require medical attention and may not require transport.
  - N/A: Priority assessment does not apply to this call (for example, no patient).

SECTION 5: Patient Demographics

Record the age, race, and gender of your patient in the Patient Demographics section.

- Age: If your patient is between 2 and 11 months old, you should mark the M response as well as responses for the appropriate number of months. Patients between the ages of 1 and 31 days old should have the D response marked along with the appropriate number of days. Leave the M and D responses blank for patients one year of age or older. REQUIRED
- Race/Ethnicity: Respondents shall select their own answers, except when it is not possible for them to do so. A form that requires identification of individuals by race includes this information for identification purposes only and may be omitted. OPTIONAL
- Gender: Mark the response that corresponds to your patient's gender. REQUIRED

SECTION 6: Vital Signs, Glucose, General Physical Exam, GCS, and Other Calculated Trauma Scores

- Vital Signs: Record the first set of vital signs based on the findings of your primary assessment of your patient. All vital signs are recorded in the same manner. REQUIRED
- Glucose Monitoring: Darken the glucometer response if you monitor blood glucose. You should note the blood glucose value elsewhere. RECOMMENDED

- Loss of Consciousness Pior to Arrival: Mark **Yes** if there are signs or testimony that your patient was unconscious prior to the arrival of your unit. Mark **No** if there were no indications of loss of consciousness. OPTIONAL
- Lung Sounds: Mark the normal response(s) for **r**ight and/or **l**eft lung(s) if your primary assessment found equal, clear breath sounds.
  - Mark the wheeze response(s) for right and/or left lung(s) if your primary assessment found whistling-type breath sounds associated with narrowing or spasm of the smaller airways.
  - Mark the rales responses(s) for **r**ight and/or **l**eft lung(s) if your primary assessment found abnormal breath sounds due to the presence of fluid in the smaller airways.
  - Mark the brhonchi response(s) for **r**ight and/or **l**eft lung(s) if your primary assessment found abnormal breath sounds due to the presence of fluid or mucus in the larger airways.
- Glasgow Coma Score: Mark the appropriate responses for Glasgow Coma Score eye, motor, and verbal responses. Verbal responses should be determined based on the patient's age.
- Safety Equipment Used: Document the use or nonuse of safety equipment by your patient if applicable. Mark all responses that apply.
- Trauma Identifier(s): Document the trauma identifier(s) that apply to your patient. Trauma identifier data should be reported for all serious injury patients independent of transportation to a designated specialty center. Mark all responses that apply.
- Mechanisms of Injury: Report all factors associated with your patient's injuries that may warrant special consideration. Trauma mechanism(s) data should be documented for all serious injury patients independent of transportation to a designated specialty center. Mark all responses that apply.

SECTION 7: Signs and Symptoms, Injury Types

This section includes a broad range of assessment information related to your patient's current need for prehospital care.

- Signs and Symptoms: Report signs and symptoms related to your patient's current condition in this section. Note that some signs and symptoms relate to both injury and medical patients. Mark all responses that apply. If your patient experienced signs or symptoms other than those listed, you should mark the "other" response and note the signs or symptoms in the blank space provided at the bottom of the form. REQUIRED

- Injury Types: Use the injury type section to report causes of injuries experienced by your patient. Mark all responses that apply. If you need to document an injury type other than those listed, mark the "other" response and note the other injury type in the blank space provided at the bottom of the form. RECOMMENDED
- Conditions: Mark the illness(es) or medical condition(s) contributing to your patient's current need for prehospital care. Mark all responses that apply. To document a condition other than those listed, mark the "other" response and note the other condition in the blank space provided at the bottom of the form. RECOMMENDED
- ECG: Document your patient's first (**F**) and last (**L**) electrocardiogram rhythms. If you need to document a cardiac rhythm other than those listed, mark the "other" response and provide a description in the blank space provided at the bottom of the form. Document whether a three-lead or twelve-lead ECG was used by marking the appropriate response. RECOMMENDED
- Circulation: Use this section to indicate attempts and successes/failures at IV lines, external jugular (EJ) lines, intraosseous (IO) lines. Record the anatomic site and needle gauge used in IV placement on the line provided at the bottom of the form. OPTIONAL
- Note: Record the amount (total mL) of intravenous fluids infused during prehospital care elsewhere on the form. REQUIRED

SECTION 8: Cardiac Arrest Witnessed (e.g., CPR)

- Cardiac Arrest Witnessed: Mark Yes if the signs and/or symptoms of cardiac arrest were witnessed at the onset. Mark No if the signs and/or symptoms of cardiac arrest were not witnessed at onset. RECOMMENDED
- CPR Start By: If CPR is initiated, identify the EMS training level of the individual providing care. In cases where multiple individuals administered CPR procedures, record the training level of the highest certified individual. You should note the time CPR was initiated in the blank space elsewhere on the form. RECOMMENDED
- AED Start By: If use of an AED is initiated, identify the EMS training level of the individual providing care. In cases where multiple individuals administered AED procedures, record the training level of

the highest certified individual. You should note the time AED use was initiated in the blank space provided at the bottom of the form. OPTIONAL

- Return of Spontaneous Circulation at ED: Darken the **Yes** response if the patient did experience return of spontaneous circulation prior to arrival at an ED. If the patient did not experience return of spontaneous circulation prior to arrival at an ED, darken the No response. RECOMMENDED

SECTION 9: Airway/ Ventilation Procedures, Other Care Rendered

- Airway/Ventilation: Document all of the airway/ventilation equipment or procedures attempted. You should write the number of liters per minute at which oxygen was administered elsewhere on the form. If you use procedures or equipment other than those listed, mark the Other response and note the procedure or equipment used.
- Procedures: Identify attempts and successes for other types of prehospital procedures. You should also identify the providers performing each procedure.
  - ET: Endotracheal tube placement attempts and successes, ET tube size and provider number.
  - NT: Nasotracheal tube placement attempts and successes, NT tube size and provider number.
  - NDT: Needle decompression thoracostomy attempts and successes, NDT catheter size and provider number.
  - DEFIB: Defibrillation attempts and successes and provider number.
  - AED attempts and successes and provider number.
  - CARDIO attempts and successes and provider number.
  - PACE attempts and successes and provider number.
  - COMBI intubation using a Combitube attempts and successes and provider number.
  - OTHER CARE RENDERED: Document all care rendered to your patient. If you provide care other then the types listed, mark the Other response and note the type of care elsewhere on the form. Note that the use of restraints should be included; this can be identified by the type of restraint; "C" for chemical, "P" for physical.

SECTION 10: Medications

Document all of the medications administered to your patient, the provider number and certification level of that provider, plus all medications administered that required medical control. These medications naturally would need to conform to local Rx formularies, availability, and other common uses and practices.

- Select which medicine(s) were given and which provider gave the medicine(s).
- Other medicines not listed here should be indicated elsewhere on the form.

SECTION 11: Hospital Codes

- Darken the hospital code numbers (from locally-derived hospital information) that correspond to the consulting, transferring, and receiving hospitals for this call. If this call requires consultation with a hospital, darken the responses that correspond to the consulting hospital's code number in the Consulting section.
- If this call is an interhospital transfer, darken the responses that correspond to the transferring hospital's code in the Transferring section. Mark the responses that correspond to the receiving hospital's code in the Receiving section.

SECTION 12: Transportation/ Communication/Special Purpose

- Transport by:
  - Mark only **one** response in the Transport By section.
  - Mark No Transport if your current call resulted in no patient transport.
  - Mark This Unit if the patient was transported by your unit.
  - Mark Other Unit if the patient was transported by another ground unit.
  - Mark Other Air if the patient was transported by helicopter. RECOMMENDED
- Reason Hospital Chosen: Document the reason a particular receiving facility was chosen for this patient. Naturally these would depend on local regulations, hospitals, and other capabilities.
  - Closest protocols and conditions allowed transport to closest hospital.
  - Spec Ref; patient required the services of a specialty referral center. These include designated centers for (where applicable):
    - Perinatal Complications/Neonatal Complications
    - Hand/Extremity Injuries/Reimplantation Hyperbaric Medicine
    - Neurotrauma/Pediatric Trauma

- Adult Trauma/Eye Trauma
- Burn Trauma
- Rerte-Alert: patient transport was rerouted because the closest hospital was on alert.
- Rerte-Consult: patient transport was rerouted because of physician consult doing transport.
- Interfacility transfer: patient transfer from one facility to another.
- Routine: Nonemergent transport according to departmental regulations.
- Patient: Patient or guardian specified receiving hospital.
- Stroke Care: identifies patients transported to a particular facility based on Stroke protocol. NOTE: Other protocols can be added here. RECOMMENDED
- **R**adio: Document the quality of the EMS radio communications for this call.
  - No Attempt: This call did not require radio communication.
  - Good: All communications were discernible.
  - Poor: Some communications were not discernible and required repeated transmissions beyond normal expectations.
  - Failed: Radio communications failed to permit proper or complete transmission of information.
  - OPTIONAL
- Special purpose
  - Mul Pat Seen: Two or more patients were assessed/treated on this call regardless of whether anyone was transported.
  - Mul Pat Trans: Two or more patients were transported from this incident.
  - Haz Mat: Hazardous materials protocols were required in response to this call.
  - Fire Rehab: Identifies this call as EMS activity related to a working fire.
  - Add Nar: Indicates an additional narrative form was completed for this patient.
  - Excep Call: Documents call that fall outside the normal standard of performance. RECOMMENDED

SECTION 13: Provider Exposure

PROV. EXP	(NS) (B) (A) (O)

- Provider exposure: Document any exposure to a potentially infectious agent by marking the appropriate responses. Mark as many responses as are applicable.

- Mark the NS (needle stick) response if any member of the crew on this unit experienced a needle stick.
- Mark the B (blood) response for exposures to blood or any body fluid. This applies to both mucous or percutaneous exposures. For example, if blood splashed in the eye, nose, or on broken skin, mark this response.
- Mark the A (airborne) response for exposure to airborne pathogens. If your patient coughed or sneezed in close proximity to any member of the crew on your unit, or if the patient exhibited other signs of respiratory illness, mark this response.
- Mark the O (other) response for exposure to other body fluids such as vomitus, urine, stool, or CSF. You should document specifics of any exposure in the narrative section of this report before leaving the receiving facility. RECOMMENDED

SECTION 14: Documentation of Care Rendered, Narrative Information, and Form Identification

Space should be provided at the bottom of the form to document the following information based on the care rendered to your patient:

- SAO_2: Record the patient's saturated oxygen value based on pulse oximetry in the boxes provided.
- ET size: Record the endotracheal tube size if you intubated the patient.
- O_2L pm: Record the liters per minute of oxygen administered to the patient.
- Total mL: Record the amount of intravenous fluids infused during prehospital care in the boxes provided.
- Glucose: If you monitored the patient's blood glucose level with a glucometer, you should record the glucose level in the boxes provided.
- Gauge/Site: Record the anatomic site(s) and needle gauge used for IV placement.
- Mileage: Record the number of miles driven for this call.
- On-Line Physician: Record the name of the physician who provided medical direction during radio consult.
- Provider: Record the name. The provider considered to be the medically responsible provider among the crew.
- Signature: He or she should sign on the provider signature line.
- Hospital: Obtain the signature of an authorized hospital employee at the time you deliver the patient.

- Sign your patient into the receiving facility. Protocols stipulate that the employee receiving the patient must be at least the same or higher level of training as the highest certified provider on the unit.
- EMS: The name of the individual reviewing the contents of the form should be recorded on the
- Reviewer: EMS reviewer line.
- PROV #: Documents which provider (1, 2, or 3) was responsible for the provision of care reported in this entry.
- TIME: Military time corresponding to the time care was provided.
- BP: Blood pressure at the time care was given.
- Pulse: Pulse at the time care was given.
- Resp: Respirations at the time care was given.
- Rhythm: Rhythm from ECG reading, if applicable.
- Care Provided: Document other care such as administering medications here.
- Amount: Use this space to document amounts of meds administered.

SECTION 15: Narrative Information

Space should be provided to document pertinent information about your call. If you require additional space, please complete an additional narrative form.

This sample patient care record is included as a template only for PCRs for other EMS systems and in other locations/regions. An ideal PCR will allow data collection and immediate availability and accessibility and would also allow data collection to be computerized and automated for future uses.

Naturally the data items collected by this form do not apply to every EMS system, and PCRs need to be formulated for specific situations, locations, regions, languages, resources, regulations, and customs.

CALCULATED DATA

Certain data are not inherently recorded on the PCRs but can be calculated using PCR data. The following are such calculated data points, which can be used for quality assessment and improvement and for focus for future improvements and development.

Time Points

Accurate recording of crucial points in time during prehospital patient care is important, as it provides vital information about the timeliness of care. Monitoring the on-scene time intervals is important, as shortening on-scene time intervals results in greater availability of the prehospital care personnel to respond to other

Table 15–1	Specific Time Points to Be Recorded

1. Time of call: The time an emergency call is received by dispatch. If a caller is transferred from one desk to another, all these times should be noted
2. Time of dispatch: This is the time an ambulance unit is called and they have confirmed the order
3. Time of ambulance arrival: The time the ambulance arrives on the scene
4. Time of departure from the scene: The time the ambulance leaves the scene
5. Time of arrival at destination: The time the ambulance has arrived at the designated destination
6. Time of offloading: The time the ambulance has offloaded the patient and is ready to receive new calls

cases. In addition, it is likely that the survival rate for major trauma cases is better when the on-scene time intervals are short and transport is rapidly facilitated (especially with penetrating trauma). The standard "target time limits" utilized in some areas of the US are 20 minutes for a medical case, 10 to 20 minutes for a trauma case, and 10 minutes for a basic life support (not requiring paramedic care) case (Table 15-1).

If more than one unit is dispatched to the scene, then six time points are recorded for each unit. Several ways of recording exist, ranging from calling dispatch on the radio to report the status through systems where the unit electronically reports on its status to fully automated systems supported by a GPS. It is prudent to record the communication between dispatch and ambulance units, as it helps greatly in quality improvement and system analysis in case of an incident.

Clearly, there are a large number of reasons for which an on-scene time interval may exceed the target time limit that had been preset. These valid reasons can be categorized as delay in access to the patient, delay in evaluation of the patient, or delay in egress with the patient (Table 15-2, Table 15-3, and Table 15-4). In the US systems that carefully monitor on-scene time intervals, it is required that documentation be provided for any case in which the on-scene time interval exceeds the target time limit.

Vehicle Data

Specifics about the scene can be of great importance to the care delivered later on in the chain of care. Infor-

Table 15–2	Some Valid Reasons for Delay in Access to the Patient

The site of the incident is located a long distance from the access road
Other vehicles block access by the prehospital personnel
Initially there is no answer at the door of the building
A crowd of people may block or limit access by the prehospital personnel
There is an unsecured scene (potential violent situation and police not present on scene yet)
Slow elevator in a high-rise multistory building.
Weather conditions such as deep snow

mation about deformity to the vehicle can provide clues to the possible injuries to a patient in a motor vehicle accident. Information can be included in the PCR or during the narrative conversation handover regarding vehicular information, including:

1. Vehicle deformity/destruction
2. Shattered front windshields or side windows
3. Airbag deployment
4. Bent, broken, or deformed steering wheel
5. Use of seatbelts

Table 15–3	Some Valid Reasons for On-Scene Time Extension Due to Delay in Patient Evaluation

Patient using the bathroom
Repeated emesis by the patient
Initial refusal of care or transport with subsequent consent to care or transport
The patient or family speaks a different language than the prehospital personnel
A situation of multiple patients but only one prehospital care crew is on-scene initially
Having to wait on another person to arrive to care for children or pets of the patient or to provide security for the residence after the patient is transported
Waiting on a psychiatric health care worker to assist in involuntary transport of a psychiatric patient

Table 15–4	Some Valid Reasons That Would Extend On-Scene Time Due to Delay in Egress of Patient

The need to move furniture for access of the stretcher

Slow elevators in a high rise multistory building to bring the patient down to the ambulance

The need to move a heavy patient down or up stairs

A long distance from the scene back to the parking location of the ambulance vehicle

Environmental conditions such as snow or ice

6. Need for extrication/"jaws of life" use and length of extrication
7. Deformity/destruction of other vehicles/property/landmarks
8. A photograph of the scene can be invaluable

Other PCR Data

Information about the home environment can point to a possible cause of illness: whether the home was cold or hot or contained any heating elements/open fires. The state of hygiene and cleanliness in the home can point to the recent state of health of the patient involved, and should be noted in the PCR. Also in many EMS systems in the US, prehospital personnel are taught and instructed to go to the patient's medical cabinets or to their bedside medication supply to document the patient's sometimes lengthy list of prescription and nonprescription medications.

Electronic Patient Care Reports

Computers are increasingly used by emergency medical services around the world. A fairly new development is that of the electronic run report. Part of the information is handed over automatically from dispatch to ambulance. This saves time and increases accuracy of data transfer. Electronically gathered data on the scene can be transmitted to a receiving hospital, which can then make necessary arrangements to receive the patient with the appropriate team. An added benefit of electronically sending information ahead is that photographs of the scene as well as ECGs and other evidence can be read by the treating physician at the hospital. These can direct care even before the patient has arrived: a cardiac intervention team can be notified and the trauma team can have more accurate knowledge about the scene even before the patient has arrived in the resuscitation area.

The development and use of new computer systems provide the opportunity for very efficient systems for QI. Computer systems, however, may not be applicable to all organizations, since sometimes the amount of personnel time and expense in entering data in such a system can be greater than simply reviewing the data "manually."[1] The main advantage of a computer-based QI system is that the recorded data on cases can be re-reviewed and re-sorted by categories conveniently and efficiently.

In a supplement to the *Journal of EMS* called "Going electronic: Prehospital patient care reports in the digital age" (*JEMS*, August 2009 Supplement), the authors concisely and systematically described the advantages and disadvantages and the insights and the lessons learned from the adoption and implementation of electronic PCRs for the prehospital environment. The publication documents the advantages of having an ePCR, including the ability to generate reports of data collected for patient care, quality, and clinical research purposes.

Other available functions of the ePCR are described in Table 15-5.

Table 15-6 shows some of the possible automated data collection and reports available on different topics for the purposes of clinical care, quality improvement, and research.

In general, the supplement offers the following main points to consider:

1. Using an electronic patient care reporting (ePCR) system at the patient's side must be quick and easy.
2. You should be able to record patient vital signs, procedures, drug dosages, and current medical history as fast as you can touch the screen with your finger.
3. Real-time data can become a form of vital signs to your EMS agency. Just like vital signs can be incorrect or misinterpreted, so can data.
4. The blanket statement that "an ePCR solution will lead to better reimbursement results" must be tested within your own department.

(Source: *JEMS*, August 2009 Supplement; http://www.jems.com/Images/ePCR%20Supp%20FINAL_tcm16-207899.pdf).

In summary, the *JEMS* report on ePCRs offers the nine points in Table 15-7 to evaluate when considering an ePCR system.

Table 15–5	**Available Functions of the ePCR (electronic Patient Care Report)**		
Function	**Description**	**Specific data**	**Downside**
Integration	Pulls together data from many different electronic modules and allows transfer of information to the hospital	Computer-aided dispatch Call intake Ambulance status and locations iSTAT and other ambulance lab tests ECGs and rhythms Time analysis Hospital status Data recovery	Can lead to "information overload" Requires extensive collaboration between ambulance and hospital information and computer systems Existing systems can be hard/impossible to integrate with new additions Start-up costs can be prohibitive
Automation	Many current functions are automatically collected, compiled, transferred, and collated to allow more efficient resource allocation	PCRs are entered directly into the IT system Billing for EMS services more automated Resource and equipment function/failure reports Automatic prompts for appropriate care, interventions, physician input and oversight	Conversion and teaching curves can be problematic and time-consuming in a system that cannot afford to be shut down while being refitted IT communication can be problematic
Administration	Allows automated oversight, quality data collection and calculation, and administrative tasks	Weekly/monthly/regular summary reports of quality and administrative data ePCR documentation completeness Protocol used documentation Vital sign documentation Skills performed documentation Skill proficiency Protocol compliance Number of ePCRs completed Continuing education hours Individual dispatch times EMD protocol compliance Controlled substance log compliance	Initial learning curve and administrator buy-in can be problematic Again, initial start-up costs can be prohibitive

Patient Handovers

Regardless of the type of patient care report used by the prehospital medical staff, when patients are brought to emergency departments, hospitals, or other health-care facilities it is necessary to impart pertinent information to the waiting medical, nursing, and health professional staff at the receiving institution.

Whether this information is delivered verbally, in handwritten form, in electronic form, or in any and all other formats, there are certain pearls and pitfalls that can and should be expected from this process.

The process of patient transfer, also called "patient handover," is a very complicated procedure. It involves many different types of communication between health professionals of differing levels of training, experience,

Table 15–6   EMS ePatient Care Reports

Individual Patient Care

Patients with no documented protocol
Patients with no documented category (Defined by NEMSIS E09-11, 12, 13, and 15)
Patients with medication complications
Patients with skill complications
Patient triage and destination plan compliance
Patient pain control

High-Risk Groups Patient Care

Frequent flyers (EMS use greater than four times per month)
Repeat patients (within 48 hours)
Deaths while in EMS care
Patients with restraint use
Patient refusals
EMS patients where EMS response was canceled by first responder
Patients with obstetric deliveries by EMS
Patients with assisted ventilation or invasive airway use
Patients who underwent drug-assisted intubation or rapid sequence intubation
Patients who underwent chest decompression
Patients who underwent cardioversion
Patients who met trauma center criteria
Patients with acute STEMI
Patients with acute stroke
Pediatric patients with acute serious illness or injury
Patients with cardiac arrest
Patients with a Glasgow Coma Score of <9
Patients with abnormal vital signs

High-Risk EMS Events Care

Physician on scene
Multiple patients
Mass gathering
Police custody
Tactical EMS
Wilderness EMS rescue

Source: *JEMS*, August 2009 Supplement; available at http://www.jems.com/Images/ePCR%20Supp%20 FINAL_tcm16-207899.pdf.

authority, education, personality, and background, and there are many steps involved in effectively delivering the necessary information in a timely, accurate, reliable, and reproducible fashion.

In a report by the World Health Organization (WHO) and the Joint Commission International called "Communication During Patient Handovers," the authors define this problem as follows:

During an episode of disease or period of care, a patient can potentially be treated by a number of health care practitioners and specialists in multiple settings, including primary care, specialized outpatient care, emergency care, surgical care, intensive care, and rehabilitation. Additionally, patients will often move between areas of diagnosis, treatment, and care on a regular basis and may encounter three shifts of staff each day—introducing a safety risk to the patient at each interval. The handover (or hand-off) communication between units and between and among care teams might not include all the essential information or information may be misunderstood. These gaps in communication can cause serious breakdowns in the continuity of care, inappropriate treatment, and potential harm to the patient. http://www.ccforpatientsafety.org/common/pdfs/fpdf/presskit/PS-Solution3.pdf.

They conclude by suggesting the following strategies to improve this process of patient handover, much of which applies to the prehospital-to-hospital handover process:

The following strategies should be considered by WHO Member States.

1. Ensure that health care organizations implement a standardized approach to handover communication between staff, change of shift, and between different patient care units in the course of a patient transfer. Suggested elements of this approach include:
   a. Use of the SBAR (Situation, Background, Assessment, and Recommendation) technique.
   b. Allocation of sufficient time for communicating important information and for staff to ask and respond to questions without interruptions wherever possible. (Repeat-back and read-back steps should be included in the handover process.)
   c. Provision of information regarding the patient's status, medications, treatment plans, advance directives, and any significant status changes.
   d. Limitation of the exchange of information to that which is necessary to providing safe care to the patient.
2. Ensure that health care organizations implement systems which ensure—at the time of hospital discharge—that the patient and the next health care provider are given key information regarding discharge diagnoses, treatment plans, medications, and test results.

Table 15–7	**The 9-Point Evaluation System When Considering Implementing an ePCR**
1. Compatible with Existing Mobile Laptops	Ensure the new ePCR program works with, and does not require major modifications to, existing hardware and software
2. IT—Existing Database and Field Connectivity	Involve the IT department in the very beginning. New and old machine/platforms should be able to communicate with each other
3. Existing Interfaces (CAD, Billing, ECG Monitor)	Ensure the new ePCR program actually meets functional expectations and has a substantial enough existing feature set to meet current and future needs (i.e., normal everyday EMS uses should be built-in as standard functions)
4. Local IT/Software Gold Standard/Clinical Data Fields	Software should meet local and national "Gold Standard" certifications, if applicable
5. Existing Features (CQI, Multiple Assessments)	Software should have a CQI module, data validation capabilities, and the ability to deal with multiple patient assessments
6. Ad Hoc and Canned Reporting	ePCR solutions that don't offer extensive reporting capabilities (including custom reports) should be rejected, as should solutions that don't offer SSL authenticated Web access, the ability to select which specific computers and users would have access or that did not provide highly detailed audit trails
7. Legal Compliance for Patient Privacy and Audit Trails	Software and hardware should be private, confidential, and protected. Data should not be available to nonauthorized individuals. Data on specific individuals, units, and procedures should be available
8. Maintenance and Support	Systems that do not offer 24/7/365 user and technical support should be rejected. Systems should also offer reasonably priced upgrades that are easy to install. Vendors should have an active program of soliciting and responding to customer input on operating issues, functionality, and feature set
9. Usability	Ensure that "users" are extensively involved in the ePCR selection process Solutions that pass the first eight criteria can still be rejected if they are deemed to be difficult to use, nonintuitive, or time-consuming Make sure that the final cost of the ePCR program is rational and in line with the benefits to be experienced

3. Incorporate training on effective handover communication into the educational curricula and continuing professional development for health care professionals.
4. Encourage communication between organizations that are providing care to the same patient in parallel (for example, traditional and nontraditional providers).

See Figure 15-2 Communication During Patient Handover.

Prehospital-to-Hospital Patient Handovers

Information about prehospital events and findings can help ensure expedient and appropriate care. Despite this, accurate information required to measure the time it takes to hand over patients from ambulance crews to hospital EDs is not yet available. While certainly there have been some positive steps to improving the handover process, the true extent to which delays occur is unclear. Handover times are not being consistently recorded because of problems with new data terminals,

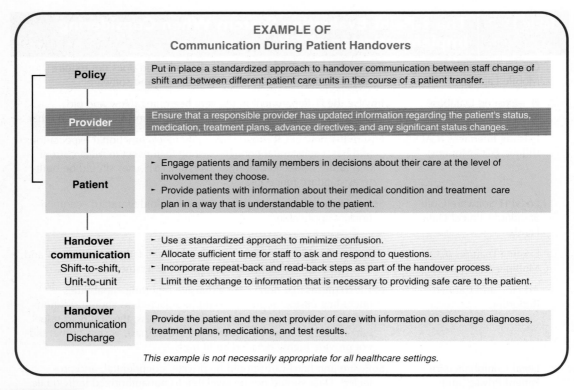

EXAMPLE OF
Communication During Patient Handovers

Policy — Put in place a standardized approach to handover communication between staff change of shift and between different patient care units in the course of a patient transfer.

Provider — Ensure that a responsible provider has updated information regarding the patient's status, medication, treatment plans, advance directives, and any significant status changes.

Patient —
- Engage patients and family members in decisions about their care at the level of involvement they choose.
- Provide patients with information about their medical condition and treatment care plan in a way that is understandable to the patient.

Handover communication
Shift-to-shift, Unit-to-unit —
- Use a standardized approach to minimize confusion.
- Allocate sufficient time for staff to ask and respond to questions.
- Incorporate repeat-back and read-back steps as part of the handover process.
- Limit the exchange to information that is necessary to providing safe care to the patient.

Handover communication
Discharge — Provide the patient and the next provider of care with information on discharge diagnoses, treatment plans, medications, and test results.

This example is not necessarily appropriate for all healthcare settings.

FIGURE 15–2

Communication during patient handover. From: http://www.ccforpatientsafety.org/common/pdfs/fpdf/presskit/PS-Solution3.pdf.

staff resistance in using them, and uncertainty over the process of recording information.

In a paper titled, "Information loss in emergency medical services handover of trauma patients," the authors wanted to study the process of EMS patient handovers and the concept of information degradation.[2] Auditors watched EMS and ED personnel interact during actual videotaped patient handovers, and information transfer of predetermined key information areas was compared on the subsequent medical record. They concluded:

Even in the controlled setting of a single-patient handover with direct verbal contact between EMS providers and in-hospital clinicians, only 72.9% of key prehospital data points transmitted by the EMS personnel were documented by receiving hospital staff. Elements such as prehospital hypotension, GCS score, and other prehospital vital signs were often not recorded. Methods of "transmitting" and "receiving" data in trauma as well as all other patients need further scrutiny.[2]

In an associated commentary on this study, Angelo Salvucci suggests the following remedies:

How can this be addressed? First, it will require a team approach involving both EMS and hospitals, and everyone needs to understand the importance of accurate and complete information transfer. Second, trauma is just part of the puzzle, as handover information loss likely also applies to other EMS-to-ED patients, especially the critically ill. And third, although this study focused on receipt of transmitted information, the authors also found that fewer than 50% of essential elements were ever verbalized by EMS—a potentially even greater concern.

Possible solutions include an abbreviated documentation using a formatted checklist that can be completed by EMS on delivering the patient and timely completion and delivery of the run report, either in the ED or electronically. EMS systems should consider evaluating their information transfer and documentation performance as a QI project.[3]

And in a similar review looking at the need for improvements in EMS patient handovers, the following suggestions were also made:

The results indicated ED staff need to appreciate that a lack of active listening skills can lead to frustration for ambulance staff. Ambulance staff must expect to repeat their handover, especially for patients in the resuscitation room. Handovers for critically ill patients should be delivered in two phases, with essential information given immediately and again thereafter to give further information when initial treatment has been undertaken.[4]

Improvements on the EMS Patient Handover Process

As suggested in the WHO/Joint Commission International publication and also in a report titled "Guidelines for Ambulance Presentations in the Emergency Department," published by the State Government of Victoria Department of Human Services (http://www.health.vic.gov.au/emergency/presentation-guide%20.pdf), there are several techniques that can be employed to decrease the amount of "information degradation," to increase patient safety, and to improve quality of the patient transfer process and ultimately the quality of care for patients. Figure 15-3 offers their suggestions during the three separate phases of prehospital-to-hospital patient transfer: normal business, alert, and escalation phases.

> The State Government of Victoria Department of Human Services report concludes by suggesting that the key message regarding patient handovers is:
> These guidelines encourage a systematic approach to the reception and handover process for ambulance patients on arrival at [a] metropolitan hospital emergency department. Timely reception and handover of ambulance patients arriving in the emergency department will impact positively on:
>
> ■ patient outcomes
> ■ patient flow in the emergency department
> ■ ambulance response times
>
> See Guidelines for ambulance presentations in the ED, State Government Victoria Department of Human Services at http://www.health.vic.gov.au/emergency/presentation-guide%20.pdf.

These guidelines provide direction for hospital and ambulance staff on the process for reception and handover of patients arriving by ambulance in Victoria's metropolitan public hospital EDs. They aim to ensure equitable and timely access to emergency care and are designed to assist with planning best-practice management and care coordination within existing infrastructure and services.

QUALITY IMPROVEMENT IN EMS

In many parts of the world, prehospital and ambulance patient care has developed without a well-structured system for quality improvement. Quality improvement (QI) represents the process by which care provided is reviewed, updated, and/or corrected with the goal of attaining and maintaining the highest quality of care possible. QI systems have to be carefully planned and operated so that they do not consume excessive amounts of resources that could better be applied to direct patient care.

The emergency physician with his/her training background, clinical experience, and professional interests occupies a natural position to be a leader in the provision of QI for prehospital care. Emergency physicians typically have more medical training and knowledge than nonphysician prehospital care providers. This allows them to better judge the evaluation and care of more complex or unusual (infrequently encountered) cases. The emergency physician also represents a "bridge" between prehospital care and inhospital care.

Since most emergency physicians receive ambulance-transported patients in the ED regularly, they have experience with direct interaction with prehospital care personnel. In the United States an additional important reason for involvement of emergency physicians in QI is the legal system structure that defines all medical care provided as ultimately the responsibility of a licensed physician. Paramedics and EMTs in the United States essentially work under the licensed authority of a physician. This oversight responsibility by the physician also means that the physician needs to have ultimate control over the care provided by the other health care workers who are essentially working under their license.

Structure of the QI System

In the ideal situation, there should be formal review by a physician of every case in which prehospital care was provided. Where this is not possible due either to financial or personnel time constraints, a sampling method (to review a predefined portion of the cases) can be successfully utilized.

Probably the most important items for the QI physician to review on a prehospital case are those items that apply to the appropriateness of the medical care provided. In most US prehospital systems, the prehospital personnel write out a narrative report of each case, and this is the main information that

	Hospital	Ambulance
NORMAL BUSINESS	**Nominated hospital representative (such as a triage nurse)**	**Paramedic**
	Activate preparation of resources appropriate to patient needs.	Pre-notify the hospital if the patient has any special health care needs.
	Facilitate access to triage.	Attend triage nurse on arrival.
	Ensure staff are allocated and available to accept patient handover.	Handover patient details to relevant clinical and clerical hospital staff.
	Provide resources appropriate to meet expected patient care requirements.	Move patient to allocated treatment or waiting area.
	Collaborate with paramedics to expedite patient transfer.	Assist emergency department staff to monitor the care needs of the patient.
	Ensure all actions to assist patient flow are implemented.	Ensure all actions to assist patient flow are implemented.
	Collaborate with ambulance paramedic/s to ensure immediate patient care needs are met.	Collaborate with emergency department staff to ensure immediate patient care needs are met.
	Advise emergency department director or nominee of any delays.	Notify MAS duty team manager of any delays.
ALERT / **20 TO 40 MINUTES**	**Emergency department director or nominee**	**Duty team manager**
	Activate internal emergency department response such as reallocation of staff.	Collaborate with emergency department director to resolve significant delays.
	Collaborate with ambulance duty team manager to resolve delays.	Document significant delays and reasons for delays.
	Ensure all action to assist patient flow are implemented.	Advise MAS group manager of significant delays and keep them informed of resolution progress.
	Advise hospital executive of significant delay and keep them informed of the progress to resolve issues.	
ESCALATION / **OVER 40 MINUTES**	**Hospital executive**	**Ambulance group manager**
	Collaborate with ambulance group manager to address issues arising from delay.	Contact hospital executive and collaborate to address issues arising from delay.
	Ensure hospital response process is activated and monitor progress.	Provide assistance to resolve delays, including coordinating attendance of a MAS manager and reviewing ambulance workload if required.
	Record major delays, reasons for the delay, and resolution.	Report and document delay to operations manager.

FIGURE 15–3

Summary of roles and responsibilities for patient transfer and escalation. Guidelines for ambulance presentations in the ED. State Government Victoria Department of Human Services. http://www.health.vic.gov.au/emergency/presentation-guide%20.pdf.

Table 15–8	The Exact Structure of Any Particular Organization's QI System Will Obviously Vary According to the Following Factors

1. The size and structure of the prehospital care system
2. The experience and training of the prehospital care personnel
3. The time and financial resources available to support QI programs
4. The overall legal system in place for the system

Table 15–9	The Main Recommended Items for the QI Physician/Committee to Focus Their Review On

1. On-scene time intervals (the length of time that the prehospital personnel spend at the scene prior to initiating vehicle transport to the hospital)
2. The validity of refusal of care or transport by a patient or family
3. The appropriateness of the medical care provided by the prehospital personnel (This is probably the most important.)
4. The adequacy of the documentation of the history of illness, the physical exam, procedures and treatments, and response to treatments provided in prehospital care
5. The timing and appropriateness of interaction of the prehospital care personnel with the receiving hospital personnel
6. The completeness and appropriateness of the history and physical exam done
7. If any abnormal vital signs were recognized and addressed
8. The correct procedures were done
9. The effects of treatment provided were noted
10. The correct cardiac rhythm sequence was identified
11. The correct destination hospital was selected for the case
12. Timing and interaction by phone or radio with a "medical command" physician or the receiving hospital facility
13. Only BLS rather than ALS was correctly provided for a particular case

is reviewed by the QI physician (Table 15-8 and Table 15-9). Quality improvement and emergency physician involvement in QI are discussed in greater detail elsewhere in this textbook.

SUMMARY

Patient care reports (PCRs) are an essential and required function of any prehospital/EMS system. PCRs should include pertinent data regarding the patient's complaint, history, physical and clinical condition, as well as documentation of any clinical changes, procedures done, or medications administered in the prehospital setting. PCRs should be automated and computerized whenever possible to aid in the collection, research, transfer, and dissemination of data as well as in quality improvement. Handover procedures from prehospital personnel to the hospital medical staff should be performed with the utmost care and precision and should be a formal, official process involving strict adherence to protocol and regulation whenever possible. Physician involvement in quality improvement for prehospital care is extremely important, as it allows monitoring of the care provided and the performance of the personnel involved. This provides an important link between the physician and the other prehospital personnel. A QI system helps to provide ongoing education for personnel and can be used to maintain interest and morale. The ideal goal of the QI system should be to carefully review the care provided for every case, although more limited reviews may be necessary because of time or financial constraints within the system.

References

1. Croskerry P, Crosby K, Schenkel S, Wears R, et al. Patient Safety in Emergency Medicine. Philadelphia, PA: Lippincott Williams & Wilkins, 2009.
2. Carter AJ, Davis KA, Evans LV, Cone DC. Information loss in emergency medical services handover of trauma patients. *Prehosp Emerg Care* 13(3): 280, 2009. http://www.emsresponder.com/online/printer.jsp?id =10176.
3. Salvucci A Jr. *EMS* Magazine Online Exclusive; http:// www.emsresponder.com/web/online/EMS-Magazine-Online-Exclusives/Information-Loss-in-Trauma-Patient-Handovers/22$10176.

4. Jenkin A, Abelson-Mitchell S, Cooper A. Patient hand-over: Time for a change? *Accid Emerg Nursing* 15: 3, 141, 2007. http://linkinghub.elsevier.com/retrieve/pii/S096523020700046X.

Additional References Recommended by Author

1. Holliman CJ, Swope G, Mauger L, et al. Comparison of two systems for quality improvement of prehospital ALS services. *Prehosp Dis Med* 8(4): 303, 1993.
2. Holliman CJ, et al. Medical command errors in an urban advanced life support system. *Ann Emerg Med* 21(4): 347, 1992.
3. Holliman CJ, Wuerz RC, Meador SA, et al: Decrease in medical command errors with use of a standing orders system. Am J Emerg Med 12(3): 279, 1995.
4. Holliman CJ, Wuerz RC, Vazquez-deMiguel G, et al: Comparisons of interventions in prehospital care by standing orders vs on-line medical direction. *Prehosp Dis Med* 9(4): 202, 1994.
5. Wuerz RC, Swope G, Holliman CJ, et al: On-line medical direction: A prospective study. *Prehosp Dis Med* 10(2): 174, 1995.
6. Swor RA (ed). Quality Management in Prehospital Care. St. Louis: Mosby Year Book, Inc., 1993, 254 pp.
7. Stewart RD: Medical direction in emergency medical services: the role of the physician. *Emerg Med Clin North Am* 5: 119, 1987.
8. Pepe PE, Stewart RD: Role of the physician in the prehospital setting. *Ann Emerg Med* 15: 1480, 1986.
9. Swor RA, Hoelzer M: A computer assisted quality improvement audit in a multi-provider EMS system. *Ann Emerg Med* 19: 286, 1990.
10. Pointer J. The advanced life support base hospital audit for medical control in an emergency medical services system. *Ann Emerg Med* 16: 577, 1987.
11. Pons PT, Dinerman N, Rosen P, et al: The field instructor program: quality control of prehospital care — the first step. *J Emerg Med* 2: 1985.
12. Holliman CJ, Swope G, Mauger L, et al. Comparison of two systems for quality assurance of prehospital advanced life support services. *Prehosp Disaster Med* Oct-Dec;8(4): 303, 1993.

CHAPTER 16

Development of an EMS Quality Improvement Program

Karen Smith, Bill Barger, Alex Currell

KEY LEARNING POINTS

- Ambulance services should implement comprehensive clinical quality improvement plans.
- Quality improvement plans are dynamic and should encompass the "plan, do, study, act" model.
- Clinical quality assurance is made up of two major components, quality improvement and risk management.
- A key area of quality improvement is the implementation of clinical indicators. Significant clinical areas that should be monitored via clinical performance measures include cardiac arrest, potential major trauma, pain, respiratory arrest, and stroke. Patient and community satisfaction should also be measured.
- Quality improvement also involves the establishment of dynamic clinical practice guidelines and clinical standards.

- Risk management can be achieved via a number of initiatives, including limited occurrence screening, clinical audit, and root cause analysis.
- Limited occurrence screening is a continuous process of retrospective screening and review of patient medical records to detect adverse patient occurrences.
- Ongoing audit of call-taking processes and dispatch rules should also form part of a comprehensive quality assurance plan. We recommend using a risk matrix approach based on consequence and likelihood ratings. This approach is also applicable to other areas of organizational risk.
- Data collection is a fundamental component of quality assurance. Where practical, data collection should be electronic and systematic. The benefit of establishing registries for key patient groups cannot be underestimated.

Better prehospital care can lead to better population health and reduce acute health care costs both pre- and in-hospital. A systematic approach to quality assurance is essential to ensure continuing improvements in care. This chapter gives an overview of the key characteristics of a quality improvement program for ambulance services. The recommendations are predominantly based on our experience and practice at Ambulance Victoria (AV), Australia, with reference to international practice where applicable.

CLINICAL QUALITY ASSURANCE

Quality improvement is one of the two major aims of clinical quality assurance. The US Institute of Medicine defines quality as the "degree to which health services for individuals and populations increase the likelihood of desired health outcomes and are consistent with current professional knowledge.[1] The quality of care component of clinical quality assurance therefore concentrates on the positive things that happen to patients.

Quality is usually perceived as having three interrelated domains (see Box 16-1 below):

Quality Service
Achieving community satisfaction by the service provided.

Quality Care
Providing clinical care to acceptable and established standards.

Quality Organization
Fostering a working culture of getting it right the first time and a commitment to doing better by participation in coordinated continuous clinical quality improvement processes.

The second major aim of clinical quality assurance in a health service is to ensure patient safety.[2] The Agency for Healthcare Research and Quality in the US defines patient safety as "the absence of the potential for, or the occurrence of, health care–associated injury to patients created by avoiding medical errors as well as taking action to prevent errors from causing injury."[3] This component of clinical quality assurance focuses on the negative things that happen to patients and taking action to ensure that they occur less frequently.

Terms and Definitions

Adverse event is defined as "an untoward patient event, which under optimal conditions is not a consequence of the patient's disease or treatment." The adverse event is then classified according to the certainty with which such an event has occurred and its severity and preventability.

Benchmarking is a structured method of measuring processes and products against each other to identify and understand the characteristics of superior performance.

Clinical performance (quality) indicators measure the standard of particular clinical activities or outcomes. They are the measurable characteristic of a product, service, or process that best represents the quality.

Clinical quality assurance is a system in which the delivery of a service or the quality of care is assessed and compared against a standard.

Clinical quality improvement is the organizational structure and procedures necessary for the ongoing review, evaluation, and continuing improvement of all facets of health care provided by EMS. The aim of the quality improvement process is not to be punitive but to foster the individual's development through training and education and organizational improvement through systematic trend analysis and development.

Limited occurrence screening (LOS) is a continuous process of retrospective screening and review of patient medical records to detect adverse patient occurrences. Histories are extracted based on the presence of one or more defined screening criteria and reviewed by clinicians for the presence of an adverse event. A similar approach is the use of audit filters to target cases for review.

Quality control refers to circumstances where quality can be objectively measured and standards set and maintained. The control criteria can be reviewed and new levels may be set by the quality assurance process to become part of the minimum standards of the EMS.

Sentinel events are relatively infrequent, clear-cut adverse events that occur independently of a patient's condition. Sentinel events commonly reflect system and process deficiencies and result in unnecessary outcomes for patients.

QUALITY IMPROVEMENT PLAN

A robust clinical quality improvement program requires a quality improvement plan, which is dynamic and organization-wide in nature, with total organizational commitment. It is an ongoing, comprehensive process, with regular evaluation of the effectiveness of patient care. The components of a comprehensive ambulance quality improvement plan, which are discussed further in this chapter, include:

1. Clinical practice guidelines and clinical standards
2. Clinical performance indicators
3. Limited occurrence screening (LOS) and clinical review
4. Sentinel events and root cause analysis
5. Call-taking and dispatch grid review

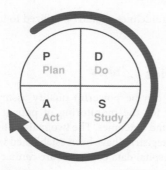

FIGURE 16–1

Plan-do-study-act cycle for quality improvement. Reprinted with permission of http://www.saferpak. com/pdsa.htm.

Philosophy of the Continuing Clinical Quality Improvement Process

The clinical quality improvement process is concerned with sustained improvement. It is an approach that challenges the status quo and insists that everything the organization does and how it does it can be done better. It reinforces to the organization the importance of getting it right the first time, of the crucial importance of the community and the community needs. The process should be one of the "plan, do, study, act" cycle (Figure 16-1).

Effective continuing clinical quality improvement cannot occur without the setting of standards and the measurement of performance against the standard.

This then allows for identifying the potential for improvement, the communication of the findings and recommendations to the relevant managers, and consequently the implementation of recommended improvements.

These are then in turn evaluated to ensure that the objectives of the process have been achieved; the emphasis is to follow through to close the loop (Figure 16-2).[2]

Quality Improvement and Patient Safety Culture

An organization's culture influences patient safety. Culture is something the organization is (the beliefs, attitudes, and values of its members) and has (the structures, practices, controls, and policies). A "safety culture" can be achieved by moving away from a system of blame to one that views errors as opportunities to improve systems and prevent harm. The reporting

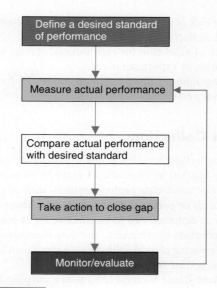

FIGURE 16–2

Basic quality improvement cycle.[2] Reprinted with permission of Wolff A, Taylor S. Enhancing patient care. A practical guide to improving quality and safety in hospitals. MJA Books Australia, 2009.

of quality improvement processes and the strength of the feedback cycle can both significantly contribute to the culture of the organization.

Challenges in the Prehospital Environment

Ambulance services are facing ever-increasing demands and quality and governance issues may be pushed into the background while "more pressing" operational factors are dealt with. It is important, however, that clinical quality improvement receives appropriate focus, as the "emergency" nature of ambulance work increases the risk of adverse events.

There are other challenges to EMS in implementing comprehensive clinical quality improvement programs, including:

1. The expanding scope of practice of EMS.
2. The difficulty in defining outcomes meaningfully (unless there is a significant risk of death).
3. The challenge of identifying the EMS contribution to outcome (given the relatively short time most patients are in the care of paramedics and the complex procedures that may be undertaken following handover at the hospital by paramedics).
4. The accuracy of data collection in the emergency setting.

5. The lack of common definitions for data elements and clinical outcome endpoints.
6. Lack of validation for each isolated clinical intervention in a spectrum of care.
7. Geographically diverse systems and workforce.
8. Privacy concerns.

Data Collection

Data collection for clinical quality assurance can be greatly assisted by clinical data entry by paramedics using electronic data capture systems, such as tablet computers or personal digital assistants. These have also been demonstrated to be effective for in-hospital data collection by clinicians. The time clinicians must spend entering clinical audit data is a significant factor in gaining their support for the activity.

Ambulance Victoria (AV) uses a purpose-built, in-field electronic data capture system and linked clinical database to capture data on all patients attended by paramedics. Victorian Ambulance Clinical Information System (VACIS) captures specific data in categories, such as case nature, patient complaint, paramedic assessment, vital signs, and management. More than 50,000 electronic patient care records (ePCRs) are collected by AV each month.

AV has made the system available without charge to other ambulance services, and all but one Australian state and territory ambulance service has joined a national collaboration that governs and funds the ongoing development of VACIS. Collaboration members have agreed to work together to achieve continuing improvement in clinical information systems throughout Australia by the development and enhancement of VACIS. The foundation block of VACIS is a standard, comprehensive, national clinical dataset that is managed by the Collaboration.

AV organizational data is stored in a data warehouse, with linked data marts for clinical, dispatch, response, finance, and workforce data. The availability of the data warehouse has allowed AV to build specific filters to assist in the identification of patient types (e.g., potential major trauma, high-acuity, potential ALS, cardiac pain). It has also facilitated the identification of cases for limited occurrence screening, which is described later in the chapter (e.g., severe unrelieved traumatic pain patients). The design of the AV clinical data warehouse was provided to the collaboration and has been incorporated into the VACIS product to promote standardized reporting of key clinical quality indicators.

Where a common data collection and reporting platform are not available for EMS, published definitions and guidelines should be utilized to inform data collection.

Registries

Registries can be powerful quality assurance tools and allow for the monitoring of patient treatment protocols and outcomes. The two main clinical groups for which registries have been established with significant prehospital data collection are cardiac arrest and major trauma patients.

Significant regional variation in survival from prehospital cardiac arrest has highlighted the importance of monitoring outcome and on good quality data collection by ambulance services.[4,5] Similarly, trauma registries have aided in establishing the quality of care of trauma patients in the prehospital setting.[6]

Victoria has government-funded, state wide registries for major trauma[6] and out-of-hospital cardiac arrest.[7] In addition, the government collects data on all patient presentations to public hospital EDs and admissions to public hospitals. These hospital minimum datasets provide an important resource for health service evaluation and monitoring of patients through the continuum of care.[8] AV also contributes to a heroin overdose registry.[9]

In the US, the National Highway Traffic Safety Administration has supported the development of a National EMS Information System (NEMSIS) that is intended to capture the entire EMS episode (activation through to patient release) and populate a national database. The majority of states in the US have agreed to support full implementation of the NEMSIS dataset into their jurisdictions.[10,11] However, it is unclear how many services will capture data electronically and whether states will set up state wide registries.

The Resuscitation Outcomes Consortium (ROC), which involves eight US and three Canadian regions, has established population-based cardiac arrest and trauma registries. These aim to capture data on all EMS–attended-9-1-1 calls for patients with out-of-hospital cardiac arrest or major trauma.[12,13]

Clinical Standards

EMS should have in place a clear set of clinical standards. These standards represent multidisciplinary consensus on the management of common prehospital emergency problems that under normal circumstances EMT and EMT-P are expected to follow. The standards include clinical guidelines or protocols, work instructions for the practical procedures and,

Table 16–1	**Types of Performance Indicators**	
Quality Indicator		
Type of Indicator	Definition	Examples
Structure	Relate to the attributes of the environment in which the care is delivered. Includes the physical setting, resources, personnel, and organization structure	Access to specific treatments or technologies (e.g., 12-lead ECG, ALS paramedics) Availability of human resources (e.g., dispatch of AED-equipped first responders, trauma team activation on admission of trauma patient)
Process	Method or process by which care is delivered	Proportion of STEMI patients who receive a prehospital 12-lead ECG Time for defibrillation for VF/VT patients
Outcome	Results of the system	Morbidity (e.g., extent of pain relief) Mortality (survival from cardiac arrest) Reattends to nontransported patients in 24 hours (also "Process") Patient satisfaction

most critically, these standards need to be supported by robust education and a continuous improvement system. Systems that include first responders and other volunteers need to have relevant standards for practice that align with the paramedic standards.

Within the EMS, the medical advisors and all operational and clinical managers are responsible for ensuring that these clinical standards are known and maintained by staff. Local adaptation within the recognized standards and quality assurance projects are also the responsibility of the medical advisors and the clinical managers. Any modification to the recognized standards for EMS local needs should only occur following consultation with, and approval of, the medical advisors.

Performance (Quality) Indicators

Background

There is increasing expectation in the health care sector that meaningful performance measures be collected and reported. Performance measures can be used to:

1. Provide continuous measurement of health care delivery.
2. Identify areas of excellence.
3. Provide a mechanism for early awareness of a potential problem and/or flag cases for review (i.e., act as an audit filter).
4. Verify effectiveness of a corrective action; and
5. Benchmark performance with other services.

A performance measure or quality indicator is a measure of clinical management and/or outcome. Generally performance indicators can be classified as structure-, process-, or outcome-based (Table 16-1).[14]

The following attributes are important considerations when defining individual performance measures:

1. Importance and relevance
2. Validity
3. Reliability
4. Usability and ability of stakeholders to understand the measure
5. Feasibility and sustainability
6. Availability of robust measures for use as minimum standards or targets

In the absence of a distinct body of literature evaluating prehospital systems and interventions, EMS performance indicators have typically been limited to the few benchmarks that have been established scientifically, such as survival from out-of-hospital cardiac arrest (OHCA). Given the lack of prehospital data, other performance measures have generally been based on measures of nonclinical endpoints and inconclusive surrogate markers such as response intervals and skill levels.

Ideally ambulance services would instigate a range of indicators, which have clearly been demonstrated to impact on patient outcome. These quality indicators would be a combination of outcome, process, and structure measures. Response intervals,

Table 16–2	Proposed Key Treatment Elements/Measures by the Consortium of US Metropolitan Municipalities' EMS Medical Directors[15]
Clinical Area	**Elements in Model**
ST-Elevation Myocardial infarction (STEMI)	Aspirin* 12-lead ECG with prearrival activation of interventional cardiology team, as indicated Direct transport to percutaneous coronary intervention (PCI) - capable facility for ECG to PCI time <90 minutes
Pulmonary edema	Nitroglycerin (NTG)* Noninvasive positive pressure ventilation (NPPV) preferred as first line of intervention over endotracheal intubation (ETT)†
Asthma	Administration of beta-agonist
Seizure‡	Blood glucose measurement Benzodiazepine for status epilepticus
Trauma	Scene time <10 minutes (nontrapped) Direct transport to trauma service for those meeting criteria, particularly for those over 65
Cardiac arrest	Response interval <5 minutes for basic CPR and automated external defibrillators

*In the absence of contraindications.
†May not be relevant when transport times are short (<10 minutes).
‡Patient with seizure activity that persists for more than 15 consecutive minutes or has two or more seizures without an intervening period of clear mental status.[15]

for instance, clearly have their place in reporting, in particular in the context of public policy and patient expectations. However, ideally they should be designed to reflect the clinical significance of timeliness (e.g., response to cardiac arrest patients, time for effective pain relief, and scene time at major trauma patients). Individual interventions also have merit as performance measures where improved outcomes have clearly been demonstrated in large-scale trials. In these instances the key issue is to report on the provision of the proven therapy and timely intervention.[15]

The US-based Emergency Medical Services Outcome Project (EMSOP), funded by the National Highway Traffic Safety Administration, has done some preliminary work in defining groups of patients where performance should be monitored.[16] EMSOP used frequency data and expert opinion to rank-order EMS conditions for children and adults based on their potential value for the study of effectiveness of care. The top five conditions identified for adults that should take precedence in EMS outcomes research

were minor trauma, respiratory distress, chest pain, major trauma, and cardiac arrest.

The Consortium of US Metropolitan Municipalities' EMS Medical Directors (2007) has also attempted to expand the list of evidence-based EMS performance measures and associated definitions and reporting standards (Table 16-2).[15] In addition, the investigators used results from published studies to predict the number needed to treat to avoid harm in each condition (Table 16-3).

In the UK, ambulance clinical indicators form part of a suite of National Health Service (NHS) performance measures.[17] For example, the Myocardial Infarction National Audit Program (MINAP) collects data on the percentage of STEMI patients who receive thrombolytic treatment within 60 minutes of call (call to needle time) plus the percentage of STEMI patients who receive primary angioplasty within 120 minutes of call (call to balloon time). The ambulance outcomes audit aims to share the MINAP data with the Ambulance Trusts and includes all patients with myocardial infarction and acute coro-

Table 16–3	Proposed Numbers Needed to Treat (NNT) by the Consortium of US Metropolitan Municipalities EMS Medical Directors		
Clinical Area	**Elements**	**NNT**	**Harm Avoided**
STEMI	Aspirin*, 12-lead ECG and direct transport to percutaneous coronary intervention (PCI) - capable facility for ECG to PCI time <90 minutes	15	Either a stroke, 2nd myocardial infarct (MI), or death
Pulmonary edema	NPPV	6	Need for ETT
Seizure	Benzodiazepine for status epilepticus	4	Persistent seizure activity
Trauma	Patients with Injury Severity Score (ISS) >15 to Major Trauma Service (MTS)	11	1 death
Trauma	Patients aged >65 years, with ISS>21 to MTS	3	1 death
Cardiac arrest	Defibrillator to scene <5 minutes rather than <8 minutes	8	1 death

*In the absence of contraindications.

nary syndrome who are admitted to the hospital by ambulance.[18]

The UK Coronary Heart Disease National Service Framework sets out national standards for emergency cardiac care, including early access to a defibrillator and the administration of aspirin and thrombolytic treatment to eligible patients with suspected heart attack. More information on UK ambulance trust performance measures can be found at the NHS Information Centre.[19]

COMMON CLINICAL DOMAINS FOR CLINICAL QUALITY INDICATORS

In this chapter, we present recommendations for clinical indicators based on our local AV clinical risk management system. The key patient groups that are covered include:

1. Time-critical patients
2. Cardiac arrest
3. Potential major trauma
4. Pain
5. Respiratory distress
6. Stroke

Where applicable we have attempted to define pediatric indicators in addition to the adult measures. We consider patients under 16 years old to be pediatric. However, there is a lack of standardized pediatric emergency care performance measures, and considerable research is still required in this area.[20]

Benchmarking

An important consideration when collecting and reporting on performance measures is the ability to benchmark performance against published results. Comparative results from other services should be used for benchmarking purposes. Benchmarks have been used historically to drive improved performance in key EMS areas (e.g., response times to urgent cases in the UK have been benchmarked against national standards).[19]

In setting benchmarks, however, it is important to account for the difference in rural, suburban, and urban EMS systems. A "call to first shock" time interval response benchmark of ten minutes might be reasonable in well-resourced communities with AED-equipped first responders. The same goal, however, may be fiscally and logistically impossible in a small rural community. For this reason we have not included benchmarks for most of the recommended performance measures.

Quality of Life Measures

EMS clinical performance measures are aimed at measuring the quality of care of patients. A key area with respect to this is the outcome of survivors in key groups of high-acuity patients. Outcome measures are concerned generally with two broad areas: function and quality of life (QOL). Function is more easily defined, while QOL is an abstract, complex, and highly individualized concept.[21,22]

When considering measuring outcomes other than survival, a clear consensus of what to measure has not been reached. However, there are a number of generic, validated QOL tools available that have been utilized in cardiac arrest research.[23-25] Functional measures are also available and provide a more comprehensive measure of outcome when used on trauma patients in conjunction with QOL measures.[21,26,27]

With the development of enhanced system integration of ambulance and hospital services for the management of trauma, cardiac arrest, stroke, and other conditions, it is likely that there will be further improvements in survival. However, it is probable that the biggest gains will come from improved function and quality of life of survivors.[21] To address this, key EMS performance measures should ideally contain some QOL outcomes.

Response Intervals

As indicated, response intervals are a meaningful component of an ambulance quality assurance program. Generally, response intervals are best presented as medians and 90th percentiles with associated confidence intervals.

Response time should measure the interval from call start at the emergency call center to arrival of the first EMS vehicle at the scene (including first responders dispatched by the EMS). This ensures that response time reflects performance from the perspective of the patient. Where possible, the timeliness of the health system (ambulance and hospital) response should also be measured.

Another useful indicator is the total time for the patient to be transferred to an appropriate level of care, from the call start time to completion of handover at the appropriate hospital. This includes response time, time at scene, time for transport to the hospital, and the time within the hospital for handover of the patient from ambulance to hospital staff. Key aspects of this measure are that it takes into account the appropriateness of the hospital destination selected and that it reflects performance at the hospital interface (as well as prehospital).

Suggested key measures are documented in Table 16-4, with other intervals presented in sections focusing on key patient groups. Note that ambulance services should monitor their performance on all the time interval components of the response process (e.g., call-taking time, time to mobilize) as part of their operational quality assurance, and the limited list presented here assumes that this more comprehensive program of monitoring operational performance is also undertaken.

Cardiac Arrest Measures

Three quarters of all deaths from myocardial infarction occur after cardiac arrest in the community.

Table 16–4	Recommended Response Performance Measures		
Area	**Measure (Median, 90th Percentile, Confidence Intervals)**
High-acuity patients	Response time to emergency cases Scene time for patients meeting time-critical guidelines (nontrauma) Time to appropriate hospital care
Potential major trauma	Scene time Total prehospital time Time to appropriate hospital care
Cardiac arrest	Response time Time to CPR (call start to first EMS CPR) ***Time to first defibrillation for VF/VT patients (call start to first shock)***

Therefore, the greatest scope to improve survival lies outside of the hospital. It is widely accepted that survival from out-of-hospital cardiac arrest is directly related to EMS performance. Such factors include response times, bystander CPR, dispatch effectiveness, and presence of ALS care.[28] If victims of out-of-hospital cardiac arrest can receive immediate and appropriate treatment, it has been suggested that they have up to a 70% chance of survival.[29,30] In addition, the value of defibrillation in reverting patients with ventricular fibrillation (VF) and rapid ventricular tachycardia (VT) has been established beyond doubt. Guidelines for routine data collection and reporting on cardiac arrest patients are available.[31,32]

EMS agencies provide patient care for many disorders, of which cardiac arrests represent only 1 to 2% of emergency calls. However, the stakes for cardiac arrest are high (i.e., patient survival). In addition, the standards of practice for other disorders are often heterogeneous, whereas for cardiac arrest they are well defined. Thus, it is appropriate to devote sufficient resources to these responses, and cardiac arrest measures must be included as key indicators of clinical performance. The American Heart Association (AHA) suggests that the treatment of out-of-hospital cardiac arrest by EMS agencies be the sentinel measure of the quality of EMS care in the community.[9]

In this light, the AHA has recently recommended that:[9]

1. Out-of-hospital cardiac arrests and their outcomes through hospital discharge should be classified as reportable events as part of a heart disease and stroke surveillance system.
2. EMS data collection should include descriptions of the performance of CPR by bystanders and defibrillation by lay responders.
3. National annual reports on key indicators of progress in managing acute cardiovascular events in the out-of-hospital setting should be developed and made publicly available.

Definition of Cardiac Arrest

An international consensus workshop classified cardiac arrest as the "cessation of cardiac mechanical activity as confirmed by the absence of signs of circulation."[31] The AHA suggests an out-of-hospital cardiac arrest would be an event in which a person is evaluated by organized EMS personnel and (a) receives external defibrillation attempts (by lay responders or EMS personnel) or receives chest compressions by organized EMS personnel, or (b) is pulseless but does not receive defibrillation attempts or CPR from EMS personnel.[9] We have adopted a similar approach with the Victorian Ambulance Cardiac Arrest Registry (VACAR) (see **box** below).

VACAR Inclusion Criteria

Patients who are pulseless at any stage in ambulance care due to any cause.
Patients who have been defibrillated prior to ambulance arrival and who have a return of spontaneous circulation.

Clinical Performance Indicators

The recommended clinical indicators for cardiac arrest patients are described in Table 16-5. Ideally, data would be sourced from an established out-of-hospital cardiac arrest registry. In the absence of hospital discharge data, survival to the ED can be used as a surrogate. It should be noted, however, that EMSs with different survival-to-hospital statistics can be found to have similar discharge statistics and vice versa, and caution should be exercised when comparing services based on ambulance data alone. Ideally patient outcome results would include the quality of life of survivors. There is currently no consensus regarding the best tools to measure quality of life in post–cardiac arrest patients. However, a number of validated general assessment tools exist, such as the Short-Form Questionnaires (e.g., SF-12) and the EQ-5D.[33,34] Outcomes for adults and children should be reported separately.

As well as reporting indicators separately for adults and children, it may be practical for some state-/province-wide services to report indicators according to geographic location of arrest and or urban/rural classification. Mapping of cardiac arrests can assist in the identification of disparities in incidence and outcomes across geographic gradients and of epidemiologic hot spots that may reflect emerging risk factors.

Benchmarks

Survival rates after out-of hospital cardiac arrest are highly variable. This observation can be partly explained by differences in patient characteristics, differences in the adequacy of prehospital systems of care, and differences in reporting definitions. While the variation in reported outcome can make benchmarking difficult, it also reemphasizes that an effective EMS system can decrease disability and death from acute cardiovascular events in the out-of-hospital setting.

Table 16–5	Cardiac Arrest Clinical Indicators
Clinical Indicator	**Measure**
Cardiac arrests (all etiologies) Resuscitation initiated by EMS*	Survival to hospital ***Survival to hospital discharge*** QOL of survivors ***Response time*** Time to first CPR ALS (EMS-P) response time
Presenting in VF/VT, resuscitation initiated by EMS	Survival to hospital ***Survival to hospital discharge*** QOL of survivors Response time ***Time to defibrillation*** At patient to first shock
EMS witnessed arrests, resuscitation initiated by EMS (includes arrests witnessed by AED-equipped first responders)	Survival to hospital ***Survival to hospital discharge*** Arrest to first shock for VF/VT

*Exclude EMS-witnessed arrests.

A recent paper described the variation in out-of-hospital cardiac arrest incidence and outcome across ten geographic regions in North America. Survival to hospital discharge ranged from 1.1% to 8.1% for all out-of-hospital arrests (EMS-assessed) and from 7.7% to 39.9% for patients presenting with ventricular fibrillation.[4] The AHA describes the median reported survival to hospital discharge rate after any first recorded rhythm as 6.4%.[9]

It is recommended that individual EMSs would set realistic benchmarks for cardiac arrest response intervals and survival after an appropriate monitoring period. Published survival data should be used as context where applicable. For services that cover wide geographic areas it might be appropriate to set different benchmarks, depending on urban status.

Potential Major Trauma

Major trauma is a leading cause of morbidity and mortality. The major rationale behind an integrated and targeted major trauma system is to achieve "early, appropriate and definitive management in major trauma,"[35] or in other words, "to get the right patient to the right hospital in the right amount of time."[36] Rapid transport of severely injured patients to a trauma center has been associated with improved outcomes.[37] As such, the essential ambulance features of an integrated major trauma system are:

1. Effective identification of major trauma; and
2. Delivery of a major trauma patient to the highest major trauma skill level hospital within one hour of an event (or 30 minutes from departure from accident site), plus efficient retrieval and transport to definitive care at a major trauma service as soon as possible.

The development of quality indicators for the care of trauma patients commenced in 1987 through the introduction of 12 audit filters by the American College of Surgeons Committee on Trauma (ASCOT).[38] The prehospital indicators are:

1. Ambulance scene time >20 minutes, and
2. Absence of ambulance record on medical record for EMS-transported patients.

Preliminary research using the ASCOT quality filters suggest that increased scene time is associated with increased length of hospital stay.[37] However, it should be noted that the impact of ambulance interventions, response intervals, and scene time on outcome for trauma patients is less clear than for cardiac arrest patients. Nearly all of the studies that suggest that the primary determinant of outcome for the trauma patient is the time interval from injury to the operating room are retrospective and provide limited evidence.[37] In addition, there is conflicting evidence regarding the risk-benefit ratio of prehospital ALS

Table 16–6	Potential Major Trauma Patients—Nontrapped
Indicator	

Number of patients meeting prehospital trauma triage guidelines*

Number (%) of patients with scene time ≤ 20 minutes
Number (%) of patients with a total prehospital time ≤ 60 minutes

Number (%) of patients directly transported to a Major Trauma Service (MTS)

Destination compliance†

Total time to appropriate care (from call start to handover at appropriate trauma service).
Number of patients defined as Major Trauma at hospital

*Included as a denominator only.
†Combined cases taken to a MTS with cases transported to the next highest level of Trauma Service where transport to a MTS is >30 minutes.

interventions in trauma patients, particularly in the area of airway management.[39] Further research into this area is required.

Clinical Performance Indicators

The recommended clinical indicators for major trauma patients are described in Table 16-6. Data should be collected for all patients meeting the prehospital potential major trauma triage criteria. This is achieved in Victoria by application of a filter to the electronic patient care data in the AV Data Warehouse. Prehospital details are also then extracted and linked via probabilistic linkage to the State Trauma Registry. This allows for the sensitivity and specificity of current triage guidelines to be monitored. Indicators for adult and pediatric patients should be reported separately.

Pain

Relief of discomfort has been identified as the most important outcome measure for the majority of prehospital conditions and also the prehospital intervention having the most potential impact for the majority of common EMS conditions.[40] A recent study of patients presenting to EDs in the US estimated that 54% of all patients had pain as a symptom on arrival and that the prevalence of moderate to severe pain in the prehospital setting was greater than 20%. In addition, inadequate pain control has been recognized in the literature as an important issue, both in the prehospital setting and the ED.[40,41] EMS oligo analgesia (underuse of analgesics in the face of valid indications) can be linked to pain underestimation, inadequate

dosing with analgesics, and withholding of analgesia.[42] Addressing such shortcomings represents a major potential for EMS to positively impact on an important outcome.

According to the Agency for Healthcare Research and Quality, the most reliable indicator for the existence and intensity of pain is patient self-report.[40] At present, the verbal numerical rating scale (VAS) appears to be the most appropriate pain measure for measuring adult pain by EMS. Either the Ouch! scale or the FACES pain scale is suitable for assessment of pain in children.[43]

A recent study of acute pain in patients post-surgery found that for patients with moderate pain (VAS= 4–6), a decrease of 2.4 units corresponded to "much improvement" according to the patient. For patients with severe pain the decrease in pain score and the percentage of pain relief had to be larger to obtain similar degrees of pain relief. The investigators also found that independent of the baseline pain severity, the minimal change in pain score that is noticeable to patients is 20%.[44] Similarly, a study of acute pain patients presenting to the ED found that a mean reduction of 30 mm on a 100-mm visual pain scale represented a clinically important difference in pain severity that corresponded to patients' perception of adequate pain control.[45] A study of acute pain in children aged between eight and 15 years in the ED found that the minimum clinically significant reduction in visual analogue score was 10 mm.[46] This information allows for clinically meaningful benchmarks to be set for prehospital management of pain. AV currently aims for a mean reduction in pain score of at least

Table 16–7	AV Inclusion Criteria for Pain Categories	
Group	**Inclusion Criteria**
Pain	Pain is selected in patient complaint or paramedic assessment or secondary survey
Ischemic chest pain	Pain case and paramedic assessment (diagnosis) is any of the following: Pain - Chest - Ischemic Acute Myocardial Infarction Acute Pulmonary Edema Angina Aortic Dissection Arrhythmia Cardiac Failure
Traumatic pain	Pain case and case nature (cause) of a traumatic nature
Medical/other pain	All pain patients who do not fall into the above two criteria

3 units along the VAS in patients presenting with moderate to severe pain.

Clinical Performance Indicators

The adequacy of pain relief in specific patient groups (e.g., ischemic chest pain and traumatic pain) following clinical practice guidelines can be used as an indicator in assessing the standard of therapy and the quality of the service overall.

In order for pain indicators to be clinically meaningful, patients should be categorized into broad categories according to the nature of the pain. Table 16-7 provides details of the categories of pain patients currently monitored by AV. In addition, work is continuing to define more precise measures around specific injuries such as burns and long bone fractures.

The recommended clinical indicators for management of pain are listed in Table 16-8. Clinical indicators for pediatric pain are similar.

At Ambulance Victoria, patients with inadequate pain relief are scrutinized further (see Limited Occurrence Screening section of this chapter).

Stroke

The advent of acute stroke therapies has highlighted the need for reliable EMS stroke identification. Through accurate diagnosis of stroke and subsequent transport with prior warning to appropriate stroke centers, paramedics are in a critical position to reduce prehospital and in-hospital delays.[47] A variety of validated prehospital stroke scales are available to assist the EMS identify stroke in the field.[48,49] The

Melbourne Ambulance Stroke Screen (MASS) was developed to assist AV paramedics to identify strokes and has been validated in the community (sensitivity 90% [95% CI:81–96%]) and specificity 74% [95% CI:53–88%]) (see Table 16-9).[46] We encourage EMS to use a tool such as MASS for all neurologically compromised patients. The recommended clinical performance measures for stroke are presented in Table 16-10.

Respiratory Distress

In the weighted priority ranking performed by EMSOP, respiratory conditions ranked in the top five priority conditions for adults and children.[11] Several specific diseases fall under the condition of respiratory distress, including asthma, chronic obstructive pulmonary disease (COPD), and congestive heart failure (CHF).

The Ontario Prehospital Advanced Life Support (OPALS) researchers found that the addition of ALS paramedics reduced mortality from severe respiratory distress by 2%. The majority of this benefit was seen in patients with pulmonary edema/CHF.[50] Also, recent studies have suggested that the use of endotrcheal intubation in pulmonary edema patients is reduced with the administration of noninvasive positive pressure ventilation.[16]

At AV, respiratory status is captured via a respiratory status assessment tool within VACIS, which classifies patients as having a normal respiratory status or mild, moderate, or severe respiratory distress. The tool is based on a number of patient parameters, including general appearance, speech, breath sounds, respiratory rate, and rhythm and conscious state. Patients with

Table 16–8	Clinical Indicators for EMS Adult Pain Management	
Patient Group	**Indicator**	
Ischemic chest pain	Number of eligible patients*	
Traumatic pain	Number of patients with pain scores available*	
Medical pain (noncardiac)	Compliance with pain scores*	
Patients receiving analgesia	Mean initial pain score, standard deviation (SD)	
	Mean final pain score (SD)	
	Mean change in pain score (SD), [range]	
	Mean percentage pain reduction	
	Proportion of all patients with a reduction in pain of ≥3	
	Proportion of severe pain patients with a reduction in pain of ≥ 3†	
	Proportion of patients with a scene time <20 minutes (ischemic chest pain patients only)	
	Mean time to treatment (at patient to first analgesic)‡	

*Exclude patients who have an initial pain score of <3, are documented as unable to rate pain, are intubated, or have a GCS<9. Included as a denominator only.
†Severe pain is initial pain score >7.
‡For patients receiving analgesic only.

moderate or severe respiratory distress are identified via a data filter and examined further. Table 16-11 and Table 16-12 describe proposed indicators around patients with respiratory distress.

Table 16–9	**MASS Assessments for a Diagnosis of Stroke**	
Assessment		**MASS**
History items:		
1. Age >45		X
2. Absent history of seizure or epilepsy		X
3. At baseline, not wheelchair-bound or bedridden		X
4. Blood glucose level between 2.8 and 22.2 mmol/L		X
Physical assessment items:		
5. Facial droop		X
6. Arm drift		X
7. Hand grip		X
8. Speech		X
Criteria for identifying stroke:		
Presence of any physical assessment item and 1–4 present		Yes

COMMUNITY FEEDBACK

It is the community, in the broader definition, that will determine whether they have received "quality service." EMS communities are patients and their relatives, hospitals and their departments, the community, and specialized organizations. Feedback of EMS performance from the people the organization serves is vital to ensure that EMS continues to meet community needs and expectations. Methods available include surveys

Table 16–10	**Clinical Indicators for Adult Stroke***
Indicators	
Number of patients†	
Number (proportion) of patients for whom a stroke screening tool is applied	
Number (proportion) of acute stroke patients transported to a stroke service†	
Total time to appropriate care (from call start to handover at stroke service)‡	

*Paramedic assessment is stroke or transient ischemic attack.
†Included as a denominator only.
‡Time of onset of symptoms is within 6 hours.

Table 16–11	Clinical Indicators for Adult Patients with Moderate/Severe Respiratory Distress*	
Groups	**Indicators**	
Respiratory distress patients (all)	*Proportion of patients who achieve normal respiratory status in EMS care*	
Asthma	Proportion of patients who receive a beta-agonist	
Acute pulmonary edema	Proportion of patients who receive NIPPV	
Severe respiratory distress	Proportion of patients with EMT-P (ALS) attendance	

*Includes patients aged >15 years whose first RSA is moderate/severe. Excludes trauma patients.

and interviews. Patient satisfaction should be included as a key indicator for EMS.

SUMMARY: KEY INDICATORS

The suggested Key EMS Clinical Performance Indicators are summarized in Table 16-13.

Monitoring and Detection of Adverse Events

The level of patient safety in ambulance services can be assessed reactively or proactively. In the reactive model, clinical activity is continuously monitored, and if an adverse event is detected, it is analyzed and appropriate action is taken to reduce the likelihood of recurrence. A proactive approach involves examination of systems of care to identify weak processes that represent an unacceptable level of risk of patients experiencing an adverse event while in EMS care. Once identified, changes are made to these processes to increase patient safety. Reducing the probability

of an adverse event's occurring is called risk management.[2]

There is considerable overlap between the quality improvement and risk management components of clinical quality assurance. An adverse event that is experienced by a patient may be detected by the risk management program but could have occurred because of poor quality of care.[2]

Adverse events are an important cause of morbidity and mortality and quality assurance plans should have a multifaceted approach to the prevention of adverse events, including:

1. Limited occurrence screening
2. Detection of sentinel events
3. Tracking of clinical variations through clinical review and audit

Limited Occurrence Screening

A form of limited occurrence screening (LOS) was developed at a regional hospital in Victoria, Australia.[51] It is a continuous process of retrospective screening

Table 16–12	Clinical Indicators for Pediatric Patients with Moderate/Severe Respiratory Distress*	
Groups	**Indicators**	
Respiratory distress patients	*Proportion of patients who achieve normal respiratory status in EMS care*	
Asthma	Proportion of patients who receive a beta-agonist	
Croup	Proportion of patients receiving nebulized epinephrine	
Severe respiratory distress	Proportion of patients with EMT-P (ALS) attendance	

*Includes patients aged <16 years whose first RSA is moderate/severe. Excludes trauma patients.

Table 16–13	**Four Key EMS Clinical Performance Indicators**	
Clinical Area	**Patient Group**	**Key Indicator**
High acuity patients	All ages combined	Response time to emergency calls
Cardiac arrest	Report adult and pediatric separately	Response time Survival to hospital discharge for all arrests with resuscitation initiated by EMS Time to defibrillation for VF/VT Survival to hospital discharge for VF/VT
Potential major trauma patients	Report adult and pediatric separately	Proportion with scene time <20 minutes Destination compliance Total time to trauma service handover
Ischemic chest pain	Adult only	Mean reduction in pain score Severe pain patients with a clinically meaningful reduction
Traumatic pain	Report adult and pediatric separately	Mean reduction in pain score Severe pain patients with a clinically meaningful reduction
Stroke	Adult only	Use of stroke screening tool Total time to stroke service handover
Respiratory distress	Report adult and pediatric separately	Proportion of patients achieving normal respiratory status in EMS care
All patients	Report adult and pediatric together	Proportion of patients who are satisfied/very satisfied with the EMS

and review of patient medical records to detect adverse patient occurrences. Briefly, histories are extracted based on the presence of one or more defined screening criteria and reviewed by clinicians for the presence of an adverse event. Categories for LOS are chosen based on areas of potential risk and not on the assumption that there is anything wrong with the management of these cases. An example of a LOS category that is used in hospitals is "unscheduled return to the operating theater."

An adverse event is defined as "an untoward patient event, which under optimal conditions is not a consequence of the patient's disease or treatment." The adverse event is then classified according to the certainty with which it has occurred and its severity and preventability.

LOS is an effective way of identifying local system problems in clinical care. In recognition of this, Ambulance Victoria has taken the hospital-based LOS model and adapted it to the EMS setting (Table 16-14).

The process of limited occurrence screening in Ambulance Victoria involves:

1. Identification of categories of patients for review (as above).
2. Auditing of patient care records for appropriateness of care and adequate documentation.
3. Referral for full clinical review of cases where clinical practice guidelines have not been adhered to and/or patient care has been compromised.
4. Tabulation and reporting of audit results.

It is expected that in the majority of cases clinical practice guidelines (CPGs) have been followed and clinical care has been appropriate. However, focusing on potentially high-risk procedures and patients allows for an efficient method of screening for adverse events. LOS involving eight screening criteria in hospitals has been shown to be effective in detecting approximately 50% of adverse patient occurrences, a much higher proportion than found by traditional medical QA programs.[51]

The Ambulance Victoria LOS system also allows for better understanding of the circumstances underpinning many of the clinical indicator results. For example, regular review of patients with unrelieved severe pain has demonstrated that in many cases that

Table 16–14	EMS Patient Categories for Limited Occurrence Screening
Clinical Area	**LOS Categories**
Reattend	Patient not transported and EMS reattend in 24 hours
Cardiac arrest	Death while in EMS care (exclude patients in cardiac arrest on EMS arrival) VF/VT patients whose "at patient" to "first shock" interval exceeds 3 minutes
Potential major trauma	Patients who are not directly transported to a Major Trauma Service, where the transport time to an MTS is estimated to be <30 minutes
Pain	Severe pain patients whose reduction in pain score is <3 Patients whose final pain score is >7
Intubation	Patients receiving intubation facilitated by sedation Patients receiving rapid sequence intubation
Tension pneumothorax	Patients treated for tension pneumothorax

patients have either received all appropriate treatment within the CPG or are comfortable despite rating their final pain level as high.

Sentinel Events

The Joint Commission on Accreditation of Health Care Organizations (JCAHO, US) defines a sentinel event as "an unexpected occurrence or variation involving death or serious physical or psychological injury, or risk thereof." Minimum judgment should be required in determining what to report as a sentinel event.[52]

Appropriate sentinel events for EMS requiring root cause analysis include:

1. Hospital admission unrelated to the original presenting condition and as a clear consequence of the actions or inactions by EMS.
2. Death of a patient as a clear consequence of the actions or inactions by EMS; and
3. A near miss of either of the preceding occurrences.

It is believed that the frequency of sentinel events is likely to be reduced by examining the settings in which they occur and identifying system changes required, which may reduce the likelihood of similar occurrences in the future.

The establishment of such a system is justified by the need to gather as much information as possible by accumulating reports of similar events from different institutions and examining them for common underlying contributing factors. This will assist in collective preventive efforts to improve patient safety. There is also the need for EMS to closely examine current prac-

tice in particular areas and critically assess processes and systems currently in place.

This approach focuses on the organization of care rather than the assignment of individual blame and is therefore likely to promote a serious approach to error reduction at all levels and is in keeping with the principles of accountability.[53]

Clinical Audit

The clinical audit process is an independent appraisal function established within an EMS to examine and evaluate its clinical activities. The objective of clinical auditing is to assist staff on the effective discharge of their clinical responsibilities. The clinical audit process is aimed at highlighting methods for improvement in task performance, ensuring compliance with standards, and effective resource utilization.

In the clinical audit process, the reviewer carries a responsibility to the paramedic, the team, management, and the organization. The overall outcomes of any clinical audit undertaken are an unwavering commitment to quality improvement.

Audits should be conducted in a variety of ways, the most common of which are detailed below.

Infield Audit (IFA)

The aim of the infield audit process is to measure and report the real time performance of paramedics on an ongoing basis. Subsequent analysis of the results will allow for the identification of areas of both high and lesser than desired outcomes. The analysis is generally intended to be at a macro level to identify organizational trends but may occur at a local or team level.

The audit looks at each step of the delivery of care by the paramedic team from receipt of case information to the conclusion of EMS care. Nonclinical matters such as driving behavior may be assessed; however, the focus is on clinical care.

It should be noted that the very fact that they are being observed may change paramedic behavior (i.e., the Hawthorne effect). However, this can be reduced by the use of multiple audits and does not outweigh the numerous advantages of IFA, including the ability to

1. Evaluate paramedics as a team.
2. Ascertain whether performance expectations are realistic in all emergency situations.
3. Offer practical solutions to procedural dilemmas as they are offered.
4. Cultivate and foster support for paramedics.

Analysis of IFA data allows for the preparation of programs to increase any areas of less than desired outcomes (e.g., Continuing Professional Education Program content or CPG) and also for the recognition of high performance.

IFA is a useful tool in reinforcing improvement in practice and accountability for clinical performance. Feedback on results of IFAs should be routinely provided to the paramedic(s), team managers, medical advisors, and quality committees.

Retrospective PCR Audit

Patient care records (PCRs) are the only written (or electronic) record of the care provided by a paramedic. They must reflect a true and accurate account of the events of the case. This is a legal document that can be subject to the provisions of Freedom of Information legislation.

A PCR Audit (chart review) allows for evaluation of:

1. Clinical management (e.g., timely, appropriate, correct sequence).
2. Clinical problem solving.
3. Adherence to clinical standards.
4. Comprehensiveness/completion and accuracy.

For example, in AV a retrospective audit of a random sample of PCRs is undertaken. AV currently audits two PCRs per paramedic per month.

Targeted Clinical Audit Activities

These are activities that target a particular procedure, protocol, or medical condition. They may be performed at a team, a group of teams, or across the EMS. These activities may be coordinated more broadly across a service or potentially with other interstate EMS.

The identification of a targeted audit may result from:

1. PCR feedback.
2. Community feedback.
3. Clinical training database.
4. Clinical infield audit.
5. Clinical information or developments.
6. Clinical review.
7. Direct request.

The data collected from targeted surveys should be analyzed, reported to the medical advisor, and acted upon as required.

Clinical Review and Exception Reporting

The clinical review process aims to foster individuals' development through training and education, to ensure that the EMS clinical standards are maintained and improved in order to deliver the best possible patient care.

Exception reporting is based on clinical standards. Performance outside the standards does not necessarily infer an individual is at fault; it may be an error of the clinical standards. However, the quality of the service has potentially been compromised and must be reviewed.

In addition to identifying potential clinical incidents from screening activities such as LOS or clinical indicators monitoring, cases for review may be identified by self- or peer reporting, complaint, or PCR audit.

Management of clinical reviews across the EMS should be done in a way that ensures that

1. The clinical review process is conducted in an appropriate manner to meet consumer and EMS needs.
2. All reviews are conducted by staff trained in undertaking an investigation.
3. All reviews are treated consistently and in a fair, timely, and equitable manner.
4. The clinical review process has structured integrity and observes the principles of natural justice.
5. A root cause analysis (RCA) methodology is used. RCA is an important tool in the assessment of major accidents in industries such as aviation and nuclear power. Similarly it can be applied to health care to investigate significant adverse events

or near misses. It generally involves the use of a multidisciplinary team to undergo an in-depth analysis of causative factors concerning the incident. The analysis would cover numerous areas such as human factors, communication, training, fatigue, or scheduling, environment, rules, procedures, barriers, and safeguards.[54]

The results of clinical reviews are then reported on an incident and trend basis. The findings of clinical reviews are often valuable input to one or more of continuing education, the review of clinical standards, and understanding the level and types of clinical risks encountered by the organization. Providing this de-identified outcome information to paramedics and their managers also promotes discussion and reflection upon clinical practice at a local level.

Communications (Call-Taking and Dispatch) Audit

The majority of EMS systems use a commercial medical call-taking system, such as the Medical Priority Dispatch System (MPDS) to categorize EMS calls by problem type and urgency.[55] The dispatch rules determined by individual EMSs specify the designated level of ambulance response to send to each call category (determinant code). Each case is assigned a determinant code based on its nature and severity. The determinant code and designated level of ambulance response are sent to the dispatcher, who generally uses computer-aided dispatch (CAD) to identify the necessary ambulance unit(s) to respond to the event in accordance with the designated level of response.

An ideal system will mobilize ambulance (and first-responder) resources in a manner that is timely and appropriate to patient acuity and has the ability to positively influence patient outcome. This needs to be balanced by rational use of resources and limiting potentially dangerous lights and sirens response.

It is widely recognized that dispatch protocols should be very sensitive (i.e., should not miss target cases) at the expense of being less specific (needing to include a larger number of nontarget cases). However, there are risks associated with over-triage, including:

1. Burden on health resources
2. Over-treatment
3. Patient dissatisfaction if ambulance attendance and/or transport was not expected or desired
4. Ambulance diversion

5. ED overcrowding
6. Longer out-of-service times
7. Paramedic dissatisfaction
8. Loss of paramedic skills by dilution of experience
9. The potential for motor vehicle accidents associated with lights and siren travel

Risks of under-triage include:

1. Under-treatment resulting in the deterioration of patient condition
2. Decreased patient and public satisfaction/confidence
3. Litigation

Regular ongoing review of data is required to validate and refine ambulance prioritization and dispatch protocols. In order for this to be effective, it should be systematic with similar methodology applied to all determinants reviewed. In addition, performance measures should be based on patient outcome as well as system outcomes as much as practicable. This will allow for decisions to be made in an evidence-based manner and aid EMS in dealings with external service providers.

The review of EMS responses should involve an assessment of three key criteria:

1. The reliability/accuracy of categorization via call-taking criteria (e.g., MPDS)
2. The accuracy of prioritization (i.e., time-critical)
3. The appropriateness of the dispatched level of care (ALS versus BLS)

Quality review of the dispatch process should include assessment of the call-taking procedures, such as address verification, review of the taped conversations, call-taking system records, the CAD data, and the subsequent event management.

Dispatch Triage Research

Investigators have examined the ability of resource systems (through dispatch triage protocols) or paramedics (through field triage protocols) to correctly assign a level of ambulance response commensurate with the "needs" of the patient. However, research to date has been limited by a number of factors:

1. There is limited clinical consensus regarding the categories of emergency calls that should be awarded a top-priority emergency response.
2. There has been limited investigation of the reliability of the decisions made based on protocols for commercially available dispatch prioritization systems.
3. The actual value of advanced life support (ALS) care or any ambulance care at all has not been

demonstrated for many conditions paramedics encounter in the field. This further complicates the issue of medical necessity: how "necessary" can an ambulance response, treatment by paramedics, or transport be if the outcome benefit has not been substantiated?

4. To evaluate the timeliness of needed care is very challenging. Timeliness is a subjective decision that includes social and medical factors and one that is difficult to assess.

A recent systematic review found a lack of high-quality literature on criteria-based dispatch protocols. Out of 64 papers identified as related to the prioritization of ambulance resources, only 20 contained original data and only 7 were deemed to be of reasonable quality research. According to the review there is very little evidence to support the effect of prioritization of emergency ambulances on patient outcome.[56]

Proposed Detailed Review Methodology for Individual Codes

AV performs regular review of the AV dispatch rules. Target determinants are identified and prioritized via review of clinical data in the AV Data Warehouse. Two filters are applied to the data warehouse cases. One, the potential high-acuity filter, identifies emergency cases based on key variables in fields related to primary survey, perfusion status, vital signs, cardiac rhythm, case nature, paramedic assessment, and management. Similarly, the second filter identifies patients who may potentially benefit from ALS care (potential ALS filter).

Detailed reviews of individual determinants may cover the following issues, depending on the focus of the review (e.g., accuracy of determinant or effectiveness of dispatch grid):

1. Rationale of review
2. Sample size and data set
3. Demographics
4. Reliability/accuracy of call-taker categorization
5. Accuracy of the allocated priority
6. Hospital data (via linkage with Government Registries)
7. Appropriateness of the level of care
8. Risk rating
9. Discussion/recommendations

Reliability/Accuracy of MPDS Categorization

The data set for the review of the accuracy of call categorization should include all cases for the time period covered by the analysis (i.e., not just those cases with the determinant of interest). This will allow for a sensitivity table to be constructed (Table 16-15).

The Accuracy of the Allocated Priority-Determinant Specific

If the urgency of the response is under review, then the analysis should provide details of the proportion of patients with the determinant of interest who are classified as high-acuity (emergency). This would form the basis of discussion regarding the accuracy of the determinant in correctly picking up high-acuity patients (for determinants with an emergency response and vice versa). The data set for this analysis would be all cases with a final event type of the determinant of interest (Table 16-16).

The Appropriateness of the Level of Care

The appropriateness of the level of care is an assessment of whether patients in the relevant call category are likely to have benefited from ALS level care. This should not be based on whether patients received ALS-specific interventions, as this would be influenced by

Table 16–15	**Example Analysis for Determinant—"Breathing Problems: Severe Shortness of Breath (SOB)"**	
	Paramedic Final Assessment	
MPDS Final Event Type	Breathing problems – severe SOB (true case)	Breathing problem but no severe SOB or no breathing problem (false case)
Breathing Problems: Severe SOB	True positive	False positive
Other code	False negative	True negative

Table 16–16	**Analysis of the Accuracy of the Allocated Priority (Urgency of Response)**	
	High-Acuity Patient	**Not High-Acuity Patient**
Emergency Response	Number (%): also provide details on cardiac arrest patients as a subset	Number (%)

more factors than the patient's clinical condition (e.g., current dispatch rules and ALS availability).

Risk Levels

Ideally, for consistency and to aid decisions regarding changes to dispatch rules, an acceptable level of risk for sensitivity regarding patient acuity and non–ALS attendance would be agreed a priori (for relevant event codes).

Establishing risk levels is hindered by a lack of consensus on acceptable level of risk for ambulance dispatch. Similarly, a further review of health and other industries has not revealed publicly available published levels of acceptable risk within industry standards. Instead organizations (such as airlines) tend to utilize a risk matrix where consequence is cross-tabulated with the likelihood of an event to provide a risk rating. This approach is in accordance with the Australian Standard on Risk Management (AS/NZS 4360:2004) and International Standards.[57] Ambulance Victoria uses a similar approach for establishing and managing organizational risk.

Risk levels need to be calculated for any change contemplated. That is a change in priority (increase or decrease urgency of response) and/or a change in the level of care (ALS dispatch). For example, the following steps would be required to review the risk of reducing the priority of a determinant:

1. Identify high-acuity patients in the sample.
2. Assess the consequence of a lower priority (less urgent) response via an expert panel.
3. Assign likelihood to each consequence value. (Note that low-acuity patients would always elicit a consequence of "one" and there may also be some high-acuity patients in this consequence group.)

For cases determined to be high acuity (as per predefined criteria), the following consequence matrix could be constructed (Table 16-17).

A similar matrix can be constructed for the appropriateness of the level of care (e.g., ALS).

Within Ambulance Victoria, a risk matrix for each element is constructed based on agreed-upon a priori levels of likelihood (Table 16-18).

Table 16–17	**Consequence Matrix for High-Acuity Patients**				
	Consequence of Lack of Emergency Response to High-Acuity Patients				
	Catastrophic	*Major*	*Moderate*	*Minor*	*Insignificant*
Consequence Rating	*5*	*4*	*3*	*2*	*1*
Description	Nonemergency response results in death or serious permanent injury/condition to patient	Nonemergency response results in a significant adverse impact on a patient's condition	Nonemergency response potentially has a moderate adverse impact on a patient's condition	Nonemergency response has minor impact on patient condition	No compromise to the patient
Number of patients					

Table 16–18	Example of Likelihood Rating		
Likelihood Description	Likelihood Rating	Criteria	Proportion of Total Annual Caseload for the Event Code
Almost certain	5	The event will occur in a one-year period	> 50%
Likely	4	The event is likely to occur in a one-year period	21 to 50%
Moderate	3	The event may occur in a one-year period	6 to 20%
Unlikely	2	The event is not likely to occur in a one-year period	2 to 5%
Rare	1	The event will occur only in exceptional circumstances	≤1%

Inherent risk is a function of the ratings for likelihood and consequence as specified by the risk matrix. As noted above, AV has adopted a risk matrix as part of its organizational risk management system. A modified version of the matrix has been developed for use in the MPDS/Dispatch Rule review (Figure 16-3).

Due to the nature of the risk review, there are likely to be multiple entries in a risk matrix for a determinant (e.g., a small number of cases identified with significant potential consequences and a larger number of cases identified with less significant consequences). The likely action arising from the risk matrix is driven by the highest calculated inherent risk for

the determinant (e.g., seven). This is then cross-referenced against the AV risk management plan where risk scores are given context (e.g., a score of "five" represents a moderate risk to the organization).

Reporting

Performance measures, LOS results, and results from audits (including resultant recommendations) should be reported to the relevant clinicians and their respective groups and throughout the EMS using standard management and committee structures. Also, key measures should form part of publicly available data.

Performance reports need to be detailed; however, they should always maintain patient privacy and confidentiality. The report should contain appropriate statistical information (e.g., percentiles, means, confidence intervals) together with simple interpretation of results for staff members without statistical training.

Regular performance reporting assists with fostering an organizational culture that embraces quality improvement.

SUMMARY

In this chapter we have provided an overview of the main things to measure in a quality improvement program for an ambulance service. The recommendations are based on our experience and practice at Ambulance Victoria and international literature. We believe they have applicability to most established EMS.

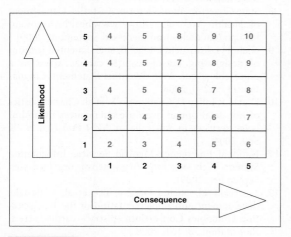

FIGURE 16–3

Modified risk matrix. Reprinted with permission of Ambulance Victoria Risk Management Framework 2009 (FRA/FCS/002).

The clinical quality improvement process is concerned with sustained improvement. It is an approach that challenges the status quo and insists that everything the organization does and how it does it can be done better.

Clinical quality assurance has two major components: quality improvement and patient safety. We have focused on the use of performance measures to monitor the quality of care and a risk management process to monitor and improve patient safety. Both rely on consistent, valid, and readily available data. The importance of data collection cannot be underestimated, and ideally EMS would implement in-field electronic data collection and associated data warehouses and registries. Data linkage is also a powerful component of health service performance review and where possible, patient outcomes should be obtained from hospital data.

In summary, the key components of a comprehensive ambulance quality improvement plan, which have been discussed in this chapter, include:

1. Clinical practice guidelines and clinical standards
2. Clinical indicators
3. Limited occurrence screening (LOS) and clinical review
4. Sentinel events and root cause analysis
5. Call-taking and dispatch rule review
6. Maintenance of appropriate structures and processes to ensure good clinical governance
7. Engendering a "safety culture"

Suggested Key Reading

Quality

Willis C, Evans SM, Stoelwinder JU, et al. Measuring quality. *Aust Health Rev* 31: 276, 2007.

Performance Measures

Myers JB, Slovis CM, Eckstein M, et al. Evidence-based performance measures for emergency medical services systems: A model for expanded EMS benchmarking. A statement developed by the 2007 Consortium US Metropolitan Municipalities EMS Medical Directors. *Prehosp Emerg Care* 12: 141, 2008.

Risk Management

Wolff A, Taylor S. Enhancing patient care. A practical guide to improving quality and safety in hospitals. MJA Books, Sydney, Australia, 2009.

Resuscitation

1. Morrison LJ, Nichol G, Rea TD, et al. Rationale, development and implementation of the Resuscitation Outcomes Consortium epistry – cardiac arrest. *Resuscitation* 78: 161, 2008.
2. Newgard CD, Sears GK, Rea TD, et al. The Resuscitation Outcomes Consortium epistry – trauma: design, development and implementation of a North American epidemiological prehospital trauma registry. *Resuscitation* 78: 170, 2008.
3. Jacobs I, Nadkarni V, Bahr J, et al. Cardiac arrest and cardiopulmonary outcome reports: Update and simplification of the Utstein templates for resuscitation registries. A statement for healthcare professionals from a task force of the International Liaison Committee on Resuscitation. *Resuscitation* 63: 233, 2004.

References

1. Lohr KN, Schroeder SA. A strategy for quality assurance in Medicare. *N Engl J Med* 322: 707, 1990.
2. Wolff A, Taylor S. Enhancing patient care. A practical guide to improving quality and safety in hospitals. MJA Books, Sydney, Australia, 2009.
3. Agency for Healthcare Research and Quality. AHRQ's Patient Safety Initiative: building foundations, reducing risk. Interim report to the Senate Committee on Appropriations. Rockville, Md: AHRQ Publications, 2003.
4. Nichol G, Thomas E, Callaway CW, et al. Regional variation in out-of-hospital cardiac arrest incidence and outcome. *JAMA* 300:1423, 2008.
5. Eisenberg M, White RD. The unacceptable disparity in cardiac arrest survival among American communities. *Ann Emerg Med* 54: 258, 2009.
6. Cameron PA, Gabbe BJ, McNeil JJ, et al. The trauma registry as a statewide quality improvement tool. *J Trauma* 59: 1469, 2005.
7. Fridman M, Barnes V, Whyman A, et al. A model of survival following prehospital cardiac arrest based on the Victorian Ambulance Cardiac Arrest Register. *Resuscitation* 75: 311, 2007.
8. State Government of Victoria, Australia, Department of Health. Web site: http://www.health.vic.gov.au/hosdata/datafields.htm [accessed September, 2009].
9. Nichol G, Rumsfeld J, Eigel B, et al. Essential features of designating out-of-hospital cardiac arrest as a reportable event. AHA Scientific Statement. *Circulation* 117: 2299, 2008.
10. Dietze P, Jolley D, Cvetkosvki S, et al. Characteristics of non-fatal opioid overdose attendances by ambulance services in Australia. *A NZ J Pub Health* 28: 569, 2004.
11. National Emergency Medical Services Information System. Web site: http://www.nemsis.org [accessed September, 2009].
12. Morrison LJ, Nichol G, Rea TD, et al. Rationale, development and implementation of the Resuscitation Outcomes Consortium epistry – cardiac arrest. *Resusitation* 78: 161, 2008.
13. Newgard CD, Sears GK, Rea TD, et al. The Resuscitation Outcomes Consortium epistry – trauma: design, development and implementation of a North American epidemiological prehospital trauma registry. *Resuscitation* 78: 170, 2008.

14. Willis C, Evans SM, Stoelwinder JU, et al. Measuring quality. *Aust Health Rev* 31: 276, 2007.

15. Myers JB, Slovis CM, Eckstein M, et al. Evidence-based performance measures for emergency medical services systems: A model for expanded EMS benchmarking. A statement developed by the 2007 Consortium US Metropolitan Municipalities EMS Medical Directors. *Prehosp Emerg Care* 12: 141, 2008.

16. Maio RF, Garrison HG, Spaite DW, et al. Emergency medical services outcomes project I (EMSOP I). Prioritizing conditions for outcomes research. *Ann Emerg Med* 33(4): 423, 1999.

17. Indicators for Quality Improvement. Full indicator list. The Health and Social Care Information Centre, Department of Health, NHS, England. 2009.

18. Horne S, Weston C, Quinn T, et al. The impact of prehospital thrombolytic treatment on re-infarction rates: analysis of the Myocardial Infarction National Audit Project. *Heart* 95: 559, 2009.

19. National Health Service Information Centre. Web site: http://www.ic.nhs.uk [accessed September, 2009].

20. Moody-Williams JD, Krug S, O'Connor R, et al. Practice guidelines and performance measures in emergency medical services for children. *Ann Emerg Med* 39: 404, 2002.

21. Cameron PA, Gabbe BJ, McNeil JJ. The importance of quality of survival as an outcome measure for an integrated trauma system. *Injury* 37: 1178, 2006.

22. Dijkers M. Measuring quality of life: methodological issues. *Am J Phys Med Rehabil* 78: 286, 1999.

23. Stiell I, Nesbitt LP, Nichol G, et al. Comparison of Cerebral Performance category score and the Health Utility Index for survivors of cardiac arrest. *Ann Emerg Med* 83: 241, 2009.

24. Wachelder EM, Mouaert VRPM, van Heugten C, et al. Life after survival: Long-term daily functioning and quality of life after an out-of-hospital cardiac arrest. *Resuscitation* 80: 517, 2009.

25. Granja C, Cabral G, Pinto AT, et al. Quality of life 6-months after cardiac arrest. *Resuscitation* 55: 37, 2002.

26. Gabbe BJ, Simpson PM, Sutherland AM, et al. Functional measures at discharge: are they useful predictors of longer term outcomes for trauma registries? *Ann Surg* 247: 854, 2008.

27. Willis CD, Gabbe BJ, Butt W, et al. Assessing outcomes in paediatric trauma populations. *Injury* 37: 1185, 2006.

28. Cummins RO, Ornato JP, Thies WH, et al. Improving survival from sudden cardiac arrest: The "Chain of Survival" concept. A statement for health professionals from the Advanced Cardiac Life Support Subcommittee and the Emergency Cardiac Care Committee, American Heart Association. *Circulation* 83(5):1832, 1991.

29. Larsen MP, Eisenberg MS, Cummins RO, et al. Predicting survival from out-of-hospital cardiac arrest: A graphic model. *Ann Emerg Med* 22(11):1652, 1993.

30. Valenzuela TD, Roe DJ, Cretin S, et al. Estimating effectiveness of cardiac arrest interventions. A logistic regression survival model. *Circulation* 96(10): 3308, 1997.

31. Jacobs I, Nadkarni V, Bahr J, et al. Cardiac arrest and cardiopulmonary outcome reports: Update and simplification of the Utstein templates for resuscitation registries. A statement for healthcare professionals from a task force of the International Liaison Committee on Resuscitation. *Resuscitation* 63: 233, 2004.

32. Zaritsky A, Nadkarni V, Hazinski M, et al. Recommended guidelines for uniform reporting of paediatric advanced life support: the paediatric Utstein Style. A statement for health professionals from a task force of the American Academy of Paediatrics, the American Heart Association, and the European Resuscitation Council. Writing Group. *Circulation* 92: 206, 1995.

33. Short Form Health Survey. Web site: http://www.sf-36.org/tools/sf12.shtml [accessed September, 2009].

34. EQ-5D. web site: http://www.euroqol.org/ [accessed September, 2009].

35. DHS. Review of trauma and emergency services Victoria 1999: Report of the Ministerial Taskforce on Trauma and Emergency Services and the Department of Human Services Working Party on Emergency and Trauma Services: Victoria Department of Human Services; 1999.

36. Esposito TJ, Offner PJ, Jurkovich GJ, et al. Do pre-hospital trauma centre triage criteria identify major trauma victims? *Arch Surg* 130(2): 171, 1995.

37. Willis CD, Gabbe BJ, Cameron PA. Measuring quality in trauma care. *Injury* 38: 527, 2007.

38. ACSCT. American College of Surgeons Committee on Trauma. Resources for the optimal care of the injured patient. Chicago: American College of Surgeons; 1993.

39. Spaite DW, Criss EA, Valenzuela TD, et al. Prehospital advanced life support for major trauma: Critical need for clinical trials. *Ann Emerg Med* 32(4): 480, 1998.

40. Maio RF, Garrison HG, Spaite DW, et al. Emergency Medical Services Outcome Project (EMSOP) IV: Pain measurement in out-of-hospital outcomes research. *Ann Emerg Med* 40(2): 172, 2002.

41. McLean SA, Maio RF, Domeier RM. The epidemiology of pain in the prehospital setting. *Prehosp Emerg Care* 6:402, 2002.

42. Thomas SH, Shewakramani S. Prehospital trauma analgesia. *J Emerg Med* 35: 47, 2008.

43. Jennings PA, Cameron P, Bernard S. Measuring acute pain in the prehospital setting. *Emerg Med J* 26: 552, 2009.

44. Cepeda MS, Afrcano JM, Polo R, et al. What decline in pain intensity is meaningful to patients with acute pain? *Pain* 105: 151, 2003.

45. Lee JS, Hobden E, Stiell IG, et al. Clinically important change in the Visual Analogue Scale after adequate pain control. *Acad Emerg Med* 10: 1128, 2003.

46. Powell CV, Kelly AM, Williams A. Determining the minimally clinically significant difference in Visual

Analog Pain Score for children. *Ann Emerg Med* 37: 28, 2001.

47. Bray JE, Martin J, Cooper G, et al. Paramedic identification of stroke: Community validation of the Melbourne Ambulance Stroke Screen. *Cerebrovasc Dis* 20: 28, 2005.

48. Kidwell CS, Saver JL, Schubert GB, et al. Design and retrospective analysis of the Los Angeles Prehospital Stroke Screen (LAPSS). *Stroke* 31: 71, 2000.

49. Kothari RU, Pancioli A, Liu T, et al. Cincinnati Prehospital Stroke Scale: reproducibility and validity. *Ann Emerg Med* 33: 373, 1999.

50. Stiell IG, Spaite DW, Field B, et al. Advanced life support for out-of-hospital respiratory distress. *N Engl J Med* 356: 2156, 2007.

51. Wolff AM. Limited adverse occurrence screening: using medical record review to reduce hospital adverse patient events. *Med J Aust* 164: 458, 1996.

52. The Joint Commission. Web site: http://www.joint commission.org/ [accessed September, 2009].

53. Clinical Risk Management Strategy 2001, Acute Health Division, Victorian Department of Human Services, July 2001.

54. Bagian JP, Gosbee J, Lee CZ, et al. The Veterans Affairs root cause analysis system in actin. *Joint Comm J Qual Improv* 28: 531, 2002.

55. Clawson JJ, Martin RL, Hauert SA. Protocols vs. guidelines...choosing a medical-dispatch program. *Emerg Med Serv* 23: 52, 994.

56. Wilson S, Cooke M, Morrell R, et al. A systematic review of the evidence supporting the use of priority dispatch of emergency ambulances. *Prehosp Emerg Care* 6: 42, 2002.

57. Australian Risk Management Standards Web Site: http://www.riskmanagement.com.au   [accessed November 2009].

CHAPTER 17

EMS Vehicles

Mark Sochor, Benjamin Sojka, William Brady

KEY POINTS OF AMBULANCE DESIGN

- Consider the environments and conditions and how people work within them.
- Consider the needs for vehicle maintenance.
- Address the ergonomic and safety needs of all personnel who will work in or around the ambulance.

- Consider the staffing model used by the agency. For how long are personnel in the vehicle at one time?
- Address any specific needs of the patient groups served (e.g., children, psychiatric patients, rural residents).

THE AMBULANCE – WHAT DEFINES AN AMBULANCE?

EMS services have always been defined and identified by the vehicles that treat patients in the field and transport them to definitive care. Napoleon's chief physician (1797–1815), Baron Dominique-Jean Larrey, developed a system of retrieval for the wounded from the battlefield. A key part of the retrieval process was a designated corps of soldiers with a distinctive hierarchy and, most importantly, a covered cart that took both medical supplies and surgeons to the battlefield as well as delivered the wounded back to the hospitals – likely the initial description of the ambulance. The EMS system in Prague (The Prague Volunteer Rescue Corps) was established in 1857, using horse-drawn vehicles. In the 1870s, New York City and Cincinnati used horse-drawn ambulances to treat the patients in "the field." Patients were identified by word of mouth or telegraph.

The importance of rapid response to trauma became evident with the experience gained from numerous armed conflicts in the 20th century.

Recording of mortality rates during the world wars and the Vietnam conflict showed a steady decrease in mortality with advances in time to definitive care for the fallen soldier. With rapid transport of the physician/medic to the wounded and/or the retrieval of the wounded, the mortality rates dropped roughly in half in each conflict (8.5% First World War, 4.5% Second World War, and 2.4% Vietnam War).

The other major milestone that highlighted the importance of rapid response by EMS utilizing specially equipped vehicles came out of Boston in the 1960s. Dr. Bernard Lown developed and constructed a portable direct-current (DC) defibrillator. Unfortunately, in the early 1970s closed-chest massage was being touted as a good "bridge" to get patients to a defibrillator. It would take many more years until the full potential of rapid delivery of care using a defibrillator in the field would be realized.

The report that finally highlighted the importance of the EMS system in terms of traumatic injury was the 1966 landmark document "Accidental Death and Disability: The Neglected Disease of Modern Society." The quote most often used from

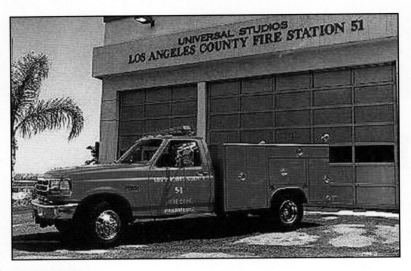

EMS response vehicle, Squad 51, popularized in the television series "Emergency" in the 1970s. Photo Courtesy of William Brady, MD.

this document is "their chances of survival would be better in the zone of combat than on the average city street." This document called many to action within local governments to actually manage the EMS system and eliminate private funeral homes as ambulance providers.[1] During this time a television show "Emergency" featuring "Squad 51" also brought the prehospital care concept to the American public, which would help drive citizens' awareness and demands for the services (Figure 17-1). Years later, the US Emergency Medical Services Systems Act of 1973 began the funding stream to purchase communications equipment and ambulances.

Current initiatives to further develop the US EMS system are contained in the 1995 "EMS Agenda for the Future" which has driven the National Highway Traffic and Safety Administration to produce "EMS Research Agenda for the Future: A Systems Approach" and the "EMS Research Agenda for the Future."[2]

BASIC AMBULANCE REQUIREMENTS

Ambulances typically have the look of a mobile Emergency Department (Figure 17-2). Other types of vehicles with "AMBULANCE" stenciled on them serve as enclosed stretcher carriers (Figure 17-3). This difference in capability is based on need and available resources. Specifically, the type of care that can be administered is based on time available and the atten-

dant's level of training as well as the funds available to purchase and equip the vehicle, not only with equipment but with personnel as well. This observation raises the question of how an ambulance should be specified. Should there be one standard for design across the globe? Should each country have a standard? Or is the delivery of care so specific that each individual system will have to derive its own creation? As is true with complex machine considerations, the answer appears to be a mixture of all of these options.

In the United States the document that has been viewed as a standard for ambulance design is the Federal Specification for "*Star of Life Ambulance*," KKK-A-1822E.[3] This document was created as a specification for the purchase of ambulances by the federal government or those agencies utilizing federal funds. The stated purpose of this document, shown below, is a good example of the basic design considerations and objectives that should be present in any specification for an ambulance.

Ambulances that are authorized to display the "*Star of Life*" symbol developed by the US National Highway Traffic Safety Association (NHTSA) (Figures 17-4, 17-5) meet minimum specifications and test parameters and meet minimum criteria for ambulance design, performance, equipment, and appearance. The objective of such standardization is to provide ambulances that are nationally recognized, properly constructed, easily maintained, and, when professionally staffed and provisioned, will function reliably in prehospital or other mobile emergency medical service.

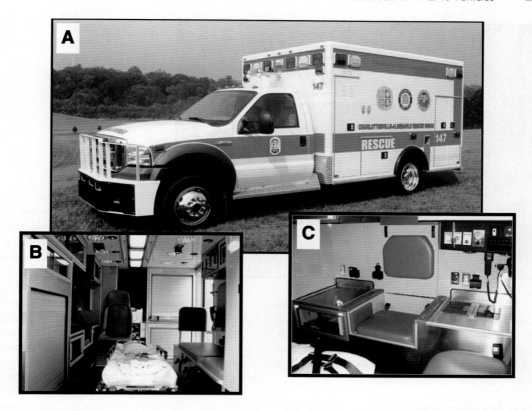

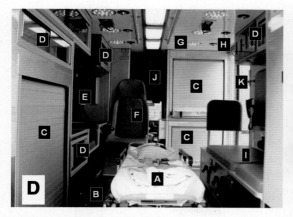

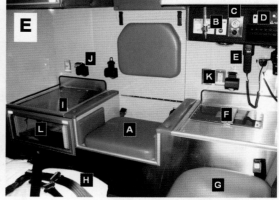

FIGURE 17–2

A, Charlottesville Albemarle Rescue Squad Ambulance 147 (Virginia, US). **B**, Interior view from the rear doors. **C**, Primary patient care area/attendant seat from the side door. **D**, Patient care interior of ambulance 147 – [A] Patient stretcher. [B] Stretcher floor bracket (secures stretcher). [C] Large equipment cabinet (medication storage box, portable monitor-defibrillator unit, portable suction, oxygen kit, supply/equipment bag). [D] Small equipment cabinet (bandages, splints, other supplies/equipment). [E] Work area detail. [F] Attendant seat. [G] Ceiling lighting. [H] Ceiling hooks (for intravenous fluids/medications and other equipment). [I] Bench /additional patient cot area (also serves as storage cabinet under bench). [J] Open area to driver compartment. [K] Side door. **E**, Patient care interior of ambulance 147 – [A] Additional attendant seat. [B] Gas exchange outlets (oxygen). [C] Suction outlet. [D] Electrical control panel for environmental and lighting controls. [E] Communications console. [F] Refuse and used needle containers. [G] Attendant seat. [H] Patient stretcher. [I] Counter surface area. [J] Straps to secure equipment during transport. [K] Electrical outlet. [L] Cabinet. Photos Courtesy of Anthony Judkins, NREMT-P.

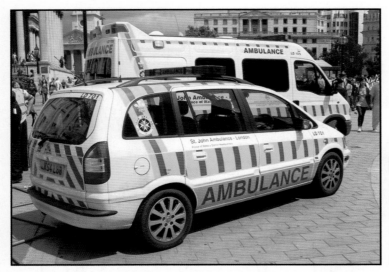

FIGURE 17–3

London Ambulance Service (St. John Ambulance – London) – EMS supervisor vehicle in foreground and ambulance in background. Photo Courtesy of William Spencer, NREMT-P.

The *Star of Life Ambulance* specification also includes the "Definition of an Ambulance," which is a concise explanation of one government's expectations of an ambulance. The ambulance is defined as a vehicle for emergency medical care which provides:

1. A driver's compartment.
2. A patient compartment to accommodate an emergency medical technician (EMT)/paramedic and two litter patients (one patient located on the primary cot and a secondary patient on a folding litter located on the squad bench) so positioned that the primary patient can be given intensive life support during transit.
3. Equipment and supplies for emergency care at the scene as well as during transport; and
4. Two-way radio communication, and, when necessary, equipment for light rescue/extrication procedures.

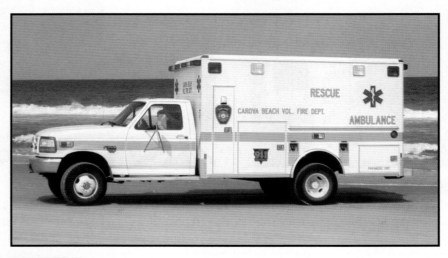

FIGURE 17–4

Carova Beach Volunteer Fire Department Ambulance 7 (North Carolina, US). This ambulance is equipped not only with four-wheel drive capability but also high-ground clearance. This ambulance has its primary response area in the northern coastal area of North Carolina; no paved roads are found in this area, necessitating response into areas accessed only via sand roadways. Photo courtesy of William Brady, MD.

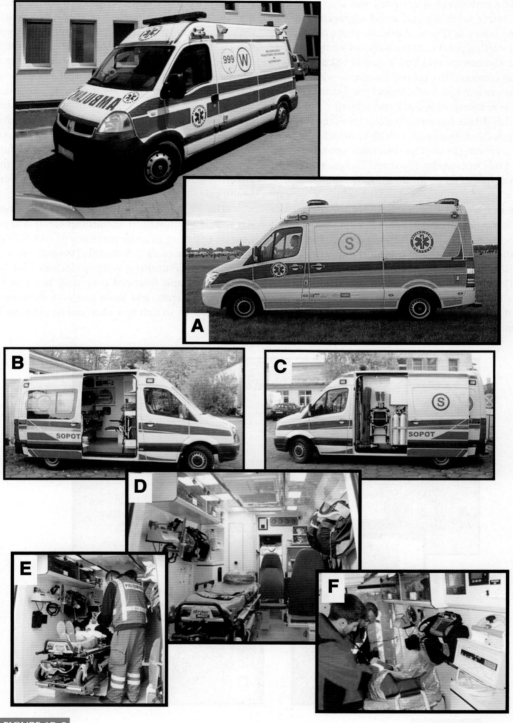

FIGURE 17–5

A, Ambulances in Poland. **B**, Side view with door. **C**, Side view with equipment compartment. **D**, Patient care interior from the rear doors. **E**, Patient care area. **F**, Patient care area. Note the equipment storage in easily accessed yet secure postings in the patient care area. Photos courtesy of Piotr Wozniak, MD.

The ambulance is designed and constructed to afford safety, comfort, and avoid aggravation of the patient's injury or illness. While the above description gives a starting point as to the basics of what an ambulance could contain and how it should be constructed, there is concern that setting standards with narrow parameters will negatively impact the industry whose goal it is to transport the sick and injured.

This debate has arrived in the US as the National Fire Protection Association (NFPA), which has commenced creating its own specifications for ambulances. While Fire Department–based ambulances account for less than half of those produced in the United States, there is concern that this standard, which it appears will be adopted in place of the *Star of Life* Ambulance Specification by the federal government, would result in larger vehicles beyond what is needed by the majority of the American patient transport industry[4] (Figure 17-6), although this debate continues.

The United Kingdom has struggled with how to ensure that the ambulances transporting those in a time of need are safe and appropriate as well. Information from the "National Health Service (NHS)

National Reporting and Learning System" illustrated that patient and staff safety was at risk as a result of ambulance design factors. As a result, a study was launched by the Royal College of Art to "Establish a design direction for future emergency ambulance and equipment development." The study included several workshops where multiple stakeholders were brought together from manufacturers to ambulance staff. From these workshops, nine design challenges were identified. By addressing these challenges using evidence-based methods, it is hoped that current and future emergency medical vehicles will be safer and more effective while operating in their role of delivering health care (Table 17-1).

The method employed by the Royal College of Art should be utilized by all agencies when designing new or updating existing machinery.[5] (Available at: http://news.bbc.co.uk/2/hi/health/7986460.stm.)

Design committees should include not only management and financial personnel but also field personnel, patients, and those from the manufacturing community so that new ideas can be implemented rapidly.

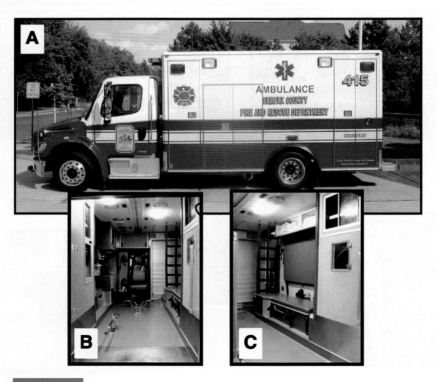

FIGURE 17–6

Fairfax County Fire Rescue 415 Ambulance (Virginia, US). **A**, Side view. **B**, Interior view from the rear doors. **C**, Interior view of bench from the rear doors. Photos courtesy of Steve Hartman, NREMT-P.

Table 17–1	Nine Ambulance Design Challenges from the Royal College of Art

1. Ensure safe and effective access and egress
2. Improve working space and layout
3. Effectively secure people and equipment in transit
4. Ensure effective communication
5. Address security, violence, and aggression
6. Facilitate effective hygiene and infection control
7. Maximize equipment usability and compatibility
8. Improve vehicle engineering
9. Humanize the patient experience

A walk-around an existing unit is often all that is needed to begin a dialogue with all of the stakeholders about changes that are desired. Often, there are reasons not known to one group as to why something exists in the state that it does. These "walk-arounds" can often quickly become a collaborative session (design *Charente*, a group of designers and users work together to draft a design) where small, workable changes can result in significant advances in safety, patient care, and patient experience.

Numerous questions must be asked in the early consideration of the ambulance design. National or state design requirements, such as the *Star of Life Ambulance* Specifications, can be utilized as a guide so that critical design questions are not overlooked. Finally, once these questions are used to stimulate a discussion and components are questioned and discussed using a standard specification as a checklist, the Nine Design Challenges from the Royal College of Art can be used as a validating tool for the decisions made. The following questions should be considered in the early design phase of ambulance creation:

1. Consider the environments and conditions that the vehicle will be used in and around and how people work within it.
2. What are the ergonomic needs of all personnel who will work in or around the apparatus?
3. Consider the staffing model used by the agency. For how long are personnel in the vehicle at one time?
4. What are the demographics of the patient groups served?
5. Are there specific needs for patient groups that should be integrated into the vehicle?

A final question to keep in mind when creating an ambulance design: Is this what is needed for our employees and our patients, or is it the design that management, and/or the builder thinks is most appropriate? Sometimes what is needed has never been created.

OCCUPANT SAFETY

Occupant safety is the most critical component of ambulance design. Seatbelts and airbags are helpful in preventing injuries but do not address all of the safety issues for the safety of the attendants and patients. Patient compartment layout and equipment mounting are critical to ensure that attendants are not put in a situation where they must decide between their own safety and caring for the patient. The environment where the unit will operate also must be considered from the safety perspective.

Is it hot or cold? Are prolonged periods of extreme cold the norm or will the unit sit in direct sun every day? Consider the heating and cooling system not only for the patient compartment but also for the operator's area. Ambulances tend to idle long periods of time. Will this affect the efficiency of these systems? Extremes of temperature can have an impact not only on the patient but also on those who call this vehicle their office. In addition, the temperature range where certain medications can be carried should be considered. Is additional equipment needed in order to successfully accomplish this task?

Urban versus rural: Does this have an impact on unit design? Of course, large units are often considered a positive element for the crew, but is this true? Tight city streets may make it difficult for large units to turn around. While a fire truck may be able to navigate a small area, it normally carries additional personnel who can assist with backing maneuvers. This is typically not the case with an ambulance once the patient is loaded. In the rural setting, narrow farm lanes may necessitate narrower vehicles and those with all-wheel drive.

Equipment placement should also be considered. If interstate operations are part of a unit's daily activity, consider how compartment layout can keep personnel away from traffic. Similarly, units that have to work on tight streets may need to have options to keep their "working width" (width when compartment doors are open) to a minimum. Special units may be developed to either deliver care on the scene without transport capabilities or with transport capabilities, depending on space limitations (Figures 17-7, 17-8, 17-9, and 17-10).

Environment doesn't just mean temperature. Do the ambulances and their crews work in areas where

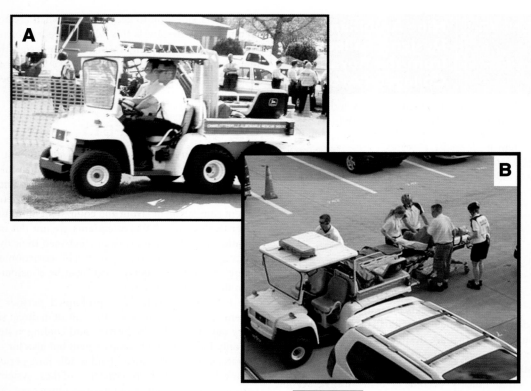

FIGURE 17–7

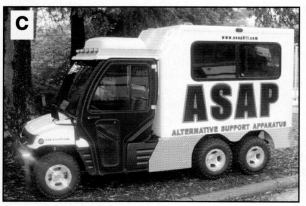

A, EMS-equipped gator capable of patient transport, Charlottesville-Albemarle Rescue Squad (Virginia, US). These patient transport vehicles are of value for short distances when traditional ambulance transport is not possible. **B**, Loading of a patient onto an EMS-equipped gator, Charlottesville-Albemarle Rescue Squad (Virginia, US). **C**, The mini-ambulance mode of patient transport. This vehicle is capable of safe patient transport in areas where congestion and/or lack of traditional paved roadways would preclude such conveyance. A and B, photos courtesy of William Brady, MD; C, photo courtesy of Benjamin Sojka, NREMT-P.

personal safety is often at risk? Carrying keys and locking the truck may not always be the answer, as this may increase the potential for personnel to be assaulted. Hidden unlock features or punch code locks may be the solution.

An easily cleanable ambulance will reduce the threat of transferring bacteria and other illnesses from an infected patient to the crew and subsequent patients. Surfaces in the patient care area should be easy to clean. That does not just mean solid, impermeable surfaces. Cleanable surfaces should be constructed so that corners do not trap dirt, and surfaces in impact areas should be of materials that will not crack or chip. All padded surfaces should be of materials that cannot harbor bacteria and that can be removed for cleaning.

ERGONOMIC NEEDS

No one wants anyone to get hurt on the job. A well-planned ambulance can have a direct impact on reducing job place injuries. Don't just think about the patient compartment. **Consider the process of**

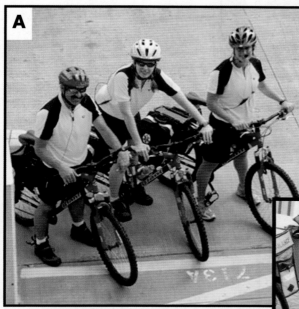

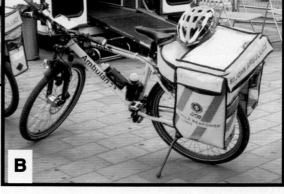

FIGURE 17–8

EMS support vehicles — "The Bike Team." Such teams are capable of rapid response over longer distances at large or mass events when traditional vehicular traffic would be inefficient. Of course, patient transport is not possible with such a "first response." **A**, Special Event Medical Management (University of Virginia)/Charlottesville-Albemarle Rescue Squad. **B**, London Ambulance Service (St. John Ambulance – London). A, photo courtesy of William Brady, MD; B, photo courtesy of Anthony Judkins, NREMT-P.

how a call is run. Does the crew get in the truck at the beginning of the call? Will the truck steps trap debris or ice that could become a slip hazard? Will required equipment such as map books result in a facial injury if the brakes are applied suddenly? Is there a good place to mount a flashlight so that it WILL be taken with the crew when they exit the truck on a dark night?

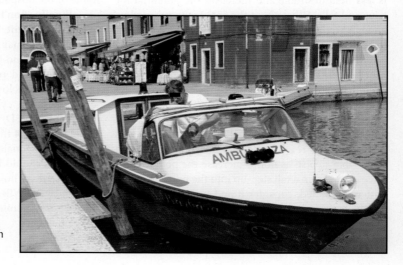

FIGURE 17–9

Water ambulance in Burano, Italy (near Venice). Photo courtesy of Jim Scuffham.

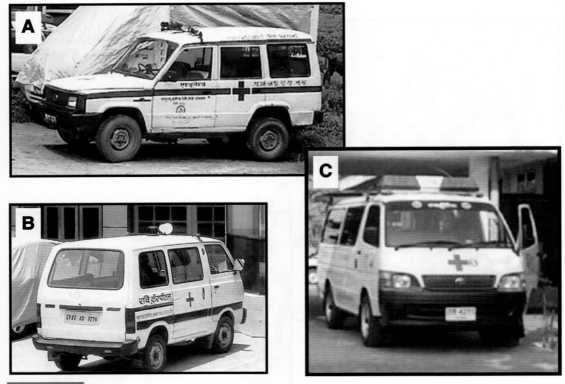

A, Ambulance (Nepal). **B**, Ambulance (India). **C**, Ambulance (Thailand). A and B, photo courtesy of Robert O'Conner, MD; C, photo Courtesy of William Brady, MD.

Once the unit arrives on scene, additional equipment needs to be quickly retrieved. Consider how the vehicle is accessed. Having to step up and into the unit is less than desirable and increases the potential for trips and falls. What about the cot? Is the vehicle low enough so that the cot can be easily removed or will the truck need to lower?

Remember, the more complex the solution, the more potential for failure. Step back and look at the overall situation. Can the unit run with shorter sidewall tires, thus reducing the load height of the cot? Once the patient is in the unit, how does the attendant get into the patient compartment? Are grab rails needed at the rear? Does the side door require a removable step so as not to increase the potential for knee injury from a tall step-up into the unit? Once the patient is loaded, consider if and how the attendant will have to ambulate in order to provide care. Are overhead grab bars in the correct locations? Consider

where items such as heart monitors are located. Can they be easily operated by the attendant while safely seated, and can they be accessed for carrying into a home or the hospital?

Finally, don't forget those who care for and maintain the unit. This may be the crew or it may be personnel at a maintenance facility. Cabinets that are easy to access and load with equipment will increase productivity and reduce the potential for errors in restocking. The location and access to compressed air and oxygen cylinders also must be considered (see Figure 17-5D, E and F). In certain applications, the placement of these cylinders is driven strongly by the desire to equally distribute weight in the vehicle. While this should be considered, thought must also be invested in how the cylinders will be removed and replaced. Will a lift be utilized? Will the lift be integral or a mobile unit that places the cylinder into the ambulance?

THE AMBULANCE IS A MOBILE OFFICE

Consider the duration of shifts when creating the work environment of the ambulance personnel. If workers will be based out of the unit for 8 to 12 hours at a time and do not typically return to a home-base facility, they must carry what they need for their work and their comfort. Cup holders are a necessity. It is not realistic to believe that people will not consume beverages in the cab of the vehicle. Cup holders should be integrated so that beverages will not spill on reference books or computers and will not increase injury potential during an accident.

Laptop computers and Global Positioning Systems are an integral part of work and recreation. Power sources should be provided both in the front and in the patient compartment so that laptops can be easily utilized.

If the ambulance will not be parked in a conditioned space when not on a call, how will the crew maintain a conditioned environment? Excessive idling is degrading to the environment and can be harmful to the life of the vehicle's engine. While a fire station is not an option to many ambulances as a place to post and await the next call, an electrical connection may be available. Shore line electrical systems can be integrated into the ambulance design so that climate control and other systems, including equipment chargers, can be operated from an appropriately sized extension cord routed to an electrical source. If a shore line is not even an option, consider borrowing technology created by the over-the-road truck industry. This industry has created highly efficient generators that can operate electronics and climate control equipment for extended periods of time when drivers sleep in their trucks.

WHO IS BEING SERVED?

When designing an ambulance, consider the community being served. Ambulances designed primarily for answering calls for service generated from citizens contacting 911 operations centers have different requirements than those that provide critical care transfers or neonatal transports. Ambulances responding to emergent calls must have the capability to carry a diverse cache of medical equipment. Some may even carry rescue equipment, including the **jaws of life** used in the extrication of victims from damaged vehicles. A critical factor in the layout of such vehicles is that routinely needed equipment must be easily accessible. Layout should be based upon what the crew needs in order to care for the patient on the majority of calls. Information regarding typically used equipment can be sourced from call reports, but staff should also be polled.

The location of the potential patient base should also be considered in ambulance design. In rural areas where long distances may need to be covered, the number of patients that can be transported in a single ambulance can become a critical factor in transport, especially with patients who have suffered traumatic injuries. While most ambulances in North America and western Europe typically have the capacity to carry one or two patients, those in other areas often carry more, especially during times of disaster. Learning and adapting successful methods from other regions should be part of the design collaboration.

Specific Needs

Certain portions of the patient base served may have needs that must be considered in the design of ambulances. For example, consider the morbidly obese patient. Typical ambulance cots have a load rating of around 500 pounds. Depending on the stretcher unit, this rating may only be valid when the cot is nearest the ground. As a result, broader and higher capacity cots will need to be integrated into the ambulance fleet. The ambulance must be designed so that the cot can be loaded into the ambulance without subjecting the crew to injury. Lifting heavy loads can be accomplished with a winch and ramp system. Such equipment should be integrated by the ambulance manufacturer so that liability for appropriate operation remains with a single entity. All of this equipment will need to be stored in the ambulance, typically resulting in this unit's being less than optimal for typical operations. A dedicated unit may not be an option and therefore ease of conversion may need to be considered for a primary ambulance.

Ambulance design and specification should be strongly based on the needs of the care providers and the patients (Figure 17-11). EMS personnel should be empowered to make suggestions during the design phase. Once vehicles are placed in service, adaptations suggested by EMS personnel should be accommodated at the factory in the future, so that underlying deficiencies either in the truck or medical system can be appropriately addressed. **Safety must be considered with every design decision.**

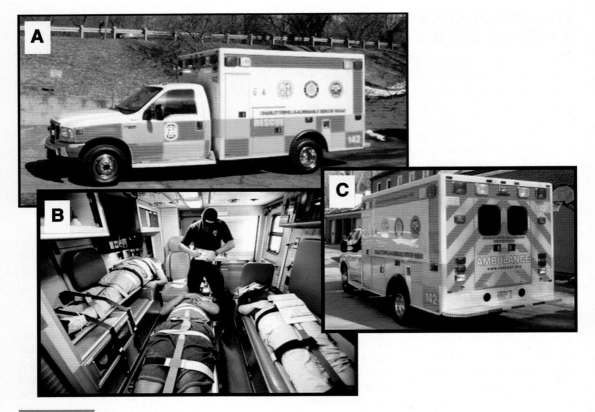

FIGURE 17–11

A, Charlottesville Albemarle Rescue Squad Ambulance 142 (Virginia, US). Side view. Note the patterned coloration for increased visibility. **B**, Interior view from the rear doors. Note the ability to transport three supine patients in safe and appropriate fashion. **C**, Rear view with high visibility coloration. Photos Courtesy of Anthony Judkins, NREMT-P.

Web Resources

1. http://www.objectivesafety.net/; accessed December 22, 2009.
2. http://www.objectivesafety.net/PDFHO.htm; accessed December 22, 2009.
3. http://www.nrls.npsa.nhs.uk/ National Reporting & Learning Services; accessed December 22, 2009.
4. http://www.saambulance.com.au/publicweb/pdf/ CAA07%20report_final.pdf; Council of Ambulance Authorities – National Patient Satisfaction Survey Results 2007; accessed December 22, 2009.

References

1. Brennan JA, Krohmer J. Principles of EMS Systems. 3rd ed., 2005. American College of Emergency Physicians, Dallas, TX.
2. http://www.nhtsa.dot.gov/people/injury/EMS/ agenda/EMSman.html; NHTSA-EMS Agenda for the Future – December 31, 2001 (accessed 12/20/09).
3. http://www.gsa.gov/gsa/cm_attachments/GSA_ DOCUMENT/ambulanc_1_R2FI5H_0Z5RDZ-i34K-pR.pdf. Federal Specifications for Ambulances KKK-A-1822E (accessed 12/20/09).
4. Mannie G. *EMS Insider* 36(1): 2009.
5. http://news.bbc.co.uk/2/hi/health/7986460.stm. Emergency Transport of the Future, Tuesday, 7 April 2009 09:54 UK, accessed Dec 22, 2009.

CHAPTER 8

Ambulance Station Design

Manuel Hernandez

KEY LEARNING POINTS

- EMS station design begins with identifying the station location that best serves community needs.
- Establishing the vision of a new EMS station and desired performance outcomes will inform the design process and provide a more responsive EMS station design.
- Understanding the needs of the EMS personnel with respect to work roles, respite needs, religious/cultural requirements, and educational/research objectives will better inform EMS station design.
- EMS station design should incorporate the need for proximity of particular areas to promote greater efficiency, comfort, and safety of personnel and visitors as well as ensuring equipment is stored safely and conveniently to areas of need.
- EMS stations have the potential to serve as a community focal point and, as such, should be designed to incorporate community meeting and education space (where appropriate).
- Sustainable design elements can be included in EMS station design to lessen the environmental impact while reducing the overall cost of station operation.

As EMS programs grow and evolve across the globe, attention has focused on personnel development through additional training and improvements in care delivery through advances in equipment and technology. While this is important, the often-overlooked aspect of designing an innovative EMS station is also important. Designing an EMS station is more than simply building a space to house vehicles and equipment. When properly designed, EMS stations can serve a wide variety of functions that not only provide a proper base for operations of EMS personnel but also serve as a community resource. As EMS station design has continued to evolve, EMS leaders, architects, and planners have begun taking an innovative look at how to make an EMS station more than a box with four walls and a roof, instead looking at how facility design can transcend its primary design to become so much more.

In many systems, realities such as stressful working conditions, personal safety, limited mobility, and irregular working hours can contribute to poor EMS personnel morale and increased challenges with recruitment and retention.[1] Where possible the facility design process should be undertaken with the intent of using the facility as a tool to mitigate the impact of these realities on EMS. EMS stations in and of themselves can serve as a magnet for EMS providers by creating a comfortable, stimulating work environment. In such situations, tasks as potentially challenging as recruiting qualified personnel in communities where a shortage of such personnel exists can be made easier. In addition, the facility, because of innovative design, pleasing interiors, and access to technologies, can serve to stimulate community interest in EMS and as a vehicle for new education initiatives. In communities that rely on all or partial volunteer staffing models, the provision of a comfortable and stimulating EMS station may potentially increase volunteer involvement and frequency of response to service requests. Increased participation in service requests translates into more frequent opportunities to utilize procedural skills, which is known to improve performance.[2]

The EMS station also has the potential to serve the vital role of educating the public about the role of EMS in accessing emergency care while instilling a sense of confidence in the professionalism and competence of EMS personnel. In many communities, information about how to access EMS services is either lacking or confusing.[3,4] Carefully thought-out EMS stations that incorporate communication education and public service activities into their function and design hold the potential to provide on-going community education regarding access of EMS services and their role in the health care system.

This chapter will take a detailed look at the many variables to consider when beginning the process of engaging in planning and design of a new EMS station. While differences in care delivery models, technologies, and financial recourses exist in EMS systems across the globe, the concepts that need to be thoroughly vetted are the same (Table 18-1). With careful planning, attention to the requirements of process, human capital, technology, and facility design, the future EMS station

Table 18–1	**Design Considerations for New EMS Stations**

Site selection
EMS staffing model
EMS transport vehicles
Equipment storage
Continuing education/new education for EMS
 providers
Supplemental uses of EMS station
Sustainable design
Physical layout/adjacent areas

Table 18–2	**Learning Objectives**

Upon completion of this chapter, readers should be able to

1. Identify important components of the site selection process
2. Articulate the impact of the personnel staffing models and the needs of EMS providers on the design of an EMS station
3. Understand how different EMS transport and nontransport vehicles will impact on how the ambulance bay must be configured
4. Discuss approaches to equipment storage as well as separation of clean and soiled storage areas
5. Consider how the educational needs of current and future EMS providers can be accommodated within the EMS station with proper understanding of the educational modalities to be employed
6. Evaluate potential supplemental uses of the EMS station and understand how these uses can enhance the EMS system and the overall quality of the community
7. Review basic concepts of sustainable design that may be included in the design of any future EMS station
8. Appreciate how, after considering all individual components to be incorporated into a new EMS station design, adjacent areas can improve the overall flow and function of a new EMS station

will serve as an innovative focal point of the emergency care system and the community. Table 18-2 shows the learning objectives for this chapter.

SITE SELECTION

The process of initiating the design process for a new EMS station begins with appropriate station site selection. Site selection is an important first consideration owing to the fact that EMS services and prehospital care are typically time-sensitive. Excessive EMS station distances and, by extension, EMS provider distances and response time to patients requiring emergent intervention for a treatable condition can have profound implications on patient outcomes and mortality (Table 18-3). This reality needs to be considered in selecting an EMS station site location and understanding its relevance to clinical outcomes.

Another consideration with respect to EMS station location is the distance from patients as it relates

Table 18–3	Examples of Time-Sensitive Medical Conditions/ Interventions Potentially Impacted by Patient Distance from EMS Station
Medical Condition	**Metric Potentially Impacted**
Trauma	Golden hour
Acute myocardial infarction	Door-to-balloon
	Door-to-needle
Acute ischemic stroke	Door-to-needle
Cardiac arrest	Onset of resuscitation
	Initial time of defibrillation for ventricular fibrillation/pulseless ventricular tachycardia
	Airway access
Active labor	Precipitous delivery in the field

to overall average response times. Benchmarks for acceptable response times by EMTs and paramedics vary by country, region, and medical condition and, as of this publication, no consensus has been reached about what constitutes appropriate response time but, clearly, longer response times by EMS professionals are considered less desirable.

While an EMS station may operate with a primary service area that ranges from as little as one square mile in diameter to hundreds of square miles, it is important to recognize that the geographic center of a service region is not always the most logical or appropriate location for an EMS station (Figure 18-1). The location of the EMS station with respect to the primary service area should consider frequency and distribution of calls within the entire service area with the express intent of locating the EMS station in such a manner that it can respond to the maximum number of calls in the least amount of time. In addition, EMS stations that provide frequent mutual aid services to a population served by another EMS station's primary service area will need to consider the frequency and impact of requests for mutual aid services into the station's secondary service area with respect to response times and patient outcomes.

While two important components of selecting the appropriate site location for an EMS station are the distribution of call volumes in the primary service area as well as response time benchmarks, another important aspect of these particular components is the access to convenient, reliable transportation corridors. Transportation corridors will vary based on the individual service area but might include surface streets, limited-access highways, and waterways. For example, if an EMS station relies heavily on a limited-access highway for responses to a significant portion of call requests, then consideration should be made to

locating the station in close proximity to this transportation corridor. Conversely, if there is a particular transportation corridor that is known for restricted access owing to obstacles such as traffic, pedestrians, floods, or other physical barriers (Table 18-4), location of an EMS station along this transportation corridor should be reconsidered.

Similarly, it is important to select an EMS site that is sheltered from potential natural or man-made phenomena that may limit response capabilities or threaten the EMS stations, its contents, and the EMS personnel. For example, in areas with unstable ground that are prone to avalanches or mudslides, EMS stations should not be placed on or at the bottom of hills. In areas with the potential for snow or ice storms, EMS stations should not be placed on hills or designed with driveways that include an incline. EMS stations should never be placed along rivers, streams, or storm runoff of channels in an effort to prevent impact from flooding. Also, EMS station driveways should be free of trees and other potential physical barrier that could become obstacles if they fell and blocked the station driveway.

Table 18–4	Potential Access Barriers Between EMS Stations and Service Requests
Flood waters	Bridge collapse
Fallen trees	Passenger/freight trains
Mudslides	Electrical wires
Rock slides	Civil disorder
Avalanches	Livestock
Ice/snow	

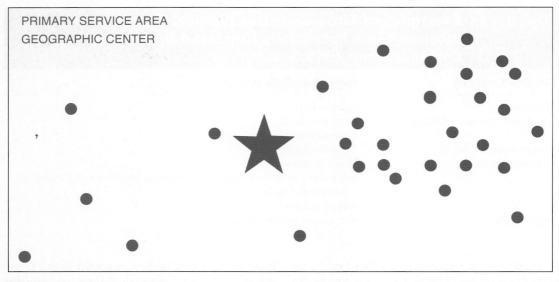

EMS CALL LOCATION

★ EMS STATION LOCATION

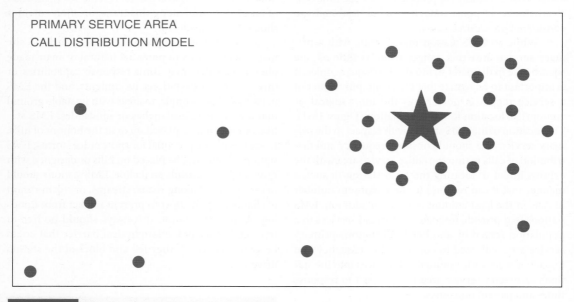

FIGURE 18–1

Approaches to EMS station location in primary service area.

Another important site selection consideration for EMS stations is the collocation of other public
service organizations such as fire, rescue, and law
enforcement. While on the surface collocation of public service organizations may not appear to be a necessary consideration, significant gains can be made with
respect to interdepartmental collaboration, mutual
education, and training exercises as well as building
rapport between EMS, fire, rescue, and law enforcement areas. In addition, collocation of public service
agencies provides the potential for establishment of
economies of scale between all organizations involved.
Examples of economies of scale include: design fees,
construction costs, shared community spaces, shared
educational spaces, and shared vehicle and station
maintenance expenses.

EMS STAFFING MODEL AND FACILITY IMPACT

During the predesign phase for any EMS station, care and attention must be given to understanding the current and any planned future staffing models that will be employed within the EMS system in which the EMS station operates (Table 18-5). Superficially, this may not seem to be an important aspect of EMS station design planning, but the unique needs of various staffing models can have profound implications on how to design an innovative and functional station. While staffing models vary across the globe, most can be broken down into a few key considerations. By gaining a thorough understanding of the staffing implications of the EMS station under consideration, planning for necessary amenities for the EMS personnel will be conducted with greater ease and foresight into personnel expectations.

When designing an EMS station, it is important to consider that the station design is not simply about creating a space to house vehicles and equipment. If

Table 18–5	Staffing Model Considerations for EMS Design
Hours of in-station staffing	
24 hours Partial in-station staffing No in-station staffing (respond to station when service request placed)	
In-station staffing duration	
<12 hours per duty rotation > 12 hours per duty rotation	
Staff compensation model	
All-paid staff All-volunteer staff Mixed compensation model	
Staff gender	
Unisex Mixed gender staffing	
Faith-based staff	
Communities with strong faith-based principles Faith-based worship/reflection requirements Faith-based holidays	

this were the case designing a simple square building with a roof, garage doors, and a door would likely suffice. In many regions of the world there is a shortage of qualified EMS providers. Where EMS employment opportunities are plentiful, personnel will frequently move about in search of the optimal working environment. The challenge to EMS operations leaders is that increased employee turnover translates into increased time and expense associated with recruitment and training as well as the very real potential of gaps in coverage. With this reality in focus it becomes easy to see how the EMS station design can not only function to create a location to base vehicles and store equipment but, in fact, the station itself can become a powerful recruiting tool for paid or volunteer EMS personnel. This is accomplished through innovative design practices that respond to the explicit, implicit, and latent needs of the EMS personnel who will be working in the station.

COMMUNICATION

Whether EMS personnel are located in-station or respond to the station once service requests are made, communication with and between EMS personnel plays a pivotal role in ensuring expedient response times. That said, the communication needs of in-station-based personnel and remote responders will vary.

Within the physical plant of the EMS station, communication technologies need to be employed in a manner that allows contextual awareness across the station. For example, if automated call notification systems such as alert tones, verbal annunciation, or electronic visual displays are used, these should be accessible in all crew areas of the building while not necessarily being accessible in areas of the building used by the community, especially if privacy is a concern.

The communication methodology employed should be designed with the specific intention of being intrusive into the activities of the personnel at any given moment. For example, communication devices placed in the garage area should be loud enough to be distinguished from ambient noise such as verbal communication, music, and vehicle engines. Visual communication modalities should be designed to be distinguishable from emergency warning lights on response vehicles and should be able to be recognized in both daylight and at nighttime. In crew lounges and sleeping quarters, communication modalities should be able to wake EMS personnel from sleep, disrupt attention being given to entertainment activities, and even reach into areas such as water closets and shower facilities.

Communication needs for EMS personnel not physically located within the confines of the EMS station are varied and should be considered independently of in-station modalities. External communication strategies should focus on accessing personnel regardless of location. With growing emphasis on wireless technologies such as mobile phones, paging systems, and 3G wireless networks, care should be taken to ensure "dead zones" do not exist. These have the obvious potential to fail and risk delayed service request response times. Conversely, if auditory warning signals are used (such as fire horns) it is important to ensure these can be heard within an appropriate proximity of the station.

STAFF WORKSPACE

EMS personnel spend considerable time on "stand-by" mode awaiting requests or service from the community. While busy urban and suburban services may have less stand-by time than some of their counterparts, there will be times when EMS personnel are in-station. During this time, EMS personnel will require dedicated space to perform administrative functions such as medical record documentation, verbal and electronic communication, and other tasks that will vary, based on their specific roles and responsibilities.

To accommodate such activity, EMS stations need to incorporate dedicated workspace for EMS personnel. Separate from staff respite and nutritional space, dedicated workspace should be designed with productivity in mind, being free of distractions typically emanating from lounge spaces and other common areas of the station.

In planning the design of dedicated workspace, it is important to understand the needs of staff, the technology implications, and the overall size of the workforce on duty at any given moment. Ideal design would enable the workspace to be an enclosed area, free from potential noise pollution from other areas of the station. Typically, technology should include computer terminals with wired or wireless Internet access if available. If EMS personnel use laptops to complete patient care records, laptop docking stations should be available and may obviate the need for dedicated desktop computers. Telephones should be provided and shared equipment such as printers, scanners, and fax machines should be centrally located within the workspace.

When planning a staff workspace, care should be taken to ensure the design of the space and that its contents are ergonomic in form and function. While many experts have addressed the ergonomics of ambulance

vehicle design,[5] similar considerations must be given to workspaces to prevent potential injury.

STAFF RESPITE SPACE

In many communities, EMS personnel spend time in stand-by mode awaiting dispatch to the next service request. During this time, personnel desire activities that provide intellectual stimulation, physical activity, entertainment, or interaction with the world at-large. While many EMS stations are not designed with staff respite in mind, creating inviting spaces that engage EMS personnel is an important design consideration (Table 18-6). Understanding the explicit, implicit, and latent needs of EMS personnel will assist in selecting the appropriate amenities to include in a lounge/respite area.

As a component of staff respite space, consideration should be given to creating a small space for private reflection. Such spaces can serve an important role for personal reflection after particularly challenging patient encounters and for stress reduction. The concept of reflection is becoming more popular in acute care hospital design, and such spaces are generally small, often consisting of nothing more than a lounge chair and lighting.

NUTRITION SPACE

EMS is a fast-paced and unpredictable work environment. In such an environment, access to nutrition is not always guaranteed, sometimes resulting in hungry, frustrated staff. In addition, in many cultures, the "breaking of bread" among colleagues and friends is an important relationship-building activity. With these considerations in mind, establishing proper nutritional space is important in EMS station design. Depending on social, cultural, staffing, and budgetary limitations, EMS station design may simply incorporate storage for food brought to the station by EMS personnel, storage for prepared and fresh foods to be consumed at the station, or even entire food preparation kitchens, commonly seen in newer EMS stations with full-time personnel working longer duty tours.

Nutritional spaces need to account for the various practical and cultural aspects of food preparation and storage. For example, EMS stations designed for personnel who have kosher nutritional practices will need to incorporate designs and facilities to support this reality. Facilities that include strict vegetarians who may work alongside of nonvegetarians need to consider if separate storage for meat and meat products will be necessary. Included in the food preparation

Table 18–6	Amenities to Consider for Inclusion in Staff Respite Space	
Amenity	**Justification**	
Comfortable, ergonomic seating	Ergonomic seating decreases risk of back injuries and discomfort	
	Community development/staff alignment	
Visual entertainment (e.g., television, DVD player)	Personnel access to external communication/information	
	Creation of training video library	
	Promotes in-station presence for volunteer staff	
Internet access	Personnel access to external communication/information	
	Access to on-line training information	
	Access to information related to research activities	
	Access to e-mail communications	
	Promotes in-station presence for volunteer staff	
Music/radio	Stress reduction	
	Entertainment	
Exercise equipment/exercise room	Strength training	
	Physical exercise/weight management	
	Promotion of healthy lifestyle	
	Stress reduction	
Games/assorted entertainment	Community development/staff alignment	
	Stress reduction	

areas should also be equipment necessary to prepare culturally or socially appropriate food items.

A design element that is often overlooked is appropriate dining environments. Since consumption of meals has specific social, cultural, and religious implications, design of dining spaces should be respectful of the unique customs associated with dining in that community.

SLEEP QUARTERS

In EMS stations housing personnel with prolonged duty tours, space will need to be dedicated to sleeping quarters. Traditionally, these consisted of rooms, typically with bunk beds, that slept two to four or more personnel. While this is efficient use of space, this model is a frequent source of dissatisfaction among many EMS personnel. Newer design of work facilities that incorporate sleep quarters are taking a more innovative and friendly approach to design, responding to changing expectations and considering often overlooked issues such as avoiding the placement of quarters directly adjacent to garage space where noise can disrupt sleep.

Designing and incorporating sleeping quarters needs to take into consideration the cultural and reli-

gious needs of the personnel, incorporating enough flexibility in design to ensure that as many unique circumstances as possible can be accommodated. Here, opportunities exist to learn from other industries such as regular hotels and the newer "micro-hotels." In the micro-hotel concept, small sleeping pods have been designed using minimal space but providing maximum comfort. Sleeping pods as small as 50 square feet can provide ample space for sleeping, changing, and basic personal hygiene activities. This is accomplished with innovative design considerations that promote design adaptability such as wall-mounted fold-down beds, sinks, and toilets that retract or fold into more compact storage spaces, pocket doors that retract into the walls, and wall-mounted communication devices. Regardless of the design model selected, enough sleep quarters should be included into EMS station design to accommodate crew needs in a manner that is respectful of their cultural beliefs with the flexibility to adapt to surges in staffing numbers.

An additional factor impacting on the design of sleeping quarters is whether or not mixed gender crews are assigned to duty tours. In this case, sleep quarter design needs to accommodate religious and cultural customs associated with opposite-gender interactions.

For example, in many cultures male and female personnel are not permitted to sleep in the same room unless they are married. In other cultures, this reality extends to items such as water closet facilities, showers, and changing rooms. These unique needs must be considered as a part of the predesign phase.

PERSONAL HYGIENE SPACE

Personal hygiene space is an important design component that is often overlooked. Crews working prolonged duty tours as well as those engaged in activities where they may have become soiled with environmental elements, body fluids, or other contaminants may wish to clean up after a service request is completed. Shower facilities should be incorporated into EMS station design. While many older EMS stations may have incorporated a single or communal shower into the station, new EMS stations have the opportunity to consider incorporating shower facilities into individual sleeping pods or into a larger "locker room" that would include showers, water closets, storage space for personal items, and areas for grooming. In any case, care should be taken to ensure gender-specific facilities are designed in stations with mixed gender personnel.

REFLECTION/ MEDITATION SPACE

EMS organizations that operate in faith-based communities or cultures with strong religious influences need to understand how religion is interwoven into the lives and daily activities of EMS personnel. In communities where this reality exists, EMS station design needs to reflect the religious and faith-based needs of personnel. For example, in Islamic cultures, attention should be given to designing spaces appropriate to and respectful of prayer activities and at the same time having awareness and understanding of requirements with respect to men and women participating in religious activities together or separately. In Buddhist cultures, EMS stations may wish to incorporate meditation spaces that provide the required balance and harmony. Equally important is the understanding of how religions in open-religion societies interact with one another and how space can be designed to be respectful of all religions and cultures contained within a community.

The extent to which personnel amenities can be provided is based not only on the available footprint of the future EMS station but also on budgetary limitations that may place restrictions on what can and cannot be incorporated into new station design. In the planning and predesign phase, including EMS personnel in the design discussions will help guide leaders and architects with respect to the priorities of the personnel staffing the station day in and day out.

EMS TRANSPORT VEHICLES

Storing and securing the vehicles used in the delivery of EMS care is one of the most important functions of any EMS station. Securing vehicles from the external environment and the elements contributes to prolonged equipment life span while minimizing risks of vandalism, damage, and theft. When designing a new EMS station it is important to understand what type of vehicles will need to be stored at the EMS stations as well as understanding the utilization frequency of vehicles. Individual vehicle types will have unique impacts on EMS station facility design (Table 18-7). Height, width, and length of vehicles impact on sizing of the individual vehicle bays. Additionally, understanding future vehicle investments and upgrades will enable planners to better create a design that is flexible and adaptable to future needs. In countries with well-established EMS systems, many stations quickly became obsolete when ambulances progressed from station wagon models to ambulance vans and then to modular box-type units that range in size from standard to very large.

When evaluating the needs of motorized transport vehicles, it's important to understand the needs of the ambulance vehicles at the various stages of use and readiness. With this understanding, EMS stations can be designed to serve all vehicular needs.

Once the needs of specific vehicles have been established, attention should turn to the logistics of placing vehicles within the EMS station. Vehicles can be staged in parallel or tandem configuration. In parallel configuration vehicles are placed side-by-side as opposed to in-line in a tandem configuration. Tandem configuration offers the benefit of reducing the number of garage doors. The disadvantage of tandem configuration is that if need arises for a vehicle parked behind the vehicle closest to the garage doors, then the forward vehicle must be moved. This can potentially delay response times to service requests. This situation can be exacerbated if the forward vehicle becomes unexpectedly inoperative which, without manual movement of the vehicle or towing, renders two vehicles out-of-service.

Flooring of the vehicle bay is something not often considered important by EMS personnel. However, appropriate or inappropriate flooring can limit fluid runoff and increase risk of injury to EMS crew from slip and fall situations. While flooring in many EMS station vehicle bays is concrete, other options exist for

Table 18–7	Vehicular Needs to Be Considered in EMS Design
Design Consideration	**Implications**
Number of vehicles	Single garage door or multiple garage doors
Dedicated service bay	Recommended for large motorized fleet Reduces out-of-service time associated with transporting vehicle to and from service location
On-site vehicle cleaning	Convenient location of cleaning equipment eases cleaning process Equipment for terminal cleaning after exposure to communicable diseases and body fluids Proper ground-level draining essential
On-site fuel source	Efficient refueling process Potential for wholesale fuel purchasing On-site environmental considerations
Floor level drainage	Runoff of water Runoff of hazardous vehicle fluids Runoff of cleaning fluids
Internal environmental controls	Climate-controlled environment prevents freezing of medical fluids in ambulances Prevention of locks, windows, and doors freezing Comfort of vehicle passenger compartments

lining either the entire ground surface or those portions most frequently traversed by EMS personnel. Whatever ground surface is selected, it should promote runoff of all fluids and reduce the risk of slip and falls.

While EMS station architects and planners frequently consider the needs of ambulances when designing new stations, attention is seldom given to the needs of nonmotorized patient transport devices, nonpatient transport vehicles, or aquatic ambulances. Each of these patient care and transport devices has unique requirements with respect to staging and maintenance (see Table 18-8 and Figure 18-2).

Table 18–8	Design Considerations for Alternative Ambulance Vehicles				
Vehicle Type	**Design Consideration**				
	Secure to Prevent Theft	Access to Air for Tire Inflation	Dedicated Storage Space to Prevent Damage	Access to Electrical Source for Battery Charging	Easy Access to Water Source (if near station)
Bicycle (with or without attached stretcher)	√	√	√		
Ambulance golf cart	√	√	√	√	
Motorized personal transport (e.g., ATV, motorcycle, Segway™)	√	√	√	√	
Ambulance boat	√	√	√		√

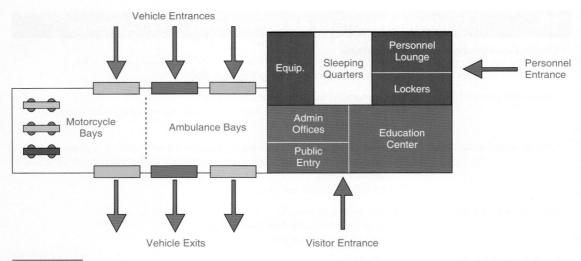

Vehicle Entrances

Equip.

Sleeping Quarters

Personnel Lounge

Lockers

Personnel Entrance

Motorcycle Bays

Ambulance Bays

Admin Offices

Public Entry

Education Center

Vehicle Exits

Visitor Entrance

FIGURE 18–2

EMS station design with multiple modality vehicle bays.

EQUIPMENT STORAGE

As with many other facility designs, equipment and supply location is commonly an afterthought in EMS station design. Commonly the reality, poor or inadequate supply location creates inefficiencies with respect to equipment restocking as well as limitations of supply availability if supply and equipment space is limited.

In any facility design supporting an industry dependent on easy access to equipment and supplies, equipment should be stationed in an area that is not only convenient but logically organized.

The ideal physical location of supplies and equipment used in the delivery of patient care or vehicle maintenance is in the ambulance bay. Centrally locating the equipment within the ambulance bay reduces the maximum distance between supplies and ambulances. This decreases the time necessary to restock ambulance supplies.

After determining equipment storage location, attention must be given to what technologies will be employed to assist with and secure all equipment and supplies. Standard storage options include supply cabinets and lockers or simply using shelves secured to the perimeter walls. While the latter provides the most economical solution, it limits the ability to secure equipment to prevent theft, limits the opportunity to develop a just-in-time restocking model, and also limits the ability to appropriately track and charge for supplies used.

Many organizations have begun the process of moving toward secured electronic supply cabinets. These cabinets provide considerable functionality with respect to securing supplies, requiring log-in informa-

tion to properly track staff access to supplies and equipment. Electronic supply cabinets, when connected to an automated inventory control system, create capabilities that can automatically submit supply orders when specific supply par levels have been breached. Electronic supply cabinets also increase revenue vis-à-vis direct connection with patient billing/revenue technologies in an effort to attribute supply use to specific patients. This is a particularly useful methodology for EMS systems that rely on patient billing and insurance reimbursement revenue to support operations.

Another added benefit of automated electronic storage cabinets is the ability to safely and securely store medications and, specifically, narcotics. Loss of medications and concerns over control of narcotic medications are challenges facing many EMS systems. Electronic storage of medications eliminate the need for a locked "narcotics box" that may be secured simply with a key that is passed from crew to crew, increasing the risk of loss of chain of custody of narcotics. In addition, electronic supply cabinets can be programmed to require medication count reconciliation each time a staff member accesses medications, again enhancing security of the medication supply.

Electronic supply cabinets are not without their limitations. First, they represent a significant upfront revenue investment for EMS systems. While the technology when properly used can help reduce waste and improve revenue collection, the return on investment is typically over years. Second, electronic supply cabinets must be protected from potential damage. Prevention of vehicle-caused damage, exposure to the elements, and damage from aggressive use must all be considered.

Table 18–9	Facility Design Implications of Soiled Storage
Soiled Product	**Facility Design Implication**
Nondisposable equipment	Cleaning decontamination station Staged areas for pre-decontamination and post-decontamination phases Decontamination cleaning agent storage Sink with running water Floor-level liquid runoff drain
Medical sharps	Dedicated space to station full sharps containers
Soiled linen (if not exchanged at hospital)	Soiled linen bins Washer/dryer (if not exchanged at hospital) Post-cleaning staging area
Biohazardous waste	Dedicated space for biohazardous waste bins Floor-level liquid runoff drain

Third, electronic cabinets require access to electrical sources. Redundant power supplies must be established to ensure access to supplies in the event of a power loss. Finally, downtime plans must be established to access supplies in the event the electronic storage cabinets fail.

Another important component of designing appropriate storage space is providing dedicated storage of biohazardous materials, contaminated and soiled linen, medical sharps, and other waste as well as providing dedicated space for cleaning and decontamination of nondisposable equipment such as laryngoscope handles and blades (Table 18-9). Soiled storage space should be distinct from other dedicated storage areas and should provide a means to provide safe shortage.

EMS STATION SAFETY AND SECURITY

Protecting the safety and security of the EMS personnel, visitors, vehicles, and equipment is a paramount consideration in EMS station design. In many parts of the globe, crime, vandalism, and terrorism are very real concerns that must be mitigated. With the potential for significant financial investment in facility design and equipment, careful planning of station security should be incorporated into the new facility.

Building Security

Providing secured access to the EMS station should be a standard component of the station design. Regardless of the staffing model employed, there will be periods of time that the EMS station is unstaffed while crews are responding to service requests or volunteer staff are awaiting service requests from home. In addition, in many regions of the world, the security of the staff stationed within the EMS station is also an important and essential consideration.

When considering techniques to secure the EMS station, an understanding of the benefits and limitations of various security measures requires a clear assessment (Table 18-10). The security measures undertaken should be reflective of the needs and levels of potential crime within the community. However, it cannot be overstated that even in historically safe communities, crime is not absent and sometimes these areas are targeted for this very reason.

CONTINUING EDUCATION/ NEW EDUCATION FOR EMS PROVIDERS

Education is an important component of all EMS systems. Education of new providers becomes an ongoing source of new personnel while continuing education of existing personnel ensures that providers remain up-to-date on the latest information on treatment modalities, rescue techniques, and equipment and other information relevant to EMS operations. Providing in-house education, both new and ongoing, is an important offering for all EMS systems. The complexity of educational offerings is largely dependent upon the needs of the providers, available technologies, and available budgets (Table 18-11). Although they are often an afterthought in facility design projects, educational objectives for EMS personnel, both current and future, need to be considered as a key component of new EMS station design.

Table 18–10	Approaches to EMS Station Security	
Security Method	**Advantages**	**Disadvantages**
Keyed lock	Inexpensive solution Easy to change	Loss of keys Unauthorized duplication
Manual-push security coded lock	Inexpensive solution Easy to change Can change regularly More secure than standard key	Repeated tries may result in discovering code Required override in case becomes jammed Single access code only
Electronic security coded lock	Easy to change Can change regularly Can track entry by individual staff	Required redundant power source (battery) in case of power failure More expensive solution Requires back-up in case system fails
Magnetic strip ID access/key fob	Can track entry by individual staff	Intentional or unintentional hand-off of access method to another person Required redundant power source (battery) in case of power failure More expensive solution Requires back-up in case system fails
Biometrics (iris scan, fingerprint scan)	Most secure option Can track individual staff access Unable to duplicate access	Required redundant power source (battery) in case of power failure Most expensive solution Requires back-up in case system fails
Remote release via smart phone technology	Easy to change Can change regularly Can track entry by individual staff	Intentional or unintentional hands-off of access method to another person Required redundant power source (battery) in case of power failure More expensive solution Requires back-up in case system fails

Focusing first on continuing education, the impact on EMS station design can range from minimal to extensive, depending on the investment with respect to technological sophistication of continuing education services.

Basic educational programming can be delivered by providing access to educational materials. Design considerations for these materials are limited and focus more on centralized storage of these materials, although facilities expecting larger utilization of these services may wish to construct a dedicated resource library that provides access to print journals, textbooks, training models, and computer-based information and training.

For EMS stations that envision providing didactic educational programming within the station, a classroom will be required. The configuration of a classroom is quite simple in that it is primarily a large room. Ideal facility designs incorporate flexibility into the classroom design that permit the segmentation of the main classroom into breakout rooms for smaller education and training sessions.

More advanced educational programming can be provided through computer and Internet-based programming that have been shown to be an effective and low-cost approach to education for EMS providers and hold the potential added benefit of enhanced education through local and international collaboration with other EMS providers.[6,7] Requirements for computer-aided and Internet-based education are more extensive and include adequate computer terminals and dedicated space that is free from distractions found in the common areas used by personnel. This area should be secured to prevent any potential loss of expensive equipment.

Decisions about inclusion of these spaces into the facility design will be driven largely by the size of the EMS station and corresponding personnel, the need

Table 18–11	Potential Continuing Education/New Education Uses for EMS Station	
Use	**Design Implications**	
Didactic education programs	Classroom space Parking for vehicle-oriented communities Bicycle racks for bicycle-oriented communities Visitor water closets Audiovisual technologies	
Hands-on skills stations	Program space (can be combined with classroom) Parking for vehicle-oriented communities Bicycle racks for bicycle-oriented communities Visitor water closets Disposal solutions for medical waste Equipment storage	
Computer-aided education	Computer stations IT workspace Computer server storage	
Simulation training	Dependent upon complexity of simulation program ranging from basic computer terminals to fully integrated robotic simulation programs	

for station-based education as opposed to partnering with local educational and health-care organizations, and the available budget.

Some highly sophisticated EMS organizations have opted to add simulation training to their educational programs. Simulation training is a technology-heavy approach that requires dedicated space for house computers and, typically, robotic patient technology as well as a control and observation rooms and necessary educational adjuncts and equipment. Simulation training is an expensive undertaking and has frequently been relegated to regional training centers, higher education facilities, and hospitals in many communities.

SUPPLEMENTAL USES OF EMS STATIONS

In many parts of the world, public service sites such as law enforcement, fire, rescue, and EMS stations serve as focal points of the community. As such, the stations frequently provide services that extend beyond simply staging equipment, vehicles, and personnel. Understanding the potential supplemental uses of EMS stations is an important component of planning appropriate EMS station design (Table 18-12). Planning around supplemental uses is not as simple as just add-

ing a large community hall. Planning requires detailed understanding of the intended uses and potential equipment and storage needs as well as potential numbers of people using the sites.

EMS Dispatch

EMS dispatch is handled in very different ways across the globe. In countries where a centralized emergency number is used such as "112" in many European countries and "911" in the United States and Canada, there is often a centralized dispatch center that controls communication with EMS, fire, rescue, and law enforcement. In communities where centralized emergency call numbers do not exist or frequent requests are made for nonemergency EMS transport or interfacility

Table 18–12	Potential Supplementation Uses of EMS Station
EMS dispatch EMS service administration Community education/wellness programs Disaster preparedness/response	

transfers, individual EMS stations may be required to maintain responsibility for incoming requests for all emergency and nonemergency transports. In this instance, the EMS station should be designed to support dispatch functions.

Planning to support dispatch functions begins with understanding the technological requirements and capabilities for dispatch within the community. Typically, initial requests for EMS services are made via telephone. However, as the utilization of portable mobile technologies continues to progress, it is likely that new modalities will emerge to request EMS services. If dispatch is to be incorporated into the facility design, this should be considered when planning the location to ensure mobile phone/wireless data reception as well as avoiding construction material that does not result in new reception dead zones being developed.

In addition to technological requirements for incoming service requests, technology to communicate with EMS units, personnel and mutual aid providers, law enforcement, and fire and rescue should be considered. Typically a combination of landline phone, wireless, and radio technologies is employed with redundancies built into the system.

When planning for dispatch capabilities in EMS station design, the dispatch area should be located in a secure portion of the facility away from public circulation. In addition, it should be away from other areas of the station where such a concentration of wireless communication technologies might interfere with the operation of other equipment or communication devices.

EMS Service Administration

In regions of the world with organized EMS services that operate as a part of larger coordinated systems or that perform financial transactions in the form of patient billing, dedicated space should be reserved in the EMS station. Spaces to support administrative functions are designed around typical administrative styles with a reception area with visitor seating and group and/or individual offices for various staff members. EMS station leadership such as the EMS chief should be located in this area as well. Location of the administrative functions typically is not required to be within the secured personnel area, although care should be taken to provide a security barrier between visitors and the administrative offices. The administrative area may also include a conference room for small to midsized staff meetings with vendors or other visitors.

Community Education/ Wellness Programs

In many communities, an EMS station serves as a focal point of the community where services well beyond simple staging of equipment, personnel, and vehicles occur. Understanding how the EMS station will be used as a community resource will drive decisions related to design implications (Table 18-13).

Table 18–13	Potential Community Education/Wellness Program Uses for EMS Station
Use	**Design Implications**
Community education programs	Classroom space Parking for vehicle-oriented communities Bicycle racks for bicycle-oriented communities Visitor water closets Internet-based learning stations (if appropriate)
Wellness and screening programs	Program space (can be combined with classroom) Parking for vehicle-oriented communities Bicycle racks for bicycle-oriented communities Visitor water closets Disposal solutions for medical waste Equipment storage
Safe baby/protection from abuse receiving center	Program/reception space Visitor water closets Necessary equipment supplies for infant care

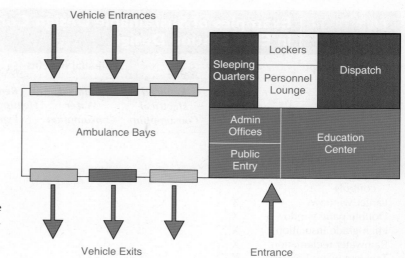

Vehicle Entrances

Ambulance Bays

Sleeping Quarters

Lockers

Personnel Lounge

Dispatch

Admin Offices

Public Entry

Education Center

Vehicle Exits

Entrance

FIGURE 18–3

Avoiding tandem parking and backing vehicles into ambulance station improves vehicle accessibility and reduces potential for accidents.

Disaster Preparedness/Response

EMS is a central component of disaster planning and response activities. Be it natural, manmade, or terror-related disasters, EMS's role in response and management is central, and any failures in planning or response can result in further harm and loss of life.

The primary role of an EMS station with respect to supporting disaster planning and response is related to storage of necessary equipment and resources to support disaster management activities. Equipment should be stored in a dedicated space that is secure and separate from other equipment storage to avoid potential diversion of the equipment and supplies for other unintended uses. EMS systems that maintain disaster response vehicles should have these vehicles housed within the ambulance bays in a secure manner. As discussed in the section dedicated to EMS vehicles, attempts should be made to avoid tandem parking schemes (Figure 18-3), and all equipment related to disaster response should be located in close proximity to the disaster response vehicles. As these vehicles and equipment are likely to be the least often used, they can safely and appropriately be located in a distant portion of the ambulance bay.

SUSTAINABLE DESIGN

Much attention has turned in facility design and architecture to concepts associated with sustainable design. Initially with a focus primarily on reducing the environmental impact of buildings, sustainable design has also demonstrated real value to building operators through reduced energy consumption, which translates into lower operating fees. While the purpose of designing an EMS station is to respond to community need for emergency medical services and access to emergency care, this author believes that sustainable design practices can easily be incorporated with a considerable return on investment (Table 18-14).

While many options exist for items to include in a sustainable design model, the items to incorporate will be based largely on the unique needs and budgets of specific EMS organizations. For example, EMS stations located in areas with limited direct sunlight may not realize benefit from inclusion of solar panel technology into the EMS station's design. Conversely, EMS stations located in an area with an abundance of wind may find significant benefit from the addition of a wind turbine to the facility design. When planned properly and with clear understanding of the available natural resources, energy consumptions hold the potential to significantly reduce or eliminate electrical consumption. Some facilities with well-planned strategies have even been able to return electricity to the power grid, resulting in a profit generation for the EMS station. Moreover, in regions of the world where reliable electricity is not available, sustainable design techniques focused on electricity consumption will likely create a more predictable energy supply for the EMS station, which is particularly important if station security is dependent on electronic access or surveillance.

STATION LIGHTING

In recent years, institutional facility design has begun looking more closely at how increasing natural lighting can not only reduce energy consumption from artificial lighting but also promote a greater sense of well-being

Table 18–14	Examples of Sustainable Design Concepts to Include in EMS Station Design				
Design Concept	**Potential Benefits**				
	Reduced Carbon Footprint	*Reduced Electrical Consumption*	*Reduced Water Consumption*	*Reduced Heating/Cooling Expenses*	*Reduced Maintenance/ Replacement Fees*
LED/Compact Fluorescent lighting	X	X			X
Motion sensor light controls	X	X			
Larger windows	X	X			
Double pane windows	X			X	
High-grade insulation	X			X	
Rainwater reclamation	X		X		
Tankless water heaters	X			X	
Flushless urinals	X		X		X
Two-flush toilets	X		X		
Low-flow shower heads	X		X		
Solar panels	X	X		X	
Wind turbine	X	X			
Geothermal system	X			X	

and maintenance of circadian rhythms. Planning of number, size, and positioning of windows is an important consideration. For example, east-facing windows will promote morning natural light, while west-facing windows enhance afternoon and evening lighting. Northern and southern directed lights have variable impact, depending on the season and geographic location (e.g., northern versus southern hemisphere, latitudes). Regardless of geographic location, abundant natural lighting versus windows should be included in EMS station design. Ample sky and wall lights in areas such as personnel lounges and ambulance bays can obviate the need for artificial lighting during periods of daylight. Personnel space with windows that provide attractive views of nature or urban landscapes can assist in providing a sense of well-being and harmony.

A quick, easy opportunity to reduce energy consumption and create a more sustainable design can be realized today with the replacement of traditional incandescent light bulbs with either compact fluorescent lights (CFL) or light-emitting diode lights (LED). Both lighting options are considered to be high efficiency with lower energy consumption and longer life spans than traditional incandescent light bulbs. In addition to their energy efficiency, both high-efficiency options generate less heat during use, a considerable benefit in warmer climates.

WATER CONSERVATION

Water conservation is a critical facility design component in areas where water is either expensive or limited in availability. Where this is the case, aggressive water conservation strategies can yield considerable results. Flushless urinals and dual-flush toilets significantly decrease water consumption. This benefit is further enhanced by installing low-flow showerheads, which can reduce water consumption from showers by over 50%. Installation of motion-activated faucets can also decrease water consumption. In areas where rainwater is plentiful, a water reclamation system can capture rainwater runoff to support nonpotable functions such as urinal and toilet flushing and lawn irrigation. In communities where water is provided from a community water supply, this can help reduce consumption and, by extension, fees. EMS stations that rely on a ground well for water will place less demand on the well when water conservation and reclamation strategies are employed.

RECYCLED MATERIALS

Another valuable component in designing and constructing an EMS station with sustainable principles is the inclusion of post-consumer (recycled) components in the facility's construction. For example, many fiberglass insulation solutions can be provided using recycled materials. The same can be said for metal support structures, even the wood or metal used to design garage doors. Recycled rubber and tires can be used to create no-slip flooring in areas where slippage and fall risks exist. This type of flooring also reduces impact from prolonged ambulation on hard surfaces, is easier to clean than carpet, and is more resistant to damage.

PHYSICAL LAYOUT/ ADJACENT STRUCTURES

When planning a new EMS station, additional benefit can be gained from understanding how adjacent or specific areas or functions can impact the workings of an EMS station and the flow of EMS personnel (Figure 18-4). With minimal effort, collocated activities that are important can be identified and incorporated into station design.

Front-Stage Versus Back-Stage Operations

The operation of any organization can be broken down into functions and activities that occur in areas where transparency and visibility to staff and visitors are important (front stage) and functions and activities that are preferentially kept out of sight (back stage). In deciding to take a front-stage–back-stage approach to design it is important to consider who should have access to each area.

For example, if visitors come to the EMS station for the purposes of visiting administrative offices, attending community events, or participating in educational programming, it is important to consider where to locate these areas so that visitors are not navigating across personnel lounge space, near respite space, or have the ability to gain access to the ambulance bays. If housekeeping services are provided at the EMS station, back-stage operations can be designed to allow access to personnel respite spaces and lounge areas without providing access to ambulance bays or other sensitive areas.

Front-stage–back-stage separation can be accomplished in a number of ways. Typically this begins with identifying primary access points to the EMS station for both personnel and visitors. Access by visitors should be provided in areas distant from access, internal or external, to the ambulance bays. Separation of front-stage and back-stage operations can also be accomplished with physical barriers such as doors with or without secure access.

Staff Respite Versus Vehicle Staging

The location of staff respite and sleep spaces as it relates to vehicle staging has the potential to impact on staff well-being. Locating staff respite spaces near vehicle staging creates the potential to disrupt staff rest and sleep owing to vehicle noise, back-up alarms, noise from garage doors, and exhaust fumes from vehicles. While it is important to position staff respite

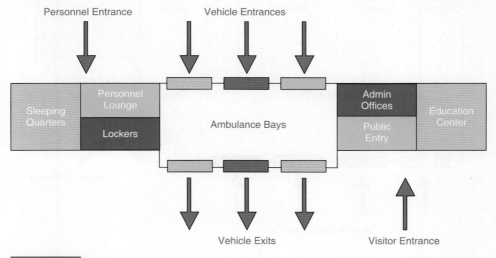

FIGURE 18-4

Separation of public and nonpublic spaces ensures greater comfort and safety of personnel; collocated areas create greater efficiency.

spaces in close proximity to vehicle staging to ensure rapid response with respect to service requests, this must be balanced against staff disruption.

Parking Versus Points of Access

Ideally, personnel and visitor parking should be separated and located in well-lit areas, free of obstacles, and in close proximity to their respective points of access. Personnel parking should be located near an access point leading directly to personnel areas of the building through a secured access site. Visitor parking should be in clear sight of a visitor access point with well-delineated signage.

Staff Respite Versus Staff Nourishment and Hygiene Spaces

All staff support spaces should be clustered as close together as possible. Sleeping quarters should be in close proximity to water closets and shower facilities. If individual sleeping rooms are selected, direct access to water closet and/or shower facilities can be provided, with each sleeping room having dedicated hygiene spaces or two rooms sharing a joint space for hygiene. While dedicated hygiene facilities are ideal, they increase design and construction costs as well as the building footprint. If communal facilities are chosen, they should be gender-specific and centrally located with respect to the sleeping facilities.

FACILITY EXPANSION

Many buildings are not designed with expansion in mind. This limits the ability to respond to future growth needs or unanticipated new technologies or vehicle designs. EMS station design should be completed with the ability to easily expand ambulance bays as well as personnel space. Ideally, these sections of the facility should become "plug and play," with the ability to simply add on to the end of the existing facility (Figure 18-5).

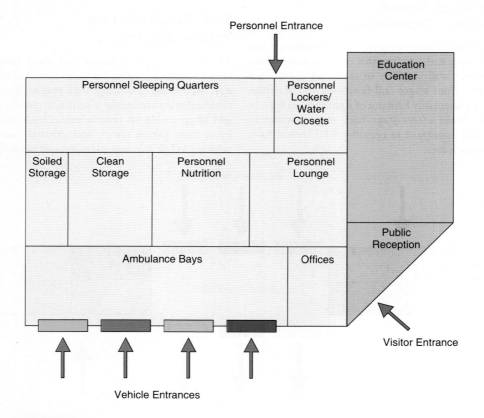

FIGURE 18–5

Nonlinear "big box" design allows easier expansion of specific areas when necessary without impacting on other areas of station.

VISIONING EMS STATION DESIGN

Developing an EMS station design that will serve the community's needs into the future is no simple task. Careful consideration and vetting are required to ensure the selected design is leading practice in its application. To accomplish this, the planning team and EMS station designers and architects will need to look beyond today's leading practices and focus on truly innovative design elements that, while not necessarily proven by others in the industry, hold the potential for truly transformative innovation (Figure 18-6).

EMS station design should be undertaken with careful attention to ensure the design is flexible and adaptable. No designer or architect can possibly plan for every future development in vehicle design, emerging technology, or new equipment. Designing a facility that is easily adaptable to support the unanticipated is an important design consideration that, while potentially resulting in greater up-front design and construction costs, will result in significant long-term savings. A new EMS station design should facilitate easy expansion, particularly of ambulance bays and personnel respite spaces and sleeping quarters. In rapidly growing communities, EMS expansion is an inevitable reality that should be planned to avoid expensive and disruptive future expansion projects that result in avoidable inefficiencies and potential safety and security issues being inserted into the facility design.

EMS station design should not be performed in a vacuum. The most successful and functional EMS station designs are those that are completed with the active and ongoing input of all parties interested in and impacted by the station's design. Through a thoughtful and deliberate collaborative planning process, an innovative, flexible, and expandable EMS station design can follow. This author advocates the use of a seven-phase design planning process that is aimed at delivering superior results while avoiding unanticipated consequences and expensive design and construction change orders (Table 18-15).

Table 18–15	EMS Station Design Planning Process
Step I:	Assemble the team
Step II:	Establish the vision
Step III:	Identify desired outcomes
Step IV:	Process mapping
Step V:	Initial design schematics
Step VI:	Mock-ups and prototyping
Step VII:	Final design

Step I: Assemble the Planning Team

When engaging in a design process, multiple methodologies can be employed that range from a grassroots-led process to processes driven singularly by either architects or a combination of architects and EMS leadership. This author recommends an inclusive process bringing together representatives from all groups that will use or work in the EMS station (Table 18-16).

Step II: Establish the Vision

Properly designing any new facility begins with identifying the vision that will drive the form and function of the EMS station and, ideally, the design as well (Table 18-17). While sometimes overlooked, the importance of defining the vision cannot be understated. The

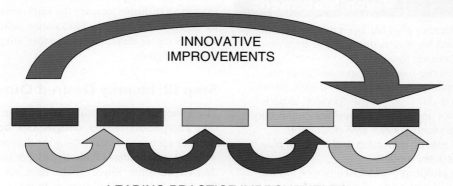

FIGURE 18–6

Innovative improvements transcend the "known" of leading practice improvements.

Table 18–16	Roles/Personnel to Include in EMS Station Design Planning Process

Role/Individual for Inclusion	Potential Insights Provided
EMS providers	Equipment locations Personnel respite space Personnel sleeping/hygiene needs Continuing education needs Vehicle stocking, storage, and decontamination requirements Station safety and security
EMS leadership	Budgetary considerations Administrative requirements Staffing models Disaster planning/response Station safety and security
Dispatch personnel (if in-station dispatch to be provided)	Technology needs Dispatch processes and facility requirements Continuing education needs
Community representatives	Potential community uses community awareness/participation
Contracted service providers (e.g., vehicle maintenance, housekeeping)	Work flow processes Equipment location Work safety

vision should tell the story of the EMS service and what it seeks to achieve. Is the vision one of "responding to our neighbors in need"? Or perhaps the vision is "to serve as an integral link in the chain of survival." Maybe

Table 18–17	Concepts to Consider When Establishing a Vision Statement

- Historically, what has been the purpose of our EMS service? Is this purpose appropriately moving forward?
- What is our role and responsibility to the community? To health care? To each other?
- What is our vision of the "perfect" experience for an EMS encounter? For community engagement? For our EMS personnel?
- What role do education and research play in our delivery model?
- Is our philosophy of service one of innovation, early adoption of new practices, or consensus adoption after new trends have been proven in the marketplace?

the vision is "to enhance the health and well-being of our community through patient care, education, and outreach in a manner that is respectful and inclusive of the community we serve." In the end, the vision should provide a litmus test to evaluate every decision made concerning the station's operations and design.

Developing the vision statement should be a process that is inclusive of EMS providers, service leaders, community members, and other important stakeholders. In approaching the vision development in such an inclusive manner, the EMS service delivery model and, ultimately, the EMS station hold the potential to bring all stakeholders together around a common set of goals.

Step III: Identify Desired Outcomes

The author's experience with facility design has shown that exceptional facility designs can be achieved through a process of establishing the desired outcomes with key stakeholders (Table 18-18). For example, one desired outcome might be to have no workplace injuries within the EMS station. In this instance, the design will need to consider workplace ergonomics and utilization of materials, surfaces, and designs that reduce the risk of injury. Another outcome might be to

Table 18–18	Example Outcomes/Performance Metrics that Might Be Incorporated into Facility Design Process
Metric	**Design Consideration**
85% of service requests-to-responding times ≤5 minutes	Proximity of personnel respite spaces to vehicles Availability of personnel sleeping quarters and respite space to promote in-station stand-by
85% of service requests-to-on-scene times ≤10 minutes	Station site selection Proximity of personnel respite spaces to vehicles Availability of personnel sleeping quarters and respite space to promote in-station stand-by
Slip and fall rate = 0%	Slip-reducing flooring in ambulance bays Appropriate liquid runoff drainage in ambulance bays Showers and water closets with slip-reducing flooring Avoid use of steps or uneven floor surfaces Avoid highly-polished flooring
Lifting injury rate = 0%	Limited height of storage spaces Lifting devices positioned near equipment and supplies
Facility energy consumption rate decreased by 25%	Sustainable design techniques
Equipment loss rate <5%	Equipment storage security features Front-stage–back-stage design
10 hours of continuing education monthly	On-site continuing education space On-site education activities
Reduce average weight of personnel by 5%	On-site fitness facilities

have 85% of service requests result in EMS personnel on scene within 10 minutes from the initial time of service request. With this outcome in mind, emphasis will be placed on appropriate site selection. Prior to beginning design schematic development, the planning team should be assembled and should engage in a process that clearly identifies in detail all outcomes and performance metrics that should be addressed by the facility design.

Step IV: Process Mapping

Once the interests of various stakeholders have been identified and desired outcomes have been established, attention should turn to engaging in process mapping exercises. The process mapping exercises form an important component of informing the architects and space planners about how various process flows are interrelated to one another. Detailed process maps should be developed for every task and function undertaken at the EMS station and should include information on involved parties and potential uses of technology and equipment.

Step V: Initial Design Schematics

Once high-level visioning and process mapping have been completed, the architects will likely develop initial design schematics. The designs should incorporate and interpret the information received in the previous steps within the budgetary realities of the overall project. Initial design schematics should be shared with the planning team established in step I. The planning team should vet the designs against processes, workflows, and desired design considerations. Tabletop exercises focused on executing processes will illustrate opportunities to improve on initial designs.

Step VI: Mock-ups and Prototyping

Once designs have advanced beyond preliminary phases, consideration must be given to the physical location of supplies, equipment, furniture, and other items within the newly designed EMS station. Use of a mock-up space will create the opportunity for the programming team to visualize how spaces will be utilized and allow for changes before construction begins, thus minimizing expensive change orders. Low-cost mock-up solutions can be employed using cardboard and stick-on notes to simulate walls and equipment and supplies, respectively.

Step VII: Final Design

Once the first five phases have been completed, architects should be well positioned to move to final design. Once final design is completed, the programming team should provide one final review prior to approving progression to the construction phase.

SUMMARY

EMS station design is a complex undertaking that extends far beyond building bricks and mortar to house equipment and vehicles. Rather, designing an EMS station is an important exercise in establishing the optimal outcomes with respect to quality, safety, efficiency, and performance and building a facility that promotes these qualities while serving as a magnet for EMS providers and a community resource for education and wellness.

Methodical in nature, the process of EMS design should begin with selecting an interdisciplinary design team. What follows should be a process of establishing the proper vision, identifying desired outcomes, and mapping flow and process to deliver the outcomes desired and vision established followed by initial design, prototyping, and final design. With the additional inclusion of design adaptability, capacity for expansion, and sustainable design, the EMS station of the future will extend far beyond the simple garages of yesteryear to the multifunctional centers of tomorrow.

References

1. Institute of Medicine. Committee on the Future of Emergency Care in the United States Health System – Emergency Medical Services: at the Crossroads. Washington, DC: The National Academies Press; 2007.
2. David G, Brachet T. Retention, learning by doing, and performance in emergency medical services. *Health Serv Res.* 2009 Jun; 44(3): 902-25. Epub 2009 Mar 5.
3. Báez AA, Giraldez E, Lane PL, Pozner C, Rodriguez J, Rogers S. Knowledge and attitudes of the out-of-hospital emergency care consumers in Santo Domingo, Dominican Republic. *Prehosp Disaster Med.* 2008 Jul-Aug;23(4):373-6.PMID: 18935954
4. Peralta LMP. The prehospital emergency care system in Mexico City: a system's performance evaluation. *Prehosp Disaster Med.* 2006 Mar-Apr;21(2):104-11.
5. McCallion T. Ambulance safety first: experts convene to discuss personal & patient safety issues. *JEMS.* 2007 Jun;32(6):44-7
6. Gershon RRM, Canton AN, Magda LA, et al. Web-based training on weapons of mass destruction response for emergency medical services personnel. *Am J Disaster Med.* 2009 May-Jun;4(3):153-61.
7. Williams B, Upchurch J. The internationalization of prehospital education: a merging of ideologies between Australia and the USA. *Emerg Med J* 2006; 23:573-577 doi:10.1136/emj.2005.030866

CHAPTER 19

EMS Equipment

David Menzies, Ian Brennan

KEY LEARNING POINTS

- Properly selected EMS equipment is essential to complement training.

- The type and quantity of equipment carried will vary depending on local circumstances and the training of the providers.

- The ideal piece of EMS equipment is small, lightweight, cheap, durable, and will not go out of date.

- Excessive amounts of equipment can pose as many difficulties as inadequate equipment.

- It is useful to consider equipment in terms of "basic" and "advanced."

- Equipment type and storage layout should be standardized throughout an EMS.

- Improvisation is possible for a variety of situations where equipment is not readily available.

INTRODUCTION

Equipment is necessary for many EMS diagnostic procedures and for the delivery of all but the most basic of EMS interventions. Equipment ranges from very basic items, such as triangular bandages, to modern multifunction defibrillators.

Appropriate equipment is necessary to supplement EMS providers' diagnostic and therapeutic training. Knowledge and skills are of no use if the EMS provider does not have the tools to implement them.

There is a huge amount of equipment that the EMS provider could potentially use in the provision of patient care. It is necessary to rationalize this vast amount of equipment according to space, effectiveness, frequency of use, and value for money.

This chapter details some of the considerations in EMS equipment selection and evaluates the most commonly used equipment using a systems approach. At the end of each section a suggested list

of "basic," "advanced," and "optional" equipment is given. The basic and advanced equipment is considered essential for the level of EMS provider concerned. The boundaries between basic and advanced care differ between different EMS systems and internationally, items that are considered advanced in one country, might be considered basic elsewhere.

The division between essential and optional equipment is somewhat arbitrary, as accepted standards of care are changing continuously; previously a defibrillator might have been considered optional and was not available on all ambulances, but now it is considered an essential piece of equipment

EQUIPMENT SELECTION

Budgetary constraints are a significant factor in EMS equipment choice. There are financial limits to what can be acquired for most EMS systems, and therefore every effort should be made to select the most appropriate equipment. Factors to consider when selecting EMS equipment follow.

Frequency of Use

How often is a piece of equipment likely to be needed? Regularly used items such as dressings and oxygen masks have to be stocked, but less frequently needed items such as vacuum mattresses might not be justifiable. Infrequently used items could be held at a central store and dispatched via an equipment vehicle as needed.

Reusable

Items that are reusable after appropriate cleaning and disinfection may offer a cost advantage over single-use items. This needs to be balanced against the costs of undertaking the cleaning and disinfection as well as the risk of infection.

Potential Benefit

Some items such as defibrillators are actually used relatively infrequently but are potentially lifesaving. These pieces of equipment would be considered more important than those that have a less significant impact on patient care.

EMS Provider Skills

EMS equipment must be sufficient to allow delivery of the standard of EMS desired. Thus, basic life support equipment is universally necessary, but more advanced equipment may not always be required. EMS equipment must match the skills of the EMS providers using it. There is little point in providing expensive sophisticated equipment if the EMS providers are not trained in its use. If an EMS has a limited number of advanced providers, for example, it may be more cost-effective to provide them with their own advanced equipment rather than stocking it on every ambulance.

There may be some relevance in carrying equipment that EMS providers are not trained to use themselves in case another more experienced provider is available (e.g., some EMS carry doctors bags on their ambulances, so that if a doctor is available at the scene, advanced interventions may be performed).

Response and Transport Times

A rural EMS with long transport times will have differing equipment requirements than an urban EMS with short transport times. Equipment needs to reflect the geography and caseload of a particular EMS.

Vehicles

The amount and type of equipment carried will vary considerably, depending on the type of vehicle used by the EMS. A standard land ambulance will be able to carry most of the equipment described here, but practitioners operating on bicycles, motorcycles, or rapid response cars will have different requirements. Similarly, EMS systems using rotary or fixed wing aircraft often carry a greater range of critical care equipment, although they too may be compromised by space restrictions. Any equipment used in air transport should be certified as safe for that environment.

Versatility

It is useful, where possible, to select equipment that has multiple uses. This has the advantage of saving space on board and reducing the number of items carried. At its most basic, this may involve carrying wound pads and crepe bandages rather than a selection of different sized individual field dressings. Similarly, a combined defibrillator-diagnostic monitor offers space-saving advantages over separate defibrillators and diagnostic sets. The disadvantage of this approach is that, if the equipment fails or is misplaced, the impact is greater.

Life Expectancy

The duration of service a piece of equipment can be expected to give before it needs replacement will be reflected in its cost. Very expensive items, which may last several years (e.g., defibrillators), can have their cost offset across a number of financial years. On the other hand, items with a shorter shelf life (e.g., sterile equipment sets) should have appropriately lower costs.

Durability

EMS equipment is generally expected to be durable enough to withstand greater forces and mistreatment than comparable hospital equipment without compromising on quality or performance. This may be achieved by the use of additional protective casing and secure fixings or by fundamentally changing the design. This may result in a higher cost for EMS equipment in comparison to similar hospital equipment.

Ongoing Costs

As well as initial start-up costs in terms of acquisition of equipment, the running costs of such equipment need to be considered. Consumables such as paper, ink, batteries, and spare parts may represent a greater cost over the lifetime of the equipment than the initial expenditure.

Servicing and Repairs

Equipment may require regular servicing or maintenance. Consideration will have to be given to what facilities are available locally to perform this and the issue of replacement equipment in the interim.

Storage and Portability

The size of equipment is relevant in terms of storage space, both at home base and on the ambulance. Similarly, equipment generally must be removed from the ambulance to treat patients and should be small and lightweight to facilitate this. Equipment that takes up too much space or is difficult to carry is not suited to EMS operations.

Standardization

EMS equipment should be standardized within an individual EMS so that providers can use equipment from any vehicle or base within that EMS and know that it will be the same. This can save time in emergencies and reduces error. It may also be advisable to try to standardize equipment with other agencies such as fire or police departments for the same reasons. Finally, if there are arrangements for a resupply of consumables with local hospitals, equipment should be standardized with them as well.

While numerous examples of current EMS equipment are given here, this chapter is not exhaustive and there are many additional examples not included here. The choice of which items to acquire will involve careful consideration of the factors discussed above but will also be influenced by local availability and operator preference. Inevitably, there will be some "trial and error" within an EMS regarding appropriate equipment choices. There may be situations when a particular piece of equipment is unavailable. It may be possible to improvise equipment when this situation arises, and such suggestions are given at the end of each section.

Equipment, bags, and the organization and layout of items should be standardized across a service so that practitioners are able to operate with equal efficacy from any vehicle or equipment bag. The use of personalized equipment or bags is to be discouraged as this inhibits the ability of practitioners to operate effectively as a team.

Equipment is categorized according to practitioner level – divided into basic and advanced. However, it is recognized that what is considered basic or advanced is not consistent across different jurisdictions, for example, supraglottic airways may be considered an advanced intervention in most areas but are available to more basic practitioners in some areas.

The equipment described here is that which is appropriate for a general EMS. However, special considerations may apply to EMS systems that wholly or largely service particular patient groups such as pediatrics or maternity. Similarly, alternative requirements may pertain to EMS systems that operate in different environments such as military, tactical, or search and rescue.

STOCK LEVELS

Most items of equipment are designed for single patient use only and should be disposed of appropriately following this. Other items require cleaning/disinfecting following use. It is not desirable to require an EMS crew to return to the station following each call in order to restock all equipment and medication used or contaminated on the previous case.

Excessive amounts of equipment can pose as many problems as insufficient equipment. While an EMS will generally wish to provide as much equipment as possible to maximize good patient outcomes, too much equipment can result in difficulties in terms of storage, staff familiarity, training, and expiration dates. It is necessary to compromise on a level of equipment that maximizes the skills of the EMS providers rather than inhibits them through an excess of choices and difficulties in maintaining current training and locating it when needed.

Some small items (e.g., oxygen masks) are used very frequently, and several should be stocked in each vehicle. Other items may be too large (e.g., spinal boards) or infrequently used (e.g., maternity kits) to require more than a single one to be carried on each vehicle. In so far as is possible, local practice and call characteristics should be used to try to predict which items are used regularly.

For each section of this chapter, a list of equipment and quantities is suggested based on a standard two-person land ambulance. This is not intended to be comprehensive or definitive, as there are many variables to consider in compiling a stock list for each individual EMS as well as the differing response levels within each EMS.

PERSONAL PROTECTIVE EQUIPMENT AND INFECTION CONTROL

It is inevitable that EMS personnel will be present at potentially hazardous situations, such as motor vehicle collisions and industrial accidents. EMS systems work closely with their colleagues in the fire and rescue services to ensure accident scenes are a safe place to work for both the providers and the patients. A safe scene should be at the forefront of the EMT's or paramedic's mind. EMS systems often provide their personnel with a range of equipment to help protect them in these potentially hazardous situations.

Personal Protective Equipment

Personal protective equipment (PPE) includes everything from boots to gloves and high visibility clothing to thermal vests.

High Visibility and Reflective Clothing

The terms reflective clothing and high visibility clothing are often used interchangeably; although the two often go hand in hand, they are actually different. It is important that EMS personnel are seen, especially at night and at dark scenes. Both reflective clothing and high visibility clothing increase the presence and appearance of EMS personnel in these circumstances. High visibility or reflective clothing is an important piece of equipment for emergency personnel; it can prevent EMS personnel from being involved in an accident by making them visible to others, including motorists and people operating heavy machinery. Clothing includes jackets, waistcoats, coveralls, and over–trousers. They are available in a range of different sizes, designs, and colors. Military and tactical EMS may not require this because high visibility is not always desirable in these situations.

High Visibility Clothing   High visibility clothing is brightly colored clothing (typically yellow, orange, or red), which is highly visible in poor light and from a greater distance than standard clothing. Such clothing is available in heavy and light material and waterproof and non–waterproof material. High visibility clothing often incorporates some or many reflective strips to make it both highly visible and reflective.

Reflective Clothing   Light that shines on reflective clothing or reflective strips is reflected back and makes the EMS personnel more visible, potentially reducing the risk of injury to the EMT. Reflective clothing may not necessarily be high visibility, but some or all of it will be highly reflective when light is shone on it. It is particularly useful at scenes involving motor vehicles, as the headlights of oncoming traffic will illuminate EMS providers on scene.

EMS systems should assess their needs for high visibility and reflective clothing based on the types of scenes and different environments they attend.

Eye Protection

Many forms of protective eyewear exist to protect EMS personnel from injury and infection. Depending on needs, EMS personnel may use or need more than one form of eye protection. When managing patients, safety glasses are available to protect the eyes against body fluid splashes or aerosol particles, such as when a patient coughs. EMS personnel should use this type of eye protection when there is a potential risk of infection. Safety glasses also exist to protect EMS personnel against injury. These glasses often protect against impacts, chemical splashes, and dust. Protective eyewear is available in different ranges, designs, and specifications. EMS systems and personnel should assess their needs for protective eyewear based on the potential risks they encounter, but it is suggested that at least one form of eye protection be offered to personnel.

Some safety eyewear is available with prescription lenses or can be designed to fit over the EMT's own glasses.

Protective Gloves

EMTs need gloves to protect against infection and injury. EMS personnel will often wear protective examination gloves several times a day. It is often a requirement of EMS systems that their personnel wear protective examination gloves with all patients. The gloves should protect against contamination and infections. It is imperative that examination gloves are worn to protect both the EMT and the patient, especially when there are body fluids or open wounds present. When choosing protective gloves EMS systems should consider the following:

1. How many different sizes are needed? The gloves are available in sizes from extra small upwards to extra large.

2. Are sterile or nonsterile gloves needed?
3. Are the gloves made of latex? Some patients and EMS providers are allergic to latex.
4. Are the gloves powdered or non-powdered? Some patients and EMS providers are allergic to the powder on the gloves.
5. What do the gloves need to protect against?
6. Do the gloves need to be made of Nitrile material? This can further reduce the risk to both the patient and EMS provider for potential allergic or hypersensitivity reactions.
7. Is the glove made of strong or light material? The type of glove required will be dependent on need and use.

Ideally, an EMS will have standardized gloves available for all personnel, which will enable staff to operate over a range of sites or vehicles. However, individual staff preferences and allergy requirements should be accommodated.

EMS personnel and systems will sometimes need gloves to protect against injury. Some potential hazards include extreme heat or cold, sharp items, and chemicals; these hazards are often experienced by EMS personnel during motor vehicle collisions when there may be broken glass and chemicals present. Like the examination gloves, rescue gloves (sometimes referred to as extrication, debris, or fire-fighting gloves) are available in a wide range of specifications and designs, depending on needs. Some of these gloves can have a very high specification, protecting personnel against fire, rope burn, puncture wounds, and chemical spills.

EMS systems should assess their needs for these rescue gloves based on types of environments, scenes attended by personnel, and potential exposure to types of hazards. Some EMS systems, with both an emergency medical and rescue response, may need a high specification glove.

Protective Headgear

EMS personnel often wear protective headwear when attending at motor vehicle collisions, industrial accidents, and fires. The headwear should protect the EMS personnel against bumps, knocks, and falling debris. Protective headwear is available in different designs and specifications. Some EMS systems prefer to opt for a fire-fighter's helmet, which is normally very tough and offers protection against most of the potential hazards that a paramedic may encounter. There are also specific rescue helmets available, quite often with integrated protective eye shields or goggles. Some EMS systems that offer a mountain/cliff rescue service opt for a lighter weight helmet that can be worn comfortably for longer periods during lengthy rescues.

Protective Face Masks

Protective face masks can protect against infection and injury. They are available in many different specifications. They can protect EMS personnel against blood and body spills, dust, oil, and water mists, chemicals, and bacterial and viral infections. Like the other forms of protective equipment, EMS systems should assess their needs based on potential hazards. There may be a high risk of infection through the inhalation of particles, such as avian or swine influenza or severe acute respiratory syndrome (SARS). EMS personnel would need the correct face masks to protect themselves and the patient in these cases. Face masks have different specifications to filter different particles and make them easier to wear for long periods. Some have an integrated shield, visor, or splash guard to protect against splashes into the health-care worker's eyes.

Whatever mask is chosen, it is important that the user is specifically fitted to ensure that the model chosen is the best fit for the individual operator. Whether an N95 respirator offers greater protection over a standard surgical face mask is a matter of debate, and current evidence is inconclusive. It is perhaps more important that the mask meets with operator approval so that it is more likely to be used regularly.

Ear Protection

Ear defenders and earplugs may be available for EMS personnel to wear if the risk exists. They are often available for EMS personnel who attend at concerts or at scenes with loud noises.

Protective Footwear

Protective footwear can protect against injuries to the foot caused by slips, excessive heat/cold, and debris falling on the foot. There are many different types of footwear available to the EMS provider, ranging from lightweight safety shoes to heavy durable waterproof boots. If the EMS system is supplies boots/shoes to their personnel, they should take into account hazards and risks that might be encountered and what standards apply to safety footwear. Many types of safety footwear comply with global safety standards such as CEN (Comité Européen de Normalisation), CSA (Canadian Standards Association), and ASNI (American National Standards Institute).

Chemical and Decontamination Suits

For specialist EMS situations full chemical and decontamination suits might be required. While these would not normally be carried on every ambulance, they should be available when needed.

Protective Clothing

EMS systems in certain jurisdictions will also supply stab and ballistic jackets to their staff if the risk of attack is present. There are many different types of ballistic jackets available that offer different degrees of protection. EMS system/personnel will have to determine which best suits their needs. Like ballistic jackets, stab jackets can offer protection against stabs, spikes, needles, and blunt trauma.

Turnout Gear

EMS personnel at scenes of motor vehicle collisions and fires often use full firefighter turnout gear. It offers protection against fires, sharp objects, and chemical spills.

Infection Control Equipment

Infection control is an important part of the EMT's duty. Varying types of infection control equipment are available for EMS personnel. The simple infection control equipment includes examination gloves, face masks, and eye protection (as mentioned above). See Table 19-1 for a suggested list of PPE and infection control equipment.

EQUIPMENT BAGS

A vital part of the kit for EMS personnel includes carrying devices for their equipment. There are multiple types of bags, boxes, and cases that can be used. When choosing which equipment-carrying devices to be used, EMS systems should consider the following:

1. If the bag, box or case is going to be stored on the vehicle, is there room for it?
2. What type of equipment is to be carried?

Table 19–1	Suggested PPE and Infection Control Equipment

Basic

High visibility/reflective jacket and over trousers
Eye protection
Examination gloves
Rescue gloves
Protective head wear
Face masks
Ear protection
Aprons
Protective Footwear
Detergent
Alcohol wipes
2 × sharps bins
Clinical waste bags

Advanced

Biochemical/decontamination suits

Optional

Disposable gowns, overshoes
Stab/ballistic protection vests

3. Does the bag need to have small or large pockets or a combination of both?
4. Is there a need for waterproof carrying devices?
5. Is there a need to carry delicate or very expensive items that could be broken if not stored correctly?
6. What level of EMS personnel will be using the bags or boxes? Paramedics, doctors, or emergency nurses may be required to carry more equipment than EMTs or first responders.
7. How heavy is the equipment that is to be carried?
8. Does the bag need to be tailor-made for the particular EMS system? Many manufacturers make bags, boxes, or cases to suit the needs of their customers. They will design the contents of the bags to the EMS system's specification, including color and EMS logos and details.
9. How far does the equipment need to be carried? For example, mountain rescue EMS teams may carry more compact bags with more padded straps for ease of carrying for long distances.
10. What are the budgetary constraints of the particular EMS system?

First-Aid Bags/ First-Response Bags

Simple first-aid/first-response bags are usually easily affordable, hardwearing, and easy to carry. They are mainly used to carry basic first aid and BLS equipment such as dressings, plasters, and gloves and basic resuscitation equipment such as a pocket face mask and oropharyngeal airways. They can be also used to carry specific equipment in an ambulance such as burn dressings, diagnostic tools, or a maternity kit. The interior is normally divided into several pouches with additional side pouches; they often include small elastic straps in which to place smaller items such as a shears or tweezers. These types of bags are extensively used by EMS systems, first-aid organizations, and sporting organizations.

Medic's Bags

These bags are bigger and have the ability to carry more equipment. They are designed for EMS systems and EMS personnel such as EMTs and paramedics. They are generally made from strong, tough, hardwearing material and have heavy-duty shoulder and carrying straps. Like all the EMS bags, these medic's bags are available in different sizes, colors, and configurations. Many EMS systems use bags like these to carry full resuscitation equipment like oxygen cylinders, basic and advanced airway management equipment, and diagnostic equipment and trauma management. Some of these bags are also able to hold an AED. They are available with many different sized pockets and pouches. Some of these pockets and pouches are made of a clear plastic material for optimal visibility and access.

Advanced Life Support (ALS) Bags

Some EMS bags are designed for use by personnel with ALS capabilities; they have specific pouches and elastic straps to secure ALS equipment such as endotracheal tubes, laryngoscopes, IV cannulas, and accessories. These bags can be stand-alone bags for a particular skill, for example intubation bags, infusion bags, pneumothorax bags, or they can be integrated within a medic-type bag.

Drug Bag

Many EMS systems use a separate bag for the storage of medications. They often include clear plastic pockets and pouches for easy medication identification. Most of these bags are designed with elastic straps to carry numerous medication ampoules and vials. They also have specific straps or pouches for storage of minijet type prefilled syringed medications. Many of these bags also have pouches for storage of needles and syringes so that they are easily accessible during medication administration. These bags should be well padded for safety and storage on the vehicle and have lockable zips for extra security. Like all bags they come in various different sizes; ampoule wallets can accommodate a few ampoules and can be easily slotted into the EMT's pocket for easy transportation or into full bags that can carry over a hundred ampoules and all the medication that a paramedic or doctor might need.

Military EMS Bags

Bags have also been designed for medics to use in the military. They are similar to normal EMS bags with multiple pockets and pouches and are available in different sizes. They are sometimes made from stronger material with extra padding; they are also available in various camouflage colours. These bags often have integrated pouches for military equipment such as maps, ammunition, and radio communication equipment.

Custom EMS Bags EMS bags can also be adopted and customized to accommodate different types of specialized equipment such as

1. Oxygen therapy: nebulizers, ventilators.
2. Sports injuries kit for EMS at sporting events.
3. Doctor's kit containing extra ALS equipment.
4. Mass casualty equipment.
5. Specialized pediatric/neonatal kits for use on EMS intensive care units.
6. Rescue equipment—ropes, cutting equipment.

Personal Protective Equipment (PPE) "Hold-Alls"

Many EMTs and paramedics carry a hold-all type bag to carry their personal equipment such as helmet, high-visibility and rescue jackets, waterproof overtrousers, and debris gloves.

Cases and Boxes

The alternative to carrying EMS bags is boxes or cases. All the equipment mentioned above can be carried in boxes or cases as an alternative. They have some advantages over bags as they are often waterproof, made of tough plastic or metal, and equipment is easily accessed and visualized in divided compartments. They can also be easily washed and disinfected in the case of spillage. Some boxes/cases can be mounted in the vehicle with brackets. The disadvantages include increased bulk and weight, making them difficult to carry. Additionally, there is no room for maneuver if an item of equipment is too bulky for the compartment. They make good storage for items that can be broken easily, for example, medication ampoules. They also make good storage compartments for sharp rescue tools.

Personal Pouches

EMS personnel often carry a personal pouch on their belt, consisting of items such as a paramedic shears, stethoscope, penlight. and artery forceps. These pouches are also available in different sizes and colors to adapt to whatever the EMT wishes to carry on his or her belt.

The benefits of carrying personal equipment on an EMT's belt include familiarity and rapid access. However, it is important not to excessively duplicate equipment carried in EMS bags. Because the belt equipment is often personal to each EMT, it is important that the same standards of quality and infection control are applied to this as pertain to standard EMS equipment.

Improvisation

Many of the EMS bags and boxes mentioned above are expensive to buy, in particular the customized bags. An inexpensive way of holding EMS equipment is to use normal bags or rucksacks and to use toolboxes or fishing tackle boxes as an excellent cheaper alternative (Table 19-2).

DIAGNOSTICS

A vital part of any EMT or paramedic training is obtaining accurate patient vital signs and observations. The more vital signs obtained, the more accurately the EMT or paramedic will be able to diagnose the injury or illness. Some vital signs, for example pulse rate, breathing rate, and skin color, can be obtained by the EMT or paramedic without the use of equipment. Other vital signs such as blood pressure, cardiac rhythms, and oxygen saturation levels can only be obtained with the use of equipment.

Table 19–2	Suggested Equipment Bags
Basic	
First responder bag Oxygen cylinder bag Splint bag Personal belt pouches	
Advanced	
Advanced life support bag Drugs bag	
Optional	
"Doctor's" bag ATLS bag Rescue equipment	

ATLS = Advanced Trauma Life Support.

BASIC DIAGNOSTIC EQUIPMENT

Basic diagnostic equipment should be available in all EMS systems and should include equipment to measure blood pressure, a stethoscope, and a penlight.

Blood Pressure Measurement

Blood pressure can be measured using a sphygmomanometer or an automatic blood pressure machine.

Standard manually operated blood pressure cuffs come in different sizes to accommodate infants, children, adults, and large adults. They can come with either one or two tubes to the 'bladder' of the cuff. The release of the pressure can be done by either a button-type release or a screw-type release. The pressure gauges vary in sizes and clarity. It is important that EMS personnel are able to easily read the gauge to obtain accurate readings. Standard blood pressure sphygmomanometers should be affordable for EMS personnel and systems.

A more expensive option to obtain blood pressure readings is to use an electronic blood pressure monitor. They vary in size, price, and functionality. They are often integrated with SpO_2 and/or cardiac monitors. They can either be wall mounted in the ambulance or used as portable devices. They offer the advantage to the EMT/paramedic of the ability to perform other treatments or procedures while the monitor is automatically obtaining the blood pressure.

Stethoscope

A stethoscope is a useful piece of diagnostic equipment. It is used by EMS personnel primarily to listen to breath sounds, arterial blood flow during blood pressure measurement, and heart sounds. They are available in different acoustic levels, the more advanced with high acoustic sensitivity. They are available in different sizes for use on both adult and pediatric patients. Some stethoscopes have two different size diaphragms on one bell, eliminating the need to carry two different size stethoscopes. Some more advanced stethoscopes are available in an electronic version to help deliver better acoustics; some of the electronic stethoscopes have built-in "Bluetooth" software to send signals to a computer for analysis. For EMTs, the basic stethoscope will usually suffice.

Penlight

Basic assessment of the patient's eyes requires a penlight or small torch to check for pupillary reaction. Penlights are also useful for oral cavity inspection and other dark recesses. They are easy to use and affordable. Some penlights are disposable, whereas others require batteries. Many that are specifically designed for medical use have a gauge on the side to determine pupil size.

ADVANCED DIAGNOSTIC EQUIPMENT

Many EMS systems carry far more than the basic diagnostic equipment, as mentioned above. The advanced diagnostic equipment may vary from service to service. The following are often used:

Oxygen Saturation Monitoring Equipment

A common piece of diagnostic equipment includes an oxygen saturation monitor. This machine measures the percentage of hemoglobin saturated with oxygen. There are many different oxygen saturation machines; each EMS system must evaluate its needs when purchasing this piece of equipment. They come in many different sizes and specificities. The most popular for EMS use would be a more portable and handheld machine or one linked to an ECG and/or noninvasive blood pressure (NIBP) machine. The SpO_2 monitors normally also display the pulse rate and pulse strength. There are different probes available to accommodate all patients, such as finger, toe, ear, and foot probes. This piece of equipment is particularly useful when treating a patient with breathing difficulties.

Thermometers

Thermometers are available in many forms, from disposable paper/tape type thermometers to electronic thermometers integrated with other electronic diagnostic equipment. Thermometers are available in oral, rectal, auxiliary, or tympanic forms. The most practical thermometers, although not always the most accurate, are those that can perform a reading in a few seconds; they are often tympanic or oral thermometers. Depending on protocols and guidelines, some EMS systems need colder or higher reading thermometers, such as if the paramedic is undertaking active cooling postcardiac arrest. Accuracy of readings should be considered for each thermometer type; it is worth testing readings in the particular clinical context before purchasing the instrument.

Blood Glucose Measuring

Some EMS systems have protocols and/or guidelines for the analysis of a blood sample for glucose levels using a glucometer. This machine can be particularly useful when managing an unconscious patient or a patient who suffers with diabetes. The glucometer is a small battery-operated machine that accepts a test strip with a drop of blood for analysis. The size of the drop of blood, or type of test strip used, will depend on the make and model of glucometer used. Lancets are used in conjunction with glucometers to prick the patient to obtain the blood sample. Glucometers have different specifications and functionality; the most important thing is that they are kept precise and accurate during their use.

Advanced Point-of-Care Testing Equipment

Some EMS systems operating in remote areas with long transport times or those operating critical care retrieval services over long distances have advanced point-of-care (POC) testing equipment. Devices are available to rapidly assess acid-base status, hemoglobin, electrolytes, and cardiac enzymes at the patient's side. The decision to carry these will be individual to each EMS. The principal criterion, however, must be that the EMS providers have protocols and equipment to act on the information obtained; otherwise the value of the equipment is negated.

End-Tidal Carbon Dioxide (ETCO$_2$) Measurement Equipment

The EMS provider sometimes requires an ETCO$_2$ measurement or continuous ETCO$_2$ measurements (capnography). It is routinely used when a paramedic has intubated a patient; it is also becoming popular when treating patients with breathing difficulties such as asthmatics and patients with chronic obstructive pulmonary disease (COPD). It can be measured by either qualitative, quantitative, or colorimetric devices. A colorimetric ETCO$_2$ device changes color when CO$_2$ is detected. They are disposable devices that attach between an ET tube and Bag Valve Mask (also known as a *BVM* or Ambu bag); they change from purple to yellow on detection of CO$_2$. This device is not always accurate and can be contaminated. A superior device would be an electronic monitor, which measures ETCO$_2$ levels continuously. These machines can be stand alone or integrated with a cardiac monitoring machine. They produce waveforms and actual measurements of both ETCO$_2$ and respiratory rate. Like all medical devices, they are available with different functions and specifications.

Carbon Monoxide Monitoring Equipment

Carbon monoxide monitoring is becoming increasingly popular with EMS systems for both paramedics and EMTs in near suicide attempts and enclosed fire situations. These devices are similar to that of the traditional SpO$_2$ monitor; in fact many of the CO monitors are integrated with SpO$_2$ monitors. They are handheld battery-operated machines with a finger probe attachment with infrared light to obtain the measurements. They can also be integrated within cardiac monitors.

Peak Flow Meters

Respiratory peak flow meters are becoming a more common EMS diagnostic tool. The peak flow meter measures the patient's maximum expiration—peak expiratory flow rate (PEFR). EMS personnel must have a chart with the normal range of PEFR for patients, depending on their sex and height. This will enable the EMT to measure the rate obtained compared to the normal expected value. A peak flow meter is an inexpensive item that uses disposable mouthpieces. It is particularly useful when assessing an asthmatic or COPD patient.

Cardiac Monitoring Equipment

Most EMS systems have cardiac monitoring abilities. They can be in the simple form of continuous cardiac monitoring through two, three, or four monitoring leads or through the capture or continuous monitoring of a 12-lead ECG. The prices, specifications, and functionality of cardiac monitoring equipment vary. Many of the modern cardiac monitors have several capabilities integrated into one machine such as SpO$_2$ monitoring, ETCO$_2$ monitoring, cardiac monitoring, 12-lead ECG, defibrillation, non-invasive blood pressure (NIBP), pacing, and modems to send information to receiving hospitals. Twelve-lead ECG transmission is becoming important with prehospital triage of patients suitable for immediate coronary artery dilatation and stenting.

Ophthalmoscope and Otoscope

Rather than the standard penlight, some EMTs prefer to use ophthalmoscopes and otoscopes. The otoscope is a useful piece of diagnostic equipment if the EMT has the ability and/or protocols to examine the inner parts of the ear. The instrument can be valuable in detecting an ear infection. Otoscopes are usually battery operated and are available with disposable ear funnels. An ophthalmoscope is also battery operated; many are available with halogen or fiberoptic bulbs for increased illumination. Some of the otoscopes and ophthalmoscopes available are integrated into one instrument, utilizing the same batteries and handle.

Portable Ultrasound Machines

Some EMS systems in the US, Australasia, and Europe are now using portable ultrasound machines to aid in the detection of injuries and illnesses. Most work has been done in the use of ultrasound in trauma patients to detect blood in the abdomen and chest. (see Table 19-3 for a list of suggested diagnostic equipment).

AIRWAY MANAGEMENT EQUIPMENT

Oropharyngeal Airways (OPAs)

OPAs – also known as Guedel airways or oral airways – are the most basic of airway management tools. A full range of sizes from 000 (preterm neonatal) to 5 (large adult) should be carried. OPAs are generally color-coded according to size. Tongue depressors are

Table 19–3	Suggested Diagnostic Equipment

Basic

Pen torch
Manual sphygmomanometer
Stethoscope
Blood glucose monitor
Thermometer
SpO_2 monitor

Advanced

Automatic NIBP cuff
Cardiac monitor
12-Lead ECG
$ETCO_2$ colorimeter/waveform capnograph
Peak flow meter

Optional

CO detector
Portable ultrasound
Ophthalmoscope
Otoscope
Advanced POC testing equipment

NIBP = noninvasive blood pressure.

useful for inserting the OPA in pediatric patients and should also be carried.

Nasopharyngeal Airways (NPAs)

NPAs – also known as nasal airways – perform a similar function to OPAs but may be more suitable for patients with a higher level of consciousness, as they often do not stimulate the gag reflex. Although they are commercially available, NPAs are obtainable in pediatric sizes but often only adult sizes (6, 7, 8) are stocked and pediatric NPAs are improvised from ETTs (see below). In addition to the NPA, it is necessary to carry a lubricating gel and a selection of safety pins (often prepacked with the NPA), which are used to determine the length to which the NPA is inserted; this is the more important factor in sizing the NPA rather than the diameter.

Magill Forceps

Magill forceps are a useful tool for the removal of oropharyngeal foreign bodies such as food boluses.

They are available in adult and pediatric sizes and are a necessary adjunct for any EMT who has clinical practice guidelines for clearing airway obstructions.

Suction Machines

Suction apparatus is necessary for clearing secretions, blood, and vomitus from the patient airway. There are a number of different types available. Handheld apparatuses are useful for initial response and are portable enough to carry in a first-response bag along with basic airway equipment. However, they generally lack the suction power necessary for clearing more than a small amount of fluid. An electric suction apparatus offers a stronger vacuum and is able to clear larger quantities of fluid. While portable enough to carry to the patient's side, they are generally not small enough to fit within most response bags and thus are kept on the ambulance at the head end of the stretcher.

Extraglottic Airways

The term extraglottic airway includes laryngeal mask airways (supraglottic) and laryngeal tube airways (retroglottic). These offer an alternative to endotracheal intubation in many patients and also act as a rescue device in the setting of a failed intubation. Both have the advantage of easy insertion and reduced training requirements in comparison to an ETT. The decision to carry an extraglottic airway will depend on local protocols and training. It is suggested that an extraglottic airway is mandatory for any EMS using endotracheal intubation (to act as a back-up airway device). Extraglottic airways may also be appropriate as an alternative to endotracheal intubation in a service that does not have the capacity for any advanced airway procedures. All extraglottic airways require a profoundly reduced level of consciousness and absence of pharyngeal reflexes in order to permit insertion.

Laryngeal Mask Airway (LMA)

The LMA is the prototypal supraglottic airway and many different commercially available options are now available. Sizes range from 1 (pediatric) to 5 (large adult). The sizes stocked should reflect what local protocols allow (e.g., pediatric LMAs may not be necessary if staff are not trained or authorized in their use).

Laryngeal Tube (LT)

The laryngeal tube represents an alternative to the LMA and may offer some advantages in terms of ease of insertion. Stock and use again depend on local protocols but it is not anticipated that both LTs and LMAs would be carried.

Combitube

The Combitube is another acceptable alternative to intubation. However, it has declined in popularity since the advent of the LMA and LT. If this is the chosen airway of the EMS, it should be stocked in both available sizes (no pediatric sizes are available).

Endotracheal Intubation

The advent of extraglottic airway devices provides a practical alternative to endotracheal intubation, but endotracheal intubation is still offered by many EMS systems, either with or without the assistance of drugs. All the equipment necessary for intubation should be carried in a single bag or case. The use of an **intubation roll** is useful in allowing all equipment to be visualized easily. Consideration should also be given to keeping pre-drawn intubation medications here as well if drug-assisted intubation is provided.

Endotracheal Tubes (ETT)

A selection of ETTs in sizes from pediatric to adult (2.0–10.0) should be carried. If these are pre-cut, this should be the standard throughout the EMS as opposed to individual preference. If tubes are carried in half-sizes, it is probably reasonable to stock a single tube of each size on the ambulance. If pediatric ETTs are used routinely to improvise nasopharyngeal airways, then extra tubes should be carried. Traditionally, uncuffed tubes have been recommended for the pediatric patient; however, recent evidence suggests that cuffed tubes may also be appropriate.

Laryngoscopes

Traditionally, laryngoscopy is performed using a hand-held laryngoscope with a curved (MacIntosh) or straight (Miller) blade. Two universal laryngoscope handles and selection of blade sizes should be carried. Ideally, two of each size blade will be stocked to allow for failure of the bulb. However, if spare batteries and bulbs are also carried, this may not be necessary. Single-use disposable laryngoscope blades are favored by many EMS systems; however, these do not always meet with operator approval in comparison to reusable stainless steel blades.

Tube Ties

Tube holders with built in bite-blocks are available for securing the tube. Alternatively, the tube may be secured with tape or a length of ribbon gauze and an Oropharyngeal Airway placed in the mouth to prevent biting on the tube. For patient transport, it is worth considering the use of a cervical collar and blocks to minimize the potential for tube dislodgement, even where spinal injury is not suspected.

Additional Equipment

Some additional equipment is necessary for ETT insertion.

- Syringes to inflate balloon
- Lubricant jelly
- Scissors to cut tubes

Bougies/Stylets

In the event of a poor laryngoscopic view, a bougie or stylet may assist in the passage of the ETT. A malleable stylet is inserted into the ETT and increases the rigidity and angulation of the tube, whereas a bougie is inserted through the cords first and the tube is subsequently threaded over the bougie. The choice of which to carry is a matter of local preference, although some gum elastic bougies have the facility for oxygen insufflation in the event that an ETT cannot be passed over the bougie.

Additional Laryngoscopic Devices

Traditionally, the MacIntosh or Miller laryngoscope was the only method of visualizing the vocal cords at intubation. There is now a wide variety of alternative devices available, including video laryngoscopes and optical laryngoscopes. The evidence base in favor of many of these devices is growing rapidly, and there is a trend toward more successful intubation and reduced cervical spine motion for many of them. While the role for prehospital intubation remains controversial, these devices may offer an alternative method for those services providing it.

Surgical Airways

In the event of a total airway obstruction where ventilation or intubation is not possible, surgical airways offer a potentially lifesaving alternative. The equipment required for these will reflect the techniques EMS staff are trained in locally. It is essential that any practitioner performing drug-assisted intubation have the training and equipment to perform at least one of these techniques.

Tracheostomy

The technique of tracheostomy is not generally suited to the prehospital environment because of the time necessary to perform the procedure and the reported increased risk of complications. Either a cricothyroidotomy or a needle cricothyroidotomy is advocated.

Cricothyroidotomy

While it is possible to perform a cricothyroidotomy with only a scalpel and a tracheostomy tube, additional equipment is usually necessary. This equipment is listed in Table 19-4. Alternatively, pre-packaged kits containing the necessary equipment for either a traditional or Seldinger approach are available. There is some evidence that the Seldinger approach may be safer, but choice of equipment will largely be affected by local training and preference.

Needle Cricothyroidotomy

Needle cricothyroidotomy is the technique of choice in the pediatric population, where the anatomy precludes surgical cricothyroidotomy. It is also an appropriate technique in adults, for whom no alternative means of oxygenation is available. Although the equipment necessary to perform a needle cricothyroidotomy is often carried on the ambulance for other purposes, it may be useful to keep a preassembled kit (Table 19-5). These can be prepared from standard stock or acquired commercially.

Detection Devices

It is essential to confirm proper placement of endotracheal tubes and Combitubes. It is also best practice to

Table 19–4	Cricothyroidotomy Equipment

Scalpel No. 15 or No. 11 blade
Tracheal dilator or spreader
2 × Artery forceps or hemostats
Scissors
Tracheal hook
Tracheostomy tube (size 5-6 for an adult)
Tie to secure tube in place
Syringe to inflate balloon

Table 19–5	Needle Cricothyroidotomy Equipment

Large-bore IV cannula
10-mL syringe
High-flow oxygen source
Oxygen tubing
Three-way tap

confirm proper placement of supraglottic airways. Placement can be confirmed using clinical assessment, but capnography and/or the use of an esophageal detector device is also necessary.

End-Tidal CO_2 Colorimeter

The most basic form of $ETCO_2$ detection is a colorimetric device that is inserted between the ETT or supraglottic airway and the BVM. A change in color (typically purple to yellow) occurs after several successful ventilations, confirming the presence of CO_2.

End-Tidal CO_2 Waveform Capnography

$ETCO_2$ waveform capnography has the advantage of providing continuous, real-time information on the quality of ventilations as well as conforming initial tube placement. $ETCO_2$ waveform capnography is useful in alerting failures of tube position or ventilation that have occurred after initial placement has been confirmed. These events may not be detected using a colorimeter. $ETCO_2$ waveform capnography is a standard or optional feature on many multifunction monitor defibrillators, but stand-alone devices are also available. $ETCO_2$ waveform capnography is mandatory for any EMS providing drug-assisted intubation.

Esophageal Detector Device (ODD)

An alternative to $ETCO_2$ monitoring is the use of an esophageal detector device. It is most compatible with the Combitube but can be used with ETTs as well. The esophageal detector device has been associated with significant false-positive and false-negative results but may be more appropriate in cardiac arrest patients in whom levels of $ETCO_2$ are too low to be detected. In the interests of simplicity, it is suggested that either an $ETCO_2$ detector or an ODD are carried but not both.

Improvisation

Nasopharyngeal airways (NPAs) can be improvised by using an ETT cut to the appropriate size and secured to the face with tape. The tube size can be selected in the same way as sizing a commercially available NPA (see **Chapter 22 Airway & Respiratory Management**). The tube diameter should correspond to the diameter of the patient's little finger and the length should measure from the corner of the mouth to the tragus of the ear. See Table 19-6 for a list of suggested airway equipment.

Table 19–6	**Suggested Airway Equipment**

Basic

2 × set of OPAs (size 000–5)
2 × set of adult NPAs (size 6–8), safety pins
Sterile lubricant gel
Tongue depressors
2 × Magill forceps (adult)
2 × Magill forceps (pediatric)
Handheld (manual) suction device
Electric suction device

Advanced

1 × set of LMAs or LT (sizes appropriate to local EMS protocols)
2 × Laryngoscope handles
2 × Set of laryngoscope blades (size and design appropriate to local EMS protocols)
2 × Set of ETTs (sizes appropriate to local EMS protocols)
2 × Stylet or gum-elastic bougie
1 × Adult and pediatric tube holder/bite-block
Ribbon gauze as alternative tube tie
2 × ETCO$_2$ colorimeter (or ETCO$_2$ capability on multifunction monitor)
Syringes appropriate for inflating LMA/LT and ETT
Needle cricothyroidotomy set

Optional

Combitube
Esophageal detector device
Video laryngoscope
Optical laryngoscope
Alternative advanced airway devices
Surgical cricothyroidotomy set

OPA = Oropharyngeal Airways; NPA = Nasopharyngeal Airway: ETT = Endotracheal tube LMA = Laryngeal Mask Airway; LT = laryngeal tube.

RESUSCITATION AND OXYGEN THERAPY

Oxygen delivery and resuscitation are cornerstones of emergency medical care. EMS should stock sufficient oxygen and appropriate delivery systems for all patients.

Oxygen

Almost all patients will benefit from oxygen administration, and there are few contraindications. This should be presumed at the beginning of a shift, and each ambulance should carry a quantity likely to be sufficient for the duration of that shift. In areas with long travel distances between ambulance bases and destination hospitals, it may be possible to have replacement arrangements with local hospitals as well.

Oxygen Cylinders

Small oxygen cylinders are suitable for treating patients at the scene and during transfer into or out of the ambulance. Once in the ambulance, patients should be transferred to the on-board oxygen supply in order to preserve portable oxygen cylinder supply. Oxygen cylinder nomenclature varies among jurisdictions. In most of Europe either a C or D cylinder is used, which supplies 170 or 340 L of oxygen, respectively. More recently a CD cylinder has been introduced that is made of a lightweight composite material and can carry 460 L. This is perhaps most suited to the prehospital environment, combining convenience with sufficient capacity to run at high flow (15 L/min) for up to 30 minutes.

On-Board Oxygen

The amount of on-board oxygen carried will depend on transport times and local geography. At a minimum, there should be sufficient oxygen to run at a high flow rate (15 L/min) for the duration of the longest potential transport encountered in a particular EMS. Ideally, more than this should be carried because to carry less would be to limit the ability of the ambulance to respond to further calls until restocked. Furthermore, the possibility of delays in transport must also be taken into account.

Oxygen Delivery Systems

Masks

For the conscious patient who is maintaining his or her own airway, supplemental oxygen via a face mask is administered for a variety of respiratory, cardiac, and other conditions. There are a variety of possible oxygen delivery systems available depending on the patient's clinical need.

Nonrebreather Face Mask

Most basic EMS providers are trained to administer oxygen at high flow via a nonrebreather face mask. The nonrebreather face mask features a reservoir bag, which fills with oxygen between patient breaths and thus allows a high concentration of oxygen to be inhaled with each breath. Side valves on the mask allow the patient to exhale but minimize the entrainment of room air in inspiration. These masks facilitate both ease of administration and treatment of hypoxia but could compromise a small number of patients relying on hypoxic drive (usually severe COPD patients). As it is a frequently used item, the EMS should carry several nonrebreather masks in adult and pediatric sizes.

Face Mask

The simple face mask allows between 6 and 15 L/minute of oxygen to be administered via a direct connection to the oxygen source. While easy to use, this provides a relatively crude regulation of oxygen delivery between 28 and 50%. Less than 6 L/minute of oxygen through this mask may result in rebreathing of exhaled CO_2.

Nasal Cannula

A nasal cannula may be better tolerated by the patient, particularly if claustrophobia or emesis is a concern. For each 1 L of oxygen administered, inhaled oxygen rises by about 4%. Flow rates of up to 6 L/minute may be tolerated, delivering oxygen concentrations of 25 to 45%, depending on the amount of mouth breathing occurring. Flow rates over 4 L/minute may cause drying and irritation of the mucous membranes, and a face mask is generally preferable in this situation.

Venturi Masks

Venturi masks use a selection of color-coded delivery valves to entrain room air with a predetermined oxygen flow, which is designed to deliver a specified oxygen concentration from 24 to 60%. These have the advantage of being interchangeable; therefore a single mask can be used on an individual patient with different valves.

Assisted Ventilation Devices

In patients with inadequate or absent respiratory effort, assisted ventilation is required. This can be delivered as mouth-to-mouth ventilation, mouth-to-mask ventilation, or bag-valve mask ventilation.

Mouth-to-Mouth Ventilation

There are concerns regarding infectious disease transmission when mouth-to-mouth ventilation is performed. While there is little evidence to suggest a high risk of disease transmission, EMS providers should try to minimize the situations where they may be in a position to provide mouth-to-mouth ventilation without some form of protective equipment. However, mouth-to-mouth ventilation can be lifesaving and each situation requires individual risk assessment.

There are barrier face shield devices available to reduce the risk of infection with mouth-to-mouth ventilation. While not specifically part of an EMS equipment list, they may be appropriate for EMS providers to carry while off duty for personal protection. These devices are small and can be carried in a purse or wallet or as a key ring.

Face Mask

An alternative to the face shield is a face mask, which is still a relatively small and portable piece of equipment for delivering artificial ventilation. This is suitable for carrying on the person and is generally compatible with BVMs (below). In addition, many have the capability to entrain supplemental oxygen via a side port.

Bag-Valve Mask

The bag-valve mask removes the need for the EMS provider to use his or her mouth to provide assisted ventilation. It combines a face mask with a self-inflating bag, which delivers a single tidal volume each time it is compressed. A valve between the bag and face mask allows the patient to exhale into the atmosphere. Most BVMs also have an oxygen reservoir bag, which should ensure that the FIO_2 is maximized with each ventilation. Different sizes of both bag and face mask are available from neonatal to adult. Currently most BVMs are single-use devices, but some services may still employ reusable BVMs. The BVM is an essential part of all EMS kits and given its lifesaving potential, at least two adult and pediatric sizes should be carried.

Anesthetic Circuit

Some EMS systems carry anesthetic circuits (e.g., Mapleson C Circuit). These are similar to the BVM in many respects but rely on a continuous flow of oxygen to operate, as the bags are not self-inflating. Most feature an adjustable PEEP valve, which can be useful in administering positive airway pressure (see below) and in preoxygenating patients prior to drug-assisted intubation. Anaesthetic circuits are generally essential for those services offering drug-assisted intubation.

CPAP Circuit

In the situation where hypoxia is still a problem despite administration of high flow oxygen, positive airway pressure may be needed. Typically, this may occur with acute pulmonary edema or severe pneumonia. Positive airway pressure can be delivered via a continuous positive airway pressure (CPAP) mask or using an anaesthetic circuit (such as a Mapleson C Circuit) with an adjustable PEEP valve. The Boussinac CPAP circuit is designed for EMS operation and attaches to a standard oxygen flowmeter.

Ventilators

Some EMS (particularly air medical services) may choose to provide a ventilator for the delivery of artificial ventilation. Typically, this is restricted to intubated patients, although use of a ventilator with a laryngeal mask airway (LMA) or face mask is possible. Ventilators used in prehospital care have to maximize value for money as well as size and durability. This may be at the expense of some features normally available on hospital ventilators.

Nebulizers

In the situation where an EMS provider is required to deliver nebulized medications, nebulizer masks must be provided. Typically these are oxygen-driven via the standard flowmeter; however, many patients with chronic respiratory diseases have electric home nebulizers that do not entrain additional oxygen. Adult and pediatric nebulizer masks should be stocked.

Special adaptations are available for delivering nebulized medications to intubated patients.

Chest Drain/Needle Thoracentesis

Advanced interventions often include the ability to perform needle decompression of a tension pneumothorax. While a standard 14 G intravenous cannula is often recommended for this purpose, there is evidence that this may not be long enough for a substantial proportion of the population. Some EMS will carry dedicated needles for this purpose. These may be merely a longer than standard cannula or encompass a device that includes one-way valves and aspiration

syringes as well as devices to secure the cannula after insertion.

Improvisation

In the case where an intubated patient is exhibiting signs of bronchospasm and a nebulizer fitting for the ETT is not available, a 50-mL Luer-Lok syringe and a handheld Salbutamol or albuterol inhaler can be used to deliver an inhaled aerosol via the ETT.

Following needle aspiration of a tension pneumothorax, it is possible to secure the cannula to the chest wall using an improvised combination of a pediatric oxygen mask, a 10-mL syringe, and the finger of a rubber glove (which acts as a flutter valve). This has the advantage of using readily available and familiar equipment as well as preventing kinking of the cannula.

Carriers (Table 19-7)

Oxygen and delivery systems are often carried in a dedicated response bag along with basic airway equipment (see above).

Table 19–7	**Suggested Oxygen and Resuscitation Equipment**
Basic	
2 × Portable oxygen cylinder (with capacity for 30 minutes of high-flow oxygen) Sufficient on board oxygen for maximum length journey on continuous high flow 5 × Adult and pediatric non–rebreather oxygen masks Selection of variable concentration oxygen masks (e.g., Venturi masks) 5 × Adult and pediatric nasal cannulas 2 × Adult and pediatric bag- valve masks	
Advanced	
2 × Adult and pediatric nebulizer masks Anesthetic circuit	
Optional	
Automatic ventilator CPAP circuit Face mask Barrier face shield	

CPAP = continuous positive airway pressure mask.

CARDIAC CARE

The provision of basic cardiac care to patients with signs and symptoms of cardiac disease and to those in cardiac arrest can often be provided using only the equipment mentioned elsewhere in this chapter, particularly in the airway and oxygen sections. Advanced cardiac care, however, requires at a minimum defibrillation for those patients suffering ventricular fibrillation or pulseless ventricular tachycardia. Automated external defibrillators (AEDs) are commonplace now, and with increasing reports of successful use by civilians with little or no training, AEDs may now be considered a basic component of emergency cardiac care.

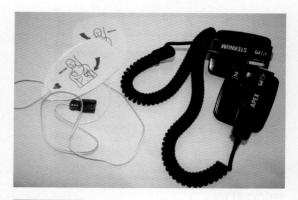

Defibrillator multifunction pads and paddles.

Defibrillators

Automatic external defibrillators (AEDs) have transformed the nature of emergency cardiac care in recent years. It is recognized that early defibrillation for patients in VF or pulseless VT maximizes the chances of survival. Given that AEDs have been successfully and safely used by civilians with little or no training, it is imperative that they are part of all EMS operations. Every EMS practitioner should have access to at least one AED.

Monophasic versus Biphasic

Most defibrillators currently available use a biphasic energy waveform, which is thought to have a greater success rate in converting VF or VT into sinus rhythm than a monophasic waveform. Any EMS acquiring new defibrillators should ensure that they use a biphasic waveform.

Screen

Manual defibrillators have a screen to display the rhythm for analysis and generally also a print function to record rhythm strips. A display screen is also a feature of some AEDs. This is not strictly necessary as the operator is not required to analyze the rhythm, but it may be useful if the AED is also to be used for monitoring patients. For both AEDs and manual defibrillators, there is often a choice between an LED screen and a backlit screen. Where available, the backlit screen is often easier to read in extremes of light and dark.

Battery Life

An important consideration for any EMS equipment, but particularly defibrillators, is the battery life and the time to recharge. All defibrillators should have easily rechargeable batteries and at least one fully charged spare battery should be carried in addition to the battery in the machine.

Multifunction Pads versus Paddles

Traditionally, defibrillators delivered the shock via a pair of paddles connected to the machine and placed apically and at the sternum of the patient. More recently, most defibrillators now have multifunction adhesive pads either as standard or as an alternative to paddles. Multifunction pads adhere to the patients' chests in the same position as the paddles and can be used to monitor rhythms, deliver shocks, and externally pace patients as necessary. Pads offer a safer form of shock delivery as the possibility of inadvertent contact with charged paddles is eliminated. In the situation where repeated shocks are delivered during a prolonged resuscitation, it may be necessary to change the pads after a number of shocks (usually specified by the manufacturer) (Figure 19-1).

Automatic External Defibrillators

AEDs can deliver an appropriate shock to patients in VF or pulseless VT with minimal input from the operator. They undertake the functions of rhythm analysis and delivery of shock. The operator is generally only required to undertake a number of steps: power the unit on, attach multifunction electrodes to the patient, confirm cardiac arrest, and press the "charge" button. As the operator is required to actually make the decision to deliver the shock, these AEDs are, strictly speaking, semiautomated defibrillators; however, the term AED is in common use to describe these devices. Most modern AEDs also provide voice prompts to guide the operator in these steps as well as in the performance of CPR (Figure 19-2).

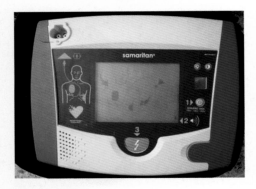

FIGURE 19–2

AED.

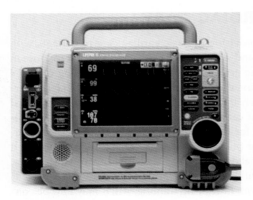

FIGURE 19–3

Manual defibrillator. Reprinted with permission from Physio-Control, Inc. http://www.physio-control.com/default.aspx.

Modern AEDs are relatively compact, lightweight, and cost-effective. There is a wide variety to choose from and individual EMS services will have differing needs depending on their patient population and the level of emergency cardiac care offered. Any AED chosen should be sufficiently durable to withstand the EMS environment. Ideally the AEDs will be easily upgraded to comply with any changes in ILCOR guidelines. AEDs, in particular, should be standardized across all EMS vehicles so that providers can seamlessly provide care wherever they are working within a service.

Manual Defibrillators

Manual defibrillators require the operator to perform all the steps required for AEDs, and the operator is additionally required to analyze the rhythm, select the appropriate energy level, and deliver the shock. Manual defibrillators are only suitable for advanced providers with appropriate training in rhythm interpretation and shock delivery. Most manual defibrillators have an AED function to enable their use by more basic providers. Additionally, most manual defibrillators for EMS use combined facilities for SpO_2, blood pressure, $ETCO_2$, and 12-lead ECG recording and transmission. Therefore these are often the models of choice for many EMS, even where they are largely used by basic practitioners (Figure 19-3).

Additional Functions

Additional functions available on some manual defibrillators include the ability to deliver synchronized shocks (e.g., to patients with a tachyarrhythmia but also a pulse) and to externally pace a patient via the same multifunction pads. Selection of these machines depends on the level of training of individual EMS crews.

Pediatric Pads

Both AEDs and manual defibrillators come with pediatric sized pads and paddles for use on pediatric patients. In the case of an AED, the machine will recognize that pediatric pads have been connected and adjust the energy of the shock accordingly. If pediatric pads or paddles are not available, it is suggested that adult pads be used on patients over 8 years old or adult paddles be used on patients over 1 year old or weighing 10 kg.

CPR Adjuncts

ILCOR guidelines have placed increased emphasis on consistent, high-quality chest compressions as the cornerstone of CPR. There is evidence to suggest that rescuers fatigue rapidly and that there is a dramatic reduction in the number of effective chest compressions delivered after only a few minutes of CPR. There are several devices currently available to augment or replace manual CPR.

External Chest Compression Assist Devices

There are a number of devices that are available either as stand-alone or integrated into defibrillators. These can deliver a combination of voice or audio prompts and visual cues to maximize efficient CPR. They may offer some advantage in ensuring adequate rate and depth of compression and ventilation but do not compensate for poor technique or rescuer fatigue.

Active Compression-Decompression Devices

Active compression-decompression CPR (ACD-CPR) describes a technique whereby the elastic recoil of a patient's chest is supplemented by a suction cup attached to the external chest during CPR. This allows maximal chest recoil and theoretically increased venous return, thus improving CPR. During the course of a prolonged resuscitation, the patient's natural elastic recoil may decline and ACD-CPR can compensate for this. ACD-CPR is, however, more fatiguing than standard CPR. There is a device that allows the rescuer to deliver ACD-CPR manually.

Mechanical CPR Devices

Recognizing that good quality CPR is fatiguing, there are several mechanical CPR devices available to take over the role of chest compressions from the rescuer. These offer the advantages that they deliver consistent, high-quality chest compressions without fatigue. They also free EMS providers to perform other tasks such as securing the airway and administering drugs. If CPR is performed in a moving ambulance, these devices may offer a more effective and safer approach. However, they are expensive and large to store or carry. They all require either a battery or compressed gas source to operate and this may have further implications for space and cost.

There are some concerns regarding the potential of these devices to cause internal injury and none of these devices has been definitively shown to be superior to standard manual CPR; however a number of prospective studies are ongoing that may soon provide high-level evidence on this matter. Three such devices, which EMS may wish to consider, are discussed here.

Thumper® The Thumper® is one of the original mechanical CPR devices. It consists of a gas-driven piston, which compresses the patient's chest against a backboard at a rate of 100 compressions per minute. It also has the additional benefit of allowing mechanical ventilation via the same device.

Autopulse® The Autopulse® is a battery-powered load-distributing band that compresses the patient's chest against a backboard at a rate of 100 per minute.

LUCAS® The Lund University CPR Assistance System (LUCAS®) is a gas-operated (either air or oxygen) piston that compresses the patient's chest against a backboard at a rate of 100 per minute. It also offers Active compression-decompression CPR via a

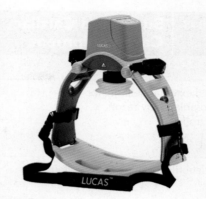

FIGURE 19–4

The Lund University CPR Assistance System (LUCAS®). Reprinted with permission from Physio-Control, Inc. http://www.physio-control.com/default.aspx.

suction cup on the end of the piston. A more recent model is battery-powered (Figure 19-4).

Impedance Threshold Devices

Impedance threshold devices (ITDs) attach to either an endotracheal or extraglottic airway and restrict the delivery of ventilations to a time period in the CPR cycle when the chest is being compressed. This reduces the delivery of ventilations when the chest is recoiling and filling with venous blood. ITDs are thought to improve venous return and thereby the quality of the CPR delivered.

Miscellaneous Cardiac Equipment

It is advisable to carry disposable safety razors to allow for removal of chest hair in patients where electrodes need to be attached for either ECG monitoring or defibrillation.

Improvisation

In a cardiac arrest situation where the presence of significant chest hair prevents multifunction defibrillator pads forming a good contact with the chest wall and a razor is not available, the multifunction pads can be used to remove the hair in a similar fashion to waxing strips! The same pads used for hair removal can be used for defibrillation, as it is not the hair attached to the pads that generally creates the barrier to proper contact but rather the air between the chest wall and the pads. Table 19-8 lists suggested cardiac care equipment.

Table 19–8	**Suggested Cardiac Care Equipment**

Basic

Automated external defibrillator
5 × Disposable safety razors
ECG electrodes

Advanced

Manual defibrillator (biphasic waveform)

Optional

Defibrillator with integrated diagnostic
    capabilities
External chest compression assist device
ACD-CPR device
Mechanical chest compression device

ACD-CPR = Active compression-decompression CPR.

VASCULAR ACCESS AND FLUID THERAPY

Venous access is essential for the delivery of fluid therapy and many medications. Generally venous access is considered an advanced skill, but increasingly basic EMS providers are administering intramuscular medications and maintaining infusions set up by advanced practitioners.

Venous Access

The standard method of obtaining venous access is using a cannula-over-needle technique. In some situations it may be necessary to use a butterfly needle (e.g., pediatrics). Some EMS systems also employ central venous access devices or rapid infusion cannulas, which are inserted using a Seldinger technique (catheter-over-guidewire). Increasingly, intraosseous access is commonplace, particularly in cardiac arrest situations.

Tourniquets

EMS providers use a tourniquet to restrict venous return from the arm or leg in order to facilitate venous engorgement and therefore easy cannulation. Traditionally, many EMS providers used their own personal tourniquet on patients. However, this approach has significant infection control concerns, particularly if blood is left on the tourniquet. Single-use disposable tourniquets are now available for this purpose.

Catheter-over-Needle Cannulas

Using a standard IV cannula, the EMS provider will be able to obtain venous access in most patients. A range of sizes should be stocked from pediatric through to large-bore 14 G or even 12 G cannulas. Typically, the 18 G and 20 G are the most commonly used sizes, and generous stocks of these should be carried. As a relatively small and inexpensive item, it is usually practical to carry large numbers. It is important to use a cannula with which EMS providers are familiar, which is compatible with the drug administration syringes, and bungs used by the EMS. Ideally, a safety cannula, which incorporates a method of automatically covering the tip of the needle, will be used, as the risk of occupational needle-stick injury in the prehospital environment is significant. Many operators will prefer a winged cannula, which is easier to hold and secure (Figure 19-5 A, B, C).

Accessories

Irrespective of which type of cannula is chosen, the following are also necessary:

1. Alcohol skin cleansing wipes.
2. Gauze pads/cotton wool.
3. Secure dressings.
4. Tape.
5. Bungs.

It is particularly important that whichever bung is chosen is compatible with any needle-free delivery system employed by the EMS.

Central Venous Access

Central venous access does not necessarily afford any advantage over peripheral venous access in the prehospital situation. However, in the circumstances where peripheral access is not available or during a cardiac arrest, central venous lines may be used by some EMS systems.

Generally, the equipment required for central venous catheter (CVC) insertion is available in pre-assembled kits using a Seldinger technique. Additionally, the operator will require:

1. Skin cleansing solution.
2. Sterile gauze pads.
3. Sterile drapes.
4. Sterile gloves.
5. Sutures to hold the line in place.

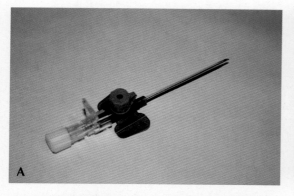

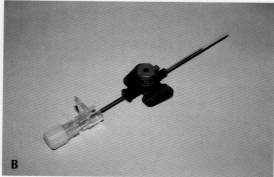

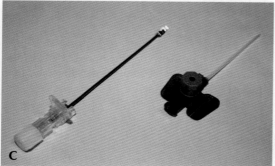

FIGURE 19-5

A, **B**, **C**, 16 G Winged catheter over needle cannula.

Rapid Infusor Cannulas

Where large-bore venous access is required, an alternative to a CVC is to use a larger bore rapid infusion cannula. Typically, these are large-bore (6–8 French) catheters, which are usually inserted into the femoral vein using a Seldinger or catheter-over-needle technique.

Intraosseous Devices

Increasingly, intraosseous devices are being used by EMS to secure vascular access in emergency situations. Intraosseous devices have the advantage of being relatively easy and quick to place, even in patients with circulatory collapse. There are a number of devices available to facilitate this. It is recommended that EMS systems consider the use of an intraosseous device as an alternative to peripheral IV access.

Intraosseous Needle The traditional intraosseous needle is driven into the bone using manual pressure and a twisting motion. While this is not technically difficult, there is potential for the device to slip or injure the operator. These devices have the advantage of being relatively low cost.

Bone Injection Gun (B.I.G.™)

The bone injection gun is a commercial device that takes over the role of delivering the intraosseous needle into the marrow via a spring-loaded device. This may also be prone to slippage during delivery but potentially is easier to handle than a manual needle.

EZ-IO®

The EZ-IO® is a handheld battery-operated drill that drives the needle into the bone in a similar fashion to that of the manual needle. It possibly offers a greater degree of control than the B.I.G.™. Needles are available in adult and pediatric sizes, and this will add to the cost of the device, which is considerably more than that of single-use intraosseous needles.

Fluid Therapy

Fluid therapy is used in the management of many acute medical and trauma situations. While the debate over the exact role of prehospital fluid therapy continues, EMS providers will undoubtedly administer fluids to patients in certain situations. Issues to consider in this regard include the type and quantity of fluid, how and where it will be stored, and how it will be administered. (**see Chapter 23 Parenteral Access**).

Fluid Storage

Intravenous fluids are generally available in soft or semirigid plastic containers. These need to be somewhat protected from outside forces, which may cause them to burst or become damaged. Fluids are often carried in drug bags, which may contain a dedicated fluids pouch. Intravenous fluids are often administered at the ambient temperature, but it may be preferable to use warmed or cooled fluids in certain clinical situations.

Fluid Warmers

Fluid warmers offer the facility to store IV fluids at a temperature higher than the ambient temperature. This may be of value in a trauma or hypothermic patient; however, there may also be implications for the shelf life of fluids that are regularly heated. As an alternative to storing fluids at a set temperature, devices are available that adjust the temperature of IV fluids as they flow from the bag into the patient. These are typically electrically powered and usually require special fluid-giving sets to administer.

Fluid Coolers

Fluid coolers are principally of value in the institution of therapeutic hypothermia after return of spontaneous circulation following cardiac arrest. Cooled fluids may also be useful in treating certain hyperthermic conditions. Unlike fluid warmers, there are unlikely to be implications for the shelf life of the coolers, which are refrigerated. Fluid coolers are usually stored in small refrigerators or cold boxes in modern ambulances.

Pressure Bags

In some situations, it is necessary to deliver a large volume of IV fluids rapidly. This can be accomplished by squeezing the fluid bag manually or by the use of a pressure bag to forcibly speed up the delivery of fluids. There are bags available for EMS use that combine fluid and vascular access equipment storage with a pressure bag feature all in one.

Fluid Delivery

Fluids require a giving set to allow delivery. Typically, these have an adjustable valve that affords a crude control of the delivery rate, measured in drops per minute. Some EMS may use automated fluid delivery sets, which deliver the fluids at a precise flow rate; these require specific giving sets. In the situation

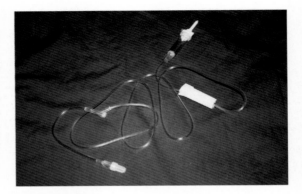

FIGURE 19–6

Giving set.

where rapid fluid delivery is required, a blood products administration set allows faster flow rates than standard giving sets (Figure 19-6, Figure 19-7, and Figure 19-8).

Hooks

Generally, ambulances have hooks or fixings in the ceiling that allow bags of IV fluids or pressure bags to be suspended above the patient in order to maximize gravitational flow.

Accessories

In addition to the above, some or all of the following may be required to assist with fluid administration:

1. three-way taps.
2. adaptors.
3. extension tubing.
4. tape.

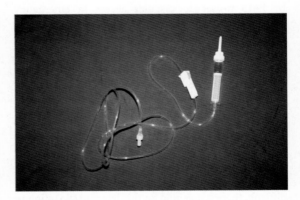

FIGURE 19–7

Blood-giving set.

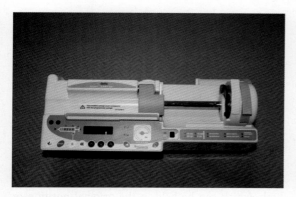

FIGURE 19–8

Infusion pump.

Improvisation

Fluids can be suspended from a variety of hooks and hangers if dedicated IV fluid stands or hooks are not available. In the patient's home, a metal clothes hanger can be bent into a simple hook, which allows fluids to be hung from a door or piece of furniture (Figure 19-9).

In the absence of a tourniquet, a latex glove can be tied around the patient's arm or leg to act in its

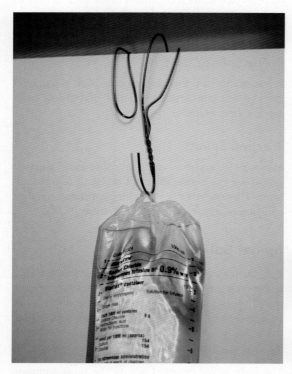

FIGURE 19–9

Improvised coat hanger IV hook.

place. This has the advantage of being a single-use item, thereby minimizing infectious disease risk. Care must be taken not to damage the skin if this approach is used, and it is suggested that the glove be tied over a shirt sleeve, for example. (Figure 19-10).

See Table 19-9 for a suggested list of vascular access and fluid therapy equipment.

SPLINTING

Many of the calls attended to by EMS personnel involve fractures or potential fractures. Some of these injuries are associated with severe pain and/or an element of neurovascular compromise; splinting is an effective method of both analgesia and restoring neurovascular status. EMS systems must ensure that there is a range of equipment available to deal with different types of fractures.

Basic Splinting

Many forms of simple splinting equipment are not only easy to use but are also cost-effective.

Triangular Bandages

Triangular bandages can be used to splint injured arms to the torso and injured legs to the uninjured leg. Triangular bandages are extremely versatile and can also be used to fashion slings and dressings.

Splinting Straps

Splinting straps with Velcro fixings are an alternative, reusable splinting material, which can be used to splint legs and arms.

Box Splints

Box splints are rigid splints covered in a tough plastic material with padding and Velcro straps to hold them in place. They are offered in different sizes to accommodate legs, arms, and children. They are also easy to

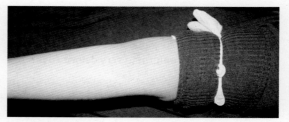

FIGURE 19–10

Latex glove as improvised tourniquet.

Table 19–9	Suggested Vascular Access and Fluid Therapy Equipment

Basic

Selection of needles and syringes for IM medication administration
5 × 2 mL syringes
5 × 5 mL syringes
5 × 10 mL syringes
10 × drawing up needles
10 × blue needles
10 × green needles

Advanced

Disposable torniquets
Selection of cannulas
5 × 24 G
5 × 22 G
10 × 20 G
10 ×18 G
5 × 16 G
5 × 14 G
Selection of bungs, dressings, etc., to use with the above
Giving sets – at least one for every bag of fluids carried
Pressure bags
Intraosseous device – with adult and pediatric needles

Optional

Blood-giving sets
Central venous catheter sets
Infusion pumps
Fluid warmers
Cooled fluids
B.I.G.™ bone injection gun
EZ-IO® device

clean and user friendly but offer relatively less immobilization compared to some other forms of splinting and cannot readily conform to very deformed limbs.

SAM® Splint System

This splint system is a lightweight cost-effective splint made of padded, flexible aluminium. It can be shaped to the injured extremity and offers a semi-rigid splinting system. It can also be easily cleaned.

Inflatable Splints

Inflatable splints are easy to use and available in different shapes and sizes; they offer good support to an injured extremity. However, they are vulnerable to puncture damage and have a limited ability to conform to deformed limbs.

Vacuum Splints

Vacuum splints consist of a bag filled with polystyrene balls, from which the air can be sucked out using a pump. This allows the splint to conform to the injured limb, which can be held in the original position or manipulated to an improved anatomic position. They are constructed from tough plastic material that can be washed and disinfected. They are available in different sizes for use on both arms and legs. In the absence of the pump, a suction unit can be used. A full body vacuum mattress is also available for full body splinting; this is particularly useful for patients with spinal injuries who must be transported over long distances.

Advanced Splinting

Advanced splinting techniques include those where there is often some realignment of the injured limb to an anatomic position. Many of these techniques are often performed by basic EMS providers.

Pelvic Splints/Straps

Pelvic splints help to stabilize open-book pelvic fractures. There are several varieties of purpose-built pelvic splints available.

Traction Splints

Many EMS systems carry purpose-built traction splints for the management of midshaft femur fractures. These devices can provide alignment, stability, and pain relief to the injured leg (Figure 19-11).

Spinal Splinting

For patients involved in motor vehicle collisions, falls, and sporting accidents, EMS personnel often carry out spinal immobilization. There are various pieces of equipment available to perform spinal immobilization.

Spinal Board

The long spinal board is one of the most common pieces of splinting equipment. It is used as both an extrication device and also as a transfer device. It is

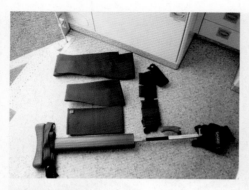

FIGURE 19–11

Femoral traction splint.

important to note that the long board was designed principally as an extrication device; even short periods spent strapped to a long board can result in pain and pressure sore formation. The long spinal board does not conform to the natural curvature of the spine, and blankets or other padding may be necessary to reduce movement and ensure comfort.

Spinal boards are available in different designs, specifications, and sizes. Many are radiolucent and are easily cleaned and disinfected. They contain holes and/or clips so that strapping and belts can be applied to hold a patient onto the board. A smaller version of the spinal board is available to accommodate a pediatric patient.

Head Immobilizer

A head immobilizer system is often used in conjunction with a spinal board; however, it is only of use if the body of the patient is also secured; otherwise, the head immobilization system will cause the neck to act as a fulcrum and actually increase movement. There are a few different types of head immobilizer systems. Variations that are more common include head blocks that are covered in a tough plastic material that is resistant to blood and attached to a Velcro base. Becoming more popular are the disposable head immobilizer systems, which are made of a tough cardboard material or plastic. From an infection control point of view, the disposable head immobilizer system may be a better option.

Cervical Collars

Extrication collars are usually employed in conjunction with a spinal board. These are available in different sizes from a baby up to an adult. Some are disposable to reduce the risks of infection. They provide some sup-

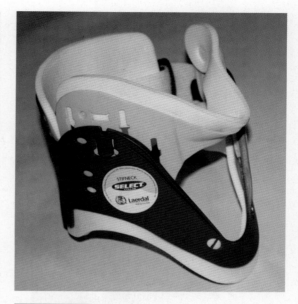

FIGURE 19–12

Adjustable cervical collar.

port to the neck during spinal immobilization; however, it is important to note that even comprehensive immobilization with a long spinal board, collar, and head straps does not completely eliminate movement at the spinal column. EMS providers should carry a full range of sizes. An alternative when space is a premium is to use adjustable collars, which are available in adult and pediatric sizes (Figure 19-12).

Orthopedic Stretcher

The orthopedic or "scoop" stretcher can be useful for either full body splinting or be used to aid in splinting an extremity. It is available in either steel or hard plastic construction and has holes to accommodate straps. This stretcher is particularly useful in extricating patients from situations in which a long spinal board cannot be used.

Extrication Devices

Extrication devices such as the Kendrick Extrication Device (KED®) offer a combination of the features mentioned above. They consist of a semi-rigid jacket, which can be strapped around the torso, and a head/neck extension, which reduces movement of the spine. There are also pelvic straps to reduce movement of the device upwards. The KED and similar devices are useful for extrication of patients from confined spaces and provide splinting support for the pelvis, spine, and head (Figure 19-13).

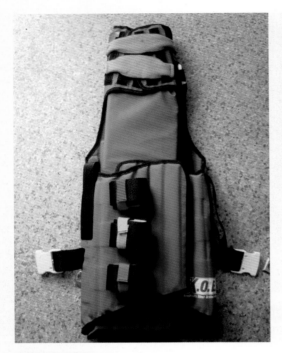

FIGURE 19–13

KED.

See Table 19-10 for a comparison of various types of splints.

Improvised Splinting

Despite the wide array of splinting devices available, the nature of patients' injuries means that a degree of creativity is always necessary in applying splints in a position of comfort. This is even more necessary if equipment is missing or defective.

Splinting can be improvised from equipment such as a newspaper wrapped in a triangular bandage, a scarf, or a tie. Patients' clothes can be used to support an injured arm by using the buttons on their jackets or

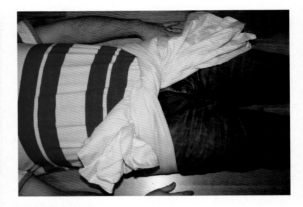

FIGURE 19–14

Improvised pelvic splint using sheet.

applying a safety pin to a jumper or shirt to form a sling.

Pelvic splints can be improvised using patient's clothing, sheets, or belts. For motorcyclists, the ideal pelvic splint may be to leave their riding leathers in situ; the splint can also be improvised using belts or sheets (Figure 19-14).

Improvised Cervical Collars

Rolled up newspaper or blankets can be used to improvise a temporary cervical collar as shown below in Figure 19-15

Improvised Head Blocks

It may often be necessary to improvise head immobilisation if head blocks and straps have been left at the receiving hospital. Rolled blankets and tape can be used to make an improvised head immobilizer; alternatively, sheets or towels rolled over bags of IV fluids can perform a similar function. Some services use solid blocks or sandbags to prevent lateral movement of the cervical spine; however, these will exert significant

Table 19–10	**Features of Different Splints**				
	Cost	Versatility	Durability	Ability to Conform to Deformities	Reusable
Triangular bandages	$	++	−	++	−
Splint straps	$	++	++	++	++
Sam splints	$$	++	+	++	+
Box splints	$$	+	+++	+	+++
Inflatable splints	$$	+	+	+	++
Vacuum splints	$$$	+	++	+++	++

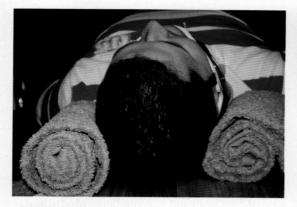

FIGURE 19–15

Improvised head blocks.

lateral pressure on the cervical spine if the patient is rolled (e.g., during vomiting) and additionally will exert significant G-forces during movement of the vehicle. It is recommended that any cervical immobilisation device — whether improvised or not — be lightweight enough to avoid this problem (Figure 19-15).

Improvised Limb Splints

Cervical collars can form a useful splinting tool for injured limbs in the absence of alternative splints. Triangular or crepe bandages can be used to secure the limb (Figure 19-16). Table 19-11 lists suggested splinting equipment.

TRAUMA AND WOUND MANAGEMENT

Much of the work of an EMS will relate to the management of trauma, bleeding, and wounds. Traditional wound management was limited to the application of pressure dressings and limb elevation. However, recent advances now afford the EMT a wide array of additional management options for wound care and the control of bleeding.

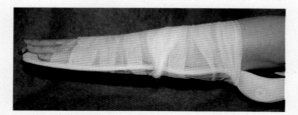

FIGURE 19–16

Improvised cervical collar forearm splint.

Table 19–11	Suggested Splinting Equipment
Basic	
10 × Triangular bandages Splinting straps Set of box splints/Inflatable splints/vacuum splints Long spinal board – adult and pediatric sizes Orthopedic scoop stretcher Set of extrication collars – adult and pediatric sizes Head immobilisation system	
Advanced	
Femoral traction splint Extrication device Pelvic splint	
Optional	
SAM® Splint	

Basic Wound Management

All EMTs are trained in basic wound management. A selection of wound dressings, wound pads, and gauze/crepe bandages will suffice for the initial management of most wounds. Some EMS systems may choose to carry "field dressings," which consist of a wound pad with gauze bandaging already attached. Alternatively, separate wound dressings and roller bandages allow greater versatility in wound management.

Accessories

The EMT will often carry a number of wound management tools in his or her personal belt pouches. Items such as trauma shears, artery forceps, and tweezers are commonly carried.

It is recommended that trauma shears are carried on the personal belt pouches of EMTs because they are employed regularly for a variety of uses, including clothing removal, seatbelt removal, and preparing dressings.

The role for artery forceps is less clear, as the technique for clamping bleeding blood vessels in the field is generally not advocated and few EMS have protocols allowing for this.

Tweezers can be useful for removal of splinters or foreign bodies and may negate the need to transfer patients with minor injuries to the hospital if they can be successfully treated in the prehospital environment.

Scalpels may be necessary in the treatment of motorcyclists who have a 'hump' built into their protective leathers. This hump needs to be removed prior to spinal immobilisation. This is normally possible by making a small incision over the top of the leathers (some brands have zip fastener here to facilitate removal).

All of the above instruments should be single-use items, as even the trauma shears have the potential to transfer bodily fluids from one patient to another at the scene of a major trauma incident. Items such as tweezers and artery forceps should also be sterile and packaged accordingly.

Advanced Wound Management

Some EMS systems may offer advanced wound management options including formal wound closure using sutures, Steri-Strips®, or tissue glue. Additional equipment and supplies relevant to the EMS individual protocols are required as indicated.

Hemostatic Dressings

There have been recent advances focused on the use of hemostatic compounds in dressings or as powder/gel that can be placed directly into a heavily bleeding wound. These have been pioneered in the military/tactical EMS initially but are starting to become more commonplace among civilian EMS systems as well.

Some of the products available include Hemcon®, Quick-clot®, and Celox®. They differ in their mode of action application and side-effect profile. It is likely that an individual EMS will only be approved for a single product and within tightly defined criteria. However, if that is the case, then it should be carried on the ambulance.

Tourniquets

Tourniquets were out of favor for many years due to concerns regarding distal neurovascular damage. These concerns still persist, but it is recognized that for *catastrophic hemorrhage*, there is a role for the application of a tourniquet. This is normally the situation following a severe crush or blast injury to an extremity. As with the hemostatic compounds, the use of tourniquets has been pioneered in the military. There are a number of tourniquets suitable for application to the injured limb that can be applied single-handedly by the injured party if necessary. Available tourniquets include the Combat Application Tourniquet (CAT®) and the Mechanical Advantage Tourniquet (MAT®). Whichever product is chosen, it is essential that it distributes enough pressure to occlude arterial supply to the affected part but also distributes this pressure over a wide enough area so that underlying viable tissue is not also damaged.

Chest Drains

Some EMS systems have protocols for the insertion of chest drains for pneumothoraces/hemothoraces. This is most likely to be the case when critical care retrieval is carried out by air and such conditions need to be stabilized prior to flight. There are a number of preprepared kits that contain the necessary equipment for the insertion of a chest drain using either a Seldinger or catheter-over-needle technique. The individual choice will depend on local protocols, and it may be preferable to assemble an individualized kit for each EMS.

Sucking chest wounds have the potential to deteriorate rapidly into a tension pneumothorax. There are one-way valves (such as Asherman® Chest Seals) that are suitable for application to the sucking wound, allowing air to exit but not to reenter. Alternatively a three-sided dressing can be fashioned to accomplish the same result.

Improvised Equipment

It is possible to use defibrillation pads as a cover for an open chest wound. Although expensive, the pads are very adherent, even in the face of active bleeding and can easily be used to occlude a sucking chest wound or provide a three-sided dressing. It is recommended that the cables are cut off any pads used for this purpose in order to avoid confusion.

In the absence of a tourniquet, a manual sphygmomanometer can be used to occlude arterial blood flow to an affected limb. This has the advantage of allowing the pressure to be recorded and also spread over a wide area to minimize damage to underlying tissue. Table 19-12 lists suggested trauma and wound management equipment.

BURNS MANAGEMENT

Burn Management Equipment

The EMT/paramedic should have some equipment to deal with the management of burn patients. The equipment required depends on the protocols or guidelines of the particular EMS. Equipment could include:

Table 19–12	Suggested Trauma and Wound Management Equipment
Basic	
Selection of wound dressings, crepe bandages, and triangular bandages Trauma shears Sterile tweezers	
Advanced	
Chest seals Wound closure products Sutures Steri-Strips Tissue glue Hemostatic dressings Torniquets	
Optional	
Chest drain set	

1. Dry sterile dressings

This inexpensive first-aid equipment is also more commonly used to treat wounds but can also be used to treat burns. The dressings can be dampened with sterile water, and sterile dressings are available in many different thickness and sizes.

2. Burn Cling Film/Bags

Another inexpensive item that can be used is cling film or simply a plastic bag. The use of cling film is an accepted way to treat burns that many EMS systems use

Table 19–13	Suggested Burns Equipment
Basic	
Dry sterile dressings Burn dressing kits/gel Cling film Sterile water Clean sheets	

worldwide. This is also a key way of improvising when managing burn patients, since cling film is widely available in many households and businesses.

3. Specialist Burn Gel

There are different types of specialized burn gel dressings available for the management of burns Figure 19-17). Many EMS systems and fire services would carry a full burn gel kit consisting of different size dressings soaked in burn gel. Some of these more advanced burn gel kits include full body dressings and dressings that can be placed over a face with cut outs for eyes, nose, and mouth. The advantages of using burn gel kits are that water is not needed and the gel will continue to cool the burn during transport to the hospital. Full burn gel kits can be expensive. See Table 19-13 for a list of suggested burn equipment.

MATERNITY

Many EMS systems will carry emergency maternity kits and equipment to manage the delivery of a baby.

In general these kits are fully disposable, minimizing the risk of infection.

Some services now have advanced protocols and standing orders for their paramedics to utilize urinary

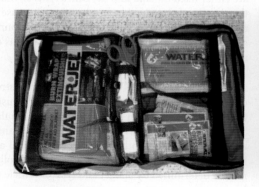
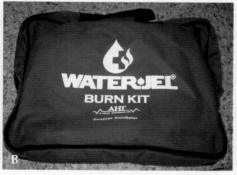

FIGURE 19–17

A, **B**, Burn gel dressings.

Table 19–14	**Suggested Maternity Equipment**

Basic

Incontinence sheets
Sterile gloves
Bulb suction
Umbilical cord clamps and scissors
Towels
Blankets/maternity pads
Clinical waste bags

Advanced

Urinary catheterization set

catheterization in certain obstetric emergencies. If these protocols exist the right equipment must be available such as different sized urinary catheters.

Table 19-14 lists suggested maternity equipment.

PATIENT LIFTING DEVICES AND PATIENT COMFORT

Patient Lifting Devices

The essence of any EMS system is to transport ill and injured people to a health-care facility. Many of the ill and injured people encountered by EMS on a daily basis are unable to walk because of the severity of their injuries and illnesses. EMS personnel must have devices that are able to assist them in the lifting of these non-ambulatory patients from the scene to their ambulances and from there into the hospital. Like other EMS equipment, there are a wide variety of lifting devices available to the EMS community. The most adequate lifting devices will depend on a number of factors, including geographical area of the EMS system, level of training received and available to EMS staff, budgetary constraints of the particular EMS system, vehicles used, and types of patients treated by the particular EMS system.

Manual Lifting Without Devices

Patients can be lifted without the use of any device if necessary. Some of those techniques include a clothes drag, one or two rescuer assist, and an extremity lift.

When EMS personnel are using any of these manual lifting/assisting techniques they should use care not to do themselves an injury by lifting patients who are too heavy or lifting improperly.

Chairs

Carrying Chairs   Carrying chairs are a common piece of EMS lifting equipment. A carrying chair will assist EMS personnel to primarily carry a patient up or down stairs and be wheeled for short distances. There are many varieties of carrying chairs, which include a simple two-wheel chair with carrying loops and handles for each EMS personnel to chairs with a triwheel or track system that can be much more easily lowered down stairs to minimize lifting. When choosing a chair, EMS systems should take into account storage space in the ambulance, budgetary confinements, load capacity of the particular chair, and type of work done by the particular EMS system. The carrying chairs with a triwheel system or tracks have the advantage of reduced manual handling for the EMS crew.

Wheelchairs   Some EMS systems may have vehicles that are able to store and accommodate standard wheelchairs. This can make it easier to move patients who are not able to walk or need assistance.

Stretchers   The majority of all EMS vehicles have some form of stretcher. Stretchers can also be referred to as gurneys, trolleys, litters, or cots.

Carrying Sheets   A simple sheet made of heavy material with handles is often used by EMS personnel. The advantages of this carry device are that it is light and easily stored, has several handles designed for team lifting, and is cheap and can be easily washed or disposed of. Some of these carrying sheets have holes to place bars to make them into a simple pole stretcher.

Emergency Stretchers/Pole Stretchers   "Field stretchers," as they are referred to because of their use on the battlefield, exist in different forms. Usually they consist of a canvas or similar material with carrying bars that are either fixed or slide into the canvas sheets. Many of these types of stretchers have advantages because they are light to carry and easily stored. EMS personnel at sporting events and in first-aid and medical tents often use them.

Ambulance Stretchers/Trolleys   Ambulance stretchers exist in many different forms; they can be used to transport a patient from the scene into the ambulance. They are fixed in the ambulance during transport and have the ability to be taken out on arrival at the health-care facility. The "best" ambulance trolley is mainly determined by budget and type of vehicle used.

Basic Ambulance Trolleys   Basic ambulance trolleys consist of a durable mattress on a frame with four wheels, carrying poles and push/pull handles. They can be manually lifted into the ambulance and locked into position. Some have the ability to adjust the position and height of the patient. Many of these trolleys require physical manual handling for the EMS crew when placing them in the ambulance and when raising them up to different positional heights. For these reason many EMS systems will opt for some type of an easy-load stretcher.

Easy-Load Ambulance Stretchers As the name would suggest, easy-load stretchers have the ability to be loaded more easily into the ambulance than the basic ambulance trolley. In general there are three different types:

1. Stretcher with a bar at the end that catches a hook on the floor of the ambulance; this takes much of the weight off the stretcher while the EMS crew loads it into the ambulance.
2. A stretcher is loaded onto a hydraulic ramp and lifted into the ambulance.
3. A stretcher from which the weight is once again taken at the head of the stretcher by the back of the ambulance; while the crew pushes the stretcher the legs collapse and the stretcher is pushed easily into position.

All of the easy-load stretchers reduce the physical manual handling for the EMS crew.

Other advantages of modern easy-load stretchers are

1. Hydraulic foot pump or battery-operated system to raise the stretcher to different height levels: reduced manual handling for EMS crew.
2. Many optional extras that include IV poles and hooks for carrying EMS bags.

Splinting Stretchers Some splinting devices also double up as stretchers for carrying patients, such as the spinal board, orthopedic stretcher, and vacuum mattress.

Rescue Stretchers There are many kinds of rescue stretchers used by EMS systems that offer a helicopter/flight service and mountain/cliff and coastal rescue service. Each of these kinds of stretchers has its benefits for the particular area of use and all have the ability to carry a lying down patient. Some of them include:

1. Basket-type stretchers: some are able to be floated on water, towed behind a vehicle over rough terrain, or towed behind a snowmobile.
2. Neil Robertson stretchers®: rescue stretcher that is suited for heights and helicopter rescue.
3. Paraguard stretcher™: used for search and rescue operations, building collapse, or confined spaces.

Patient Comfort and Disposable Hygiene Equipment

In addition to EMS patient lifting devices, equipment should be used to make the patient more comfortable.

Blankets

Blankets can be used to keep a patient warm and comfortable and can be also used to preserve a patient's modesty during procedures that require exposure. Light or heavy blankets can be used depending on environment. Disposable or reusable blankets are also available.

Sheets and Pillows

Standard reusable sheets can be used on stretcher mattresses for hygiene and patient comfort and are a useful device for making it easier to transfer a patient from an ambulance trolley to a hospital trolley. Disposable stretcher sheets are also available.

Incontinence sheets can be used where there is a possibility of soilage from the patient. Some EMS systems may require incontinence pads for patients for longer journeys.

Pillows are often used to make the journey for the patient more comfortable; disposable or reusable pillowcases can be used in conjunction with the pillows. When choosing a pillow, EMS systems should choose one that can be wiped clean and disinfected. Pillows can also be used for supporting or padding an injured limb.

Table 19-15 is a suggested list of patient handling equipment.

Table 19–15	Suggested Patient Lifting and Patient Comfort Equipment	
Basic		**Optional**
Carry chair		Splinting stretchers
Carry sheet		Rescue stretchers
Ambulance trolley		
Blankets		
Pillows		
Drinking water		
Emesis bowls		
Urinal bowls/bottles		
Incontinence pads		
Stretcher covers		

SUMMARY

There is a wide variety of equipment available to assist the EMS provider in the provision of patient care. The requirements of individual EMS systems differ depending on patient characteristics and staff training. There is no "one size fits all" approach—the choice of equipment for each individual EMS and vehicle requires consideration of factors specific to the regional health system, geography, surrounding health-care institutions, finance, training of health professionals, and caseload.

It has not been possible to discuss all available equipment within the confines of this chapter, but the equipment discussed provides a starting point for EMS teams to consider optimal equipment for their particular circumstances.

It should be remembered that equipment alone does not lead to improved outcomes. The choice of equipment and the integration of new equipment should only occur as part of a comprehensive patient care package, including training.

CHAPTER 20

Financing of EMS Systems and Cost-Effectiveness

Gerard O'Reilly

KEY POINTS

- The major sources of funding for EMS are government and private insurance/subscription.

- Most developed nations have a centralized, government administered, predominantly publicly funded EMS.

- In many countries, volunteers provide the core functions of EMS.

- Most nations have no formalized EMS system.

- First-aid and BLS training can augment the effectiveness of an underdeveloped EMS, at minimal cost.

A formal EMS is accessible to less than half of the global population.[1] As nations have developed economically and politically, the demand for a high quality and equitable EMS has increased. Similarly, in developed nations, as the standards and capacity of EMS systems increase, the financial support by which such advances can be sustained in an equitable fashion continues to be scrutinized.

This chapter aims to provide an overview of EMS financing, considering the relative costs for various components and levels of EMS and the various methods used to finance these resources.

Furthermore, some consideration will be given to the cost-effectiveness and sustainability of various approaches to EMS financing.

OVERVIEW

This chapter necessarily builds upon the framework used in Chapter 4 to describe the structures of different national EMS systems. Each domain or element of the EMS structure — administration; resources; processes — will be considered under the new heading of *Costs*. Having broadly identified the element of cost, the chapter will examine the current *approaches* to funding, using examples, and consider the cost-effectiveness and sustainability of different approaches. This second, and larger, part of the chapter is titled *Financing*. The matter of EMS financing can be considered through the subheadings of administrator; source; and distribution.

As noted in Chapter 4, the characteristics of different nations, when viewed from the perspective of *Costs* and *Financing*, can vary enormously. Again, while it would be unwise to attempt to consider EMS financing in every nation — and every community of every nation — some broad determinants of costs and financing can again be listed as follows:

LEVEL OF NATIONAL DEVELOPMENT

1. Developed.
2. Developing.
3. Least developed.

FACTORS *WITHIN* LEVEL OF NATIONAL DEVELOPMENT

1. Sociopolitical framework.
2. Health system priorities.
3. Geography.

As noted in Chapter 4, for many nations the approach to EMS financing may broadly match and can be predicted by the characteristics of other domains of EMS structure, namely *Authority* and *Agency*.

EMS FINANCING

Ideally, EMS financing, and therefore EMS system development, depends upon and is planned according to the perceived (or measured) cost-effectiveness of EMS. Historically, however, such analyses are complex, and the pattern of EMS development and financing has been founded in the absence of a guiding evidence-base.[2] Moreover, there is a paucity of literature that addresses the cost and economic value of prehospital care.[3,4] It is more likely to be in retrospect that the cost-effectiveness of an EMS system is considered.

Measuring effectiveness is dependent upon the perspective of the observer and defined objectives. Objectives, in turn, will vary according to who defines them: the "community" (including patient and family) versus the EMS staff; the Ministry of Health versus the Ministry of Finance; the private EMS company versus the volunteer brigade. Furthermore, measuring effectiveness of a single item or intervention (paramedic; helicopter; dispatch center; operational procedure; triage model) against a whole-of-nation system objective is notoriously difficult. Cost, on the surface at least, *might* more easily be estimated.

COSTS

For each of the elements of EMS structure described in Chapter 4, there are corresponding costs. While it would be impractical to determine the contemporary real costs of all EMS systems in dollars and cents, the following section revisits the main "sources" of cost in an EMS system and broadly considers the relative financial burden of these items.

Administration

Managing a system can be costly. For an EMS system to be efficient and effective, the following administrative components are necessary:

1. Operational director.
2. Management team, including senior advisors on policy and operations.
3. Clinical director.
4. Clinical team, guiding standards and providing oversight.
5. Ancillary staff (e.g., human resources, secretarial staff).
6. Administrative center.

The level of responsibility and oversight of this managerial team will be determined by its jurisdiction. While the big-ticket transport and communication items of an EMS system (listed below) will incur the bulk of the start-up and intermittent costs, senior salaried staff in a workable facility will contribute to considerable recurrent costs.

Resources

Operational resources are the visible costs (and obstacles) of an embryonic EMS system. The components can be classified into hardware and human resources.

Equipment

EMS Transport   Within the range of potential EMS transport utilized in any EMS system, there are extremes in cost (Figure 20-1).

In many developing countries, EMS transport is largely inaccessible if it exists at all. The most basic EMS "system" is provided as a transport operation only (see Chapter 4). In many communities of India, for example, most patients arrive at the hospital by private transport or taxi. Similarly, in Ghana, most injured people who make it to a hospital are transported by taxis and minibuses

In a more formalized EMS system, there exists, at the very least, patient transport vehicles. Four-wheeled

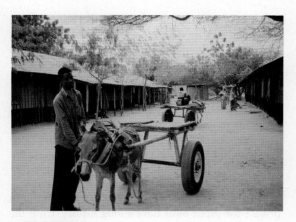

FIGURE 20–1

There is a wide range of EMS transport, with extreme differences in cost. For example, a donkey cart is used at a hospital in Kenya.

patient transport vans, the core vehicle of most EMS systems, are expensive.

Motorcycles are considerably cheaper but need to be accompanied by an EMT rather than a "driver" to be of any value, as they arrive in advance of a patient transport vehicle.

As EMS transport becomes equipped to provide ALS, the expense increases considerably; monitors, defibrillators, and ventilators, if present, will incur the greatest cost. The cheapest of stretchers, on the other hand, may still be functional. Unique EMS transport capabilities may increase costs considerably; armored ambulances, for example, are not unusual in Israel (see **Chapter 4** Structures of Different National EMS Systems).

Helicopters and fixed-wing aircraft clearly provide rapid patient access and transport but are purchased at great expense. De Wing and coworkers described a seven- to eight-fold increase in charges for helicopter transport compared to ground transport.[5] Only developed nations have sustainable, nationwide access to these vehicles. Austria, Germany, and Australia report a proportion of air ambulance use of greater than 30%.[6]

In addition to purchase, the ongoing maintenance of such vehicles, particularly to ensure the safety of aircraft, continues to incur a high price. It is not unusual to find discarded road ambulances in developing nations unable to keep abreast of vehicle maintenance costs.

Communications   Communication systems vary across EMS systems. Basic communication systems utilize radio and/or mobile phones. In developed nations, central dispatch requires a much more costly communication system, combined with computer-based algorithms and transport-tracking devices to enable timely and prioritized dispatch.

Consumables   Most medications and fluids used as part of EMS protocols are relatively inexpensive and consumables largely include gloves, syringes, suction apparatus, intravenous cannulas, and tubing, oxygen masks, dressings, and occasionally endotracheal tubes. While providing a recurrent cost, such consumables have a relatively low cost impact when compared with ALS-functional EMS transport.

Human Resources

Staffing   The cost of staffing on EMS transport will depend upon the level of development of EMS and the operational model, that is, Anglo-American versus Franco-German (see Chapter 4).

Of course, as EMS staffing level ranges from driver, to EMT-BLS, to EMT-ALS, to mobile intensive care ambulance paramedic, to physician, so do the costs increase. From this perspective, in isolation, the Franco-German model of staffing EMS with physicians would be expected to be more costly than the paramedic-staffed Anglo-American model.

A developed EMS system demands coverage 24–7, and unsociable shift work magnifies the of late hours.

It makes sense that where *volunteers* can provide a comparable standard and coverage of EMS, costs will be much less (see Finance: Human Resources).

Education   As the level of EMT expertise increases, so does the level of education needed. This is at a relatively smaller incremental cost.

Processes

The EMS approach to triage and dispatch is also a determinant of EMS cost. Integrated EMS systems (such as the trauma system illustrated in Chapter 4) will bypass the closest hospital in order to deliver patients to the nearest appropriate urban center. Such systems are reliant on rapid, medium-distance transport such as helicopter, which is inherently expensive.[7-9]

The different approaches to EMS delivery may have some impact on costs for EMS. The "scoop and run" approach would be more likely to shift costs to the receiving hospital than the "stay and play" approach, where time and resources are deployed more in the prehospital arena (see Chapter 4).

Triage-decision support systems resulting in limited dispatch and/or more efficient dispatch would be expected to reduce costs. France and the Netherlands utilize such aggressive triage in their EMS systems (see Distribution, below).

FINANCE

The components of EMS financing can be classified under the headings of Administrator; Source; Distribution. The following sections will provide examples of current practices and options.

Administrator

In general, in developed nations, the funding model of EMS in each country or region matches the national or state-based approach to EMS authority and provision. That is, EMS will be financed either publicly through a government body (national, state, municipal), privately through companies (either by insurance/subscription or fee-for-service), or a mix of both.

In turn, as described in Chapter 4, the government or company will either administer EMS directly, through a government agency or outsource EMS through another agency (e.g., Red Cross, St John Ambulance, S.O.S, private EMS organization). Examples of EMS fund-administration models in developed nations are provided below.

Most Australian states fund government-administered emergency service transport. Non-emergency transports are often managed differently, through private companies. That is, a public agency provides salaried paramedics and is funded primarily by the state government. Additional funding is also provided through direct patient billing, private subscriptions, and insurance agencies such as accident compensation bodies. In Western Australia and the Northern Territory, however, the service provider (St John Ambulance) is contracted to the state government. Similarly, in Canada, the province or territory provides funding; but the extent of coverage is more variable across jurisdictions.

In the UK, the Trusts of the NHS fund government-based agencies, or in some cases, contract private companies. In Poland, the government-based EMS agency is the local hospital. Similarly, in France, EMS is predominantly government-funded through the hospital-based EMS agency (SMUR).

In Norway, EMS is again funded by the government, but commonly outsourced, often to transportation companies operating a variety of types of service. In Iceland, EMS is predominantly government-funded but there is a small charge to the individual as a "deterrent" fee.

In the Netherlands, the government funds EMS but contracts private companies to provide the agency. Interestingly, Dutch law forbids EMS systems to earn any profit; any surplus revenue is required to be directed to additional improvements to the system, including training, equipment, and vehicles.[10]

Across a number of other developed nations, the approach to EMS funding is not uniform.

In Italy, the level of EMS provision is driven in large measure by what the community can afford.

In the US, ambulance services operating on a private-for-profit basis have a long history. Until the early 1970s, one of the most common providers of EMS in the US was a community's local funeral home. Over decades, many EMS companies merged and there remain several large enterprises that continue to operate either on a fee-for-service basis to the patient or by means of contracts with local municipalities. Alternatively, some EMS systems in the US are operated and funded directly by the municipality they service.[10]

Few developing countries have managed to reach a point where the majority of EMS funds are held and managed publicly at government level. In those communities where a formalized EMS exists, funding is managed by private insurance or payment schemes. Examples of this approach are common in some regions of India, where there is a "gross discrepancy seen in prehospital services "between paying and nonpaying patients"[11] Community financing, including through loan funds, have been used in some African contexts, especially for emergency obstetric transport.[12]

Source

The source of funds to allow *private* access to EMS is relatively clear: the individual. Individuals pay either via a private insurance scheme, membership with a private EMS company, or they are billed directly (or indirectly through family) upon the utilization of a private EMS company.

The source of funds to allow for government-subsidized or government-paid EMS depends upon *public* funds. "Universal" health care exists, to a variable extent, in the socialized health systems of numerous developed nations, including the U.K, France, Sweden, the Netherlands, Australia, New Zealand, and Canada. Methods by which the government accrues public funds can vary. Commonly, a proportion of income tax is directed to public health care, and this will often include EMS. Other "tax" or "levy" options have been used, and even in those countries with so-called universal health care, EMS may be privately subsidized through a copayment. In Australian states, for example, to avoid the cost of utilizing an ambulance, the user is required to pay a small annual subscription.

In developed nations, the steady development of a structured trauma system over recent decades has allowed trauma funding to similarly be streamlined in some settings. For comprehensive trauma care in Australia, for example, road users' vehicle registration is pooled to fund a no-fault comprehensive health insurance. Other sources for EMS funding have included property tax. In Canada, the degree to which EMS utilization is subsidized by provincial health insurance (up to 100%) varies by province and may be supplemented by either partial fee-for-service or from the property tax revenues of local municipalities operating such services.

Another funding source is donation. In Taiwan, EMS is provided by both governmental and privately supported services. The main funder of public EMS is taxation, but other important sources are the donations from Taoist and Buddhist temples. In turn, ambulances and equipment bear the names and logos of donating temples or charities.[13]

The greatest perceived obstacle to the establishment of EMS in many developing countries is funding. This was a major consideration for the WHO publication[14] that focused on the "most promising interventions and components of pre-hospital trauma care systems, particularly those that require minimal training and relatively little in the way of equipment or supplies...regardless of the level of resources available." The key premise guiding financial considerations according to Sasser and colleagues is that access to a potentially life- or limb-saving service should not be restricted only to those who pay for it. Nevertheless, reasonable efforts to recover costs will ensure the financial viability of EMS.[14]

Regarding emergency care–based projects in developing countries, Doney and coworkers noted "EMS development" as having one of the most difficult paths to obtaining funding.[15] It makes sense that innovative EMS financing options need to be considered for developing nations, where in the absence of surplus funds, there is an increased imperative to prioritize cost-effective EMS interventions and financing alike. Funding, using trauma care as the example, might be sourced from highway construction budgets; vehicle registration; traffic fines; and fuel tax.[14]

In India, the country with the greatest burden of injury, Fitzgerald and associates have widely advocated a compulsory vehicle registration–based tax to fund no-fault, comprehensive trauma care (including EMS).[16,17]

Distribution of Funds

EMS Transport

A key component and cost of an EMS system is transport. However, most low-income countries, including many regions in Africa and South Asia, have minimal access to EMS transport. Again, innovative methods for the provision of EMS transport in these low resource settings is a global imperative.

EMS transport initiatives in the least-resourced settings are illustrative of the global EMS resource disparity. In Tanzania, where maternal mortality rates are high, the communities developed a variety of transport systems, including canoe, tricycle, and ox-cart.[18]

Mock and coworkers demonstrated how a low-cost six-hour basic training course for commercial (taxi and bus) drivers in Ghana led to considerable improvements in the provision of first aid. The authors concluded that in the *absence* of formalized EMS transport, improvements in prehospital care are possible by building on existing, informal patterns of prehospital transport.[19]

An alternative approach was reported by Marson and Thomson in Brazil, where a *new* EMS system (including ambulances) was started along a major, crash-prone, highway, with a resulting decreased mortality rate.[20] Hauswald and Yeoh offered a sobering contrast by calculating the potential cost-effectiveness of instituting a formal EMS along high-income country models in Kuala Lumpur, Malaysia. They estimated a cost of $2.5 million per annum (in 1997), with a saving of seven additional lives.[21]

Studies in settings with an existing basic EMS (Mexico, Trinidad) have demonstrated, using mortality as the outcome, the cost-effectiveness of widespread BLS training (as compared to more costly ALS training).[22,23] Some authors question whether the more costly prehospital ALS provides *any* benefit to injured patients in terms of either mortality or morbidity.[24]

At the very least, it would appear that widespread first-aid training for non-EMTs and BLS training for existing EMTs are cost-effective methods for financing an improved EMS in low-resource settings. In the mined rural areas of Kurdistan and Cambodia, both approaches were utilized. A two-tier program provided first-aid training to lay first responders and BLS to existing EMTs (without ambulances). Mortality from landmine injuries decreased from 40% to 9%.[25]

Human Resources

In the majority of countries, there is no formalized EMS. Since most emergencies start at home, any system to promote the early recognition of emergency conditions should be based in the community. In Mexico, the training of mothers and first-level health care workers led to care being sought more rapidly with a significant reduction in child mortality.[26] In fact, many of the benefits of prehospital emergency care could be realized with minimal cost by teaching community volunteers simple but vital interventions.[27]

For the same number of staff in some countries, there will be dramatically less cost if the EMTs provide a voluntary workforce. While many developing nations are dependent upon a predominantly volunteer-based EMS, examples in developed nations are less common. Commonly, volunteers (e.g., St John Ambulance, Red Cross) have a minimal role in the core EMS system.

In New Zealand, St John Ambulance provides the majority of EMS, and the rural EMS staff is largely volunteer-based. In South Africa, in addition to the paid responders, the government system is supplemented in many areas by unpaid volunteers (South African Red Cross and St John Ambulance). In Italy, volunteer organizations, including the Italian Red Cross, are the primary EMS providers. In the US, outside of large cities and in many colleges and universities, EMS is often provided by volunteers. In fact, without the presence of dedicated volunteers, many small communities in the US, might be without local EMS systems.

Magen David Adom, which provides EMS in Israel, is staffed by approximately 90% volunteers, many of them foreign-born (Table 20-1).[28]

Another common approach to cost-saving and efficiency for EMS is cross-training. Rather than being provided by stand-alone organizations, the EMS may be operated by the local fire or police service. This is particularly common in rural areas, where maintaining a separate service may not be as cost-effective. In the US, for example, the EMS system may be integrated into the operations of another municipal emergency service, such as the local fire and police departments. In the case of full integration, the EMS staff may be fully cross-trained to perform the entry-level function of the other emergency services.

A novel method of improving EMS delivery in Minnesota, US, involved financial incentives. Whyte and Ansley found that financial motivation improved targeted quality measures in a rural EMS.[29] The sustainability of such an approach is questionable.

Table 20–1	Role of Volunteers in EMS Financing in Selection of Developed Systems		
Nation	**Government**	**Volunteers**	**Private**
UK	✓		
Australia	✓		
Canada	✓		
France	✓		
Hong Kong	✓		
Israel		✓✓	
Italy		✓	✓
Netherlands	✓		
New Zealand		✓	
US		✓	✓

Major funding sources.

As noted in the above section regarding EMS transport, BLS training can be a very cost-effective method of improving EMS delivery in under-resourced systems. There are a number of short courses available for this purpose; Primary Trauma Care (PTC), for example, can be provided at no formal cost to the trainee.[12]

Processes

Different models of triage and dispatch can be employed to minimize costs. Equity and efficiency need to be balanced in order to ensure that all patients needing EMS receive it rapidly and effectively, at the least cost.

As mentioned previously, the French philosophy for medical emergencies allows the reanimation units to be dispatched only in life-threatening cases. Because of aggressive triage, as few as 65% of requests for ambulance service may actually receive an ambulance response.[30]

Similarly, in the Netherlands, the call is triaged using computed decision support, and in approximately 40% of cases there is no ambulance response.[10]

In other contexts, the approach to reduce *unnecessary* patient transport, with an implied impact on efficiency, has been a transport payment. Ting and colleagues (Brisbane, Australia) concluded that abolishing direct patient cost (in 2004) stimulated "inappropriate" ambulance use.[31] Similarly, a study on transport cost in Japan concluded that the introduction of a user charge for EMS may improve system efficiency.[32]

In addition to augmenting the training of EMTs, Mexico established an increased number of ambulance stations, reducing response times and contributing to a mortality decrease (from 8.2% to 4.7%). There was a 16% increase in the EMS budget, but this proved to be sustainable within the local economy.[33]

In Malawi, motorcycle ambulances placed at rural health centers were found to be a more effective method of reducing referral delay for obstetric emergencies when compared with ambulance cars at the district hospital. Operating costs were also reduced.[34]

In addition to effective EMS transport, timely dispatch requires an effective communication system. At a basic level, this need not be expensive. In Sierra Leone, equipping traditional birth attendants with radios linked to local hospitals reduced maternal deaths.[35] The global development of a cellular mobile phone infrastructure has increased exponentially over the last decade; this clearly improves the access of isolated communities to EMS at relatively low cost.[12]

SUMMARY

Globally, EMS financing is critical to sustaining equitable access to effective emergency care. In the majority of countries, the costs of accessing the available elements of an EMS system appear prohibitive. In these contexts, acute illness or injury "forces individuals and families to choose between risking financial ruin because of medical expenses or risking death or lifelong disability attributable to a lack of medical care."[36] In the absence of an equitable funding approach to EMS provision, both outcomes of such a choice may have a catastrophic long-term impact.

At the basic level, efforts to improve emergency care need not lead to increased costs.[12] Nevertheless, sustainable EMS development beyond a community-based response requires significant political and financial investment. In almost all developed nations, EMS financing and health care funding in general have progressed *toward* a centrally administered and funded model. For the majority of countries where there is no formalized EMS system, the ultimate goal would be to initiate sustainable public financing of an efficient EMS.

Finally, key components to ensuring a cost-effective and sustainable EMS are stakeholder participation and integration into the wider health system, including public health and hospital-based emergency care. EMS development needs to be linked with general societal expectations, and effective prehospital resuscitation must be matched with similar standards of care across the chain of survival pathway.

References

1. Mock C, ed. International approaches to trauma care. *Trauma Quart* 14(3): 191, 1999.
2. Dixon S. What will be the costs of a quality emergency service? *J R Soc Med* 94(S39); 54, 2001.
3. Lerner EB, Maio RF, Garrison HG et al. Economic value of out-of-hospital emergency care: a structured literature review. *Ann Emerg Med* 47: 515, 2006.
4. Lerner EB, Nichol G, Spaite DW, et al. A comprehensive framework for determining the cost of an Emergency Medical Services system. *Ann Emerg Med* 49: 304, 2007.
5. De Wing MD, Curry I, Stephenson, E, et al. Cost-effective use of helicopters for the transportation of patients with burn injuries. *J Burn Care Rehabil* 21: 535, 2000.
6. Roudsari BS, Nathens, AB, Arreola-Risa C, et al. Emergency Medical Service (EMS) systems in developed and developing countries. *Injury* 38: 1001, 2007.
7. Harrington DT, Connolly M, Biffl WL, et al. Transfer times to definitive care facilities are too long. A consequence of an immature trauma system. *Ann Surg* 241(6): 961, 2006.
8. Moyer P, Ornato J, Brady W, et al. Development of systems of care for ST-elevation myocardial infarction patients: the emergency medical services and emergency department perspective. *Circulation* 116(2): e42, 2007.
9. Acker JE, Pancioli AM, Crocco T, et al. Implementation strategies for emergency medical services within stroke systems of care: a policy statement from the American Heart Association/American Stroke Association expert panel on emergency medical services systems and the Stroke Council. *Stroke* 38(11): 3097, 2007.
10. The CIA World Fact Book, https://www.cia.gov/library/publications/the-world-factbook/index.html (accessed & verified March 2010)
11. Joshipura MK. Trauma care in India: current scenario. *World J Surg* 32: 1613, 2008.
12. Kobusingye OC, Hyder AA, Bishai D, et al. Emergency medical systems in low- and middle-income countries: recommendations for action. *Bull World Health Organ* 83: 626, 2005.
13. Chiang W-C, Ko PC, Wang HC. EMS in Taiwan: past, present and future. *Resuscitation* 80: 9, 2009.
14. Sasser S, Varghese M, Kelleram A, Lormand JD. Prehospital Trauma Care Systems. Geneva, World Health Organization, 2005.
15. Doney MK, Smith J, Kapur B. Funding emergency medicine development in low- and middle-income countries. *Emerg Med Clin North Am* 23: 45, 2005.
16. Fitzgerald M, O'Reilly G, McKenna C. Emergency Medical Assistance. Kerala State Transport Project – Road Safety Action Plan. Vic Roads International; 2005.
17. Fitzgerald M, Dewan Y, O'Reilly MJ, McKenna C. India and the management of road crashes:

Towards a national trauma system. *Ind J Surg* 68(4): 237, 2006.

18. Schmid T, Kanenda O, Ahluwalia I, et al. Transportation for maternal emergencies in Tanzania: empowering communities through participatory problem solving. *Am J Public Health* 91(10): 1589, 2001.

19. Mock CN, Tiska M, Adu-Ampofo M, et al. Improvements in pre-hospital trauma care in an African country with no formal Emergency Medical Services. *J Trauma* 53: 90, 2002.

20. Marson A, Thomson J. The influence of prehospital trauma care on traffic accident mortality. *J Trauma* 50: 917, 2001.

21. Hauswald M, Yeoh E. Designing a prehospital system for a developing country: estimated costs and benefits. *Am J Emerg Med* 15: 600, 1997.

22. Arreola-Risa C, Mock C, Herrera-Escamilla A, et al. Cost-effectiveness and benefits of alternatives to improve training for pre-hospital trauma care in Mexico. *Prehospital Disaster Med* 19: 318-325, 2004.

23. Ali J, Adam RU, Gana TJ, Williams JI. *J Trauma*. 1997 Jun;42(6):1018-21;discussion 1021

24. Liberman M, Roudsari BS. Prehospital trauma care; what do we really know? *Curr Opin Crit Care* 13(6): 691, 2007.

25. Husum H, Gilbert M, Wisborg T, et al. Rural prehospital trauma systems improve trauma outcome in low-income countries: a prospective study from North Iraq and Cambodia. *J Trauma* 54: 1188, 2003.

26. Guiscafre H, Martinez H, Palafox M, et al. The impact of a clinical training unit on integrated child health care in Mexico. *Bull World Health Organ* 79: 434, 2001.

27. Vargehese M. Technologies, therapies, emotions and empiricism in prehospital care. In: Mohan D, Tiwari G, eds. Injury Prevention and Control. London & New York: Taylor and Francis, 249-264; 2000.

28. MDA Training website. At www.mdais.org; accessed December 2009. http://translate.google.com/translate?hl=en&sl=iw&tl=en&u=http%3A%2F%2Fwww.mdais.org%2F (verified March 2010)

29. Whyte B, Ansley R. Pay for performance improves rural EMS quality: investment in prehospital care. *Prehosp Emerg Care* 12: 495, 2008.

30. National SAMU website, at www.samu-de-france.fr/en, accessed December 2009. http://www.samu-de france.fr/en/System_of_Emergency_in_France_MG_0607 (updated & verified March 2010)

31. Tin JY, Chang AM. Path analysis modeling indicates free transport increases ambulance use for minor indications. *Prehosp Emerg Care* 10: 476, 2006.

32. Ohshige K, Kawakami C, Kubota K. A contingent valuation study of the appropriate user price for ambulance service. *Acad Emerg Med* 12: 932, 2005.

33. Arreola-Risa C, Mock C, Vega F, et al. Evaluating trauma care capabilities in Mexico with the World Health Organization's Guidelines for Essential Trauma Care. *Pan Am J Public Health* 19: 94, 2006.

34. Hofman JJ, Dzimadzi, Lungu K, et al. Motorcycle ambulances for referral of obstetric emergencies in rural Malawi: do they reduce delay and what do they cost? *Int J Gynaecol Obstet* 102: 191, 2008.

35. Samai O, Sengeh P. Facilitating emergency obstetric care through transportation and communication, Bo, Sierra Leone. *Int J Gynaecol Obstet* 59(S2): 157, 1997.

36. Razzak JA, Kellerman A. Emergency medical care in developing countries: is it worthwhile? *Bull World Health Organ* 80: 900, 2002.

Part 3

Protocols and Procedures

CHAPTER 21

EMS Clinical Care Protocols

Douglas F. Kupas

KEY LEARNING POINTS

- EMS clinical care protocols allow standardization of care across different EMS units within larger EMS systems.
- EMS protocols need to be carefully designed to have some flexibility to allow for unusual situations that may be faced by EMS personnel.
- All "levels" of EMS personnel should have input into the formulation and the review and updating of EMS protocols.

Many EMS systems use protocols as a means of formalizing the expected care that the system's EMS personnel provide the individual patients of the system. Depending upon regulatory requirements and system preferences, EMS protocols span a continuum from mandated requirements that may not be exceeded to general guidelines that may be altered by EMS providers for each individual patient. EMS protocols can take many structures, covering:

- Large EMS systems (country, state, province, or region) OR small EMS agencies with few personnel and transporting resources.
- Comprehensive patient illnesses and EMS situations OR focused on a few common patient complaints.
- All patient ages and subpopulations OR focused on a small subset of the patient population.
- All levels of EMS providers within a system OR applying only to a subset of providers.

- All aspects of patient triage, treatment, and transport OR isolated to a single segment of patient care.

No matter how the protocols are structured, physician oversight of the process of protocol development and quality improvement review for appropriateness of protocol use is essential. Simply, EMS protocols can be viewed as the preapproved specific physician order or orders for treatment provided by EMS personnel.

Protocols are more likely to be used to standardize and guide the care provided by nonphysician EMS personnel and are more likely to be used for nonphysician EMS personnel who provide advanced level skills (e.g., paramedics), but they can be also beneficial in standardizing care in EMS systems that use physicians as out-of-hospital EMS providers.

This chapter will provide an overview of EMS protocols, including advantages and disadvantages to care by protocol, considerations when developing protocols, examples of protocol use, and resources for EMS protocols.

DEFINITIONS

Standing Orders versus EMS Protocols

Standing orders generally refer to written orders for specific medical conditions that define the treatments that may be provided by EMS personnel without any additional contact or consultation with a physician. These orders may be written by a specific patient's physician and tailored for that patient, for example, transport orders written before an interfacility transport, or standing orders may be prewritten by physicians providing general oversight for an EMS system and covering general patient conditions and situations that are expected to be encountered by the service's EMS personnel. EMS protocols may include standing orders, but protocols are conceptually broader and may also include additional resources like educational information, options, and performance measures. EMS protocols are a form of off-line medical control. (See Chapter 1 for additional definitions.)

Bypass

The situation where EMS personnel do not take the patient to the closest medical facility but instead to a medical facility farther away either because of the relative care capabilities of the facilities or the request by a facility that it not be brought any new patients (usually due to overcrowding).

Off-Line Medical Control

These are the components of medical supervision and administration of an EMS organization or system that do not involve the direct management of care for a patient. This would include clinical care protocol development, standing orders, review of written reports of care provided, and required Continuing Medical Education. Off-line medical control includes prospective elements (relevant legislation, policy and procedure manuals, protocol development, and research) and retrospective elements (review of ambulance transport reports, statistical reviews, education conferences, and counseling "feedback" sessions by management personnel for the patient-care EMS personnel).

On-Line Medical Control

The direct (either in-person or by electronic communication such as telephone or radio) supervision and direction of medical care in the prehospital or out-of-hospital environment. Usually this would be a physician supervising or directing EMTs. This term could also be considered synonymous with "on-line medical direction."

Outpatient

A patient who receives medical care but does not stay overnight for further care or evaluation in a medical facility.

Protocols

The overall steps in patient care that are to be undertaken at every patient encounter, or the sequence of prehospital care measures that prehospital personnel are allowed to perform when they are unable to contact their on-line medical control or direction. Protocols may encompass Standing Orders but additionally present recommendations for further care to be carried out after the Standing Orders are completed for a particular patient.

Standing Orders

The established list of prehospital care measures or items that prehospital personnel may perform prior to contact with their on-line medical control or direction. Standing Orders often constitute part of EMS protocols.

ADVANTAGES OF EMS PROTOCOL USE

The institution of EMS protocols leads to several potential benefits. These include standardization of care, evidence-based care, and improved disaster preparedness.

Standardization

The Institute of Medicine Reports on Emergency Care, Emergency Medical Services, and Emergency Care for Children all recommended increased regionalization of care. Successful regionalization of care requires that care be standardized and uniform over the geographic area involved in the "region."

Standardization of care has obvious advantages in reducing medical errors related to unnecessary variation in the health-care system and allows easier analysis and review of care provided.

Standardized EMS protocols are more easily linked to benchmarks or performance measures for quality improvement. This allows EMS systems to compare care across various EMS systems and in conjunction with receiving hospitals that interact with several EMS services.

In some countries and regions, it is not unusual for an EMS provider to either work or volunteer for several EMS agencies within a geographic region. Uniformity in care among services within a geographic region also has benefits when EMS personnel work with several different EMS agencies or services.

Standardizing protocols in large systems, like states or provinces, has the added benefit of providing uniformity with EMS provider scope of practice, education and continuing education programs, procedural skill credentialing, and medication/equipment lists.

Evidence-Based

There is increasing interest in assuring that EMS protocols are based upon the best scientific evidence related not only to emergency medical patient care but also specific to out-of-hospital emergency patient care when that evidence exists. Although scientifically rigorous evidence does not specifically exist for much of the care provided by EMS personnel, when evidence is lacking, EMS protocols should be developed using the consensus of medical experts with expertise spanning the breadth of EMS care. When international or national guidelines are available (such as those promulgated for cardiac care by the American Heart Association and the European Resuscitation Council), these are important resources for EMS protocol development.

A truly evidence-based process for protocol development is a huge undertaking. The process of the International Liaison Committee on Resuscitation that is used to develop the guidelines that update the recommendations for CPR and cardiac resuscitation care is an example of the tremendous amount of effort that is required to develop evidence-based consensus guidelines that cover even a small portion of the patients encountered by EMS.

An example of an advanced attempt to provide evidence-based EMS protocols is the process used by the Canadian province of Nova Scotia. The Nova Scotia EMS protocols are developed with a structured,

evidence-based process that includes defined levels of evidence, classes of recommendation, and references to the scientific evidence used within each protocol. These Canadian Prehospital Evidence Based Protocols are done in conjunction with the Nova Scotia Emergency Health Services and Dalhousie University, and they can be found at http://emergency.medicine.dal.ca/ehsprotocols/protocols/toc.cfm.

Disaster Preparedness

The threat of terrorism and recent natural disasters has led to the need to prepare for and at times mobilize medical teams from broad geographic areas to provide specific medical care in affected areas. When EMS providers from outside of an affected area arrive in different teams, there are advantages to these "outside" teams following similar protocols.

When considering terrorism-related mass casualty events, there are predictable threats that are rare outside of these specific terrorism-related events. If multiple unrelated EMS agencies from a region respond to care for victims of these specific terrorism related threats, the use of identical treatment protocols will improve the ability of these EMS agencies to work in concert while providing similar care. Examples of these specific situations include cyanide and nerve agent exposure, radiation exposure, and blast injury.

In considering more typical mass casualty incidents such as a transportation accidents (e.g., bus or train crash), when EMS services from multiple municipalities follow similar mass casualty protocols for triage, operations, use of air medical transport services, and destination protocols, this can bring order and efficiency to the response. In contrast, if multiple responding agencies follow many differing protocols, this can lead to chaos and of course poor patient care.

Additionally, when a natural disaster requires that EMS resources from outside of the geographic area respond in groups, many of these groups are formed from EMS providers from multiple agencies that are expected to work together as a team at the disaster location. Following the same protocols makes the responding groups more uniform in their equipment, patient care, and patient transport.

DISADVANTAGES TO EMS PROTOCOLS

Some may argue that standardizing care creates a "cookie cutter" approach to treating patients that does not consider the variations in patients' clinical presentations or treatment needs. Others challenge whether the specific steps within an EMS protocol are the "ceiling" or the "floor" as related to the expected care rendered by an EMS system. Another frequently cited fear of protocolized care is that EMS providers will not learn to use their own judgment or think for themselves but instead will provide "cookbook" type care without developing the skills to recognize which patients require deviations from the protocol.

All of these potential disadvantages can be overcome with an approach to protocol use that encourages the development and use of judgment while taking advantage of a standardized approach that minimizes unwarranted variation. Treatment protocols that minimize unwarranted variation are increasingly recognized as valuable—even for high-end in-hospital surgical procedures such as coronary artery bypass and angioplasty — and improved standardization of EMS care would likely have similar benefits to patient outcome.

EMS PROTOCOL ORGANIZATION

EMS protocols in different countries are organized in many differing formats. One of the most controversial decisions in system protocol development is establishing consensus on the format or template that will be used for each protocol. Individuals responsible for developing EMS system protocols would be wise to begin with a consensus process that uses broad-based input to establish the protocol template early in the process. The aesthetics and style that a set of protocols takes is secondary to choosing a template that is embraced by those who will use the protocols.

Generally, protocols fall into one of two categories: (1) those that follow an algorithmic design with decision points that lead to separate branches of differing patient care, and (2) those that follow a stepwise narrative format. Systems that use more general protocol titles, such as "Tachycardia," may find the algorithmic approach more useful, while systems that use a larger number of specific protocols may find success with the narrative format.

EMS protocols are often separated into those related to pediatric care and those related to adult care, while other systems cover the pediatric and adult differences in care within the same protocol. The state of Maryland in the US includes adult and pediatric protocols together within each protocol, but uses a "Teddy Bear" symbol to draw attention to pediatric treatments or medication doses (see the web site list at the end of this chapter).

Each system must also determine how to differentiate between pediatric and adult patients. Ages chosen for this differentiation vary, and different systems have chosen an age as low as 8 and as high as 18 for this distinction. There are some physiologic and logistic benefits to considering a patient who is 14 years of age or below for pediatric care within protocols. For those patients whose age cannot be directly determined by EMS, using the presence of secondary sexual characteristics (axillary hair in boys and developing breasts in girls) is a good indication of puberty and potentially an indication to then use adult treatment protocols.

One consideration related to the discussion of pediatric versus adult protocols is that of medication dosing. With wide variations in even adult body weights in today's societies, protocol developers should consider the use of weight-based rather than fixed drug dosages when appropriate, even for adults.

Protocols are also frequently organized by the level of the EMS provider. Some systems provide mandated protocols for basic level providers such as basic EMTs while providing more latitude to advanced level providers (such as paramedics or physicians) or agencies, while other systems use the opposite. Many systems use protocols for all levels of providers. In these instances, the system must determine whether to separate the protocols (for example, separate BLS and ALS protocols) or whether to cover all levels of provider within a protocol, distinguishing parts that apply to each provider by using a color code or some other symbol. Examples of this include the North Carolina (US) protocols that use color to distinguish the treatments provided by each level of provider.

Additionally, EMS systems that use protocols need to determine their scope. Protocols can be limited to covering medical conditions and their applicable treatments or can include sections that standardize performance steps for procedures (for example, chest needle decompression or intraosseous access), operational aspects of patient care (for example, triage and bypass for individuals who require a level of care that is higher than that provided by the closest hospital), or administrative issues (for example, infection control procedures). See Table 21-1 for examples of possible EMS protocol topics.

Systems must determine whether protocols are true protocols that mandate a certain expected care or represent guidelines that set "best practice" with options for liberal variation at the agency or individual EMS provider level.

Most importantly, there must be a general understanding of when an EMS provider must consult

Table 21–1 | List of Possible Protocol Topics

EMS systems can structure individual protocols to cover the general or specific topics listed below. These are examples. Some protocols cover topics that are not listed here, and most do not cover all of these topics

1. Resuscitation

Cardiac Arrest
Cardiac Arrest: Asystole
Cardiac Arrest: Hypothermia
Cardiac Arrest: Pulseless Electrical Activity
Cardiac Arrest: Trauma
Cardiac Arrest: Ventricular Fibrillation/Pulseless Ventricular Tachycardia
Termination of Resuscitation
Dead on Arrival (DOA)
Do Not Resuscitate (DNR)
Newborn/Neonatal Resuscitation
Postresuscitation Care

2. Cardiovascular

Bradycardia
Chest Pain
    Suspected Acute Coronary Syndrome/Cardiac Chest Pain
        ST-Elevation Myocardial Infarction (STEMI)
Congestive Heart Failure/Pulmonary Edema
Tachycardia
Narrow Complex Tachycardia
Supraventricular Tachycardia
Atrial Fibrillation
Wide-Complex Tachycardia
Ventricular Tachycardia
Ventricular Ectopy (included for completion but not an evidence-based topic)

3. Respiratory

Airway
Airway: Failed
Airway Obstruction
Airway: Paralytic (Rapid Sequence Induction)
Airway: Sedation-Assisted (Nonparalytic)
Confirmation of Endotracheal Tube/Advanced Airway Placement
Respiratory Distress
    Asthma/Reactive Airway Disease
COPD
Croup
Suspected Pneumonia

4. Obstetrics/Gynecology

Gynecologic Emergencies
Newly Born/Newborn Care

Obstetric Emergencies
Childbirth/Labor/Delivery
    Postpartum Hemorrhage
Vaginal Bleeding
    First Trimester Vaginal Bleeding
    Third Trimester Vaginal Bleeding

5. Behavioral/Poisoning/Exposure

Behavioral
Agitated/Violent Behavior
Patient Restraint
Poisoning/Toxic Exposure
Exposure: Airway Irritants
Exposure: Biological/Infectious
Exposure: Blistering Agents
Exposure: Chemicals to Eye
Exposure: Cyanide
Exposure: Inhalation
    Carbon Monoxide Poisoning
    Smoke Inhalation
Exposure: Nerve Agents
Exposure: Radiologic Agents
Exposure: Riot Control Agents
Overdose: Ingestion/Injection/Drugs of Abuse

6. Medical

Abdominal Pain
Allergic Reaction/Anaphylaxis
Altered Mental Status
Diabetic Emergency
Hypoglycemia
Hyperglycemia
Back Pain (Nontrauma)
Diarrhea
Epistaxis
Fever
Hypertension (included but may not be evidence-based)
Hypotension/Shock (Nontrauma)
Influenza-like Illness/Upper Respiratory Infection
Nausea/Vomiting
Seizure
Eclampsia
Seriously Ill–Appearing Patient
Steroid-dependent Patient
Stroke/TIA
Syncope

(continued)

Table 21–1 | **List of Possible Protocol Topics** *(Continued)*

7. Trauma

Amputation
Bleeding/Hemorrhage Control
Crush Syndrome
Electrical Injuries
Extremity Trauma
Eye Trauma
Explosive/Blast Injury
Head Trauma
Impaled Object
Multisystem Trauma/Traumatic Shock
Spinal Cord Trauma
Tooth Avulsion/Fracture/Dental Injury

8. Environmental

Altitude Sickness
Aquatic Emergencies
Diving Injury
Dysbarism
Near Drowning
Bites and Envenomations
    Insect or Spider Envenomation
    Snakebite
    Wild Mammal Bite
Burns
Cold Exposure
Frostbite/Cold Injury
Hypothermia
Hyperthermia
Heat Exhaustion
Heat Stroke

9. Operations

Air Medical Transport Indications
Cancellation of Response/No Patient Found
Refusal of Treatment/Transport
Triage to Specialty Facility
STEMI Triage Scheme
Stroke Triage Scheme
Postcardiac Arrest Triage Scheme
Trauma Triage Scheme

10. Patient Assessment

Abuse and Neglect
Child Abuse
Domestic Violence
Elder Abuse
Body Substance Isolation/Infection Control
Cardiac Monitoring
    12-Lead ECG Use
Pain Control
Respiratory Monitoring
    Capnography
    Co-oximetry/Carbon Dioxide Monitoring
    Pulse Oximetry Use
Universal Patient Care/Initial Patient Contact

11. Procedures

Alternative/Rescue Airway Use
Cardioversion
Defibrillation
Synchronized Cardioversion
Chest Needle Decompression
Confirmation of Airway Placement
Cricothyrotomy
Endotracheal Intubation
Intraosseous Access
Intravenous Access
Personal Protective Equipment (PPE) Use
Spinal Immobilization

12. Special Circumstances/Considerations

Crime Scene Preservation
Individualized Patient Protocol (Some systems
    permit EMS providers to recognize individu-
    alized protocols that are written for a specific
    patient. In these instances, the patient may
    carry the protocol and any specific personal
    medication that may be administered by EMS
    personnel. This may be helpful for patients
    with rare illnesses that require a specific,
    time-sensitive treatment.)
Indwelling Devices
Device Malfunction
On-Scene Physician
Interfacility Transport Protocols

with a higher level provider (for example, an on-line physician) to exceed or vary from the standing orders within a protocol. Some protocols specifically list when on-line medical direction must occur, and other systems permit variation or deviation from a protocol by an EMS provider as long as the variation is justified in the patient care report or other documentation. Variations from protocol can be used as triggers for automatic quality improvement or peer review of a specific case.

EMS PROTOCOL SECTIONS

EMS protocols differ in the sections that they contain, but there are general themes to these sections:

Title

Each protocol within a set of EMS protocols has a name or title, and these can vary significantly. For example, some protocols use general individual titles such as "Respiratory Distress," while others may be more specific with separate protocols for "Asthma," "Congestive Heart Failure," "Chronic Obstructive Pulmonary Disease," and "Croup." Table 21-1 provides examples of common illness-related protocols that include both generalized and specific possibilities for protocol titles.

Inclusion Criteria

While many protocols ignore this concept, some include more specific information related to patient inclusion or entry criteria that are to be used to identify patients to whom the protocol applies. For example, a generic chest pain protocol could lead to inappropriate care if it is used by a novice provider to administer nitroglycerin to a 20-year-old with pleuritic chest pain. In contrast, entry criteria that identify specific indications for the use of a "Suspected Acute Coronary Syndrome" protocol that includes more specific symptoms and age criteria may lead to better application of the protocol. It could be argued that this is micromanaging the protocol process and that the education of the EMS provider is responsible for teaching the provider to use good judgment in determining which protocol to follow.

Exclusion Criteria

These criteria are related to the entry or inclusion criteria, but alternatively, they suggest specific symptoms or patient criteria that should exclude the use of the protocol. In the chest pain example, young age or pleuritic quality to chest pain could be used to exclude care that includes providing nitroglycerin to a patient with chest pain.

System Requirements

Some protocols only apply to certain EMS providers or services that have specialized equipment or education that is necessary to safely provide certain care. An example of this would be special requirements for additional monitoring equipment or personnel if doing a procedure such as rapid sequence induction or sedation-facilitated endotracheal intubation. Protocols can also be used to remind EMS providers of the level of personal protective equipment (PPE) that should be used when dealing with situations like toxic or infectious substances.

Treatments

This section of protocols generally describes the allowable treatment(s) for the medical condition covered by the protocol. It is critical that all protocol users understand that appropriate use of the protocol requires good judgment, and no treatment should be given if there is any concern that it may not be appropriate for the specific patient. The treatment section generally is organized in either a stepwise, sequential narrative flow or an algorithmic flow with decision branch points as discussed in the preceding section on protocol organization.

Possible On-Line Treatment Orders

Some protocols include only care that is provided by standing orders, while other protocols include care that may be provided by EMS personnel beyond the point of on-line consultation in the event that there is communication failure that prohibits on-line consultation. Additionally, some protocols include treatments that may only be done after on-line consultation with a physician, but these treatments are still included in the protocol to educate the EMS providers about potential orders so that they can anticipate them.

Footnotes

It is difficult to cover the many nuances of patient care while keeping a sequential narrative or algorithmic protocol streamlined enough for easy use; therefore many protocols use footnotes to provide clinical pearls or other specific information related to steps within the protocol that address important points or considerations based upon patient variations.

Performance Measures

A few systems include performance measures or quality improvement parameters within their protocols.

By including these benchmarks, EMS providers are educated in the system expectation for best practices. These performance measures also serve as a resource to small systems and novice quality improvement officers to assist them in determining important parameters for quality improvement reviews. In the US, the state of North Carolina has embedded performance parameters into protocols by highlighting these points with the color red within their protocols, and as another example, the state of Pennsylvania adds a separate section of "Performance Parameters" to each protocol.

Appendix 21-1 at the end of this chapter presents an example BLS protocol from the (US) state of Pennsylvania regarding body substance isolation considerations.

SUMMARY

In many EMS systems, the use of EMS protocols that define the expected treatment(s) for common patient presentations leads to standardization of care, with a decrease in unwarranted variability. When the same EMS protocols are used by larger geographically associated EMS agencies (for example, national, statewide, or province-wide), the economies of scale permit the protocols to be more evidence-based and more easily updated across all agencies. In addition to directing expected patient treatments, protocols can be used to integrate with scopes of practice, medication lists, procedural credentialing, and quality improvement initiatives. Some examples of US state protocols can be found on the web links listed in Table 21-2.

Table 21–2	Examples of State EMS Protocols Web Sites from Various States Within the US
Arkansas	www.healthyarkansas.com/ems/bls_protocols.pdf
Iowa	www.idph.state.ia.us/ems/protocols
New Hampshire	www.nh.gov, http://www.nh.gov/safety/divisions/fstems/ems/advlifesup/patientcare.html
New Jersey	www.state.nj.us/health/ems (then click regulations tab)
New York	www.health.state.ny.us/nysdoh/ems/protocolsnew.htm
North Carolina	www.ncems.org, http://www.ncdhhs.gov/dhsr/EMS/trauma/guidelines.html
Maine	http://www.maine.gov/dps/ems/legal.html
Maryland	www.miemss.org/home/default.aspx?tabid=106
Massachusetts	www.mass.gov/dph/oems
Pennsylvania	www.health.state.pa.us/ems,http://www.portal.state.pa.us/portal/server.pt/community/emergency_medical_services/14138
Vermont	www.vermontems.org, http://healthvermont.gov/hc/ems/protocol.aspx

Web links verified and updated March 2010.

Example of a Protocol for Body Substance Isolation Guidelines

Pennsylvania Department of Health Operations 103 - BLS–Adult/Peds Effective 09/01/2004 103-

INFECTION CONTROL/ BODY SUBSTANCE ISOLATION GUIDELINES

Criteria

A. These guidelines should be used whenever contact with patient body substances is anticipated and/or when cleaning areas or equipment contaminated with blood or other body fluids.

B. Your patients may have communicable diseases without you knowing it; therefore, these guidelines should be followed for care of all patients.

System Requirements:

A. These guidelines provide general information related to body substance isolation and the use of universal precautions. These guidelines are not designed to supersede an ambulance service's infection control policy [as required by EMS Act regulation 28 § 1005.10 (l)], but this general information may augment the service's policy.

B. These guidelines do not comprehensively cover all possible situations, and EMS practitioner judgment should be used when the ambulance service's infection control policy does not provide specific direction.

Procedure:

A. **All patients:**

1. Wear gloves on all calls where contact with blood or body fluid (including wound drainage, urine, vomit, feces, diarrhea, saliva, nasal discharge) is anticipated or when handling items or equipment that may be contaminated with blood or other body fluids.

2. Wash your hands often and after every call. Wash hands even after using gloves.
   a. Use hot water with soap and wash for 15 seconds before rinsing and drying.
   b. If water is not available, use alcohol or a hand-cleaning germicide.

3. Keep all open cuts and abrasions covered with adhesive bandages that repel liquids (e.g., cover with commercial occlusive dressings or medical gloves).

4. Use goggles or glasses when spraying or splashing of body fluids is possible (e.g., spitting or arterial bleed). As soon as possible, the EMS practitioner should wash face, neck, and any other body surfaces exposed or potentially exposed to splashed body fluids.

5. Use pocket masks with filters/one-way valves or bag-valve masks when ventilating a patient.

6. If an EMS practitioner has an exposure to blood or body fluids,[1] the practitioner must follow the service's infection control policy and the incident must be immediately reported to the service infection control officer as required. EMS practitioners who have

had an exposure[2] should be evaluated as soon as possible, since antiviral prophylactic treatment that decreases the chance of HIV infection must be initiated within hours to be most effective. In most cases, it is best to be evaluated at a medical facility, preferably the facility that treated the patient (donor of the blood or body fluids), as soon as possible after the exposure.

7. Preventing exposure to respiratory diseases.
   a. Respiratory precautions should be used when caring for any patient with a known or suspected infectious disease that is transmitted by respiratory droplets (e.g., tuberculosis, influenza, or SARS).
   b. HEPA mask (N-95 or better), gowns, goggles, and gloves should be worn during patient contact.
   c. A mask should be placed upon the patient if his/her respiratory condition permits.
   d. Notify receiving facility of patient's condition so appropriate isolation room can be prepared.

8. Thoroughly clean and disinfect equipment after each use following service guidelines that are consistent with Centers for Disease Control recommendations.

9. Place all disposable equipment and contaminated trash in a clearly marked plastic red Biohazard bag and dispose of appropriately.
   a. Contaminated uniforms and clothing should be removed, placed in an appropriately marked red Biohazard bag, and laundered/decontaminated.
   b. All needles and sharps must be disposed of in a sharps receptacle unit and disposed of appropriately.

Notes:

1. At-risk exposure is defined as "a percutaneous injury (e.g., needle stick or cut with a sharp object) or contact of mucous membrane or nonintact skin (e.g., exposed skin that is chapped, abraded, or afflicted with dermatitis) with blood, tissue, or other body fluids that are potentially infectious." Other "potentially" infectious materials (risk of transmission is unknown) are CSF (cerebrospinal fluid), synovial, pleural, peritoneal, pericardial, and amniotic fluid, semen, and vaginal secretions. Feces, nasal secretions, saliva, sputum, sweat, tears, urine, and vomitus are not considered potentially infectious unless they contain blood.

From: Pennsylvania Department of Health Operations 103 - BLS – Adult/Peds Effective 09/01/04 103-2 of 2

CHAPTER 22

Airway Management

*Kenneth H. Butler, Benjamin J. Lawner,
Daniel L. Lemkin*

It can be difficult to detect poor respiratory effort and inadequate ventilation. For thorough respiratory evaluation, unclothe the patient's chest and observe the rate, pattern, and depth of breathing; note the use of accessory muscles; detect abnormal sounds; and identify signs of injury. Prehospital care providers should understand the concepts and procedural techniques of airway management that are described in this chapter.

The three fundamentals of airway management are (1) to ensure a patient airway, (2) to provide supplemental oxygen, and (3) to institute positive-pressure ventilation when spontaneous breathing is inadequate or absent.

OPENING THE AIRWAY: MANUAL MANEUVERS

Upper airway obstruction most commonly occurs when a patient is unconscious or sedated. Under such conditions, the upper airway musculature relaxes, and the tongue falls backward and obstructs the larynx. Basic emergency positioning maneuvers of the head, neck, and jaw or insertion of a nasal or an oral pharyngeal airway will provide patency of the upper airway. Experienced personnel may perform the triple airway maneuver (mouth opening, head extension, and jaw-thrust) in patients without suspected cervical spine injury.

In basic airway management, two positioning maneuvers improve airflow: head-tilt/chin-lift and jaw-thrust.

Head-Tilt/Chin-Lift

Purpose

To open the airway by displacing the obstructing tongue anteriorly and opening the laryngeal inlet.

Patient Selection

Head-tilt/chin-lift is the primary airway opening maneuver if cervical spine (c-spine) injury is not a concern.

Technique

Use two hands to extend the patient's neck and open the airway. While one hand applies downward pressure to the patient's forehead, the tips of the index and middle finger of the second hand lift the mandible at the mentum, which lifts the tongue from the posterior pharynx (Figure 22-1). Lifting the mandible moves the tongue anteriorly and opens the airway. When lifting, apply pressure to the bony prominence of the mandible and not to the soft tissue, so as to not to increase the obstruction being caused by the tongue. Lift the chin cephalad and toward the ceiling and open the airway.

Jaw-Thrust

Purpose

The jaw-thrust maneuver moves the tongue anteriorly with the mandible, decreasing airway obstruction. The jaw-thrust may be all that is required in a

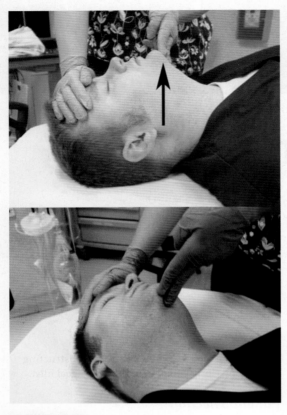

FIGURE 22-1

Head-tilt/chin-lift maneuver. Lifting the mandible opens the airway by lifting the tongue. Photos courtesy of Jim Burger, www.burgerphoto.com.

patient who has an upper airway foreign body or one who has lost consciousness.

Patient Selection

The jaw-thrust maneuver is preferred for unresponsive patients with inadequate or absent breathing in whom c-spine injury is a concern. It can be performed with a cervical collar in place.

Risks and Precautions

Do not allow the patient's mouth to close. **The mouth must remain open so air can move in and out.**

Most airway maneuvers are associated with some movement of the c-spine. Regardless of the maneuver chosen, stabilize the c-spine in order to minimize head and neck movement in any patient with a possible c-spine injury. **Failure to stabilize the neck is associated with a 7- to 10-fold increase in spinal cord**

injury.[1] If sufficient personnel are present, use manual in-line stabilization rather than cervical collars or spinal immobilization devices to stabilize the c-spine during initial assessment and prior to transport. Cervical collars can interfere with airway maneuvers and can even cause increased intracranial pressure (ICP) from partial obstruction of jugular venous outflow. During basic airway management, collars may be removed provided that manual in-line stabilization is maintained continuously. If the collar is left in place, open or remove the front half to permit basic airway management. Spinal immobilization devices, however, are necessary during transport.

Technique

With the patient supine and the clinician standing at the head of the bed, place the heels of both hands on the parieto-occipital areas on each side of the patient's head, then grasp the angles of the mandible with the index and long fingers and displace the jaw anteriorly. **The jaw thrust is the safest first approach to opening the airway of a patient with a suspected neck injury** because, properly performed, it does not result in neck extension.

If the patient has fallen to the ground, kneel above his or her head and use the following sequence to open the airway:

- Determine if the victim has partial or complete airway obstruction. If the patient can cough or speak, allow him or her to attempt to clear the obstruction naturally. Stand by, reassure the victim, and be ready to clear the airway.
- If a cough is not successful, use your finger to quickly sweep the victim's mouth clear of any foreign objects, broken teeth, dentures, or sand.
- Using the jaw-thrust method, grasp the angles of the victim's lower jaw and lift with both hands, one on each side, moving the jaw forward (toward the ceiling in a patient lying supine) (Figure 22-2). For stability, rest your elbows on the surface on which the victim is lying. If the lips are closed, gently open the lower lip with your thumb.
- *Look* for the chest to rise and fall. *Listen* for air escaping during exhalation. *Feel* for the flow of air on your cheek.

Triple Airway Maneuver

In patients without suspected c-spine injury, the three components of head-tilt, chin-lift, and jaw-thrust can be combined to open the airway (Figure 22-3).

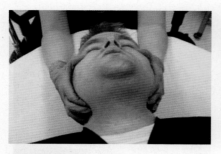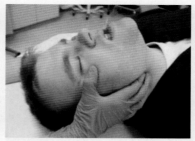

FIGURE 22-2

Jaw-thrust maneuver. By moving the jaw forward (upward in a supine patient), the tongue is lifted to open the airway. Photos courtesy of Jim Burger, www.burger photo.com.

ARTIFICIAL AIRWAYS

After the airway has been opened, many patients require an artificial airway to facilitate spontaneous breathing or bag-valve mask ventilation. It must be emphasized that neither device is a substitute for a definitive airway.

Purpose

Artificial airways keep the oral and pharyngeal airways open by displacing the tongue inferiorly and keeping it from falling back and obstructing the airway. They provide a conduit for air to travel into the airway.

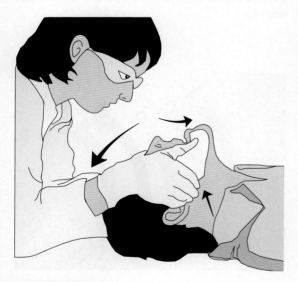

FIGURE 22-3

Triple airway maneuver. From Publitek, Inc., Waukesha, Wisconsin.

Patient Selection

An artificial airway is required in an obtunded or semiconscious patient. The nasal airway is less likely to induce vomiting in those with an intact gag reflex.

Oral Pharyngeal Airway (OPA)

The OPA is a curved, firm, hollow tube with a rectangular aperture that is used to maintain a conduit between the mouth and the glottis and to prevent obstruction by the patient's tongue and other soft tissue. OPAs have a flange that, when properly inserted, rests against the patient's lips to prevent inadvertent slippage into the mouth. This flange does not interfere with the formation of a good seal from a face mask. A line between the posterior angles of the mandible approximates the plane of the posterior oropharynx. **Therefore, a rough method for choosing the correct OPA size is to hold the airway beside the patient's mandible, orienting it with the flange at the patient's mouth and the tip directed toward the angle of the mandible** (Figure 22-4A, B). The tip of an appropriately sized device should just reach the angle of the patient's mandible.

Technique

An OPA is inserted by either of the following procedures, based on individual preference:

1. Insert the airway upside down along the patient's hard palate (Figure 22-4). When the airway is in the patient's mouth, rotate it 180 degrees and advance it fully into the hypopharynx.
2. Open the mouth fully, using a tongue blade to displace the tongue. Insert the OPA right side up, into the correct position. No rotation is needed.

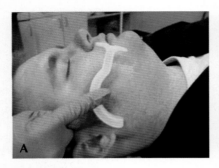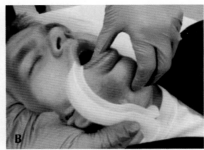

FIGURE 22–4

A, Method for approximating proper size of an oral pharyngeal airway. See text.
B, Insertion of oral airway. Photos courtesy of Jim Burger, www.burgerphoto.com.

Complications

- Pushing the tongue posteriorly worsens airway obstruction.
- Using a device of the wrong size.
  - A device that is too small is ineffective and can be lost in the oropharynx, possibly causing obstruction.
  - A device that is too large can press against the epiglottis and obstruct the larynx.
- Catching the tongue or lips (usually the lower lip) between the airway and the teeth injures the soft tissue.
- Using the device in a patient with intact airway reflexes might induce vomiting. If protective reflexes return, the OPA must be removed.

Nasopharyngeal Airway (NPA)

The NPA or nasal trumpet (Figure 22-5) is a soft rubber or plastic hollow tube that is passed through the nose into the posterior pharynx. Patients tolerate NPAs more easily than OPAs, so NPAs can be used when the use of an OPA is difficult, such as when the patient's jaw is clenched or the patient is semiconscious and cannot tolerate an OPA.

Nasopharyngeal airways are sized based on internal diameter. The larger the internal diameter of the airway, the longer the tube. A length of 8.0 to 9.0 cm is used for large adults, 7.0 to 8.0 cm for medium adults, and 6.0 to 7.0 cm for small adults. Selecting NPAs based on length rather than diameter improves accuracy.

A rough method for choosing the correct NPA size is to hold the airway beside the patient's mandible, orienting it with the flared end at the tip of the patient's nose and the distal tip directed toward the angle of the mandible. The tip of an appropriately sized NPA should just reach the angle of the patient's mandible.

Technique

First coat the NPA with water-soluble lubricant or anesthetic jelly. Contact time is insufficient for anesthetic jelly to make insertion more comfortable, but the anesthetic property of the jelly may improve tolerance of the device after it is placed. Gently insert the device along the floor of the nostril, perpendicular to the patient's face, in the direction of the occiput (not cephalad) and into the posterior pharynx behind the tongue. Note that the floor of the naris inclines in a caudal orientation by approximately 15 degrees. Advance the NPA fully until the flared proximal tip is at the nasal orifice. If resistance is encountered, rotate the tube slightly or attempt the insertion via the other nostril.

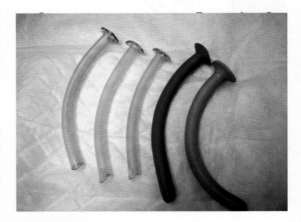

FIGURE 22–5

Nasal pharyngeal airway (nasal trumpet). Photo courtesy of UNC Training Center, Jennifer Stoeppler & Barbara Steckler, instructors.

Precautions

- Nasal or facial fractures.
- Using an airway that is too long may cause the tip to enter the esophagus, increasing gastric distention and decreasing ventilation during rescue efforts.
- Injury to the nasal mucosa causes bleeding in 30% of insertions and can lead to aspiration of blood or clots.

BAG-VALVE MASK VENTILATION

Bag-valve mask (BVM) ventilation is the most important technique in emergency airway management. This basic procedure allows oxygenation and ventilation of patients until a more definitive airway can be established and when endotracheal intubation or other definitive control of the airway is not possible.

Successful BVM ventilation depends on three conditions: a patent airway, an adequate mask seal, and proper ventilation (i.e., proper volume, rate, and rhythm). Preplacement of an oral and nasal airway aids with ventilation by relieving physiologic obstruction and opening the hypopharynx.

Patient Selection

BVM ventilation is appropriate for patients who are hypoxic and unable to breathe on their own.

Risks and Precautions

Vomiting and aspiration are risks, but providing oxygenation and ventilation is always the first priority. Bag-mask ventilation is more difficult in men with beards, patients with body mass index >26 kg/m^2, patients who do not have teeth, and in those older than 55 years of age.[2] A tight seal on a bearded man can usually be attained by applying a liberal amount of lubricant on the mask. The only relative contraindication to BVM ventilation is in patients with deforming facial trauma in whom a tight seal is impossible to attain.

Equipment

Masks come in adult sizes of small, medium, and large. Choosing the appropriate size helps to create a good seal and therefore aids in delivering effective ventilation. Bags for BVM ventilation also come in different types. Newer bags are equipped with a pressure valve. Some bags have one-way expiratory valves to prevent the entry of room air. One-way expiratory valves allow delivery of more than 90% oxygen to ventilated and

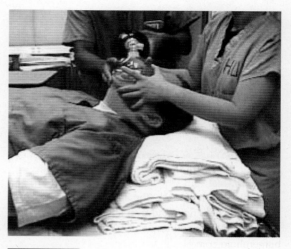

In preparation for bag-valve mask ventilation, use towels to raise the patient's head so that the external auditory canal of the ear aligns with the sternal notch. Photo courtesy of Jim Burger, www.burgerphoto.com.

spontaneously breathing patients. **Bags without a one-way expiratory valve deliver a high concentration of oxygen during positive-pressure ventilation but only 30% oxygen during spontaneous breaths.**[3]

Positioning

Place towels under the patient's head to position the ear level with the sternal notch (Figure 22-6). This opens the pharyngeal and laryngeal axes, providing optimal patency of the upper airway.

Technique

If there is no contraindication, place two nasal trumpets before performing BVM ventilation to keep the tongue from obstructing the airflow.

Once the airway is open, the next step is to correctly position the mask on the patient's face (Figure 22-7). Detach the bag from the mask prior to positioning it. Do not let a large, heavy bag pull on one end of the mask and displace it from the proper position. Spread the nasal portion of the mask slightly and place it on the bridge of the patient's nose. Then place the body of the mask onto the patient's face, covering the nose and mouth. **The three facial landmarks that must be covered by the mask are the bridge of the nose, the two malar eminences, and the mandibular alveolar ridge.** Do not put any pressure on the patient's eyes. Neither the provider's wrists nor the mask cushion should rest on the patient's eyes during

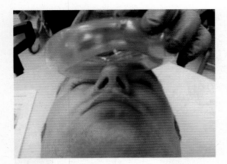

FIGURE 22–7

Initial placement of mask. The apex should cover the bridge of the nose and then fall down to cover the mouth. Photo courtesy of Jim Burger, www. burgerphoto.com.

bag-mask ventilation because this can cause a vagal response or damage to the eyes.

There are two methods for holding the mask in place: the *single-hand* (one-hand/one-person) hold and the *two-hand* (two-hand/two-person) hold. The two-hand hold is most effective but it requires a second clinician, so it is important to be comfortable with both techniques. When ventilation with a one-hand/one-person technique is unsuccessful, despite oral and nasal airway placement, use a two-hand/two-person technique.

The procedure for the single rescuer using a one-hand technique is described below:

1. Open the airway.
   a. Perform the head-tilt/chin-lift maneuver or the jaw-thrust. In patients with suspected cervical spine injury, do not tilt the head; rather, perform a jaw-thrust maneuver.
2. Position the mask.
   a. Place the mask on the patient's face before attaching the bag.
   b. Cover the nose and the mouth with the mask without extending it over the chin.
   c. Change the size of the mask, as appropriate, to create a good seal.
   d. Hold the mask in place using the one-hand C-E technique (described as follows) (Figure 22-8).
      1. Use the nondominant hand.
      2. Create a C-shape with the thumb and index finger over the top of the mask and apply gentle downward pressure.
      3. Hook the remaining fingers around the mandible and lift it upward toward the mask, creating the E.

e. The procedure for the two-hand technique is described below:
   1. If a second person is available to provide ventilation by compressing the bag, a two-hand technique can be used.
   2. Create two opposing semicircles with the thumb and index finger of each hand to form a ring around the mask connector, and hold the mask on the patient's face. Then lift the mandible with the remaining digits.
   3. Alternatively, place both thumbs opposing the mask connector, using the thenar eminences to hold the mask on the patient's face while lifting the mandible with the other fingers (Figure 22-9).
   4. No matter which technique is being used, avoid applying pressure on the soft tissues of the neck and on the eyes.

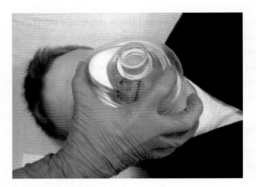

FIGURE 22–8

The one-hand E-C technique done in preparation for bag-valve mask ventilation. Photo courtesy of Jim Burger, www.burgerphoto.com.

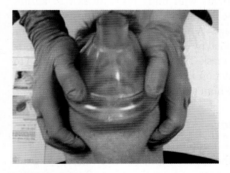

FIGURE 22–9

One option for the two-hand technique: use the thenar eminences to hold the mask on the patient's face with the thumbs while lifting the mandible with the fingers. Photo courtesy of Jim Burger, www.burgerphoto.com.

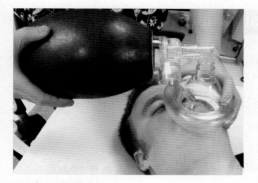

FIGURE 22-10

One-handed technique used for ventilation. Photo courtesy of Jim Burger, www.burgerphoto.com.

5. Place the web space of the thumb and index finger against the mask connector.
6. Push downward with gentle pressure.
7. Wrap the remaining fingers around the mandible and lift it upward.
3. Ventilate the patient (Figure 22-10).

Attach the bag-valve mask device to a supplemental O$_2$ source at a rate of 15 L/min to avoid hypoxia. Determine the effectiveness of ventilation and oxygenation by chest rise, breath sounds, pulse oximetry reading, and CO$_2$ monitoring, if available.

- For an adult of average size, provide a volume of 6 to 7 mL/kg per breath (approximately 500 mL).
- For a patient with a perfusing cardiac rhythm, ventilate at a rate of 10 to 12 breaths/min.

Ventilation Volumes, Rates, and Rhythm. After the airway is open and a good mask seal has been established, connect the bag to the mask and ventilate the patient. Use a volume just large enough to cause chest rise (no more than 8 to 10 cc/kg). During cardiopulmonary resuscitation (CPR), even smaller tidal volumes are adequate (5 to 6 cc/kg) owing to the patient's reduced cardiac output. **The ventilatory rate should not exceed 10 to 12 breaths per minute.** These important concepts are based on multiple randomized controlled studies in animals and observational studies in humans. The studies showed that the use of larger tidal volumes and higher ventilation rates increase intrathoracic pressures and decrease coronary and cerebral perfusion pressures.[4]

Complications. Three critical errors should be avoided:

- Giving excessive tidal volumes.
- Forcing air too quickly.
- Ventilating too rapidly.

Cricoid Pressure

There is little evidence to support the widely held belief that the application of cricoid pressure reduces the incidence of aspiration during rapid-sequence intubation (RSI).[5] Overly aggressive cricoid pressure can cause tracheal compression and prevent ventilation or require higher bag pressures. Cricoid pressure does not reliably protect against regurgitation in situations of poor mask ventilation and gastric distention.[6,7] Properly performed mask ventilation is the best way to prevent regurgitation by using low volumes delivered with low pressure and slow insufflation times.

ENDOTRACHEAL INTUBATION AND RAPID-SEQUENCE INTUBATION (RSI)

Endotracheal intubation is the most reliable means of ensuring a patent airway, providing oxygenation and ventilation and preventing aspiration. This procedure should be performed only by trained personnel with continuous experience.[8] **RSI is the administration of a potent *induction agent* (sedative or anesthetic) followed by a rapidly acting *neuromuscular blocking agent* (paralytic) to induce unconsciousness and motor paralysis to facilitate tracheal intubation.** Maintain oxygenation throughout the intubation process. Proper placement of an endotracheal tube provides oxygen to the patient and allows mechanical ventilation. Paralytics produce apnea and dampen the respiratory drive. Even patients with a Glasgow Coma Scale score of less than 3 have airway reactivity (gag and cough reflexes). Intubation without RSI is associated with more complications such as failed intubation, aspiration, airway trauma, hypoxia, and esophageal intubation compared with intubation with RSI.[9,10] Thus, RSI is the gold standard for emergency intubation.

Patient Selection

The indications for prehospital endotracheal intubation are correction of hypoxia or hypoventilation when bag-mask ventilation or supraglottic devices (e.g., a laryngeal mask airway [LMA]) fail. Paramedic expertise in intubation is associated with a robust training program and frequent clinical experience with endotracheal intubation.[11]

The decision to intubate is sometimes difficult to make and requires clinical experience to recognize signs of impending respiratory failure. Patients who

Table 22–1	**Indications for Endotracheal Intubation**

- Failure to maintain airway patency
  - Swelling of upper airway, as in anaphylaxis or infection
  - Facial or neck trauma with oropharyngeal bleeding or hematoma
  - Decreased consciousness and loss of airway reflexes
  - Failure to protect airway against aspiration; decreased consciousness that leads to regurgitation of vomit, secretions, or blood

- Failure to ventilate (i.e., deliver air to the lungs/alveoli)
  - Result of failure to maintain and protect airway
  - Prolonged respiratory effort that results in fatigue or failure, as in status asthmaticus or severe COPD
  - Chest wall trauma

- Failure to oxygenate (i.e., transport oxygen to pulmonary capillary blood)
  - Result of failure to maintain and protect airway or failure to ventilate
  - Diffuse pulmonary edema
  - Acute respiratory distress syndrome
  - Large pneumonia or air-space disease

- Anticipated clinical course or deterioration (e.g., need for situation control, tests, procedures)
  - Uncooperative trauma patient with life-threatening injuries who needs painful procedure (e.g., insertion of chest tube)
  - Stab wound to neck with expanding hematoma
  - Septic shock with high minute ventilation and poor peripheral perfusion
  - Intracranial hemorrhage with altered mental status and need for close blood pressure control
  - Hemorrhagic shock*
  - Cardiogenic shock*

*In these shock states, even though the patient may be able to breathe on his/her own, decreasing the work of breathing and the oxygen demand will improve the outcome of resuscitation.
COPD = Chronic Obstructive Pulmonary Disease.
Based on Lafferty DA, Kulkarni R. Tracheal intubation, rapid sequence intubation. Available at http://medicine.medscape.com/article/80222-overview. Accessed on December 28, 2009.

require intubation have at least one of the following indications (Table 22-1):

1. Inability to maintain airway patency or protect the airway against aspiration.
2. Inability to ventilate because of thoracic or respiratory compromise.
3. Failure to oxygenate.
4. Anticipation of a deteriorating course that will eventually lead to the inability to maintain airway patency or protection, ventilate, or oxygenate.

The fourth indication is most often the most difficult to predict. Astute clinical practice is required to recognize the subtle signs of early respiratory failure.

Endotracheal intubation of a patient who is completely unconscious does not require pretreatment, induction, or paralysis.

Risks and Precautions

Improper placement of the tube into the esophagus will result in hypoxia or hypercarbia. There is no clinically reliable substitute for direct visualization of the tube passing through the vocal cords. Hence, the adage, "*When in doubt, take it out.*"

Absolute and relative contraindications to endotracheal intubation are listed in Table 22-2.

Equipment

To prepare for a clean intubation, use the **S-O-A-P ME** mnemonic:

- **Suction device:** Rigid Yankauer suction tube attached to vacuum, with the tip placed under the right side of the stretcher.

Table 22–2	**Contraindications to Endotracheal Intubation**

- Absolute
  - Total upper airway obstruction, which requires a surgical airway
  - Total loss of facial landmarks, which requires a surgical airway

- Relative
  - Anticipated "difficult" airway, in which endotracheal intubation may be unsuccessful, resulting in reliance on successful BVM ventilation to keep an unconscious patient alive. In this scenario, techniques for awake intubation and difficult airway adjuncts can be used
  - The "crash" airway, in which the patient is in an arrest situation—unconscious and apneic. In this scenario, no time is available for preoxygenation, pretreatment, or induction and paralysis. BVM ventilation, intubation, or both should be performed immediately without medication

Based on Lafferty DA, Kulkarni R. Tracheal intubation, rapid sequence intubation. Available at http://medicine. medscape.com/article/80222-overview. Accessed on December 28, 2009.

- **Oxygen:** Ambu bag and mask attached to high-flow oxygen source (15 L/minute).
- **Airway Equipment (Rule of 2s).**
  - Two nasal airways.
  - Laryngoscope with two blades—a MacIntosh and a Miller (confirm that light source is working prior to intubation).
  - Endotracheal (ET) tubes, two sizes: 8.0 and 7.0, with stylet preloaded.
  - Syringe, 10 mL (to inflate tube cuff).
- **Pharmacologic Agents.**
  - Intravenous access.
  - Induction agents and paralytic agents.
- **Monitoring Equipment.**
  - Pulse oximeter.
  - Blood pressure cuff with gauge.
  - Cardiac monitor.
  - Carbon dioxide detector or end-tidal CO_2 monitor.

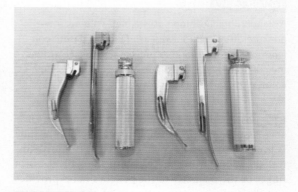

FIGURE 22–11

Standard adult MacIntosh (curved) and Miller (straight) blades with appropriate handles. Photo courtesy of Jim Burger, www.burgerphoto.com.

Laryngoscope Blades

The two basic blade designs for direct laryngoscopy are curved (MacIntosh) and straight (Miller) (Figure 22-11). The choice of blade is based on personal preference. The tip of the *straight blade* goes under the epiglottis and lifts it directly. The *curved blade* goes into the vallecula and indirectly lifts the epiglottis. Each blade has advantages and disadvantages. The straight blade may be a better choice in patients with a long larynx or a floppy epiglottis (children). The wider curved blade may be better in providing tongue displacement, allowing more room for passing the tube in the oral pharynx and laryngeal inlet. The curved blade may also be used as a straight blade if it is large enough to directly lift the epiglottis, which elim-inates the need to change blades during the procedure. Illumination provided by the laryngoscope can make significant differences in the ability to visualize the laryngeal structures in out-of-hospital as well as in-hospital intubation.[12]

Tracheal Tubes

The standard endotracheal tube (ETT) measures approximately 30 cm in length (Figure 22-12). Tube size is printed on the outside of the device and reflects the internal diameter. Also printed on the outside is a scale in centimeters that indicates the distance from the tube's distal tip. Adult males generally accept 7.5- to 9.0-mm ETTs, whereas women can be intubated with 7.0- to 8.0-mm tubes (Figure 22-13). Generally accepted practice is to place the largest

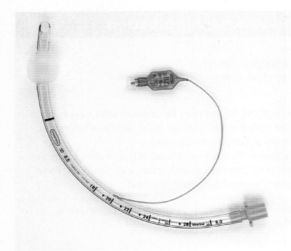

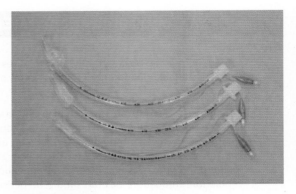

FIGURE 22–13

Cuffed endotracheal tubes, sizes 6.0, 7.0, and 8.0. Photo courtesy of Jim Burger, www.burgerphoto.com.

FIGURE 22–12

A standard tracheal tube uses a high-volume, low-pressure distal cuff to avoid aspiration of gastric contents into the lungs and to prevent air leakage around the cuff to aid in positive-pressure ventilation. Photo courtesy of Barb Steckler, EMT-P.

ETT possible to avoid the increase in airway resistance associated with smaller tubes. A 7.5-mm tube is usually appropriate for most adults. In most clinical situations, using the width of the patient's fifth finger or the diameter of the patient's nares provides a sufficiently accurate estimate of the appropriate tube size. Proper tube depth is calculated by multiplying the tube size times three. For example, when using an 8.0 ETT, the proper depth would be 24 cm at the patient's lip.

Stylets and Stylet Configuration

A stylet shapes the ETT into a preferred configuration. The stylet must not extend beyond the distal end of the ETT during oral intubation. A stylet is not used during nasal intubation.

The stylet is threaded through the ETT to stiffen it; to allow it to be bent to a more advantageous angle; and to improve maneuverability, visibility, and control during tube insertion. Endotracheal tubes should be "preloaded" with a stylet before performing RSI.

The configuration of a stylet can greatly enhance first-pass success.[13] A "straight-to-cuff" or hockey stick configuration (Figure 22-14) with a distal end angle of 35 degrees will facilitate intubation. In this configuration, as the tube is passed on the right side of the patient's mouth, the long axis of the tube enhances visibility. The straight-to-cuff shape aids in maneuver-

ability, as the tube can be tilted backward and forward. This configuration is most advantageous when the epiglottis is obstructing the laryngeal inlet. The upward angle of the tip can be maneuvered under the epiglottis and then passed into the glottic opening.

Technique

Patient Positioning

Often in prehospital settings patients are not in an ideal position, and therefore adjustments have to be made to visualize the larynx. If the patient is on a stretcher, adjust the height of the stretcher so that the patient's face is at the level of the intubator's xiphoid cartilage.

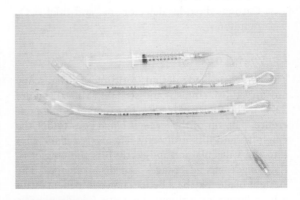

FIGURE 22–14

Endotracheal tube with stylet inserted in a hockey stick configuration with the cuff inflated and checked for air leaks. Photo courtesy of Jim Burger, www.burgerphoto.com.

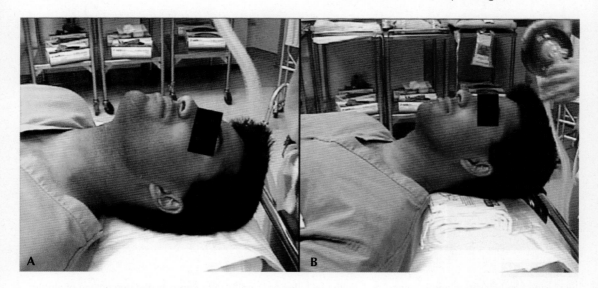

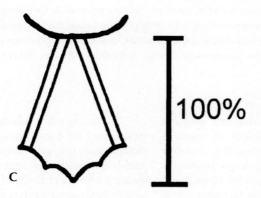

FIGURE 22–15

A, Standard supine position. **B,** Optimal positioning for laryngoscopy elevates the head to align the ear with the sternal notch. **C,** The percentage of glottic opening (POGO) score represents the portion of the glottis visualized. It is defined anteriorly by the anterior commissure and posteriorly by the interarytenoid notch. The score ranges from 0% when none of the glottis is seen to 100% when the entire glottis, including the anterior commissure, is seen. From Levitan R, Mickler T, Hollander JE. Bimanual laryngoscopy: a videographic study of external laryngeal manipulation by novice intubators. *Ann Emerg Med* 40[1]: 30, 2002. Used with permission from Elsevier.

Elevating the patient's head about 10 cm with pads under the occiput and extending the head at the atlanto-occipital joint (sniffing position), align the oral–pharyngeal–laryngeal axis so that the passage from the lips to the glottic opening is almost a straight line. This position permits better visualization of the glottis and vocal cords and allows easier passage of an ETT (Figure 22-15).[14]

The standard "sniffing position" may actually hinder the view in certain patients, especially those who are morbidly obese.[14-16] Align the external auditory meatus and the sternal notch of the patient. This alignment can be achieved by placing blankets or other devices under the patient's head and shoulders, which will align the laryngeal axis and increase the laryngeal view during direct laryngoscopy (Figure 22-16). The head is flexed relative to the chest, reproducing the position used by patients in respiratory distress, but with a supine orientation.

This position maximizes upper airway patency; improves the mechanics of ventilation with both spontaneous breathing and mask ventilation; and significantly improves the percentage of glottic opening (**POGO**) score. The position also lengthens

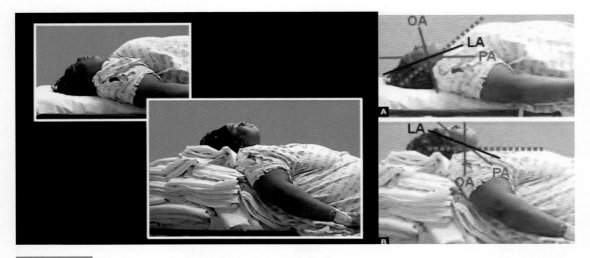

FIGURE 22–16

Increasing head elevation and laryngoscopy angle (neck flexion) significantly improves the percentage of glottic opening (POGO) scores. In comparison with the standard "sniffing position **A**, the "ramped" position **B**, is superior for direct laryngoscopy in morbidly obese patients. This position opens the laryngeal axis (*LA*) into view and provides better diaphragmatic excursion during respiration. *OA*, oral axis; *PA*, pharyngeal axis. From Levitan RM, Kinkle WC. *The AIRWAY•CAM Pocket Guide to Intubation*, 2nd edition. Wayne, PA: Airway Cam Technologies, Inc., 2007.

the apneic time to critical hypoxia and shortens the time needed with mask ventilation to return to normal oxygen saturation. In addition, this 25-degree "back-up" or head-elevated laryngoscopic position is better than the supine position for tracheal intubation. Dynamic lifting of the head during laryngoscopy is impossible in very large patients.

Pharmacologic Agents

RSI is predicated on the administration of medications in a specific sequence. The three phases of medication administration are *preoxygenation, induction,* and *paralysis.*

Preoxygenation   Preoxygenation with high-flow oxygen by a non–rebreather mask for 5 minutes prior to intubation results in supersaturation of oxygen in the tissues and displacement of nitrogen (nitrogen washout). This takes place in the functional residual capacity (FRC) of the lung. It allows the patient to maintain blood oxygen saturation during the apneic period of paralysis and allows more time for successful intubation. Nitrogen washout can also be achieved by having the awake patient take eight vital capacity (i.e., maximal) breaths.

In healthy adult volunteers who have been pre-oxygenated for 3 to 5 minutes, the average time to desaturation (oxygen saturation <90%) is approximately 8 minutes. This time is significantly shorter in patients who are critically ill and have a much higher metabolic demand for oxygen.[17]

Patients most prone to rapid desaturation are remembered by the acronym **POPS**:

- **P**ediatric: Children's metabolic rate at baseline is greatly increased and therefore so is their utilization of oxygen.
- **O**bese: In obese people, a reduction in functional residual capacity exacerbated by the supine position might decrease the effectiveness of preoxygenation and tolerance of apnea. Preoxygenation in a sitting position significantly extends an obese patient's tolerance of apnea compared with preoxygenation in the supine position.
- **P**regnancy: The affinity of fetal hemoglobin for O_2 is greater than that of maternal hemoglobin; therefore the fetus "steals" oxygen from the mother. Oxygen consumption and carbon dioxide production are increased 20 to 40% at term.
- **S**moke Inhalation: Carbon monoxide and cyanide affect affinity for oxygen and oxygen utilization, increasing the patient's risk for hypoxia. Laryngeal

Table 22–3	Common Induction Agents				
Drug	**Adult Dose**	**Onset of Action**	**Duration of Action**	**Advantages**	**Cautions**
Etomidate	0.3 mg/kg IV bolus, normal adult dose about 20 mg	0.5-1 min	3-10 mins	Does not alter hemo-dynamics or ICP; no histamine release	Myoclonus
				Useful for multiple trauma or hypoten-sive patients	Adrenal suppres-sion (typically no clinical sig-nificance)
				Generally no apnea	No analgesia
Ketamine	1-2 mg/kg slow IV bolus with bolus rate <0.5 mg/kg/min	0.5-1 min	3-10 mins	Bronchodilation	Reported to increase ICP
				Protective Airway reflexes intact	Increases mVO$_2$; avoid in cardiac ischemia
				Useful for hypotensive patients	Emergence delir-ium
				Provides analgesia and amnesia	Hypertonic muscle movements
Propofol	1-3 mg/kg IV bolus	15-45 sec	5-10 mins	Decreases ICP	Apnea
				Anti-emetic	Hypotension
				Quick onset of action	No analgesia
Sodium Thiopental	2-3 mg/kg IV bolus	<1 min	3-10 min	Quick onset of action but extremely potent	Hypotension and myocardial depression
				Decreases ICP, cere-broprotective	Apnea
				Useful in status epilepticus	Histamine release and bronchospasm

ICP = intracranial pressure; mg = milligrams.

edema develops rapidly as the pharynx and the hypopharynx take most of the heat absorption. The presence of particulate matter in the lungs decreases gas exchange.

Patients identified by **POPS** and critically ill patients have an increased risk of hypoxia when apnea is produced during RSI.

Induction and Paralysis The concept of RSI is based on the near simultaneous intravenous administration of a *rapidly acting induction agent* and a *neuromuscular blocking agent* (paralytic). Agent selection and dosing are aimed at producing a state of deep sedation and muscular relaxation quickly. The dose of each agent is precalculated to achieve the desired effect. Doses are not titrated to effect. Onset of action after administration is variable depending on the agent chosen, but the goal is to achieve intubation-level paralysis and sedation 45 to 60 seconds after the drugs are given by IV bolus.

Induction Agents Induction agents (sedatives) (Table 22-3) are integral to the performance of RSI. They provide amnesia, blunt sympathetic responses, and improve intubating conditions. Induction agents provide a rapid loss of consciousness that facilitates ease of intubation.

If a paralytic agent is used for intubation without sedation, the patient is fully aware of the environment and experiences pain but is unable to respond. In addition to its inhumanity, this circumstance allows

Table 22–4	**Choice of Induction Agent Based on Underlying Condition**

Head Injury/Elevated Intracranial Pressure (ICP)

- Etomidate or ketamine
  - Maintain adequate cerebral perfusion pressure to prevent secondary brain injury
- Ketamine should be avoided in patients with significant hypertension and those with ICP elevation caused by spontaneous cerebral hemorrhage

Status Epilepticus

- Thiopental or midazolam
  - Reduce the dose in the unusual circumstance of seizure with hypotension
- Etomidate may be used when the patient manifests hemodynamic compromise
- Ketamine should NOT be used because of its stimulant effects

Severe Bronchospasm with Stable Blood Pressure

- Ketamine or propofol
- Etomidate and midazolam are acceptable alternatives
  - In hemodynamically unstable patients with severe bronchospasm, ketamine or etomidate

Cardiovascular Compromise

- Etomidate because of its hemodynamic stability

Shock

- Ketamine or etomidate
  - If etomidate is used in a patient with sepsis and hypotension refractory to treatment with fluid resuscitation and a vasopressor, a corticosteroid may be indicated

Awake Intubation

- Ketamine or propofol

Based on Caro D. Sedation or induction agents for rapid sequence intubation in adults. Available at www.utdol.com/home/content/topic.do?topicKey=ad_resus/5167#. Accessed on December 28, 2009.

potentially adverse physiologic responses to airway manipulation, including tachycardia, hypertension, and elevated intracranial pressure (ICP). Sedative use prevents or minimizes these effects. Select an induction agent that both facilitates RSI and does not worsen the patient's underlying condition (Table 22-4).

Use of sedatives may also improve the laryngoscopic view. During RSI, the clinician must perform laryngoscopy during the earliest phase of neuromuscular paralysis. Sedatives improve laryngoscopy in part by supplementing the incomplete relaxation provided by the paralytic.

Etomidate Etomidate is *the most hemodynamically neutral of the sedative agents used for RSI.* It is cardioprotective and neuroprotective, as it is not associated

with a significant drop in blood pressure or a significant rise in intracranial pressure (ICP). The hemodynamic stability associated with etomidate makes it the drug of choice for the intubation of hypotensive patients as well as an attractive option for patients with intracranial pathology, in whom hypotension must be avoided. Etomidate decreases cerebral blood flow and cerebral metabolic oxygen demand while preserving cerebral perfusion.

Etomidate is given in a dose of 0.3 milligrams/kg IV. It has a rapid onset, with a time to effect of 15 to 45 seconds and a short duration of action (3–12 minutes). When etomidate is given without a supplemental paralytic agent, myoclonus (generalized muscle jerking, much like a seizure) can result. It may take a few minutes for myoclonus to stop. Consequently, during intubation, etomidate is followed by administration of a paralytic agent.

Midazolam This medication has fallen out of favor in North America in recent years because of its delayed time to induction, predilection for creating hypotension, and prolonged duration of action. However, it is still used for out-of-hospital sedation in many countries. The induction dose for midazolam is 0.1 to 0.3 milligrams/kg IV bolus, with a time to effect of approximately 30 to 60 seconds and a duration of action of 15 to 30 minutes. Like all benzodiazepines, midazolam does not provide analgesia but does possess anticonvulsant effects, making it an effective agent for RSI in patients with status epilepticus. Midazolam causes moderate hypotension, with an average drop in mean arterial blood pressure in healthy patients of 10 to 25%.[18,19] This tendency to induce hypotension limits midazolam's usefulness in the setting of hypovolemia or shock. If midazolam must be used in such patients, the suggested dose is 0.1 milligrams/kg, which will somewhat delay the speed of onset and the depth of sedation achieved but should not severely compromise intubation conditions.

Sodium Thiopental Sodium thiopental, administered in a dose of 3 to 5 milligrams/kg IV, is a very rapidly acting induction agent and has a short duration of action (5–30 minutes). It causes venodilation and has a negative cardiac inotropic effect, so it can induce profound hypotension. It is not a drug of choice in hemodynamically unstable patients and in patients prone to hypotension, such as the elderly. Reductions in ICP are caused by its actions of decreasing cerebral perfusion pressure and reducing arterial pressure. Because of its rapid onset and the decrease in ICP, sodium thiopental may be indicated for a patient in status epilepticus. This drug causes histamine release and can induce or exacerbate bronchospasm; therefore, it should be used with caution in patients with asthma or chronic obstructive pulmonary disease (COPD).[20]

Ketamine Ketamine, administered in a dose of 1 to 2 milligrams/kg IV, is unique among sedative agents in that it possesses all three properties desired in an induction agent: analgesia (by exciting opioid receptors), amnesia, and sedation. It stimulates catecholamine receptors and release of catecholamines, producing an increase in heart rate, cardiac contractility, mean arterial pressure, and cerebral blood flow. Because it has a quick onset of action and preserves respiratory drive, ketamine is a good choice for "awake" intubation attempts. It is also an attractive choice for hypotensive patients requiring RSI because it induces sympathetic stimulation. However, it can worsen cardiac ischemia in patients with severe coronary disease.

Controversy persists regarding the use of ketamine in patients with head injury based on concerns about elevating ICP. It increases cerebral perfusion, which may benefit patients with neurologic injury.

Propofol The induction dose for propofol is 1.5 to 3 milligrams/kg IV. This drug has a time to effect of 15 to 45 seconds and a duration of action of 5 to 10 minutes. Sedation occurs through direct suppression of brain activity. Amnesia appears to result from interference with long-term memory creation.[21,22] Propofol reduces airway resistance and can be a useful induction agent for patients with bronchospasm undergoing RSI. Propofol is also a good choice for awake intubation. Its neuroinhibitory effects make propofol a good induction agent for patients with intracranial pathology, provided they are hemodynamically stable. Propofol suppresses sympathetic activity, causing myocardial depression and peripheral vasodilation. Therefore, use the lower dose or decrease the dose to 1.0 milligrams/kg IV in hypotensive, head-injured, and elderly patients.

Paralytic Agents

Administer the paralyzing agent immediately after giving the induction agent. Paralytics are given as part of RSI to paralyze skeletal muscle and facilitate laryngoscopic intubation and mechanical ventilation. Paralytics do not induce sedation, analgesia, or amnesia, so the administration of a potent induction agent is important.

As neuromuscular blocking agents, paralytics block neuromuscular transmission at the neuromuscular junction, causing paralysis of skeletal muscles. They act either presynaptically by inhibition of acetylcholine synthesis or release or postsynaptically at the acetylcholine receptor. Neuromuscular blocking agents agents (Table 22-5) are divided into two classes based on their mechanism of action: *depolarizing* or *nondepolarizing*.

Succinylcholine is the only *depolarizing agent* used for RSI. **Because of its rapid onset (muscle relaxation in 30 seconds; total paralysis in 45 seconds) and ultrashort duration of action (7–10 minutes), it is commonly used to induce paralysis during RSI.** The dose is 1.5 milligrams/kg in adults and 2 milligrams/kg in children younger than 5 years.

Several *rare* but severe adverse effects are associated with the administration of succinylcholine.

Table 22–5	**Paralytic Agents**				
Drug Name	**Adult Dose**	**Onset of Action**	**Duration of Action**	**Advantages**	**Cautions**
Succinylcholine	0.3–2 mg/kg IV bolus (average dose, 1.5 mg/kg)	1 minute	4–6 mins	Depolarizing NMBA Rapid onset (<60 sec) Brief duration of action	Increased serum potassium Muscle fasciculation Malignant hyperthermia Cardiac arrest in children with muscular dystrophy Dysrhythmia with multiple doses
Rocuronium	1 mg/kg IV bolus	1 minute	30–45 mins	Nondepolarizing NMBA No risk of hyperkalemia	
Vecuronium	0.3 mg/kg	>1 minute	60–120 mins	Nondepolarizing NMBA No risk of hyperkalemia	Prolonged duration of action

mg = milligrams; NMBA = neuromuscular blocking agent.
Based on Lafferty KA, Windle ML. Tracheal intubation, medications. Available at http://emedicine.medscape.com/article/109739-overview. Accessed on December 28, 2009.

Situations predictive of the emergence of its adverse effects can be very difficult to identify in the prehospital setting. Succinylcholine may increase serum potassium levels by as much as 0.5 mEq/L. The risk of an exaggerated release is amplified in certain chronic disease states or after the acute phase of certain injuries or conditions. Therefore, its use in patients with the following high-risk conditions is discouraged:[23]

- Suspicion of hyperkalemia.
- Missed hemodialysis.
- Burns over a large surface area.
- Multisystem trauma with crush injury.
- Spinal cord and other denervating injuries.
- Extensive muscle necrosis (e.g., large crush injuries).
- Neuromyopathies.
- Crush injuries more than 7 days old.

One of the important considerations with the use of induction and paralytic agents is operator familiarity with drug doses and their effects. For this reason, succinylcholine remains the most commonly used paralytic agent. If the adverse effects associated with succinylcholine, a depolarizing agent, are of concern, a short-acting nondepolarizing agent (rocuronium or vecuronium) can be used. One strong advantage of this class of paralytics is that they pose no risk of inducing hyperkalemia.

Rocuronium is a muscle relaxant structurally related to vecuronium, but its onset of action is three times as rapid, making it the fastest acting nondepolarizing agent. With sufficient dose (1.0–1.2 milligrams/kg IV), its onset is 60 to 90 seconds (similar to that of succinylcholine). A common concern about the use of rocuronium in RSI is that its duration of action is "intermediate," lasting 30 to 45 minutes. This length of time may be an advantage because the patient remains paralyzed, allowing a second intubation attempt if necessary. But the duration of action may be a disadvantage because it prevents neurologic examination in the ED until the effect of the drug has worn off.

Vecuronium is an alternative to rocuronium for RSI. In its typical application in the operating room, vecuronium is administered as a muscle relaxant prior to elective surgery, as a priming dose of 0.01 milligrams/kg given 3 minutes before a higher dose of 0.15 mg/kg. Intubation-level paralysis is achieved in 75 to 90 seconds. In the emergency RSI situation, this time until onset is too long. If vecuronium is given at a higher dose, 0.3 mg/kg, without a priming dose, its onset of action is approximately 60 seconds, with a duration of 45 minutes.[24]

Reversing Agent (Sugammadex)

Sugammadex is the first agent designed to reverse the neuromuscular blocking action of rocuronium and vecuronium.[25] The European Union approved its use on July 29, 2008. It can reverse drug-induced neuromuscular blockade in approximately 3 minutes, apparently without side effects.

Technique

Bimanual Laryngoscopy

External laryngeal manipulation (Figure 22-17) can greatly improve the intubator's view during laryngoscopy. While holding the laryngoscope in the left hand, place the right hand over the thyroid cartilage, manipulating it backward, upward, or side-to-side to optimize the view of familiar structures and the laryngeal inlet. This should not be confused with cricoid pressure or other maneuvers done by assistants, which can actually hinder the intubator's view.

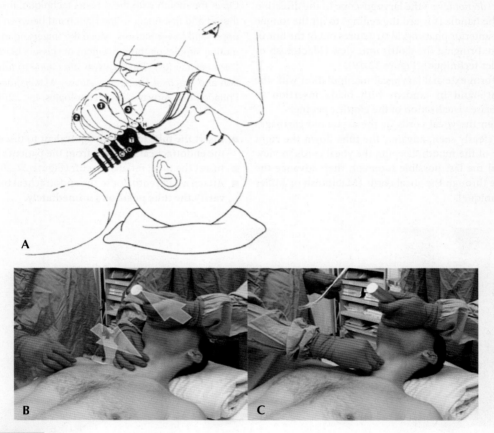

FIGURE 22–17

Bimanual laryngoscopy (external laryngeal manipulation). **A,** Manipulation of larynx to maximize laryngeal view. T, thyroid cartilage; C, cricoid cartilage; H, hyoid bone, 1, index finger; 2, movement of hand; 3, thumb. **B,** While looking into the patient's mouth, the intubator manipulates the larynx to increase the view of familiar structures and the glottic opening. *Arrows* indicate that the force on the neck is opposite the direction of lift by the laryngoscope. **C,** Once that maximized position is found, an assistant can maintain the position to free the intubator's right hand for tube passage. **B,** and **C,** from Levitan RM. *The AIRWAY•CAM Guide to Intubation and Practical Emergency Airway Management.* Wayne, PA: Airway Cam Technologies, Inc., 2004.

Direct Laryngoscopy

- Optimize patient position.
- Preoxygenate the patient.
- Verify effect of induction and paralytic agents.
- With suction available at hand, hold the laryngoscope in the left hand.
- Open the patient's mouth with a right-handed scissors technique (Figure 22-18).
- Slide the laryngoscope blade down the tongue, with the goal of visualizing the epiglottis.
- To find the epiglottis, direct the laryngoscope blade downward, toward the patient's feet, to lift the epiglottis off the posterior pharyngeal wall.
- Advance the blade tip into the vallecula to open the laryngeal inlet and bring the vocal cords into view.
- *Lift* (*do not lever*) the laryngoscope in the direction of the handle (toward the ceiling) to lift the tongue and anterior pharyngeal structures out of the line of sight, bringing the glottis into view (MacIntosh or Miller technique) (Figure 22-19).
- Perform external laryngeal manipulation with the right hand in tandem with blade insertion to increase visualization of the glottic opening.
- When the vocal cords or the arytenoid cartilages are clearly seen, advance the tube down the right side of the mouth, keeping the vocal cords in view until the last possible moment; then advance the tube through the vocal cords (MacIntosh or Miller technique).

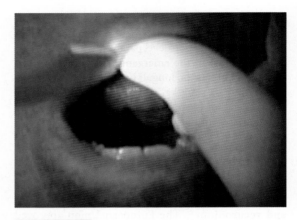

FIGURE 22–18

Open the mouth with the scissors technique. Insert the thumb and first finger of the right hand between the upper and lower incisors. Move the fingers apart, in a motion simulating the movement of scissors blades. From Levitan RM. *The Airway•Cam Guide to Intubation and Practical Emergency Airway Management.* Philadelphia, Airway Cam Technologies, Inc., 2004.

- Insert the tube to a depth equivalent to three times the endotracheal tube size from the patient's lip.
- Insert the tube; inflate the cuff (Figure 22-20).
- Attach a bag ventilator to the endotracheal tube and **verify the tube position's immediately.**

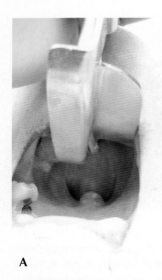
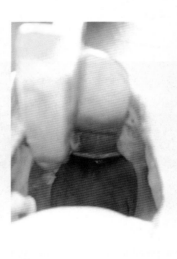
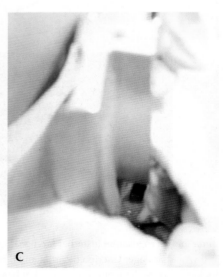

A   **B**   **C**

FIGURE 22–19

Blade insertion. **A,** Insert the laryngoscope to displace the tongue until the epiglottis is visualized. **B,** Insert the blade gently into the vallecula. **C,** With minimal lifting of the posterior structures, the laryngeal inlet and vocal cords come into view. Photos courtesy of Jim Burger, www.burgerphoto.com.

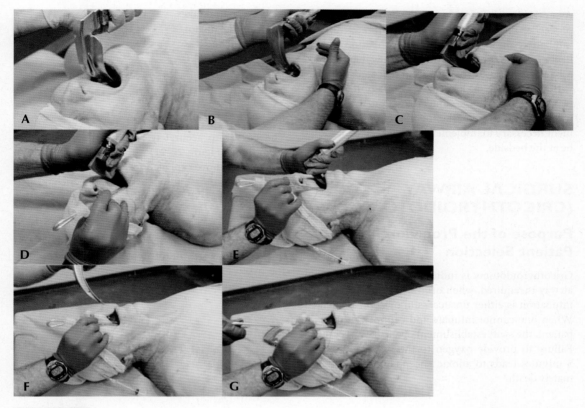

FIGURE 22–20

Sequence of direct laryngoscopy. **A**, Insert the laryngoscope blade into the patient's mouth. **B** and **C**, Insert the blade down the tongue and lift it toward the ceiling until the epiglottis is in view. Then perform external laryngeal manipulation to increase the view of the laryngeal inlet. **D** and **E**, Preload the endotracheal tube with the stylet in a straight-to-cuff configuration (hockey stick). Insert the endotracheal tube from the right side of the patient's mouth and pass it through the vocal cords. **F** and **G**, Remove the laryngoscope blade and stylet. Inflate the endotracheal cuff. Photos courtesy of Jim Burger, www.burgerphoto.com.

- Attach a CO_2 detector to the tube or use an endtidal CO_2 monitor to verify return of carbon dioxide with each breath.
- Listen for breath sounds over the epigastrium (one breath), then to each hemithorax in the midaxillary line (one breath on each side).
- Secure the ETT in position and request a chest film to confirm it.
- Ensure proper attachment of the tube to a mechanical ventilator and review the ventilator settings.
- Consider ongoing sedation, particularly if the induction agent may wear off before the effects of the paralytic agent.

Complications of Laryngoscopy

- Cannot intubate, but can ventilate with mask – continue mask ventilation until a more experienced laryngoscopist arrives; defer intubation or consider alternative technique, such as fiberoptic intubation.
- Can't intubate, can't ventilate – see surgical airway.
- Aspiration.
- Trauma from laryngoscope.
  - Damage to teeth – avoidable with proper technique.
  - Injury to soft tissues (bleeding) – usually avoidable with proper technique.
  - Edema – usually caused by repeated attempts to intubate; key is to optimize something with each new attempt, not simply repeat procedure without addressing a possible reason for failure.
- Equipment failure – verify that everything works before beginning the procedure.

A critical and often overlooked part of this initial phase of RSI is preparation for unanticipated difficulty.

Assess airway difficulty before the decision is made to proceed with RSI. Even if no indicators of difficult intubation are identified and the intubation appears likely to be routine, **the airway manager must have a back-up plan** to manage unanticipated problems with intubation or bag-mask ventilation. Back-up plans will vary with the clinical situation, the availability of devices, and the training of the provider. Equipment necessary to implement the back-up plan should be at the bedside.

SURGICAL AIRWAY (CRICOTHYROIDOTOMY)

Purpose of the Procedure/Patient Selection

Cricothyroidotomy is indicated when an emergency airway is required, when orotracheal or nasotracheal intubation is either unsuccessful or contraindicated. When one cannot intubate and cannot ventilate the patient, the swift establishment of an airway is crucial. Failure to provide oxygen to the brain within 3 to 5 minutes leads to anoxic encephalopathy and ultimately death.

Risks and Precautions

The risks of cricothyroidotomy include those listed below:

- Hemorrhage.
- Misidentifying the cricothyroid membrane.
- Making the incision above the thyroid cartilage.
- Lacerating the thyroid cartilage, cricoid cartilage, or tracheal rings.
- Perforating the posterior trachea.
- Unintentional tracheostomy.
- Passage of the tube into an extratracheal location (i.e., creating a false passage).

Cricothyroidotomy is absolutely contraindicated when the patient can be intubated safely either orally or nasally. Other absolute contraindications include complete transection of the trachea, laryngotracheal disruption with retraction of the distal trachea into the mediastinum, and a fractured larynx.

Equipment

- No. 10 or 20 scalpel blade loaded on a handle.
- No. 6.0 cuffed endotracheal tube.
- Two tracheal rakes.
- Trousseau dilator.
- Tracheal hook.
- Ambu bag.

Technique

Identify Landmarks

The goal is to accurately identify the cricothyroid membrane (Figure 22-21). First, palpate the sternal notch, then move cephalad toward the patient's chin. You will feel a "first bump," which is the cricoid cartilage (Figure 22-22). Immediately thereafter in this cephalad movement, the "first depression" is the cricothyroid membrane. In approaches advocated in the past, palpation started at the mandible and moved downward; unfortunately in this technique, the hyoid bone was often misinterpreted as thyroid cartilage, and the incision was made above it. Patients

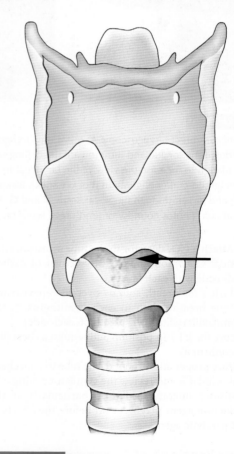

FIGURE 22–21

Location of cricothyroid membrane (*arrow*).

deteriorated and died as a result of clinicians' inability to find the larynx.

In morbidly obese patients and in patients with subcutaneous emphysema in the neck, an alternative means of identifying the desired landmark is to place the four fingers of the operator's right hand in the patient's sternal notch while standing on the patient's right side. Orient the fingers vertically up the anterior midline of the neck; the index finger will typically lie over or very nearly over the membrane.

In most scenarios, the cricoid membrane is easily palpated, allowing use of the rapid four-step technique. The open technique is usually performed in patients in whom anatomic landmarks are difficult to palpate and thus need to be visualized.

Rapid Four-Step Technique

The rapid four-step technique can be done quickly and requires only a scalpel (preferably No. 20), a tracheal hook with a large radius, and a cuffed tracheostomy tube. For this technique, stand above the patient's head, in the same position as when performing endotracheal intubation. Perform the following four steps in sequence:

1. Identify the cricothyroid membrane by palpation (Figure 22-23).

2. Make a horizontal stab incision through the skin and cricothyroid membrane with the scalpel (Figure 22-24).

3. Stabilize the larynx by placing the handle of the scalpel (or a tracheal hook, if available) under the cricoid cartilage. This marks a significant change from the standard method in which the tracheal hook or the handle of the scalpel is placed under the thyroid cartilage.

4. Insert the endotracheal tube and ventilate the patient using a bag-valve mask (Figure 22-25).

Standard (Open) Technique

1. Prepare the skin of the anterior neck with an antiseptic solution.

2. Immobilize the larynx and palpate the cricothyroid membrane. Immobilize the larynx with the nondominant hand and perform the procedure with the dominant hand. The procedure is largely tactile, so proper finger position is essential. Place the thumb and long finger of the nondominant hand on either side of the thyroid cartilage to immobilize the larynx. Palpate the thyroid cartilage with the index finger and then move caudally 1 to 2 cm until a small depression inferior to the thyroid cartilage is encountered. This is the cricothyroid membrane.

3. Incise the skin vertically. After palpating the cricothyroid membrane, make a midline vertical

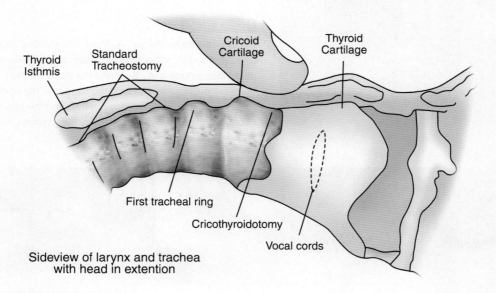

Thyroid Isthmis
Standard Tracheostomy
Cricoid Cartilage
Thyroid Cartilage
First tracheal ring
Cricothyroidotomy
Vocal cords

Sideview of larynx and trachea
with head in extention

FIGURE 22–22

Tracheal anatomy, showing location of cricoid cartilage.

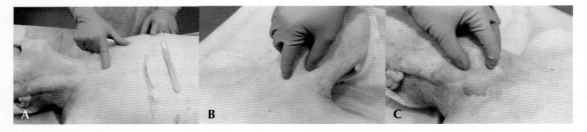

FIGURE 22–23

Cricothyroidotomy. **A,** Palpate the sternal notch. **B,** Moving in a cephalad direction, you will feel a bump and then, immediately thereafter, the first depression, which is the cricoid membrane. **C,** Using the nondominant hand, stabilize the trachea using the thumb and the third finger. With the index finger, palpate the cricothyroid membrane before making the incision. Photos courtesy of Jim Burger, www.burgerphoto.com.

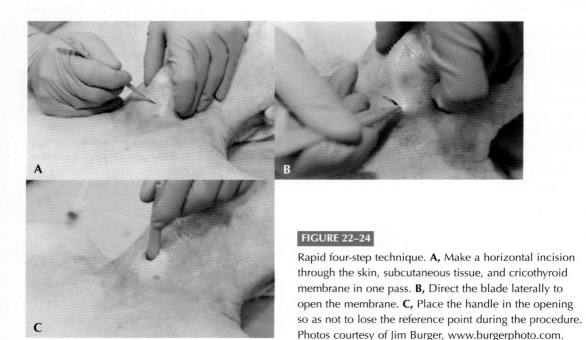

FIGURE 22–24

Rapid four-step technique. **A,** Make a horizontal incision through the skin, subcutaneous tissue, and cricothyroid membrane in one pass. **B,** Direct the blade laterally to open the membrane. **C,** Place the handle in the opening so as not to lose the reference point during the procedure. Photos courtesy of Jim Burger, www.burgerphoto.com.

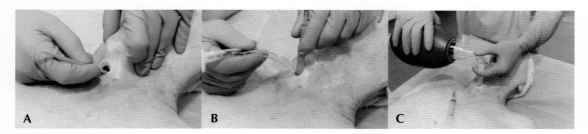

FIGURE 22–25

With the handle in the cricothyrotomy opening, insert a 6.0 endotracheal tube and inflate the cuff. Ventilate the patient using an Ambu bag. Photos courtesy of Jim Burger, www.burgerphoto.com.

incision, 3 to 5 cm long, through the skin overlying the membrane. A midline incision avoids the vascular structures that are located laterally. The vertical orientation also allows extension of the incision superiorly or inferiorly if the initial location is too high or too low or provides inadequate access to the cricothyroid membrane.

4. Incise the pretracheal fascia, which covers the cricothyroid membrane, horizontally. Make a 1-cm horizontal incision through the cricothyroid membrane. This incision should be made through the caudad part of the membrane to avoid the vasculature running across the cephalad portion.

5. Once you have made the incision in the cricothyroid membrane, keep the tip of the index finger of the nondominant hand in the entry to the incision so as not to lose the opening. Continue to immobilize the larynx firmly, maintaining a triangle formed by the thumb and middle finger on opposite sides of the larynx and the index finger in the incision in the cricothyroid membrane. It is crucial not to let go at this point, because significant bleeding usually obscures the view of the membrane.

6. Insert the tracheal hook. Place the tracheal hook under the thyroid cartilage and ask an assistant to provide upward traction.

7. Insert a Trousseau dilator and open it to enlarge the incision vertically. Squeeze the handles of the dilator to open its jaws. Leave the dilator in place until the tube is inserted; if the dilator is removed, the thyroid and cricoid cartilages will spring back into place. If a Trousseau dilator is not available, turn the scalpel around and use the handle to enlarge the incision.

8. Insert the endotracheal tube and inflate the cuff.

PRINCIPLES OF MECHANICAL VENTILATION

"Ventilation" refers primarily to the amount of oxygen and carbon dioxide exchanging at the alveolar level. Factors that influence this process include the gas exchange surface area and diffusion rate and the amount of gas that can be moved in and out of the lungs. The two goals of mechanical ventilation are appropriate oxygenation and appropriate ventilation

Patients who need ventilatory assistance tend to have conditions such as pneumonia, pulmonary embolism, high levels of blood carbon dioxide (hypercapnia), low levels of blood oxygen (hypoxia), thoracic trauma, traumatic brain injury, or stroke. Basically, the patient cannot get enough oxygen to the blood or breathe on his or her own. The patient needs to have an endotracheal tube inserted and attached to a ventilator.

The ETT serves as an artificial airway, particularly when the patient is not awake enough to protect his or her own airway. The ventilator has settings for *breaths per minute*, *volume of air per breath*, and other parameters. The machine also has modes of breathing, depending on whether the critical care physician feels the machine must do all the work of breathing for the patient or some of the work as back-up for the patient's own efforts to breathe. Oxygenation is affected by several factors: the inspired oxygen concentration (F_{iO2}), mean airway pressure (MAP), and the area of and diffusion across the gas exchange surface. Patients will require proper sedation, analgesia, and often paralysis for the ventilator to provide proper gas exchange. Patients not given these medications will "fight the ventilator and hinder ventilation or gas exchange. Fighting increases the work of breathing and may cause further lung injury.

Emergency medical services/transport ventilators offer time-cycled, volume-constant operation. They are built for the rigors of prehospital care. They are typically fast to deploy and easy to use. They use intuitive tidal volume and rate controls. They can accommodate the basic needs of ventilator-dependent transport patients and are suitable for emergency ventilation. Some now also include a continuous positive airway pressure (CPAP) function, which expands versatility.

Basic Ventilator Parameters

F_{iO2}

■ Fractional concentration of inspired oxygen delivered expressed as a percentage ranging from 21 to 100.

Breath Rate (f)

■ The number of times over a 1-minute period that inspiration is initiated (reported as breaths per minute [bpm]).

Tidal volume (VT)

■ The amount of gas that is delivered during inspiration, expressed in milliliters or liters. It is reported as inspired or exhaled.

Flow

■ The velocity of gas flow or volume of gas per minute.

Ventilator settings are tailored to specific patient abnormalities

- For a patient without preexisting lung disease, the tidal volume and rate are traditionally selected by using the **12–12 rule**. A tidal volume of 12 mL for each kilogram of lean body weight is programmed to be delivered 12 times a minute in the assist-control mode.
- For patients with COPD, the tidal volume and rate are slightly reduced to the 10–10 rule to prevent overinflation and hyperventilation. A tidal volume of 10 mL/kg lean body weight is delivered 10 times a minute in the assist-control mode.
- In acute respiratory distress syndrome (ARDS), the lungs may function best and volume trauma is minimized with low tidal volumes of 6 to 8 mL/kg.

Tidal volumes are preset at 6 to 8 mL/kg of lean body weight in the assist-control mode. These lowered volumes may lead to slight hypercarbia. An elevated P_{CO2} is typically recognized and accepted without correction, leading to the term "permissive hypercapnia."

Initial settings for ventilation may be summarized as follows (Table 22-6).

- Assist-control mode.
- Tidal volume set depending on lung status.
  - Normal = 12 mL/kg ideal body weight.
  - COPD = 10 mL/kg ideal body weight.
  - ARDS = 6 to 8 mL/kg ideal body weight.
- Respiratory rate of 10 to 12 bpm.
- F_{IO2} of 100%.
- PEEP may be added.

Complications

The transport provider must be aware of the settings and monitor the patient. Many ventilators will give alarms and these may be unimportant or can be a sign of a real technical or mechanical problem. Don't be the one who turns off the alarm settings during transport only to find your patient has died during transport.

Remember, the ventilator will still keep doing its job, even if the patient has no pulse.

Most ventilators have an alarm that signals when there is an abnormality within the ventilator circuit. An easy mnemonic to remember is **DOPE:**

 D Dislodgement of the endotracheal tube
 O Obstruction
 P Pneumothorax
 E Equipment

PREHOSPITAL CAPNOGRAPHY AND CAPNOMETRY

Purpose

The measurement of exhaled carbon dioxide (CO_2) is an important technologic achievement that directly influences patient outcomes. Capnography is the noninvasive monitoring of exhaled CO_2. Exhaled CO_2 is represented via a continuous waveform display. Capnometry more specifically focuses on the presence or absence of carbon dioxide in exhaled air. The widespread adoption of capnography makes good clinical sense in that it assists prehospital care providers in assessing respiratory failure and confirming placement of advanced airway devices. In contrast to colorimetric CO_2 devices, capnography provides ongoing measurement of another "vital sign." Colorimetric end-tidal CO_2 detectors yield singular answers with respect to the presence of exhaled carbon dioxide. **Analysis of waveform capnography, in contrast, provides paramedics with ongoing information about a patient's respiratory status.** Monitoring devices that provide emergency medical services (EMS) personnel with numeric measurements of end-tidal CO_2 have similar utility. These devices do not have waveform display capability. Rather, they provide a continuous numeric readout of end exhaled CO_2 in millimeters of mercury (mm Hg). This section focuses on the utility

Table 22–6	Initial Ventilator Settings Based on Patients' Conditions				
	Tidal Volume	Respiratory Rate	I/E Radio	PEEP	F_{IO2}
Normal lungs	8	10–12	1:2	4	1.0
Asthma/COPD	6	5–8	1:4	4	1.0
ARDS	6	10–12	1:2	4–15	1.0
Hypovolemia	8	10–12	1:2	0–4	1:0

ARDS = adult respiratory distress syndrome; COPD = Chronic Obstructive Pulmonary Disease.
From Amitai A, Sinert RH, Joyce DM. Ventilator management. Available at http://emedicine.medscape.com/article/810126-overview. Accessed on December 28, 2009.

of end-tidal CO_2 monitoring for patients undergoing prehospital tracheal intubation. The connection of a CO_2 detector in line with an endotracheal tube is technically described as "mainstream" capnography as opposed to "sidestream" monitoring.

The work of Dunford, Ochs, and Davis catapulted prehospital capnography into the spotlight. In their "San Diego study," paramedics performed RSI on head-injured patients. Patients arriving at the ED were profoundly and inadvertently hyperventilated; this correlated with increased mortality.[26,27] Conversely, patients intubated and subsequently transported by air medial crews capable of monitoring end-tidal CO_2 demonstrated an increased likelihood of survival.[28] Organizations such as the American College of Emergency Physicians (ACEP) and the American Heart Association (AHA) support the adoption of end-tidal CO_2 monitoring as a prehospital standard of care.[29] A recent ACEP position statement states that "End-tidal CO_2 detection, either qualitative, quantitative, or continuous, is the most accurate and easily available method to monitor correct endotracheal tube position in patients who have adequate tissue perfusion."[30]

Patient Selection

■ Measurement of end-tidal CO_2 should be considered in all intubated patients and in unintubated patients with severe respiratory distress.

Equipment

■ Monitor or defibrillator with end-tidal CO_2 waveform display and attached sensor (Figure 22-26).

■ Handheld or portable capnometer with attached sensor (Figure 22-27).
■ Additional batteries for portable handheld devices.
■ Additional CO_2 sensors.

Procedural Monitoring

Current literature confirms the association between hyperventilation and increased mortality. Paramedics performing endotracheal intubation on patients with traumatic brain injury can utilize the end-tidal CO_2 waveform to appropriately guide positive-pressure ventilation. For patients without immediate evidence of central nervous system herniation, target ventilations to an end-tidal CO_2 of approximately 35 to 40 mm Hg.[28] Proper placement of an endotracheal tube results in either the digital display of end-tidal CO_2 or the generation of an appropriate waveform (Figure 22-28). Loss of a CO_2 waveform or digital readout may indicate apnea or dislodgement of the tracheal tube (Figure 22-29).

The end-tidal CO_2 waveform is regular and trapezoidal in appearance. The start of the waveform coincides with the onset of exhalation when the level of exhaled CO_2 is at zero (Figure 22-30). As patient exhalation continues and airway dead space is cleared, the end-tidal CO_2 rises rapidly. The end of exhalation correlates with stable and maintained concentrations of end-tidal CO_2. This appears as a plateau on the waveform display (Figure 22-31). The plateau is never absolutely horizontal because alveoli are active in gas exchange and continually eliminating carbon dioxide. The actual end-tidal CO_2 reading comes from the end of exhalation (Figure 22-32). As inhalation begins, the level of CO_2 rapidly returns to zero (Figure 22-33).

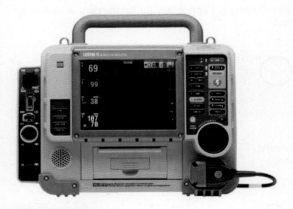

FIGURE 22–26

Defibrillator/monitor with waveform capnography capability (the Lifepak 15 from MedTronic PhysioControl). Reprinted with permission from Physio-Control, Inc. http://www.physio-control.com/default.aspx.

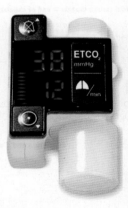

FIGURE 22–27

Portable capnometer with attached sensor.

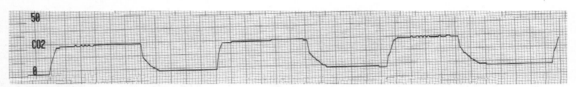

FIGURE 22–28

Normal end-tidal CO_2 waveform. Courtesy of Peter Canning, Capnograpy for Paramedics, available at: http://emscapnography.blogspot.com/2006/05/welcome.html.

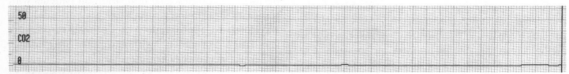

FIGURE 22–29

Loss of end-tidal waveform. Courtesy of Peter Canning, Capnograpy for Paramedics, available at: http://emscapnography.blogspot.com/2006/05/welcome.html.

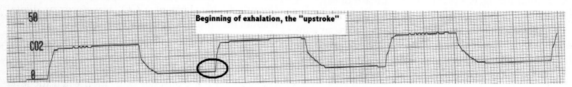

FIGURE 22–30

Onset of exhalation. Courtesy of Peter Canning, Capnograpy for Paramedics, available at: http://emscapnography.blogspot.com/2006/05/welcome.html.

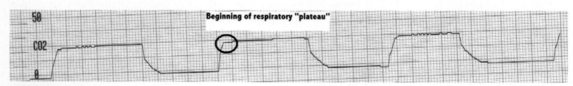

FIGURE 22–31

The plateau on the end-tidal CO_2 waveform. Courtesy of Peter Canning, Capnograpy for Paramedics, available at: http://emscapnography.blogspot.com/2006/05/welcome.html.

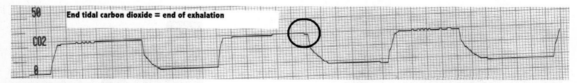

FIGURE 22–32

End of exhalation and end-tidal CO_2. Courtesy of Peter Canning, Capnograpy for Paramedics, available at: http://emscapnography.blogspot.com/2006/05/welcome.html.

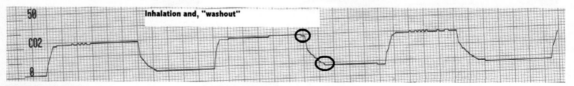

FIGURE 22–33

Inhalation and washout of CO_2. Courtesy of Peter Canning, Capnograpy for Paramedics, available at: http://emscapnography.blogspot.com/2006/05/welcome.html.

Step-by-Step Technique

- Confirm with traditional methods of direct visualization, auscultation of lung sounds, and visualization of chest rise.
- Attach end-tidal CO_2 sensor to monitoring device.
- Wait several seconds for device calibration.
- Observe either generation of waveform or digital readout of end-tidal CO_2 on monitor display.

Outcomes Assessment

The singular most important outcome of end-tidal monitoring is confirmation of endotracheal tube position. The out-of-hospital environment poses many challenges to patient care; among them is endotracheal tube displacement. **Always reconfirm tube location after patient movement or change in condition.** Visualization of the CO_2 waveform or measured end-tidal CO_2 in mm Hg is evidence of effective ventilation. Loss of waveform or digital readout at any time should prompt rapid troubleshooting and immediate patient reassessment. Though disappearance of the end-tidal CO_2 waveform can result from faulty batteries or equipment, it should be interpreted as endotracheal tube displacement until proven otherwise.

Out-of-hospital care providers should adhere to local protocol when monitoring and documenting end-tidal CO_2 data. Successful endotracheal intubation should result in the generation of the classic end-tidal CO_2 waveform. Target ventilation according to protocol. **Generally speaking, desirable levels of end-tidal CO_2 range from 35 to 40 mm Hg.** Critically ill patients may require adjustments to their mechanical ventilation plan. Care providers engaged in critical care transport should guide ventilation accordingly; this may involve the utilization of additional data such as arterial blood gases.

AEROSOLIZED MEDICATION

Purpose

Aerosolization is a rapid, effective, noninvasive method for administering medications. The inhalation route provided by aerosolized medications is preferred to IV/IM routes because it is effective at delivering medication while producing fewer systemic side effects. A majority of applications in the prehospital environment are directed toward the treatment of respiratory symptoms and disease. Indications include exacerbations of asthma or chronic obstructive pulmonary disease (COPD) and croup (laryngotracheobronchitis). Aerosolization is also used as adjunct therapy in anaphylaxis[30-32] and in patients in whom IV access cannot be established.

Patient Selection

All patients who require bronchodilator therapy can benefit from aerosolized medications. The methodology will differ, however, based on the patient's level of consciousness, respiratory effort, and severity of symptoms. Aerosolized medications may be delivered via a metered dose inhaler (MDI) and spacer (Figure 22-34), an oxygen-driven nebulizer device (Figure 22-35), or an MDI injection into a ventilator or a bi-level positive airway pressure (BIPAP) circuit. In alert compliant patients, MDI therapy is faster and more effective than nebulizer therapy.[31] Given their smaller size and self-contained nature, MDIs are ideally suited for prehospital care.

A syringe atomizer (Figure 22-36) has become a popular method for prehospital administration of intranasal medications (e.g., naloxone, a reversing agent for opioid overdose) and for inducing nasopharyngeal anesthesia prior to nasotracheal intubation or nasogastric tube insertion. This device creates a fine mist to coat the mucosal surfaces, facilitating rapid systemic absorption as well as localized effects for anesthetics (Figure 22-37).

Risks and Precautions

In any patient receiving aerosolized therapy, frequently assess vital signs (heart rate, respiratory rate, oxygen saturation, end-tidal CO_2 [if available]) and monitor the patient for fatigue and pending respiratory failure. Follow local guidelines for the dosing and dilution of aerosolized medications.

Equipment

- For administration.
  - Peak flow meter.
  - Medication (albuterol/salbutamol, terbutaline, racemic epinephrine) as inhalation solution for nebulization or prefilled MDI.
  - Large volume spacer for MDI.
  - Nebulizer apparatus with oxygen supply at 10 to 12 L/min.

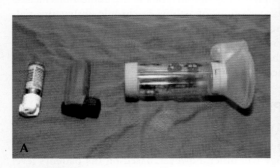
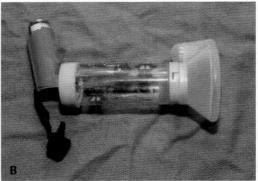

FIGURE 22–34

A, Metered-dose inhaler (MDI) and spacer—disassembled. **B**, MDI—assembled. Photos courtesy of Jim Burger, www.burgerphoto.com.

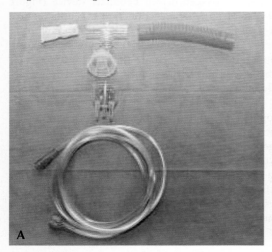
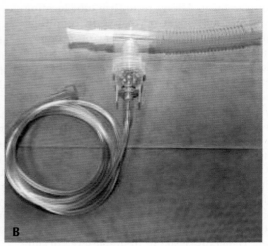

FIGURE 22–35

A, Air/oxygen nebulizer—disassembled. **B**, Nebulizer—assembled. Photos courtesy of Jim Burger, www.burgerphoto.com.

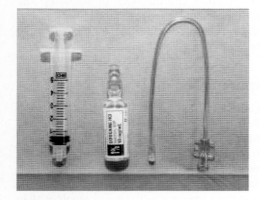

FIGURE 22–36

Syringe atomizer assembly. Photo courtesy of Jim Burger, www.burgerphoto.com.

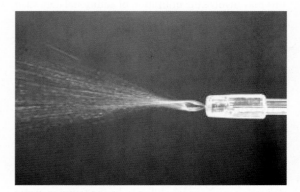

FIGURE 22–37

Fine mist created by a syringe atomizer. Photo courtesy of Jim Burger, www.burgerphoto.com.

- For patient assessment.
  - Stethoscope.
  - Blood pressure cuff.
  - Pulse oximeter.
  - End-tidal CO_2 monitor.
  - Peak-flow monitor.
- Atomizer assembly (atomizer device, syringe, medication).

Patient Positioning

As with all respiratory conditions, patients will be able to ventilate more effectively and with less effort while sitting upright. If no contraindication exists, they should be placed in a position of comfort, sitting upright.

Anesthesia and Procedural Monitoring

Patients receiving aerosolized therapy should be monitored closely for response to therapy. If they do not respond to initial aerosolized medications, the care providers should consider more aggressive interventions such as intubation and parenteral β-agonists or epinephrine. Routine monitoring includes vital sign assessment and pulse oximetry. If available, end-tidal CO_2 monitoring will provide a quantifiable measure of respiratory effectiveness. Always monitor the patient's clinical appearance and watch for fatigue, intercostal retraction, accessory muscle use, and pending respiratory failure.

Step-by-Step Technique

Assess Peak Flow

If the patient is not in extremis, obtain a peak expiratory flow rate (PEFR) reading prior to initiation of therapy. Peak flow is not a good test for assessing disease, but it has a role in determining response to therapy. If a patient's baseline nonsymptomatic PEFR is known, the response to therapy can be assessed with serial PEFR measurements. Record the baseline PEFR and the value during therapy. A goal >60% baseline is desired in response to initial therapy.[33]

MDI Administration

Inform the patient regarding the procedure you are about to perform. Insert a metered dose inhaler into the proper end of the spacer. Provide the device to the patient and have him or her place the mouthpiece in the mouth. For pediatric patients, apply the face mask to the child's face so it achieves a seal (Figure 22-38). Depress the MDI so the spacer fills with aerosolized medication. Instruct the patient to take a deep inspiration. One-way flap valves in the spacer should draw the medication into the lungs upon inspiration and divert exhalation away from the spacer chamber. Have the patient take a few breaths to clear the chamber before actuating the MDI again. Consult local protocols for dosing guidance.

Nebulizer Administration

Assemble the plastic nebulizer device. Add medication to the chamber. It is less likely to spill when added via the output port, as opposed to adding medication before final assembly of the device. Connect the nebulizer to an oxygen source and provide oxygen at a rate of 10 to 12 L/min. This rate produces finer atomization of the medication, resulting in greater distribution of medication to the bronchioles and smaller airways.[30]

Atomizer Administration   Draw the medication into a syringe of appropriate size (3–5 mL). Consult local protocols for guidance on permitted medications and doses. Connect the atomizer to the syringe. Position the patient upright. If the patient is alert, advise him or her that some of the liquid may run down the back of the throat. Insert only the tip of the atomizer into the nasal orifice. Aim the atomizer tip straight back as you would a nasal trumpet (airway). Briskly compress the syringe

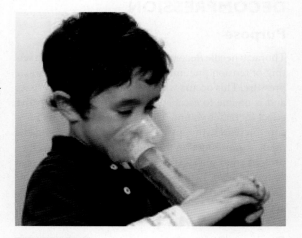

FIGURE 22–38

Self-administered metered-dose inhaler with pediatric mask. Photo courtesy of Jim Burger, www.burgerphoto.com.

to administer the medicine. If you are administering naloxone, spray it in both nares to increase surface area for mucosal absorption.

Outcomes Assessment Reassess the patient's vital signs, oxygen saturation, $ETCO_2$ if available, and clinical response to therapy. Patients who demonstrate worsening respiratory failure (fatigue, hypoventilation, diminished breath sounds, tripoding, or accessory muscle use) require immediate intervention, which may include intubation and mechanical ventilation.

Complications

This procedure is fairly simple, and complications are uncommon. Be alert for equipment failure, such as a faulty MDI or an empty or leaking nebulizer chamber. Be cognizant of the oxygen supply. Monitor the patient for worsening respiratory function.

Follow-up and Patient Instructions

Most patients who require atomization therapy in the field should be transported to a hospital for continued treatment and monitoring. A window of 2 to 3 hours is required to determine the effectiveness of initial treatments.[30] Patients should be observed for sustained improvement in respiratory function, measured by improvement of PEFR to >60% of baseline, and corresponding clinical improvement.[30,33]

THORACIC NEEDLE DECOMPRESSION

Purpose

Thoracic needle decompression is indicated in the setting of tension pneumothorax to relieve intrathoracic pressure. This occurs when air enters the pleural space and is unable to escape. The resulting one-way valve effect increases volume with each breath.[34,35] As pressure increases, the ipsilateral lung collapses and the mediastinum shifts to the contralateral side. Increased pressure and physical compression result in reduced venous return, hypotension, and hypoxemia. Needle decompression is a lifesaving technique when applied appropriately.

Patient Selection

Patients with suspected tension pneumothorax based on clinical findings should undergo needle decompression. This procedure is not indicated in the field for spontaneous pneumothoraces or stable patients with penetrating chest trauma. Findings suggestive of tension pneumothorax include the following:[34]

- Chest pain.
- Dyspnea.
- Anxiety.
- Tachycardia.
- Tachypnea.
- Hyper-resonance on affected side.
- Diminished breath sounds on affected side.
- Hypotension.
- Hypoxia/cyanosis.
- Distention of neck veins (jugular venous distention).
- Tracheal deviation toward contralateral side.

Risks and Precautions

Bloodborne pathogen precautions should be employed when performing this procedure. Landmarks must be identified to reduce the potential for injury to the internal thoracic artery. Placement of a catheter creates a pneumothorax. Patients who undergo needle decompression and are placed on positive-pressure ventilators will require tube thoracostomy with suction to prevent iatrogenic tension pneumothorax.

Equipment

- Personal protective equipment (gloves, gown, mask).
- Antiseptic cleaner (Betadine or chlorhexidine).
- 16- or 14-gauge IV catheter (>8 cm length).[36]
- Flutter valve (commercial [Heimlich™] or makeshift).
- Adhesive tape.

Patient Positioning

Patients undergoing this procedure are generally victims of trauma and should be positioned according to trauma protocols with full spinal immobilization. Be aware of respiratory difficulty when the patient is supine. Support ventilation and oxygenation as required. Monitor for emesis and potential airway obstruction.

Anesthesia and Procedural Monitoring

Monitor the patient's clinical appearance, mental status, and vital signs in accordance with standard trauma protocols. If assisting ventilations with a bag-valve mask or ventilator, monitor for increased ventilatory resistance, which can indicate tension pneumothorax or a dislodged decompression catheter.

Step-by-Step Technique

If patient is alert, advise him or her of the procedure prior to beginning. Apply 100% oxygen via non–rebreather mask.[36] Verify the proper side for tube insertion by auscultation, percussion, and other findings listed above in the section on patient selection. Locate the second/third intercostal space at the mid-clavicular line (Figure 22-39). Prepare the site with antiseptic (Figure 22-40). Insert a 14- or 16-gauge IV catheter perpendicular to the chest wall (Figure

22-41). The needle should pass just superior to the third rib, avoiding the vasculature running inferior to the second rib. The thickness of the chest wall varies, depending on the patient's musculature; the typical range is 2 to 6 cm.[36]

Slowly advance the catheter until you hear a rush of air or loose resistance from the chest wall. Advance the catheter to the hub while holding the needle securely in place (Figure 22-42). Remove the needle. Depending on your IV catheter, you may not get air return until the needle is removed. Apply a flutter valve,[37] which can be crafted from the finger of a pliable latex glove (Figure 22-43). An alternative method is to apply a three-sided occlusive dressing used for sucking-chest wounds (Figure 22-44). The dressings must prevent air from being drawn into the pleural

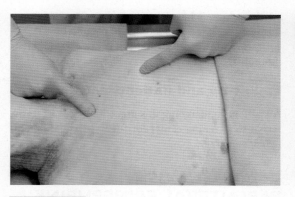

FIGURE 22–39

Locate second–third intercostal space, mid-clavicular line. Photo courtesy of Jim Burger, www.burgerphoto.com.

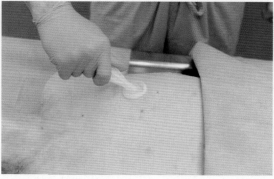

FIGURE 22–40

Prepare site with antiseptic. Photo courtesy of Jim Burger, www.burgerphoto.com.

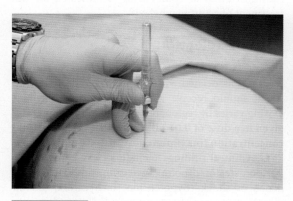

FIGURE 22–41

Insert a 16- or 14-gauge catheter perpendicular to the chest wall until a rush of air is felt/heard or chest wall resistance ceases. Photo courtesy of Jim Burger, www.burgerphoto.com.

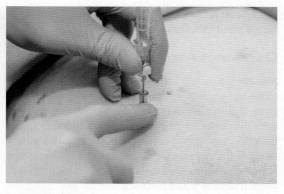

FIGURE 22–42

Advance the catheter to its hub while holding needle securely in place. Photo courtesy of Jim Burger, www.burgerphoto.com.

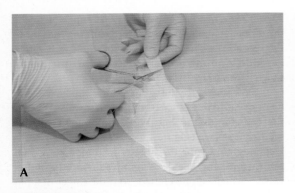
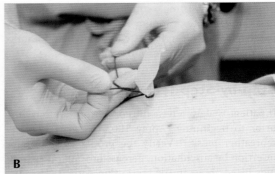

FIGURE 22–43

A, Create a one-way flutter valve with a finger clipped from a glove. **B**, Secure flutter valve to catheter with suture or string. Photos courtesy of Jim Burger, www.burgerphoto.com.

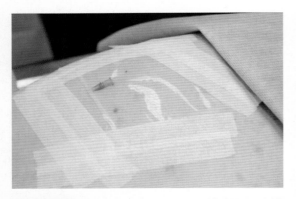

FIGURE 22–44

Alternative one-way valve with three-sided occlusive dressing. Photo courtesy of Jim Burger, www.burger photo.com.

space upon patient inspiration and must permit air to escape upon exhalation.

Outcomes Assessment

Monitor the patient for clinical improvement in mental status and respiratory effort. Continue to monitor vital signs. If the patient does not improve with therapy, consider the possibility of bilateral pneumothoraces and, if indicated, repeat the process on the contralateral side.[38] Monitor the catheter for displacement and recurrence of tension pneumothorax. If the catheter becomes dislodged, remove it and place another catheter using the same technique as described above.

Complications

Injury to the internal thoracic artery can result in hemorrhage and hemothorax. Placement without proper

sterile technique has the potential to cause infection. Positive-pressure ventilation without chest tube thoracostomy and decompression can cause tension pneumothorax.

Follow-up and Patient Instructions

All patients undergoing this procedure must be transferred to a trauma center for further evaluation and management.

ANAPHYLAXIS – PARENTERAL EPINEPHRINE ADMINISTRATION (EPIPEN®)

Purpose

Administration of epinephrine is indicated for the treatment of acute anaphylaxis.

Patient Selection

Patients with acute IgE-mediated hypersensitivity reactions associated with respiratory and/or signs of shock should receive intramuscular epinephrine.[39] Dosing varies by region, but **epinephrine is generally given in a dose of 0.01 milligrams/kg IM of a 1:1000 concentration (maximum dose, 0.3–0.5 milligrams/ kg).**[39] Clinical findings include airway compromise (stridor, stertor, drooling, wheezing, apnea) and evidence of shock (hypotension, tachycardia, altered mental status, poor tissue perfusion).[40]

Risks and Precautions

Epinephrine is lifesaving in acute anaphylaxis. Higher mortality is associated with delayed administration of epinephrine in anaphylaxis.[39] However, if used inappropriately, it can result in serious morbidity and mortality.[41] Elderly people and patients with underlying cardiac disease are at higher risk for iatrogenic cardiac arrhythmias and coronary ischemia resulting from epinephrine administration. This is especially true when 1:10,000 solutions are given intravenously. There are no absolute contraindications to using epinephrine for acute anaphylaxis. Use is guided by the patient's acuity level and risk of untoward effects.

Equipment

- **EpiPen® or a comparable autoinjector** (0.3 or 0.15 milligrams per dose) (see Figure 22-45).
- 25-gauge needle and syringe for manual administration of 1:1000 epinephrine.

Patient Positioning

Place the patient in a position of comfort to facilitate respiration or in a supine position if he or she is hypotensive.

Anesthesia and Procedural Monitoring

Patients receiving epinephrine are in extremis and should receive advanced monitoring. Provide 100% O_2 via non–rebreather mask. Place an IV line (18 gauge or larger) for fluid resuscitation and connect the patient to a cardiac monitor. Monitor blood pressure and oxygen saturation with a pulse oximeter. Do not delay the administration of epinephrine while establishing an IV line or connecting the patient to monitoring devices.

Step-by-Step Technique

Advise the patient you are about to administer epinephrine and that it will likely make his or her heart race and cause a feeling of anxiety. Wipe the injection site with an alcohol swab. Inject the initial dose of epinephrine intramuscularly. Dosing should follow local prescribing guidelines. Reassess the patient's vital signs every few minutes and observe for response to therapy.

Outcomes Assessment

Observe the patient for improvement in vital signs and respiratory status. Patients who respond to therapy generally experience improvement within a few minutes after epinephrine administration. Failure to respond (i.e., continued shock or respiratory distress) should prompt repeat dosing either intramuscularly[39] or intravenously,[42] according to local protocol.

Complications

Observe the patient for adverse effects, such as tachyarrhythmia, cardiac arrest, or acute coronary syndromes. Obtain a 12-lead electrocardiogram and follow Advanced Cardiac Life Support guidelines as indicated. Avoid the use of β-blockers in patients with acute anaphylaxis because they can worsen respiratory distress.[39]

Follow-up and Patient Instructions

All patients who receive epinephrine should be transported to the hospital for further evaluation and monitoring of their anaphylaxis.

Acknowledgments

The authors express their appreciation to Richard Levitan, MD, for sharing his expertise in airway management techniques and for providing illustrations used in this chapter. They also gratefully acknowledge the photographic skills of Jim Burger (www.burgerphoto.comj). The manuscript was copy edited

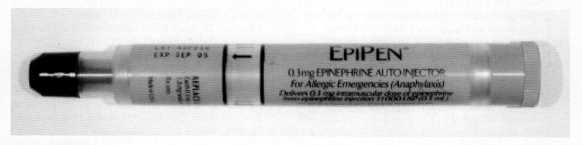

FIGURE 22–45

EpiPen™—epinephrine autoinjector. Photo courtesy of Jim Burger, www.burgerphoto.com.

by Linda J. Kesselring, M.S., E.L.S., the technical editor in the Department of Emergency Medicine at the University of Maryland School of Medicine.

References

1. Reid DC, Henderson R, Sabol L, et al. Etiology and clinical course of missed spine fractures. *J Trauma* 27: 980, 1987.
2. Kheterpal S, Martin L, Shanks AM, Tremper KK. Prediction and outcomes of impossible mask ventilation: a review of 50,000 anesthetics. *Anesthesiology* 110(4): 891, 2009.
3. Walls RM, Murphy MF. *Manual of Emergency Airway Management.* 3rd ed. Philadelphia, PA: Lippincott Williams & Wilkins; 2004:43–51.
4. Aufderheide TP. Hyperventilation-induced hypotension during cardiopulmonary resuscitation. *Circulation* 109(16): 1960, 2004.
5. Sellick BA. Cricoid pressure to control regurgitation of stomach contents during induction of anaesthesia. *Lancet* 2: 404, 1961.
6. Brimacombe JR, Berry AM. Cricoid pressure. *Can J Anaesth* 44(4): 414, 1997.
7. Smith KJ, Dobranowski J, Yip G, et al. Cricoid pressure displaces the esophagus: an observational study using magnetic resonance imaging. *Anesthesiology* 99: 60, 2003.
8. Nolan JP, Deakin CD, Soar J, et al. European Resuscitation Council guidelines for resuscitation 2005. Section 4. Adult advanced life support. *Resuscitation* 67(suppl 1): 539, 2005.
9. Lockey D, Davies G, Coats T. Survival of trauma patients who have prehospital tracheal intubation without anaesthesia or muscle relaxants: observational study. *BMJ* 323(7305): 141, 2001.
10. Li J, Murphy-Lavoie H, Bugas C, et al. Complications of emergency intubation with and without paralysis. *Am J Emerg Med* 17(2): 141, 1999.
11. Warner KJ, Carlbom D, Cooke C, et al. Paramedic training for proficient prehospital endotracheal intubation. *Prehosp Emerg Care* 14:(1): 103, 2010.
12. Levitan RM, Kelly JJ, Kinkle WC, Fasano C. Light intensity of curved layrngoscope blades in Philadelphia emergency departments. *Ann Emerg Med* 50(3): 253, 2007.
13. Levitan RM, Pisaturo JT, Kinkle WC, et al. Stylet bend angles and tracheal tube passage using a straight-to-cuff shape. *Acad Emerg Med* 13(12): 1255, 2006.
14. Levitan RM. Head-elevated laryngoscopy position: improving laryngeal exposure during laryngoscopy by increasing head elevation. *Ann Emerg Med* 41(3): 322, 2003.
15. Schmitt HJ, Mang H. Head and neck elevation beyond the sniffing position improves laryngeal view in cases of difficult direct laryngoscopy. *J Clin Anesth* 14(5): 335, 2002.
16. Collins JS, Lemmens HJ, Brodsky JB, et al. Laryngoscopy and morbid obesity: a comparison of the "sniff" and "ramped" positions. *Obes Surg* 14(9): 1171, 2004.
17. Benumof JL, Dagg R, Benumof R. Critical hemoglobin desaturation will occur before return to an unparalyzed state following 1 mg/kg intravenous succinylcholine. *Anesthesiology* 87(4): 979, 1997.
18. Blumer JL. Clinical pharmacology of midazolam in infants and children. *Clin Pharmacokinet* 35(1): 37, 1998.
19. Nordt SP, Clark RF. Midazolam: a review of therapeutic uses and toxicity. *J Emerg Med* 15(3): 357, 1997.
20. Hirota K, Hotomo N, Hashimoto Y, et al. Effects of thiopental on airway calibre in dogs: direct visualization method using a superfine fibreoptic bronchoscope. *Br J Anaesth* 81(1): 203, 1998.
21. Veselis RA, Reinsel RA, Feshchenko VA, Johnson R Jr. Information loss over time defines the memory defect of propofol: a comparative response with thiopental and dexmedetomidine. *Anesthesiology* 101(4): 831, 2004.
22. Veselis RA, Feshchenko VA, Reinsel RA, et al. Propofol and thiopental do not interfere with regional cerebral blood flow response at sedative concentrations. *Anesthesiology* 102:26, 2005.
23. *Drug Facts and Comparisons.* Philadelphia: Wolters Kluwer Health, Inc. 2008. http://www.wolterskluwer.com/WK/Press/Latest+News/2010/Feb/pr_3Feb10b.htm
24. Koller ME, Husby P. High-dose vecuronium may be an alternative to suxamethonium for rapid-sequence intubation. *Acta Anaesthesiol Scand* 37(5):465, 1993.
25. de Boer HD. Neuromuscular transmission: new concepts and agents. *J Crit Care* 24(1): 36, 2009.
26. Dunford JV, Davis DP, Ochs M, et al. Incidence of transient hypoxia and pulse rate reactivity during paramedic rapid sequence intubation. *Ann Emerg Med* 42: 721, 2003.
27. Ochs M, Davis D, Hoyt D, et al. Paramedic-performed rapid sequence intubation of patients with severe head injuries. *Ann Emerg Med* 40: 159, 2002.
28. Davis DP, Idris AH, Sise MJ, et al. Early ventilation and outcome in patients with moderate to severe traumatic brain injury. *Crit Care Med* 34(4): 1202, 2006.
29. Nagler J, Krauss B. Capnography: A valuable tool for airway management. *Emerg Med Clin North Am* 26: 881, 2008.
30. Heinrich W. Status asthmaticus in children: a review. *Chest* 19(6): 1913, 2001.
31. Rodrigo G, Rodrigo C, Jesse Hall H. Acute asthma in adults: a review. *Chest* 125: 1081, 2004.
32. Liberman D, Teach S. Management of anaphylaxis in children. *Pediatr Emerg Care* 24(12): 861, 2008.
33. Brenner BE. Asthma. Emedicine.medscape.com. Article 806890. July 2009.
34. Bjerke HS. Tension pneumothorax. Emedicine.medscape.com/article/432979-overview. May 2009.
35. Rankine J, Thomas A, Fluechter D. Diagnosis of pneumothorax in critically ill adults. *Postgrad Med J* 76: 399, 2000.
36. Mabry R, McManus J. Prehospital advances in the management of severe penetrating trauma. *Crit Care Med* 36(7 suppl): S258, 2008.

37. Baumann M, Strange C. Treatment of spontaneous pneumothorax: a more aggressive approach? *Chest* 112(3): 789, 1997.

38. Peek G, Morcos S, Cooper G. The pleural cavity. *BMJ* 320(7245): 1318, 2000.

39. McLean-Tooke A, Bethune C, Fay A, Spickett G. Adrenaline in the treatment of anaphylaxis: what is the evidence? *BMJ* 327(7427): 1332, 2003.

40. Kaplan AP. Angioedema. *World Allergy Organization* Journal. 1(6):103-113, *June 2008*

41. Johnston S, Unsworth J, Gompels M. Adrenaline given outside the context of life threatening allergic reactions. *BMJ* 326(7389): 589, 2003.

42. Lane RD, Bolte RG. Pediatric anaphylaxis. *Pediatr Emerg Care* 23(1): 49, 2007.

CHAPTER 23

Parenteral Access: IV, IO, IM, Rectal, Nasal

Terry Mulligan (IV, IM, Rectal, Nasal, Intraosseous sections)
Harm van de Pas (IV section)
Larry J. Miller (Intraosseous section)
Scotty Bolleter (Intraosseous section)
Judith Tintinalli (Rectal, Nasal sections)

INTRODUCTION

There are multiple situations that require the delivery of medications to patients in the prehospital setting. Fortunately, there are many routes for drug and fluid administration that we can use, including the IV, intraosseous (IO), IM, rectal, and nasal routes (Table 23-1).

Which route(s) are used depends on many different factors, including the patient's individual needs and complaints, the type and degree of injury or disease, the hemodynamic state, any specific allergies or other contraindications, as well as the medication(s) that one wishes to administer.

This section addresses the advantages, disadvantages, indications, and contraindications for each method of drug delivery.

PERIPHERAL VENOUS ACCESS (IV)

Purpose of Procedure

To establish secure parenteral access using a peripheral vein for patients needing fluid resuscitation or intravenous medication.

Risks and Precautions

In general, there are no contraindications for IV access when necessary and indicated. However, consider the following when selecting the site and consider alternate sites with the following conditions:

- Fracture proximal to the proposed IV access site.
- Skin or deep-tissue infection at the IV access site.
- Fracture or dislocation/burned/contaminated tissue at the IV access site.
- No pulse in the extremity at the potential IV access site.
- Latex and tape allergies to gloves and taping when applying and securing the IV line.

Equipment and Supplies

1. Tourniquet.
2. Gauze with skin disinfectant.
3. For peripheral IV sites with generous or excessive hair, apply sterile lubricant or even topical antimicrobial to slick the hair to the side. Do not shave the hair, as this could cause skin microlacerations and abrasions and increase the risk of infection.
4. IV cannula (with IV saline lock/cap, and/or IV line connected to IV fluids and primed if necessary).

Table 23–1	**Comparison of Several Routes for Prehospital Drug and Fluid Administration Not Including Central Venous Access, Transendotracheal, Subcutaneous, Intrathecal, and Others**	
Delivery Method	**Advantages**	**Disadvantages**
Oral	■ Painless, easy to use ■ Many medications in oral form	■ Slow onset of action
Rectal	■ Painless, could be uncomfortable	■ Variable bioavailability ■ Onset of action slower than IV ■ Many common medications not available for rectal administration
Buccal/sublingual	■ Painless, easy to use ■ More bioavailability than oral and rectal administration	■ If swallowed, some advantages are lost ■ Impaired children may not comprehend sublingual administration ■ Many common medications not available for sublingual administration
Intranasal	■ Painless ■ High bioavailability compared to oral and rectal administration ■ Easy and fast administration	■ Limited types of medications that can be delivered intranasally and nasal atomizer needed ■ Many medications are not adequately concentrated to achieve ideal dosing volumes, creating possible dosing errors ■ Mucosal health impacts absorption; sneezing and resistance to nasal atomization can be problems in children
Intramuscular	■ Generally known method ■ Many medications available for IM administration	■ Painful ■ Requires training for proper technique ■ Variable onset of action and bioavailability ■ Infection and neurovascular risk to patient ■ Needle stick risk to health-care provider
Intravenous	■ Generally known method ■ Many medications available for IV administration ■ High bioavailability ■ Rapid and predictable onset of action	■ Painful to establish IV access ■ Requires training ■ Infection risk to patient ■ Needle stick risk to health-care provider
Intraosseous (IO)	■ Easy to establish IO access ■ Technique is simple to teach ■ Multiple sites in pediatric and adult patients ■ All drugs and fluids that can be given by peripheral IV can be given IO	■ Requires special IO needles and insertion equipment ■ IV fluids must be given with pressure bag ■ Hand-driven, spring-loaded and powered devices can be cost-prohibitive ■ IO needle must be changed within 24 hours ■ If IO access is lost, that site no longer viable for IO access

Table courtesy of Dr. Terry Mulligan.

5. Fixation material: tape and gauze or prefabricated fixation tapes.
6. NS or other IV fluid.
7. Syringe 2, 5, or 10 mL, filled with NS for flush.
8. Blood collection tubes if necessary, with container/bag.
9. Sharps container.
10. Nonsterile gloves.

Patient Preparation

1. Inform the patient.
2. Always use universal precautions, including gloves. Sterile gloves are not necessary.

Veins of the Dorsal Hand

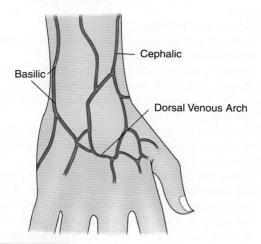

FIGURE 23–1

Veins of the dorsum of the hand. Location is variable, but veins become evident when distended from the tourniquet.

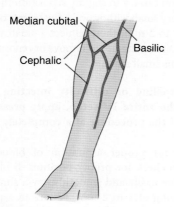

FIGURE 23–2

Veins of the forearm and antecubital fossa.

3. **Site selection hints**: Learn and use anatomic landmarks for selection of best vein for venipuncture.
   - Veins at the back of the hand or preferably larger veins on the forearm are particularly suitable for IV cannulation (Figure 23-1, Figure 23-2).
   - Large-bore cannulas are more easily inserted in the antecubital fossa than in the hand or forearm, but the arm must be kept straight and extended to prevent kinking of the IV tube and occlusion of flow.
   - Large-bore cannulas can also be inserted more easily in the dorsum of the foot if upper extremity veins are not accessible (Figure 23-3).
   - The external jugular vein (Figures 23-4, 23-5) can be cannulated (with proper training). Do not attempt venipuncture of the neck in a patient with a bleeding disorder (e.g., hemophiliac). Obviously, no tourniquet is used for this site.
4. Clear insertion site of clothing, and remove jewelry at or distal from the insertion site.
5. Apply the tourniquet (Figure 23-6) proximal to the insertion site, and tighten. To avoid overcompression and to make sure the tourniquet does not prevent arterial circulation, put one of your fingers underneath the tourniquet when tightening.
6. If needed, use sterile lubricant to move excessive hair growth aside.

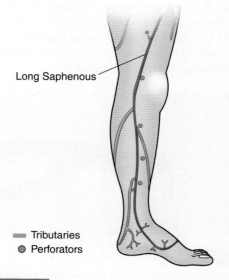

FIGURE 23–3

Veins of the lower extremity and dorsum of the foot.

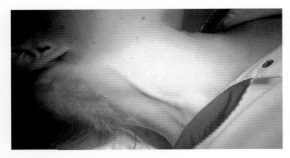

FIGURE 23–4

An external jugular vein suitable for cannulation.
The vein can be even more distended by placing the
patient in the Trendelenburg position by tilting the
stretcher so the level of the head is a few angles below
the level of the pelvis or by gently compressing the
vein near the clavicle so that it fills from above.
Photo courtesy of Harm van der Pas.

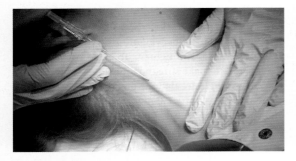

FIGURE 23–5

Compress the external jugular vein above the clavicle
so it distends, and then direct the needle into the distended vein. Since the skin of the neck can be surprisingly tough, skin puncture should be gentle but direct.
Photo courtesy of Harm van der Pas.

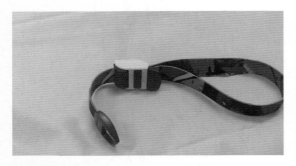

FIGURE 23–6

Tourniquet with easy release feature. Press the tab to
release the tourniquet. Photo courtesy of Harm van
der Pas.

7. Have the patient flex his or her wrist or make a fist
   a few times.
8. Mild tapping of the insertion site might engorge
   the vein, improving visualization and locali-
   zation.

Procedure

1. Pull the skin tight to fix the vein (Figure 23-7).
2. Enter the skin at an angle of 45 degrees. Puncture
   the skin and introduce the catheter into the vein a
   few millimeters until you see a "flash"—this is a
   small amount of blood that enters the back end of
   the cannula (Figure 23-8).
3. Pull back the needle a bit, holding the cannula in
   place.
4. Release the tourniquet.
5. Advance the cannula over the needle into the vein
   while holding the needle in place.
6. Fixate the cannula with tape (Figure 23-9).
7. Remove the needle from the cannula and put it
   in the sharps container immediately. Save the
   end-cap.
8. Close the end of the cannula with the end-cap of the
   needle, or place the prepared saline-lock on the
   cannula.
9. Check the correct position of the cannula using
   the following techniques: Test for proper fluid
   injection with 1 to 2 mL NS to verify that the
   catheter is in place. This should be effortless, and
   no skin swelling should appear. If you observe a
   swelling or a collection of fluid outside of the
   vein or under the skin surface, or if the amount
   of strength used to inject is not very smooth and
   easy, the IV most likely is not in the vein. In this
   case, you can try to slightly reposition the catheter
   with very small withdrawal adjustments of no more
   than 1 to 2 mm, then reinject a small volume of
   fluid. Do not attempt to remove or reposition more
   than this small amount.

   **If swelling or difficulty injecting persists,
   remove the entire IV setup, apply pressure, and
   reattempt the procedure at a completely different
   site.**
   Test for proper aspiration of blood with a
   syringe to check for proper position. If blood does
   not aspirate easily and smoothly, try a similar small
   repositioning of 1 to 2 mm. Failure to aspirate can
   imply that the cannula is not in the correct position;
   therefore remove the cannula and access another
   venous site.

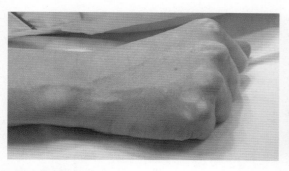

FIGURE 23–7

Veins on the dorsum of the hand, distended with a tourniquet in place. Photo courtesy of Harm van der Pas.

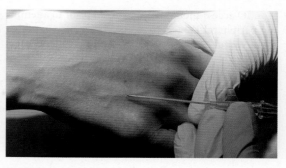

FIGURE 23–8

Insert the needle bevel up. Photo courtesy of Harm van der Pas.

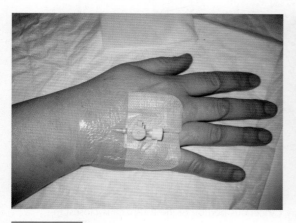

FIGURE 23–9

Securely tape the IV cannula in place. Photo courtesy of Harm van der Pas.

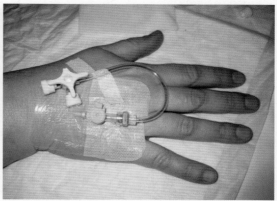

FIGURE 23–10

Saline lock to keep the IV open. Photo courtesy of Harm van der Pas.

Postprocedure Care

Secure the IV and saline lock (Figure 23-10) with appropriate dressing, gauze, tape and/or commercially available kits.

INTRAOSSEOUS ACCESS

Purpose

Intraosseous access (IO) is an immediate, reliable, and safe treatment tool for the rapid administration of lifesaving medications and fluids. IO is the emergent vascular access gold standard in pediatrics and is the first alternative to a difficult or impossible peripheral IV in adults. IO anatomy is seen in Figures 23-11, 23-12, and 23-13.

Patient Selection

Patients who should be considered for IO access are those in need of immediate *vascular access* for administration of intravenous medications or fluids and those in whom peripheral access is either difficult or impossible. These include patients who present with an emergency such as

1. Any medical or traumatic condition where fluids or medications are urgently needed.
2. Respiratory compromise (Sa_{O2} 90% *after appropriate oxygen therapy* or respiratory rate of <10 or >40 minutes).
3. Hemodynamic instability (systolic BP of <70 mm Hg).
4. Altered mental status (Glasgow Coma Score of 8 or less).

IO access should be considered prior to attempting peripheral IV access in any emergency in which rapid vascular access is critical and peripheral veins are judged to be difficult:

1. Cardiac arrest (medical or traumatic).
2. Profound hypovolemia with altered mental status.
3. Patient in extremis with immediate need for delivery of medications and/or fluids.

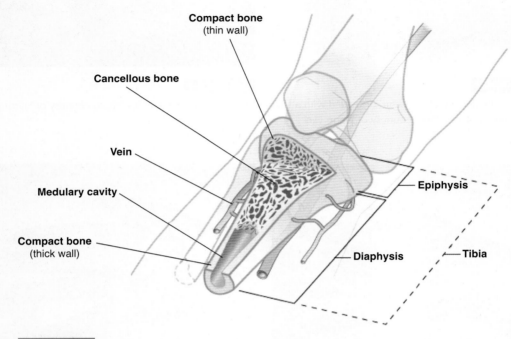

FIGURE 23–11

Anatomy of adult long bones. Note that the spongy cancellous portion of the IO space is closest to the ends of the diaphysis. Reprinted with permission of Dr. Larry Miller.

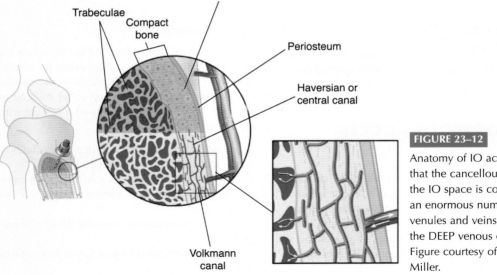

FIGURE 23–12

Anatomy of IO access. Note that the cancellous portion of the IO space is connected by an enormous number of small venules and veins directly to the DEEP venous circulation. Figure courtesy of Dr. Larry Miller.

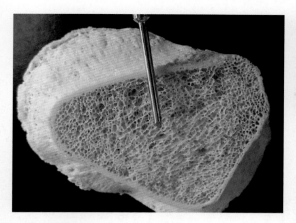

Cross-section of the proximal tibia in a 26-year-old male. This is the proper position for IO needle insertion for the proximal tibial site (more on this below). Note the very large luminal diameter of the cancellous IO space; this "target" lumen is much larger compared to the diameter of the IO needle versus the luminal diameter of an IV catheter versus a typical peripheral vein. Reprinted with permission of Dr. Larry Miller.

Risks and Precautions

IO access has an extremely low complication rate. Table 23-2 lists contraindications and relative contraindications to IO placement. Since some contraindications would apply to only one potential IO site, review all potential IO access sites before abandoning the procedure. IO sites include the sternum, humerus, distal femur, and the proximal and distal tibia. These locations have the most accessible IO fluid flow rates. **Specifically developed sternal access needle sets must be used for the sternal approach to avoid penetration of the mediastinum or heart. Sites that are not considered routine are the distal radius, clavicle, and anterior pelvis.** Do not attempt a second IO in the same bone within 24 hours of a previous attempt because this could result in extravasation of fluid or blood through the previous IO puncture site.

IO access requires specially developed devices. At present there are several US Federal Drug Administration (FDA) and Conformité Européene (CE)–approved devices used to obtain IO access, including but not limited to (see Table 23-3):

- Jamshidi®.
- Illinois Sternal®.
- Cook®.

Table 23–2	**Relative and Absolute Contraindications to Intraosseous Infusion**

1. Acute fracture of the bone selected for IO infusion
2. Excessive tissue at the insertion site with the absence of palpable landmarks
3. Recent significant orthopedic procedures near the insertion site, such as total knee replacement
4. Limb prosthesis or hardware
5. Infection at the site selected for IO insertion
6. IO placement in same limb within 24 hours

Table original by Dr. Terry Mulligan.

- F.A.S.T. 1/Pyng®.
- B.I.G.–Bone Injection Gun®.
- EZ-IO® (battery-powered drill).

Equipment

- Appropriate IO needle set (refer to Table 23-3).
- Chlorhexidine or alcohol swabs.
- IV extension set.
- 10-mL syringe.
- IV NS (or suitable sterile fluid).
- Pressure bag or infusion pump.
- 2% lidocaine (must be preservative-free).

Patient Positioning

IO access can be accomplished in the most difficult environments and awkward positions. The position of the patient is not as important as the position/accessibility of the presenting IO site. Understanding and identifying the access sites will prevent complications when geographic or anatomic challenges are present.

Anesthesia and Procedural Considerations

Commercial IO devices come in various lengths for different applications. Depending on the IO device, needles tend to come in *pediatric* and *adult* sizes, or in *small, medium,* and *large* sizes. **Be sure to select the correct length for the correct patient.**

Table 23-3	Intraosseous Devices			
Intraosseous Device Name	Photo of Device	Other Equipment Needed	Overview of Insertion Technique	Details/Comments
Cook™		– IV line – IV fluid – Pressure bag for higher pressure fluid infusion – 10-mL syringe for initial FLUSH – 2% lidocaine for infusion pain control – securing device/equipment	Oval portion of handle fits into palm and needle is twisted or screwed in by hand	Mostly used for pediatrics since adult bones are harder and more difficult to manually introduce needles
Monoject (Jamshidi)™		– IV line – IV fluid – Pressure bag for higher pressure fluid infusion – 10 mL syringe for initial FLUSH – 2% lidocaine for infusion pain control – securing device/ equipment	Curved portion of handle fits into palm and needle is twisted in or screwed in by hand	Mostly used in pediatrics since adult bones are harder and more difficult to manually introduce needles
Illinois Sternal™		– IV line – IV fluid – Pressure bag for higher pressure fluid infusion – 10 mL syringe for initial FLUSH – 2% lidocaine for infusion pain control – securing device/equipment	Round portion of handle fits into palm and needle is twisted in or screwed in by hand	Mostly used in pediatrics since adult bones are harder and more difficult to manually introduce needles

Table 23–3 Intraosseous Devices (Continued)

Intraosseous Device Name	Photo of Device	Other Equipment Needed	Overview of Insertion Technique	Details/Comments
F.A.S.T. 1, - Pyng™		– IV line – IV fluid – Pressure bag for higher pressure fluid infusion – 10-mL syringe for initial FLUSH – 2% lidocaine for infusion pain control – special securing device/equipment – special removal device is needed	– Device is pushed into manubrium at 90-degree angle – ring of needles acts as probe to ensure that center IO needle enters at proper depth – removal requires special device	– Designed for adult sternum – Manually inserts 10 probes and one IO needle at once
B.I.G. - Bone Injection Gun™	 	– IV line – IV fluid – Pressure bag for higher pressure fluid infusion – 10-mL syringe for initial FLUSH – 2% lidocaine for infusion pain control – securing device/equipment	– Shoots a needle into IO site via a high tension spring	–Used for adults only

(Continued)

Table 23–3   Intraosseous Devices (Continued)

Intraosseous Device Name	Photo of Device	Other Equipment Needed	Overview of Insertion Technique	Details/Comments
EZ-IO (Battery Powered Drill)™	Vidacare G-3 driver LD (45 mm) IO needle set attached 	– EZ-IO power driver – IV line – IV fluid – Pressure bag for higher pressure fluid infusion – 10-mL syringe for initial FLUSH – 2% lidocaine for infusion pain control – securing device/equipment	– Needles are selected based on patient size (small, medium, or large) – Device powers a hollow catheter into the medullary space	– Used in adults and children
EZ-Connect and Stabilizer: – For proximal humerus in adults and for all pediatrics IOs™				

Original by author and photos courtesy of Dr. Larry Miller.

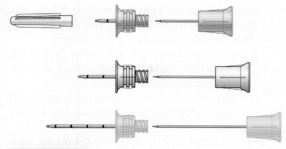

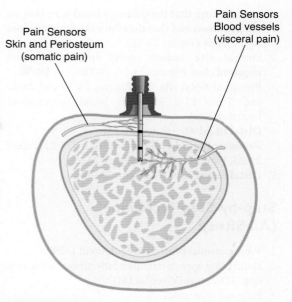

FIGURE 23–14

Shown are the three sizes/lengths of needles to be used with the EZ-IO® device. Note that the needles are marked at 5-mm divisions and have stylets that need to be in place when inserting the needle; they also need to be removed after insertion. Reprinted with permission of Dr. Larry Miller.

For most patients under 39 kg, a pediatric needle is appropriate. For most patients over 39 kg, a standard adult needle is appropriate. However, longer needles are preferred for use in the humerus and in any patient with excessive tissue over the insertion site (Figure 23-14).

Insertion of an IO device in unconscious patients causes mild to moderate discomfort, but this is usually no more painful than a peripheral IV placement. No subcutaneous or surface anesthesia is necessary for *IO insertion in a comatose patient or one with decreased mental status.*

However, ***IO infusion* for *conscious patients*** causes severe discomfort. Pain is usually registered by the patient as a deep ache or poorly localized discomfort, sometimes accompanied by nausea and/or sweating. This is due to the nature of somatic and visceral nociceptors (pain and pressure receptors) in the skin and in the medullary/IO space (Figure 23-15).

To alleviate the pain and discomfort of *IO infusions* after the IO has been inserted (step-by-step instructions for IO insertion are below):

■ Prior to IO syringe flush or continuous infusion in alert patients, slowly (over 30 to 60 seconds) administer lidocaine 2% (preservative-free) through the IO catheter. *Make sure that the patient has no allergies or sensitivity to lidocaine.*

■ For adult patients slowly administer 40 to 60 milligrams lidocaine 2% (preservative-free) into the intramedullary space.
   ■ Repeat an additional 20 milligrams of lidocaine IO after the syringe flush if necessary for further pain control.

FIGURE 23–15

Physiology of pain sensation with an IO device/ needle regarding insertion and infusion. The skin, superficial tissues, and periosteum are innervated by somatic pain fibers, which register well-localized pain sensation; this is very minimal in IO insertions compared with IV insertion. However, since the intramedullary space and the associated outflowing venous plexus are innervated with visceral pain fibers that register poorly localized, "deep aching" pain, the higher pressures and IV-pressure bags in IO infusions tend to cause conscious patients moderate to severe discomfort. Figure courtesy of Dr. Larry Miller.

■ For children, slowly administer 0.5 mg/kg lidocaine 2% (preservative-free) into the intramedullary space. Because of the small volume required, use a 1-mL syringe. **Or, dilute 1 mL of 2% lidocaine into 19 mL of saline. The resulting 20 mL specimen contains 1 milligram of lidocaine per milliliter.**

■ Titrate to effect. **Do not exceed 3 milligrams/kg lidocaine.**

FDA-approved intraosseous sites:

1. **Proximal humerus:** The **proximal humerus insertion** site is located directly on the most prominent aspect of the greater tubercle (see Table 23-4).

Make sure that the patient's hand is resting on the abdomen and that the elbow is adducted close to the body (Figure 23-16).

2. **Sternal site (adults only, specific product required)** (see Figures 23-17, 23-18).
3. **Proximal tibial site** (see Figures 23-19 and 23-20 and Table 23-5 Proximal Tibial Intraosseous Insertion Site).
4. **Distal tibial site** (Figure 23-21).
   Pediatric Considerations (see Figure 23-22, Figure 23-23, Figure 23-24, and Figure 23-25).
5. **Distal femur site** (see Figure 23-26).

Step-by-Step Technique (All Sites):

1. Wear personal protective equipment (PPE).
2. Determine appropriate indication/need for access (e.g., IO versus IV versus IM).
3. Rule out contraindications.
4. Locate appropriate insertion site (*consider all suitable locations prior to selection*).
5. Prepare insertion site using aseptic technique.
6. Prepare the appropriate needle set. NOTE: These needle sets are shown earlier in Table 23-3.

   Refer to the specific product instructions for further information. In general, these will include:

   - the IO needle.
   - the IO needle driver/handle.
   - a connector to an IV line, similar to a saline lock.
   - a securing device, where applicable/necessary.
   - aseptic wipes/dressing gauze.

7. Stabilize site and insert appropriate needle set.
8. Hold the hub with nondominant hand to stabilize the needle.
9. Remove stylet from catheter and place in approved sharps container.
10. Connect primed extension set (*prime extension set with lidocaine for conscious patients.*)
11. Confirm placement by noting that.
    - IO is firmly in position (avoid rocking or manipulation of the catheter).
    - Aspiration of blood/marrow is possible.
    - Ease of flushing.
    - Ease of intravenous flow (ensure placement of a pressure bag).
    - No evidence of extravasation into surrounding soft tissues.

12. Slowly administer appropriate dose of lidocaine 2% (preservative-free) IO to conscious patients; titrate to effect in the appropriate dosage.
    - For adult patients slowly administer 40 to 60 mL of lidocaine 2% (preservative- free) into the intramedullary space.
      - Repeat an additional 20 mL of lidocaine IO after the syringe flush if necessary for further pain control.
    - For children slowly administer 0.5 mL/kg lidocaine 2% (preservative-free) into the intramedullary space.
      - Because of the small quantity required, a 1-mL syringe should be used.
      - Or dilute 1 mL of 2% lidocaine into 19 mL of saline. The resulting 20-mL specimen contains 1 milligram of lidocaine/mL.
13. Syringe bolus (flush) the IO catheter with the appropriate amount of normal saline (3–5 mL; repeat as needed).
14. Begin infusion with pressure (syringe bolus, pressure bag, or infusion pump) when applicable.
15. Stabilize needle set with a commercial stabilizer, such as the EZ-stabilizer, or secure the needle with gauze padding and tape. Be sure not to place the tape circumferentially around the extremity.
    - Not every commercial IO needle requires or comes with a stabilizer.
    - The IO is usually firmly embedded in the bone and is not easy to dislodge, depending on the type of device used to insert the IO needle.
16. Monitor IO site and patient condition. Proper monitoring includes frequently watching for signs of swelling and extravasation, checking pulses, and measuring the circumference of the extremity.
17. Remove catheter within 24 hours.

   Important note: Safe use of an IO infusion system requires training. Become familiar with your system protocol AND have access to the specific training materials accompanying the device you intend to employ.

   AS WITH EVERY MEDICAL PROCEDURE, DO NOT ATTEMPT IO INSERTION UNTIL PROPERLY TRAINED BY A QUALIFIED INSTRUCTOR USING APPROPRIATE TRAINING EQUIPMENT AND SIMULATORS.

Table 23–4	**The Proximal Humeral Insertion Site for the Intraosseous Needle Insertion**

A. The photograph to the right shows the gross external anatomy of the shoulder and a graphic depiction of the hidden internal anatomic orientation of the humeral head (circle) and the humeral shaft (thick dashed line). The thin dashed lines can be used as a visual approximation of the deltoid/shoulder into *anterior, posterior,* and *middle* deltoid lines. Note that the greater tubercle and humeral head are both anterior to the middle deltoid line. The X marks the spot where the IO needle should be introduced—into the greater tubercle, anterior to the middle deltoid line

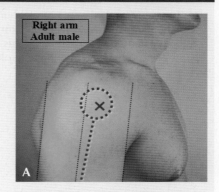

B. Another photograph showing the anterior/lateral position of the greater tubercle on the humeral head

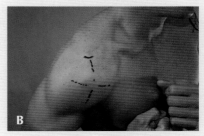

C. In a patient in the prone position, the humeral head and the greater tubercle can be located in the following fashion:
1. with one hand, grasp the acromioclavicular joint and the posterior shoulder
2. the humeral head is located in-between the fingers when the shoulder is grasped in this fashion

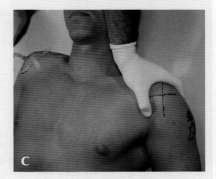

D. This photograph shows a graphic representation of the humeral head (the round part of the drawing), the greater tubercule (the intersection of the dotted lines), and the bicipital groove/biceps tendon (the thick line on the anterior portion of the humeral head). NOTE: This biceps tendon is more anterior than the greater tubercle and should be avoided. The insertion site is lateral to this groove

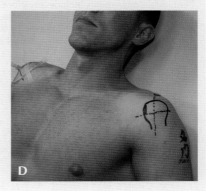

(Continued)

Table 23–4	**The Proximal Humeral Insertion Site for the Intraosseous Needle Insertion** *(Continued)*

E. This photograph shows a model humerus placed into proper anatomic relationship with this prone patient. NOTE: Since the greater tubercle of the humerus is anterolateral, the proper approach is from the anterolateral position

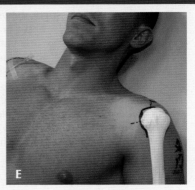

F. This renders the proximal humeral site as a preferable or acceptable site for IO access when the patient is in a confined space, such as in this military helicopter

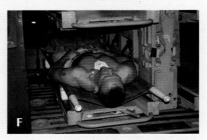

G. The medic shown here is placing an IO needle in the proximal humeral site, using the EZ-IO® device. However, any of the other (nonsternal) devices can be used at this site

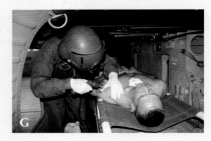

NOTE: When the proximal humeral site is used for IO access, the upper arm must then be secured to prevent any abduction (away from the body movement) or the IO needle can be forced out of its position by this movement. Permissible movements include any elbow, forearm, or hand motions or any minor upper arm motions that do not cause the humerus to force the IO needle into the glenoid lip (such as raising the arm over the level of the shoulder/head), thereby forcing the needle to come out of the bone.
Table original by Dr. Larry Miller. Photos courtesy of Dr. Larry Miller.

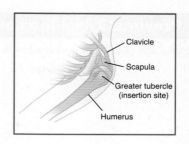

FIGURE 23–16

Insertion site for proximal humerus. Slide thumb up the anterolateral shaft of the humerus until you feel the greater tubercle, proximal to the surgical neck of the shaft of the humerus. The insertion site is 1 cm below the greater tubercle (which is approximately 1 cm above the surgical neck). Reprinted with permission of Dr. Larry Miller.

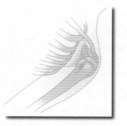
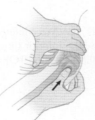
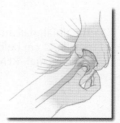

FIGURE 23–17

The sternal site is in the midline of the manubrium approximately 2 cm inferior to the sternal notch. Reprinted with permission of Dr. Larry Miller.

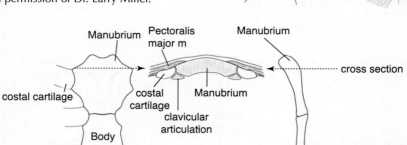

FIGURE 23–18

The sternal site is actually on the manubrium portion of the sternum. Note that the angle of the manubrium in most patients is not parallel to the floor or bed when the patient is lying prone but is instead at an angle when compared to the body of the sternum and to the anterior chest wall. This angle must be noted and appreciated when using a sternal device, since the IO needle needs to be inserted into the manubrium at a 90-degree angle to the *manubrium*, not at a 90-degree angle to the sternal body or to the anterior chest wall. Reprinted with permission of Dr. Larry Miller.

Table 23–5 | Proximal Tibial Intraosseous Insertion Site

1. Locate the patella and put two finger-breadths below the bottom tip

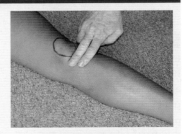

2. The tibial plateau is ALWAYS MEDIAL and inferior to the patella, 2 cm below the inferior tip of the patella and 1 cm medial. REMEMBER: BIG TOE = IO

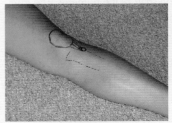

3. The tibial plateau is 2 cm inferior and 1 cm medial to the inferior tip of the patella. In this photograph, the X marks the IO insertion spot. NOTE: Since the tibial plateau is always MEDIAL, this must be the patient's LEFT LEG

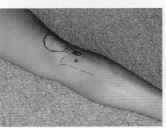

NOTE: This is a very good, reliable technique for finding the tibial plateau, especially in obese patients or in pediatric patients whose anatomic landmarks may be hard to palpate.
NOTE: No adverse effects or consequences result from placing the IO needle through the tibial tuberosity; however, the bony prominence is harder and considerably thicker. More lateral placement of the IO needle increases the chance of accidental dislodgement due to the proximity to caregivers and runs the risk of penetrating the fibular head and/or the proximal tibiofibular joint complex.
Original by author and photos courtesy of Dr. Larry Miller.

FIGURE 23–19

The proximal tibia insertion site is through the tibial plateau. NOTE: The tibial plateau is always MEDIAL. A useful mnemonic to remember on which side to insert the IO needle is "**BIG TOE = IO**"; that is, the big toe is always medial, on the same side of the tibia as the tibial plateau, which is where the IO must be inserted. Reprinted with permission of Dr. Larry Miller.

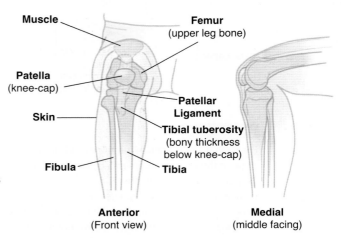

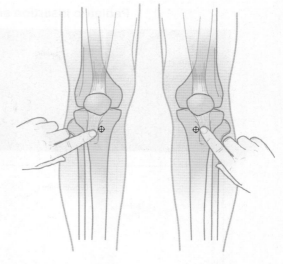

The **proximal tibia** insertion site. In adults, the tibial plateau is approximately 2 to 3 cm BELOW the patella and approximately 2 cm MEDIAL to the tibial tuberosity. In pediatric patients, the distances listed here must be adjusted downward depending on the size of the patient—see more information on this below. **NOTE: The tibial plateau is always MEDIAL.** Reprinted with permission of Dr. Larry Miller.

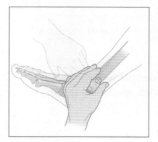
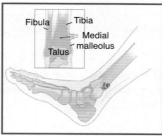
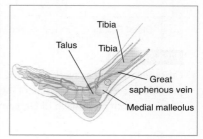

The distal tibial insertion site is located approximately 3 cm proximal to the most prominent aspect of the medial malleolus. The technique for locating this site is as follows: (1) locate the MEDIAL malleolus (remember the mnemonic "BIG TOE – IO"); and (2) three finger breadths or 3 cm PROXIMAL to the MEDIAL malleolus is the proper spot. NOTE: it is very important to insert the needle 3 cm proximal to the medial malleolus to avoid any insertion of the IO needle through the tibial-talar/mortise joint. Reprinted with permission of Dr. Larry Miller.

Pediatric IO Access

Potential IO access sites for children. While all of these sites are potentially acceptable, the proximal tibia is often the site of first choice because of the similarity of approach and landmarks to the adult patient. As always with any learned procedural skill, it is helpful for the practitioner to build his or her sensorimotor skills through laboratory and simulation practice for neonates, infants, and small pediatric patients. AS WITH EVERY MEDICAL PROCEDURE, YOU SHOULD NOT ATTEMPT IO INSERTION UNTIL PROPERLY TRAINED BY A QUALIFIED INSTRUCTOR USING APPROPRIATE TRAINING EQUIPMENT AND SIMULATORS. Reprinted with permission of Dr. Larry Miller.

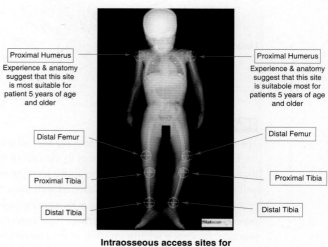

Intraosseous access sites for the pediatric patient

Pediatric Insertion sites: WITH IO needles

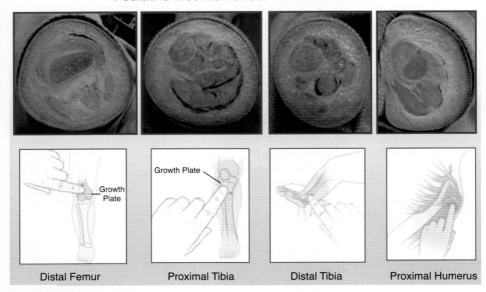

Distal Femur	Proximal Tibia	Distal Tibia	Proximal Humerus

FIGURE 23–23

Cross-sections of cadaveric pediatric IO insertion sites. From these two comparison figures, it is possible to see the relative size of the IO needle versus the intraosseous/intramedullary space. Reprinted with permission of Dr. Larry Miller.

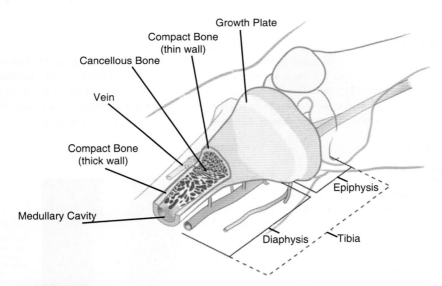

FIGURE 23–24

The location of the epiphyseal growth plate in relation to the tibial tuberosity. NOTE: the epiphysis is much more proximal to the end of the bone and to the joint space than the tibial tuberosity. Using the above techniques to locate the tibial tuberosity will ensure that the IO needle is inserted well away from the epiphysis. While the practice of inserting the IO needle at or near/through the epiphysis should be avoided, several studies have revealed that there have been no lasting complications of this practice. Reprinted with permission of Dr. Larry Miller.

The pediatric growth plate

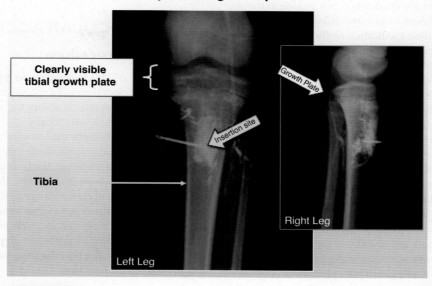

Clearly visible tibial growth plate

Growth Plate

Insertion site

Tibia

Right Leg

Left Leg

FIGURE 23–25

Position of IO needle in relation to pediatric epiphysis/growth plate. The needle is at least 2 to 3 cm away from the growth plate. NOTE: These x-rays show how IO injected contrast exits immediately into the deep central venous circulation, revealing that IO fluids and medications do not stay in the medullary space.

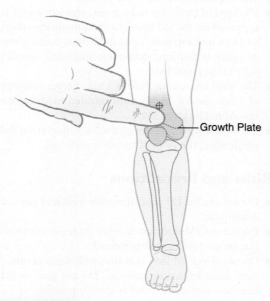

Growth Plate

FIGURE 23–26

The distal femur insertion site is located approximately 2 cm proximal to the patella and 1 cm medial, as shown. This site can be used in infants and pediatric patients only.

Outcomes Assessment

To confirm placement:

- IO is noted to be firmly in position (avoid rocking or manipulation of the catheter).
- Aspiration of blood/marrow is possible.
- Ease of flushing.
- Ease of intravenous flow (ensure placement of a pressure bag).
- No evidence of extravasation into surrounding soft tissues.
- Positive effect of medications (i.e., cardiac or RSI medications have desired effect).

Due to the anatomy of the IO space, flow rates may be slower than those achieved with an IV catheter.

- Always administer a rapid SYRINGE FLUSH with 10 mL of normal saline prior to infusion.
  - **"NO FLUSH = NO FLOW".**
- Repeat syringe flush (bolus) as needed.
- To improve continuous infusion flow rates, always use a syringe connected to an extension tube, pressure bag, or infusion pump.

Complications

Complications are uncommon but include extravasation, compartment syndrome, dislodgement, fracture, inability to infuse medication or fluids, and infection. Pain is an issue but not considered a complication.

Fluid extravasation into the surrounding soft tissues is usually the result of poor insertion technique (wobbling the needle set into position), complete perforation of the bone, or treatment-related manipulation of the catheter.

Compartment syndrome is a very rare complication almost exclusively related to placement in the proximal tibia. Compartment syndrome can develop if the catheter tip is placed into a muscle compartment followed by the introduction of fluids through the IO needle into the compartment. This complication would also be the direct result of a lack of appropriate monitoring both at and distal to the insertion site.

Dislodgement occurs if the catheter is not well secured or is manipulated after placement.

Fracture is very rare but has been reported in children if extreme force is used during insertion.

Absent or poor flow through the IO catheter is either related to poor site selection and placement, unrealistic flow expectations, not utilizing pressure to infuse fluids or (most frequently) failure to flush the IO site with 10 to 20 mL of NS before beginning infusion.

Infection rates are minimal when using appropriate technique and are not higher than those seen with peripheral IVs. Use sterile technique when placing the IO needle, and do not use IO access for more than 24 hours in order to minimize the risk of cellulitis or osteomyelitis.

Pain occurs with IO infusion if intramedullary anesthesia has not been provided. In conscious patients, consider supplementary parenteral narcotic analgesia. Recent studies have shown that humerus sites offer higher flow rates with less discomfort than other sites.

Follow-up and Patient Instructions

Most of the IO needles can be removed by attaching a 10-mL syringe to the embedded needle and twisting with the wrist while pulling outward in line with the shaft of the needle. NOTE: **Some IO devices such as the F.A.S.T. 1 (Pyng®) should not be removed in this fashion and require a special removal device. Please check the manufacturer's suggestions for removal of each type of device.**

After the IO catheter is removed, apply antibiotic ointment to the site and cover with a clean, dry bandage or dressing. Bleeding should be mild and controlled with direct pressure.

INTRAMUSCULAR ACCESS

Purpose of Procedure

An intramuscular (IM) injection is an injection given directly into the central area of a specific muscle. Blood vessels supplying that muscle absorb the injected medication and distribute it systemically.

Absorption is faster by the IM route than the subcutaneous route, and muscle tissue can often hold a large volume of fluid. However, the IV route provides a faster onset of action than the IM route. IM injection is used for the delivery of certain drugs if other routes are not available. Certain drugs (some benzodiazepines and antiepileptics) may not be well absorbed IM. Check product pharmacology before giving a drug by the IM route. **Make sure that the drug you are giving is approved for IM injection.**

Patient Selection

Nearly all patients of all ages are eligible to receive IM injections. The selection of patients and medications depends on the following:

- The clinical condition of the patient.
- The type of medicine to be given, and whether it is approved for the IM route. Certain medicines must be given into a muscle, most medicines can be given in multiple fashions, and some medicines should NEVER be given IM.
- The ideal amount of fluid is 1 mL. Larger volumes of medicines or highly concentrated medications should not be given IM.
- If the patient requires an immediate effect from the medication, the IV or IO route is preferred.

Risks and Precautions

- Do not use the IM route if muscle bulk and size are inadequate.
- Do not use IM injection if other routes of administration are sufficient or preferred.
- Do not select IM injection sites with signs of infection, acute injury, or scarring. Do not give an IM injection into an area that is already painful.

Equipment

- Alcohol wipe or other skin-cleansing gauze.
- One clean and dry small gauze and/or cottonball swab.

- Tape and/or adhesive bandage/dressing.
- 1- to 3-mL syringe.
- Sterile saline or sterile distilled water if medication needs to be dissolved.
- Large-bore needle for withdrawing medication from ampule or bottle.
- 23-gauge/25-mm needle or 25-gauge/16-mm needle for preterm babies 2 months or younger. The needle must be more than 3.8 cm (1½ inches) long.
- Sterile or nonsterile gloves for the health-care provider.
- Sharps container.
- Medication ampule, bottle, or syringe prefilled with medication.
  - If withdrawing from an ampule, shake the ampule before breaking to make sure all medication is in the base of the ampule before withdrawing it. Double check that the dose is correct.
  - If withdrawing from a sterile bottle, remove the sterile cap. Remove the cap from the needle, and aspirate a volume of air equivalent to the amount of liquid you will withdraw from the bottle. Using sterile technique, hold the bottle upside-down and inject air into the bottle. Then aspirate the correct dose from the syringe. **Do NOT reuse the syringe or needle. Do not use the same bottle of medicine for multiple patients.**

Patient Positioning

Preparation

Make sure the patient is lying down or sitting. Verify the proper dose and medication name, and prepare the medication from the vial or ampule.

Locate the correct area for injection using the guidelines below. **Make sure you hold the needle perpendicular to the injection site.**

- Shoulder.
- Middle third of anterior thigh.
- Upper outer quadrant of buttock.

Shoulder

Give the IM injection in the center of an upside-down triangle that is bounded at the top by the acromion, about 5 cm or 2 inches below it (Figure 23-27 A, B). **Do not use the deltoid muscle in infants and young children.**

Middle Third of Anterior Thigh

The vastus lateralis muscle is on the anterolateral aspect of the thigh. This muscle is usually well formed in all age groups, and the area does not contain any major arteries or nerves. Give the injection in the middle third of the muscle on the outside of the thigh (Figure 23-28). **This is the preferred site of IM injection in children.**

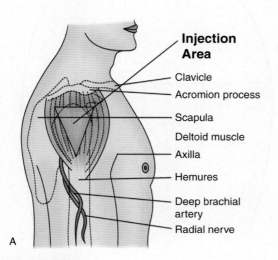

Injection Area
- Clavicle
- Acromion process
- Scapula
- Deltoid muscle
- Axilla
- Hemures
- Deep brachial artery
- Radial nerve

A

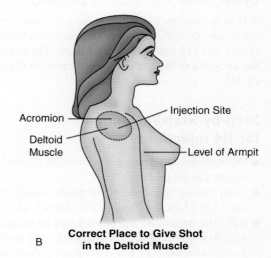

- Acromion
- Deltoid Muscle
- Injection Site
- Level of Armpit

B

Correct Place to Give Shot in the Deltoid Muscle

FIGURE 23–27

A and **B**, Intramuscular injection site for deltoid muscle, with surrounding anatomy. The preferred location is the center of the marked triangle.

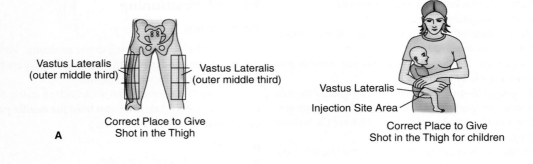

Vastus Lateralis
(outer middle third)

Vastus Lateralis
(outer middle third)

A

Correct Place to Give
Shot in the Thigh

Vastus Lateralis

Injection Site Area

Correct Place to Give
Shot in the Thigh for children

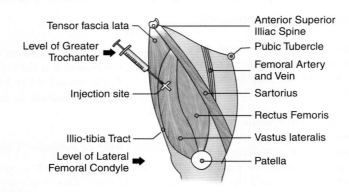

Tensor fascia lata

Level of Greater
Trochanter

Injection site

Illio-tibia Tract

B   Level of Lateral
Femoral Condyle

Anterior Superior
Illiac Spine

Pubic Tubercle

Femoral Artery
and Vein

Sartorius

Rectus Femoris

Vastus lateralis

Patella

FIGURE 23-28

A and **B**, Location of middle third of the vastus lateralis muscle in adults and children.

Upper Outer Quadrant of Buttocks

It is important to make sure you locate the upper outer quadrant of the buttocks. Injections outside of this area can injure the sciatic nerve. **Do not use the buttocks in infants and young children** (Figure 23-29).

Step-by-Step Technique for IM Injections

- Wear gloves and prepare the site with alcohol or iodine. Let the area dry.
- Grasp the syringe, directing the needle straight into the desired location (Figure 23-30, Steps 1-4).
- After the needle has entered the skin and muscle, withdraw on the plunger to make sure you are not in a blood vessel. If no blood is aspirated, then inject the medication.
- Remove the needle and syringe, place in a sharps container, and place a bandage over the injection site.

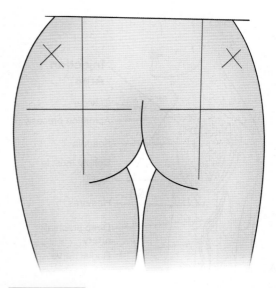

FIGURE 23-29

IM injections in the buttocks should always go in the UPPER OUTER QUADRANT (X marks the spot).

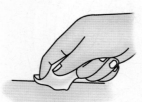

1. Use an alcohol swab to clean the skin where you will give yourself the shot.

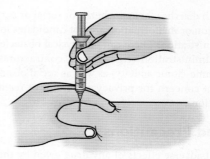

2. Hold the muscle firmly and insert the needle into the muscle at a 90° angle (straight up and down) with a quick firm motion.

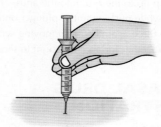

3. After you insert the needle completely, release your grasp of the muscle.

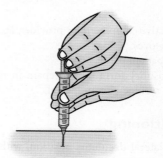

4. Gently pull back on the plunger of the syringe to check for blood. (If blood appears, withdraw the needle and gently press the alcohol swab on the injection site. Start over with a fresh needle.)

FIGURE 23–30

Technique for IM injection, Steps 1-4:
Step 1. Cleanse desired area.
Step 2. Grasp the muscle and insert the needle at a 90-degree angle into the skin and into the muscle.
Step 3. Release your grasp of the muscle.
Step 4. Aspirate for blood. If no blood appears, inject the medication.

Outcomes Assessment

Check for localized redness, swelling, or bleeding at the injection site. Observe the patient for at least 15 minutes following the injection for signs of possible drug reaction.

Complications

Expect minor discomfort for a short period after the injection. Pain should resolve within a few hours. If pain lasts longer, advise the patient to seek medical attention. Local infection, abscess, or scar formation is an unusual complication. Neurovascular injury is avoided by selecting the proper site for injection.

RECTAL ADMINISTRATION

Purpose of Procedure

Several drugs can be administered in the form of rectal suppositories. The commonest drugs given in this form are are antiemetics, benzodiazepines for seizure control (e.g., diazepam), and antipyretics. Most studies involve rectal benzodiazepines. The onset of action with the rectal route (5 to 10 minutes) is typically longer than that with intranasal or intravenous administration.[1-3] Rectal administration may not be as effective as other routes of administration.[3]

Patient Selection

The rectal route is used if other routes are unavailable and if the drug is available in rectal suppository form.

Patients with diarrhea, hematochezia, or rectal or perineal infection or malformation are not candidates for rectal administration. There can be physical obstacles to rectal administration (e.g., obesity, contractures, continual tonic-clonic activity) as well as social obstacles (patient concern for privacy or refusal of rectal administration).

Risks and Precautions

Allergy and adverse effects of any drug given by this method, such as respiratory and cardiac depression from rectal diazepam.

Equipment

- Personal protective equipment for provider, including protective gloves.
- Location with patient privacy.
- Drug in suppository form; or diazepam in rectal formulation as syringe-containing gel.

Patient Positioning

Place patient in lateral decubitus position, with top knee brought to knee-chest position.

Step-by-Step Technique

1. Select proper drug dose. Rectal diazepam is supplied as 5 mg/mL with total doses of 2.5, 5, 10, 15, and 20 milligrams.
2. Remove cap with pin from diazepam (Figure 23-31).
3. Apply lubricant to syringe tip.
4. Place syringe tip into the rectum (Figure 23-32).
5. Slowly inject over a count of three; hold syringe in place for another count of three.
6. Remove syringe and grasp buttocks closed over anus for another count of three.

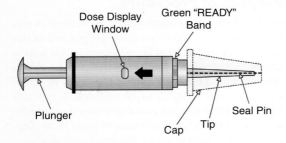

FIGURE 23–31

Device for rectal diazepam insertion. Select proper dose. Remove cap with pin, then apply lubricant jelly to tip.

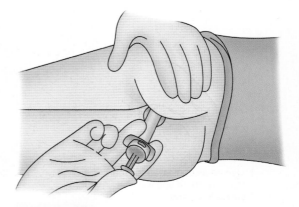

FIGURE 23–32

Insert syringe tip up to the rim, into the anus, and count to three while pushing in the plunger until it stops. Count to three again before removing syringe. Hold buttocks together for another count to three.

INTRANASAL DRUG ADMINISTRATION

Purpose of Procedure

Intranasal drug delivery results in rapid transmucosal absorption of some medications. It is a common method for treating symptoms of rhinosinusitis with antihistamines, corticosteroids, or decongestants. Currently, analgesics, benzodiazepines, and naloxone are drugs amenable to intranasal delivery in the prehospital setting.[4–12] The nares are accessible entry points for drug administration: the surface area of the nasal mucosa is large and the nasal mucosa is well vascularized, allowing for good systemic absorption (Figure 23-33).

Patient Selection

Children >3 years old and adults in whom emergency drug administration is needed and no other parenteral access is available. Conditions include acute seizures or status epilepticus, narcotic overdose, acute pain control, or procedural sedation.[4–8]

Do *not* give intranasal medication if there is epistaxis or excess mucus in the nose, if there is concern for facial or nasal fracture, or if there is underlying anatomy or disease of the face or nose, which would preclude intranasal administration.

In adults, do *not* use intranasal administration if the patient uses intranasal cocaine.

Do *not* use the intranasal route if topical vasoconstrictors have been recently used.

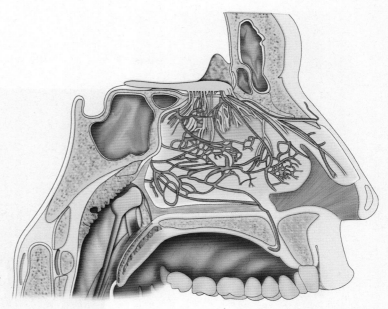

FIGURE 23–33

Cross-section of the nares with highly vascular mucosa.

Risks and Precautions

Medications are given as a **mist**, not as drops.

Medications selected for intranasal delivery must be water-soluble.

Most medications are not FDA (or regulatory agency) approved for intranasal use, so follow local EMS and hospital protocols when using the intranasal route of drug administration.

Medications must be concentrated for reasonable dosing volumes. Be very careful to administer the correct dose to avoid dosage errors. Give half the total calculated dose into each nostril.

Drug dose may need to be increased to allow for drug loss during nasal administration. For example, the intranasal dose of **fentanyl** for children is 1.5 micrograms/kg, as opposed to the standard IV dose of 1.0 micrograms/kg. The higher dose may result in an increased likelihood of hypotension and respiratory depression.

The IV formulation of benzodiazepines has a low pH and can be irritating to the nasal mucosa. However, the IV form of **midazolam** (5 milligrams/mL) has been successfully used for pediatric sedation and pediatric seizure control. The recommended dose is 0.2 to 0.4 milligrams/kg with a maximum dose of 10 milligrams.[9–11]

For adults, the intranasal dose of **naloxone** is 2 milligrams total (1 milligram/nare). For children, the dose is 0.1 milligram/kg if the child is <10 kg.[12]

Equipment

Many commercially available devices are now offered for the intranasal administration of drugs. However, if these devices are not readily available for use in the prehospital setting, the following pieces of equipment will allow appropriate prehospital intranasal drug administration when indicated:

1. Drug to be administered, in liquid form.
2. Small size syringe, 2.5 mL or less.
3. NS or other appropriate solute.
4. Airway and suction equipment, cardiac monitor, and pulse oximeter, as dictated by the clinical situation.
5. Atomized pump.

The atomized pump is the best nasal delivery system because it gives a constant dose and a very good mucosal distribution[13] (Figure 23-34).

Step-by-Step Procedure

1. Use the most concentrated form and lowest volume of the medication available – ideally 0.3 mL/nare.[7] Use both nostrils to double the absorptive surface area. **If both nares are used, give half the drug into each nare.**
2. Attach the syringe containing the drug to the atomizer, place the atomizer at the nare, and then depress the plunger firmly.

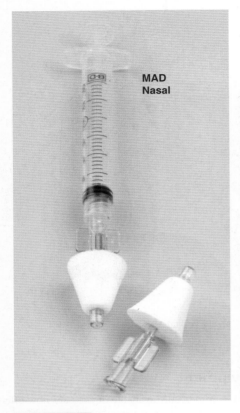
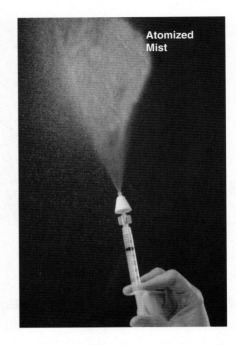

FIGURE 23–34

A, Mucosal atomization device. **B,** Mist from mucosal atomization device. Reprinted with permission from Wolfe Tory Medical.

Outcomes Assessment

Monitor blood pressure, oxygen saturation, and respirations according to standard protocol or policy.

References

Rectal Administration Section

1. Fisgin T, Gurer Y, Tezic T. Effects of intranasal midazolam and rectal diazpam on acute convulsions in children: Prospective randomized study. *J Child Neurol* 17; 123, 2002; DOI 10.1177/088307380101700206.
2. deHaan GJ, van der Geest P, Doelman G, et al. A comparison of midazolam nasal spray and diazepam rectal solution for the residential treatment of seizure exacerbation. *Epilepsia* Oct 8: 1, 2009 (e-pub ahead of print) DOI 10.1111/j.1528–1167.2009.02333.x.
3. McIntyre J. Safety and efficacy of buccal midazolam versus rectal diazepam for emergency treatment of seizures in children: a randomized controlled trial. *Lancet* 366:205, 2005.

Intranasal Administration Section

4. Wermeling, DP. Intranasal delivery of antiepileptic medications for treatment of seizures. *Neurotherapeutics* 6(2): 352, 2009.
5. Cole J, Shepherd M, Young P. Intranasal fentanyl in 1-3-year-olds: A prospective study of the effectiveness of intranasal fentanyl as acute analgesia. *Emerg Med Australas* 23: 395, 2009.
6. Pires A, Fortuna A, Alvs G, et al. Intranasal drug delivery: how, why, and what for?' *J Pharm Pharm Sci* 12(3): 288, 2009.
7. Dale O, Hjortkjaer R, Kharasch ED. Nasal administration of opioids for pain management in adults. *Acta Anaesthesiol Scand* 46(7): 759, 2002.
8. Moodie JE, Brown CR, Bisley EJ. The safety and analgesic efficacy of intranasal ketorolac in patients with postoperative pain. *Anesth Analg* 107: 2025, 2008.
9. Lane RD, Schunk JE. Atomized intranasal midazolam use for minor procedures in the pediatric emergency department. *Ped Emerg Care* 24(5): 300, 2008.

10. Fisgin T, Gurer Y, Tezic T, et al. Effects of intranasal midazolam and rectal diazepam on acute convulsions in children: prospective randomized study. *J Child Neurol* 27: 123, 2002; DOI 10.1177/088307 380201700206.

11. Harbord MG, Kyrkou NE, Kyrkou MR, et al. Use of midazolam to treat acute seizures in paediatric community settings. *J Paediat Child Health* 40: 556, 2004.

12. Robertson TM, Hendey GW, Stroh G, et al. Intranasal naloxone is a viable alternative to intravenous naloxone for prehospital narcotic overdose. *Prehosp Emerg Care* 13(4): 512, 2009.

13. Mygind N, Vesterhauge, S. Aerosol distribution in the nose. *Rhinology* 16(2): 79, 1978.

Other Useful Resources

1. Sarkar PK, Pan GD, Biswas SK, Mukherjee PK. Ideal technique and sites for intramuscular injection in infants and children *Pediatr Surg Int* 4: 140, 1989; available at: http://www.springerlink.com/content/v054x576t8w5284n/fulltext.pdf.

2. The Australian Immunisation Handbook. National Health and Medical Research Council. 7th ed. Canberra: Australian Government Publishing Service; 2000, available at: http://www.rch.org.au/nets/handbook/index.cfm?doc_id=63.

CHAPTER 24

Cardiac Defibrillation and External Pacing

Marcus E. H. Ong

DEFIBRILLATION

Purpose of Procedure

Defibrillation is the application of electricity to terminate nonperfusing ventricular fibrillation or pulseless ventricular tachycardia and allow the resumption of coordinated contractions.

Patient Selection

Defibrillation is performed for ventricular fibrillation (VF) (Figure 24-1) and pulseless ventricular tachycardia (VT) (Figure 24-2). Defibrillation should not be attempted for asystole, pulseless electrical activity, sinus rhythm, a conscious patient with a pulse, or where water in the environment or on the patient poses a danger to the operator or other caretakers.

Risks and Precautions

Defibrillation can induce ventricular fibrillation if the electric shock occurs during the relative refractory portion of the cardiac cycle[1]; therefore be prepared to repeat defibrillation if needed.

Verify Ventricular Fibrillation

First check the patient and verify the rhythm to be sure that defibrillation is indicated. Movement artifact or loose leads may be mistaken for ventric-

ular fibrillation. To make sure that an automated external defibrillator (AED) does not mistake movement for ventricular fibrillation, stop patient transport and confirm cardiac arrest before initiating analysis mode.

Avoid Carelessness

Make sure that no one touches the patient or any devices are attached to the patient when a shock is delivered. The operator should loudly state "stand clear" and also look to make sure no assistants or bystanders are in contact with the patient at the time of defibrillation. If the patient is on a wet surface, move the patient to a dry area and dry the body before defibrillating.

To avoid accidental defibrillation of a bystander or assistant when using manual defibrillation paddles, move the paddles quickly from the defibrillator cradle to the patient's chest. Point the paddles downwards but not toward each other in order to prevent inadvertent discharges and 'sparking,' which can occur when the paddle surfaces are close to each other.

Prepare the Patient for Defibrillation

Lay the patient on his or her back. Remove any metallic objects (necklaces, chains) and nitroglycerin patches from the patient's chest to avoid transmission of electrical energy across the skin. This could result in skin burns. Check for any

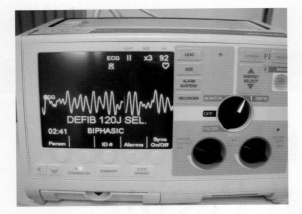

FIGURE 24-1

Ventricular fibrillation. Photo courtesy UNC Training Center, Jennifer Stoeppler EMT-P and Barbara Steckler.

sources of oxygen flow (portable oxygen tanks) and shut off the oxygen to avoid combustion and fire.[2,3]

If the chest is very hairy, defibrillation pads may not stick onto the chest, and it may be necessary to quickly shave parts of the chest hair. (If shaving is needed, stop chest compressions only for the shortest possible time.) If the chest is sweaty, wipe it dry. Sweat or moisture on the chest will impair contact and adhesion of the defibrillator pads or paddles.

Place defibrillation paddles/pads in the proper location. Paddles require the application of conducting gel. If using paddles, keep the conducting gel more than 5 cm (2 inches) from the other paddle. If you palpate a pacemaker battery on the patient's chest, keep the paddles/pads at least 12.5 cm (5 inches) from the pacemaker before defibrillating.

Allow Only Minimal Pauses from Chest Compressions

Prolonged pauses from chest compression while preparing for or performing defibrillation lower the likelihood of successful resuscitation. The 2005 International Liaison Committee on Resuscitation (ILCOR) guidelines[4] recommend only the shortest interruption of CPR for rhythm analysis. Give a single shock instead of three "stacked" shocks, and immediately resume chest compressions without a pulse or rhythm check after defibrillation.

Equipment

- Manual, semi- or fully automated external defibrillator.

FIGURE 24-2

Ventricular tachycardia on electrocardiogram.

- Defibrillators should be properly maintained and in a constant state of readiness.
- Use checklists[5] to make sure batteries are effective and to anticipate defibrillator malfunction. Identify individuals who are trained to use checklists and who perform checks routinely and frequently (as often as every shift).
- Paddles or defibrillation pads.
- Conductive gel or gel-pads for defibrillation paddles.
- Additional resuscitation equipment as appropriate, such as a bag-valve mask, other airway adjuncts, suction, intravenous cannulation, and drugs.

STEP-BY-STEP TECHNIQUE

Placement of Paddles/Pads

Several positions can be used for paddle or pad placement. Proper placement is important to maximize current flow through the heart rather than through the skin of the chest.

Preferred Placement: Anteroapical Position

Place one paddle/pad to the right of the upper half of the sternum (breast bone), just below the patient's right clavicle (collar bone) and place the other pad just below and to the left of the left nipple (in the axilla). With a female patient, place it just below and to the left side of the breast. Do not place the paddle or pad over the breast (Figure 24-3).

Anteroposterior position

Place one pad/paddle on the chest at the left lower sternal border and the posterior pad/paddle on the back, below the left scapula (shoulder blade).

Apex–posterior position

Place one pad/paddle on the chest just below and to the left of the left nipple and the other posterior pad/paddle on the back, below the left scapula (shoulder blade).

Prepare defibrillator paddles (Figure 24-4), by applying conducting gel or gel pads directly to both

One pad on right upper half of sternum (breastbone) below right clavicle (collarbone)

One pad just below and to the left of the nipple

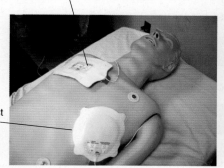

FIGURE 24-3

Anteroapical positioning of defibrillation pads. Photo courtesy of UNC Training Center, Jennifer Stoeppler EMT-P, and Barbara Steckler.

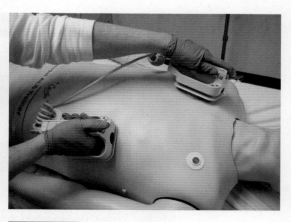

FIGURE 24-4

Anteroapical positioning of defibrillation paddles in an adult. Photo courtesy of UNC Training Center, Jennifer Stoeppler EMT-P and Barbara Steckler.

paddles. Apply the paddles firmly to the chest wall using 11 kg (25 lb) of pressure.

Press defibrillator pads firmly and gently to the chest, making sure there is good contact with the skin at around all edges of the pads. Good contact is needed for effective defibrillation. In the AED mode, the "Check Electrodes" message will be transmitted if contact is not adequate for defibillation. Large pads (12 cm) seem to be more effective than smaller pads (8 cm and smaller).[4]

MANUAL DEFIBRILLATION

1. Prepare the patient and equipment as described above. Continue CPR with no or minimal interruptions.
2. Verify that the rhythm is VF or pulseless VT.
3. Set the defibrillator to unsynchronized mode.
4. Select the appropriate energy level. For biphasic defibrillators, use the manufacturer's recommendation (150–200 joules with biphasic truncated exponential waveforms and 120 joules for rectilinear biphasic waveforms). For monophasic defibrillators, use a 360-joule shock.[4]
5. Apply the paddles with gel or gel pads and charge the defibrillator (Figure 24-4).
6. Call out "stand clear" and look to make sure no one is touching the patient or there are no devices attached to the patient.
7. Discharge the defibrillator (shock the patient).
8. Continue CPR and follow your local resuscitation protocol. The ILCOR universal cardiac arrest algorithm is shown in Figure 24-5.[6]

AUTOMATED EXTERNAL DEFIBRILLATION

1. Prepare the patient and equipment as described above. Continue CPR with no or minimal interruptions.
2. Open the package containing the defibrillation pads with the attached cable and connector. With the patient's chest prepared, carefully pull off the protective backing from the pads. Place the pads on the chest, or alternate positions as described above.
3. **Turn On** the device (follow the voice prompts according to your device). The defibrillator will not function unless it is **TURNED ON**.
4. Stop all patient movement and start rhythm analysis. If a shock is indicated, the defibrillator will automatically charge up to a preset level.
5. Call out "stand clear" and look to make sure no one is in contact with the patient and there are no devices attached to the patient.
6. Wait until the shock is discharged. Fully automated defibrillators do not require any operator action to discharge a shock.
7. Continue CPR and follow your local resuscitation protocol. The ILCOR universal cardiac arrest algorithm[6] is shown in Figure 24-5.

PEDIATRIC DEFIBRILLATION

Ventricular fibrillation is rare in children, and respiratory arrest usually precedes cardiac arrest. Therefore, support ventilation to prevent cardiac arrest. To treat ventricular fibrillation, use 2 joules/kg body

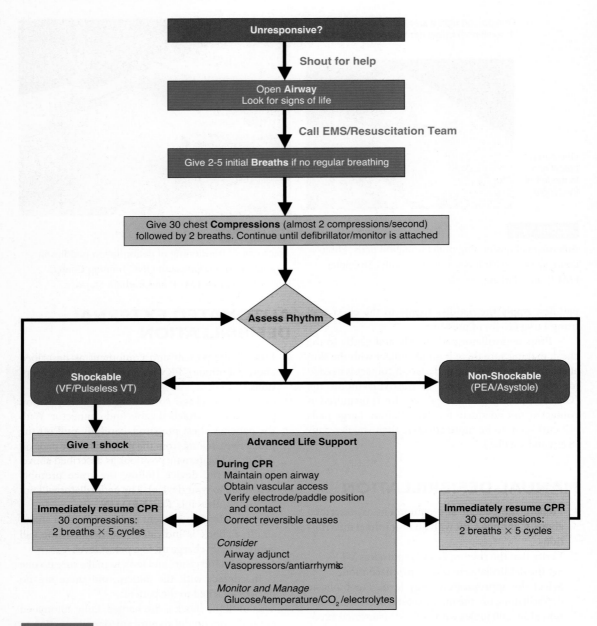

FIGURE 24–5

International Liaison Committee on Resuscitation (ILCOR) Universal Cardiac Arrest Algorithms.[6]

weight intially, and if unsuccessful, increase energy to 4 joules/kg.

In children with ventricular tachycardia with a pulse, cardiovert with 0.5 to 1 joules/kg *synchronized*. Increase energy to 2 joules/kg if unsuccessful. Use special pediatric paddles or pads. In an infant or small child, it is possible to defibrillate with the patient propped on his or her side using an anterpos-

terior paddle placement (Figures 24-6A, 24-6B, 24-6C, and 24-6D).

Outcomes Assessment

The aim of defibrillation is restoration of a normal perfusing rhythm. After defibrillation, continue CPR until the cycle is completed for a pulse and rhythm

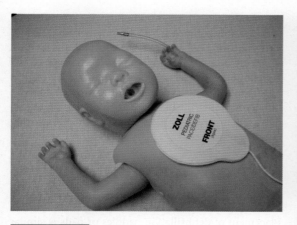

FIGURE 24–6A
Anteroposterior positioning of defibrillation pads in an infant (front).

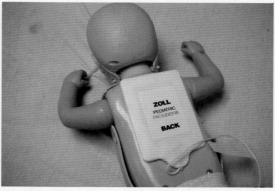

FIGURE 24–6B
Anteroposterior positioning of defibrillation pads in an infant (back). Photo courtesy of UNC Training Center, Jennifer Stoeppler EMT-P and Barbara Steckler.

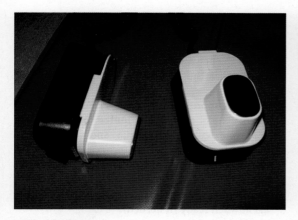

FIGURE 24–6C
Pediatric defibrillation paddles.

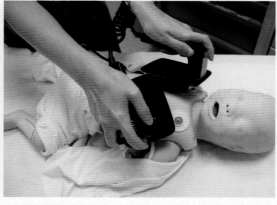

FIGURE 24–6D
Anteroapical positioning of defibrillation paddles in an infant. Photo courtesy of Children's Emergency, KK Women's and Children's Hospital, Singapore.

check (do not pause immediately for a pulse check). If the patient is in persistent ventricular tachycardia or ventricular fibrillation, continue with the local resuscitation protocol. The ILCOR universal cardiac arrest algorithm[6] is shown in Figure 24-5. Once spontaneous circulation returns, apply the usual postresuscitation care.

CARDIOVERSION

Purpose of Procedure

Cardioversion is the application of electricity to terminate a hemodynamically unstable but still perfusing rhythm (e.g., ventricular tachycardia with a pulse, supraventricular tachycardias including atrial arrhythmias) to allow a normal sinus rhythm to restart. Cardioversion is not used for a patient in cardiac arrest.

Patient Selection

Cardioversion is indicated for a hemodynamically unstable patient with ventricular tachycardia, supraventricular tachycardia, atrial flutter, or atrial fibrillation. Signs of hemodynamic instability include hypotension (systolic blood pressure <80 mm Hg), change in mental status, and chest or pulmonary edema.

Risks and Precautions

All the precautions for defibrillation apply to cardioversion. Because cardioversion can induce ventricular fibrillation, it is a procedure reserved for health-care personnel who perform at the ALS level or higher.

A patient may continue to deteriorate or may develop cardiac arrest as a result of cardioverson. Therefore cardioversion is only indicated for a patient who is hemodynamically unstable. There is no role for elective electrical cardioversion for a stable patient in the field. A patient who is able to maintain consciousness, a palpable pulse, and a blood pressure should be cardioverted in the ED or ICU, where procedural sedation, parenteral analgesia, monitoring, and stand by resuscitation equipment is available. The operator should be skilled in endotracheal intubation or other equivalent advanced airway techniques and pharmacologic therapy in case a patient deteriorates.

Cardioversion should be *synchronized*, which means the equipment senses the patient's intrinsic QRS complexes and applies the electric shock at the appropriate interval (to avoid the R- on T- phenomenon) to minimize the risk of inducing ventricular fibrillation.

Equipment

- A manual external defibrillator is required for cardioversion.
- Paddles or self-adhesive defibrillation pads.
- Conductive gel or gel-pads for defibrillation paddles.
- Related resuscitation equipment (e.g., bag-valve mask device, airway devices, suction, intravenous cannulation, and drugs (e.g., oxygen, sedation, analgesia).

Patient Positioning and Preparation

Prepare the patient and place in a position the same as that for defibrillation (see previous section).

ANESTHESIA AND PROCEDURAL MONITORING

Procedural sedation and analgesia, and cardiac, blood pressure, and pulse oximetry monitoring are necessary. Airway equipment, suction, and oxygen should be immediately available. Place an IV line. Obtain informed consent if possible (according to local protocols).

Etomidate (0.2–0.6 milligrams/kg IV), propofol (0.5–2.0 milligrams/kg IV) or midazolam (1.0–5.0 milligrams/kg IV) are used for procedural sedation. These are dose ranges only, and local protocols should be followed when selecting the drug dose. If possible, restore intravascular volume prior to procedural sedation to minimize the likelihood of hypotension or cardiovascular collapse. Continue patient monitoring after the procedure.

STEP-BY-STEP TECHNIQUE

Placement of Paddles/Pads

Placement of defibrillation paddles or pads is similar to that for defibrillation (see previous section).

CARDIOVERSION

1. Prepare the patient and equipment as described above. Provide cardiorespiratory monitoring and have resuscitation equipment at hand.
2. Check the patient and the rhythm.
3. Check that the defibrillator is on *synchronized mode.*
4. Select the appropriate energy level. For monophasic defibrillators, start at **50 joules** for paroxysmal supraventricular tachycardia and atrial flutter, **100 joules** for ventricular tachycardia and atrial fibrillation. For biphasic defibrillators, follow the manufacturer's recommendations.
5. Begin procedural sedation with an appropriate agent when ready (if needed).
6. Apply the paddles or pads (may be applied beforehand) and charge.
7. Check that no one is in contact with the patient or devices and call out "stand clear."
8. Discharge the shock.
9. Continue to monitor and manage the patient according to local protocols.

Outcomes Assessment

The aim of cardioversion is termination of the abnormal rhythm and restoration of a normal perfusing rhythm. Monitor for rhythm and level of consciousness.

Complications

Possible complications include skin burns, inadvertent electric shock to others, and myocardial damage. Failed cardioversion can also result in cardiac arrest.

Complications associated with sedation also include hypotension, depression of consciousness, loss of airway reflexes, aspiration, and cardiac arrest.

EXTERNAL CARDIAC PACING

Purpose of Procedure

External cardiac pacing or transcutaneous cardiac pacing is the therapeutic use of an electrical stimulus to cause electrical depolarization and subsequent cardiac contraction by the use of external cutaneous electrodes. Transvenous, transthoracic, transesophageal, or epicardial pacing are not used in the out-of-hospital setting.

Patient Selection

Indications for external cardiac pacing are the treatment of hemodynamically significant bradycardias unresponsive to pharmacologic management or for the treatment of hemodynamically significant bradycardias when pharmacologic therapy is not immediately available. Signs of hemodynamic instability include hypotension (systolic blood pressure <80 mm Hg), change in mental status, angina, or pulmonary edema. External cardiac pacing is often used as a temporary bridge until transvenous pacing can be initiated at the hospital or the underlying cause of bradycardia can be reversed.

Emergency pacing may also be indicated for patients with bradycardia-dependent or pause-dependent escape (ventricular) rhythms. Patients with severe bradycardia may develop wide-complex ventricular escape beats that precipitate ventricular tachycardia or ventricular fibrillation. Pacing may eliminate these escape rhythms.

Overdrive pacing can also be used to terminate malignant supraventricular and ventricular tachycardias. Overdrive pacing is performed by pacing the heart for a few seconds at a rate faster than the tachycardia, then stopping pacing to allow an intrinsic rhythm to return.

Finally, pacing has been used for pulseless patients with bradycardia, although results are mixed. Transcutaneous pacing is no longer recommended for asystolic cardiac arrest.[6]

External cardiac pacing is contraindicated for a conscious patient with a hemodynamically stable bradycardia. However it is reasonable and practical to attach pacing electrodes to such a patient and to stand by for the possibility of deterioration during transport.

Severe hypothermia with bradycardia is a relative contraindication for cardiac pacing. The bradycardia may be physiologic, and attempts to pace may lead to ventricular fibrillation. Treatment of bradyarrhythmias due to hypothermia is rewarming.

Risks and Precautions

All the precautions listed in the previous section on defibrillation regarding the use of electrical energy also apply to pacing.

In a conscious patient, appropriate sedation and analgesia may also need to be given before pacing. In all cases in which pacing is attempted, the operator should be adequately trained and prepared to handle a resuscitation in case a patient deteriorates. This includes securing the airway with endotracheal intubation or other equivalent advanced airway techniques. Thus cardiac pacing should be a procedure reserved for ALS personnel.

Equipment

- A defibrillator or pulse generator (Figures 24-7, 24-8): This should have an appropriate cardiac pacing module (fixed/demand modes).
- Cardiac pacing electrodes or self-adhesive defibrillation pads.
- Conductive gel or gel-pads for defibrillation paddles.
- Related resuscitation equipment (e.g., bag-valve mask device, airway devices, suction, intravenous cannulation, and drugs (e.g., oxygen, sedation, analgesia).

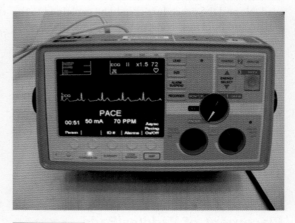

FIGURE 24-7

Transcutaneous cardiac pacing monitor.

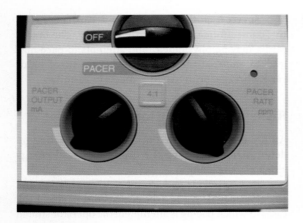

FIGURE 24–8

Transcutaneous cardiac pacing module (close up).

Defibrillators should be properly maintained and in a constant state of readiness.

Patient Positioning

The patient should be placed in a similar position as that for defibrillation (see previous section).

Anesthesia and Procedural Monitoring

For cardiac pacing, adequate anesthesia and procedural monitoring is essential. The patient should be monitored with resuscitation equipment, including cardiac, blood pressure, and pulse oximetry monitoring. Airway equipment, suction, and oxygen should be immediately available. An intravenous line must be available and the procedure should be explained to the patient and informed consent obtained where possible (according to local protocols). Once preparations are completed the patient should be sedated with an intravenous agent like etomidate, propofol, or midazolam and an analgesic agent (e.g., fentanyl, 0.5–2 micrograms/kg IV). Keep in mind that such agents may aggravate hypotension and precipitate cardiovascular collapse. Use with caution and in titrated doses. Close attention should be given to monitoring the patient during the procedure.

STEP-BY-STEP TECHNIQUE

Placement of Paddles/Pads

Placement of defibrillation paddles or pads is similar to that for defibrillation (see previous section).

EXTERNAL CARDIAC PACING

1. Identify the cardiac rhythm and indications for pacing.
2. Prepare the patient and equipment as described above.
3. Obtain intravenous access, apply oxygen, set up monitoring of pulse oximetry, electrocardiogram, and blood pressure.
4. Attempt pharmacologic management (atropine 0.5 mg IV) as appropriate.
5. Apply the pacing electrodes, assemble equipment, and connect to the pacing device (Figure 24-9).
6. Give analgesia and sedation as appropriate.
7. Set the pacing rate between 60 to 100 beats/minute as appropriate (Figure 24-10), for example, start at 80 beats/minute.

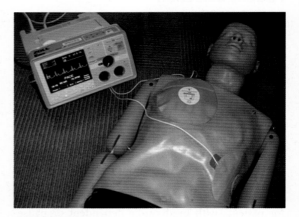

FIGURE 24–9

Transcutaneous cardiac pacing (pad placement).

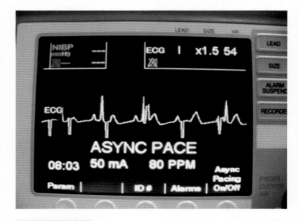

FIGURE 24–10

Transcutaneous asynchronized cardiac pacing with pacer spikes seen on monitor.

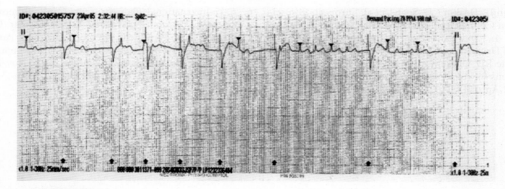

FIGURE 24–11

Electrocardiographic cardiac pacing with electrical capture. Reprinted with permission from Life Support Training Center, Singapore General Hospital, Singapore.

8. For symptomatic bradycardia, adjust the pacing output upwards until electrical and mechanical ventricular capture occur. **Electrical capture is characterized by a widening of the QRS complex and a broad T wave following a pacing spike** (Figure 24-11). Mechanical capture is indicated by the hemodynamic (pulse/blood pressure) response. Assess the pulse at the right carotid or right femoral artery to avoid confusion with the muscle contractions caused by pacing. **Start with a fixed pacing mode** and switch later to demand pacing if appropriate.

9. For bradycardic arrest, start at maximal electrical output, then decrease to the minimal level once capture is achieved.

10. Once capture has occurred, maintain pacing at a slightly higher output (10%) than the threshold for electrical capture.

11. Continue to monitor for efficacy of mechanical capture and conscious level. Titrate analgesia and sedation as appropriate.

Outcomes Assessment

Failure to capture may be related to electrode placement or patient characteristics. Patients with barrel-shaped chests and large amounts of intrathoracic air may be refractory to transcutaneous capture. Likewise a large pericardial effusion, cardiac tamponade, or recent thoracic surgery may affect capture. Other routes of cardiac pacing will need to be considered in this setting.

Complications

Possible complications include painful skeletal muscle contractions, skin burns, and electrically induced myocardial damage. However, the more important complication is a failure to capture during pacing, leading to a deterioration in the patient's condition.

Other theoretical complications are the failure to recognize underlying treatable ventricular fibrillation due to the size of pacing artifacts and induction of pacing arrhythmias or ventricular fibrillation. In practice these seldom occur with modern pacing devices.

On arrival at the hospital, temporary or permanent transvenous pacing may be required.

Acknowledgments

The author would like to thank:
Dr. Tham Lai Peng, Senior Consultant, Children's Emergency, KK Women's and Children's Hospital, Singapore.

Ms. Madhavi Suppiah, Manager, Life Support Training Center, Singapore General Hospital, Singapore.

Ms. Susan Yap, Research Nurse, Department of Emergency Medicine, Singapore General Hospital, Singapore.

Mr. David Yong, Research Assistant, Department of Emergency Medicine, Singapore General Hospital, Singapore.

References

1. Lown B. Electrical reversion of cardiac arrhythmias. *Br Heart J.* 1967 Jul;29(4):469–489. PMID: 6029120
2. Fires from defibrillation during oxygen administration. *Health Devices.* 1994 Jul;23(7):307-308. PMID: 7852078
3. Miller PH. Potential fire hazard in defibrillation. *JAMA.* 1972 Jul 10;221(2):192. PMID: 5067634

4. Nolan JP, Deakin CD, Soar J, et al. European Resuscitation Council guidelines for resuscitation 2005. Section 4. Adult advanced life support. *Resuscitation.* 2005 Dec;67 Suppl 1:S39-86. PMID: 16321716

5. White RD, Chesemore KF. Charge! FDA recommendations for maintaining defibrillator readiness. *JEMS.* 1992 Apr;17(4):70-72, 82. PMID: 10117528

6. 2005 International Consensus on Cardiopulmonary Resuscitation and Emergency Cardiovascular Care Science with Treatment Recommendations. Part 4: Advanced life support. International Liaison Committee on Resuscitation. *Resuscitation.* 2005 Nov-Dec; 67(2–3):213-47. PMID: 16324990

CHAPTER 25

Therapeutic Hypothermia After Out-of-Hospital Cardiac Arrest

Conor Deasy

KEY LEARNING POINTS

- Therapeutic hypothermia improves outcome after resuscitation of selected patients.

- The goal of therapeutic hypothermia is a decrease in core body temperature to 33 degrees C for 24-24 hours, for patients who remain comatose after cardiac resuscitation.

PURPOSE OF THERAPEUTIC HYPOTHERMIA

Much of the mortality and morbidity after hospital admission is caused by the anoxic brain injury sustained during the cardiac arrest.[1] Therapeutic hypothermia (TH) induced after resuscitation improves neurologic and overall outcomes.[2,3]

PATIENT SELECTION

The American Heart Association now recommends TH (33°C for 12–24 hours) for patients who remain comatose after resuscitation from cardiac arrest and whose initial cardiac rhythm is ventricular fibrillation.[4] It is reasonable to cool patients who had asystole/Pulseless Electrical Activity (PEA) out of hospital cardiac arrest who also remain comatose. Therapeutic hypothermia can also be applied to children and neonates.[5,6]

RISKS AND PRECAUTIONS

Overcooling can predispose to arrhythmias and interfere with blood coagulation.

EQUIPMENT

- 2 L of crystalloid at 4°C.

■ Commercial devices such as Arctic Blast® Intravenous Fluid Chiller (Medivance, Colorado, USA) are available. This device is TGA/FDA approved (http://www.accessdata.fda.gov/cdrh_docs/pdf8/K080899.pdf) and cools 2000 mL of saline to approximately 4°C as it is infused over 20 minutes.

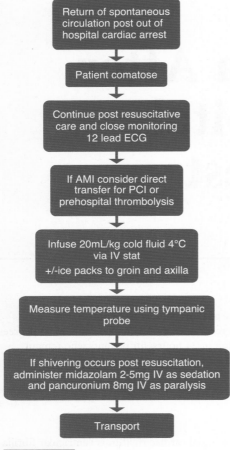

FIGURE 25–1

Step by Step Procedure for therapeutic hypothermia.

■ Ice packs applied to groin and axillae can be used.
■ Tympanic temperature probe.

ANESTHESIA AND PROCEDURAL MONITORING

■ Maintain electrocardiogram, oxygen saturation, and noninvasive blood pressure monitoring.
■ If shivering occurs, administer sedation (midazolam 2–5 milligrams IV) and a paralytic agent (pancuronium 8 milligrams).

STEP-BY-STEP PROCEDURE (FIGURE 25-1)

References

1. Oddo M, Ribordy V, Feihl F, et al. Early predictors of outcome in comatose survivors of ventricular fibrillation and non-ventricular fibrillation cardiac arrest treated with hypothermia: a prospective study. *Crit Care Med.* 2008 Aug;36(8):2296-301.PMID: 18664785

2. Bernard SA, Gray T, Buist MD, et al. Treatment of comatose survivors of out-of-hospital cardiac arrest with induced hypothermia.*N Engl J Med.* 2002 Feb 21;346(8):557-63.PMID: 11856794

3. The Hypothermia After Cardiac Arrest Study Group. Mild therapeutic hypothermia to improve the neurological outcome after cardiac arrest. *N Engl J Med* 2002 Feb 21;346(8):549-56. Erratum in: *N Engl J Med* 2002 May 30;346(22):1756. PMID: 11856793

4. ECC Committee, Subcommittees and Task Forces of the American Heart Association. 2005 American Heart Association Guidelines for Cardiopulmonary Resuscitation and Emergency Cardiovascular Care. *Circulation.* 2005 Dec 13;112(24 Suppl):IV1-203. Epub 2005 Nov 28. PMID: 16314375

5. Topjian AA, Nadkamium, Berg RA, Cardiopulmonary Resuscitation in Children. *Curr Opin. Crit Care* 2009 Jan 15(3):203.

6. Hall NJ, Eaton S, Peters MJ et al 'Mild Controlled Hypothermia in preterm infants with advancing necrotizing enterocolitis' Pediatrics 2010 Feb; 125 (2):e-300-8, epub 2010 Jan 25, 2010

CHAPTER 26

ECG Interpretation

Conor Deasy

FUNDAMENTALS OF ECG INTERPRETATION

The electrocardiogram or ECG is a way of measuring the electrical activity of the heart.

ECG Lead Placement

There are ten wires on an ECG machine that are connected to specific parts of the chest and limbs. These wires break down into two groups: six chest leads and four limb or peripheral leads. The six chest leads are positioned as in (Figure 26-1).

The six chest leads are labeled as "V" leads and numbered V_1 to V_6. They are positioned in specific positions on the rib cage. To position them accurately, it is important to be able to identify the "angle of Louis" or "sternal angle."

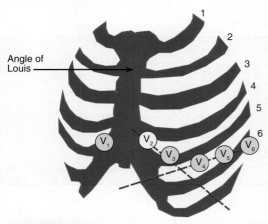

FIGURE 26–1

Chest Lead Placement.

The angle of Louis is most easily found when the patient is lying down, as the surrounding tissue is tighter against the rib cage.

The angle of Louis corresponds with the second intercostal space. From this position, run your fingers downward across the next rib and the next one. The space you are in is the fourth intercostal space. Where this space meets the sternum is the position for V_1. The corresponding intercostal space on the left is the position for V_2.

From this position, slide your fingers downward over the next rib and you are in the fifth intercostal space. The position for V_4 is in this space, in line with the middle of the clavicle (midclavicular). V_3 sits midway between V_2 and V_4. Follow the fifth intercostal space to the left until your fingers are immediately below the beginning of the axilla or underarm area. This is the position for V_5. Follow this line of the fifth intercostal space a little further until you are immediately below the center point of the axilla, (midaxilla). This is the position for V_6.

The limb leads have standardized colors so the **R**ed lead goes to the **R**ight wrist, the ye**LL**ow to the **l**eft wrist. The mnemonic "**Ride Your Green Bike**" is helpful in reminding the practitioner of lead placement, progressing clockwise from limb to limb commencing at the **r**ight wrist with the **r**ed lead, the **l**eft wrist with the **y**ellow, the green lead to the left ankle and the black lead to the right ankle (Figure 26-2). ECG machines often have a diagram printed on them indicating appropriate placement of leads.

Make sure that the electrocardiograph has been properly calibrated so that the standardization mark is 10 mm tall (1 mV = 10 mm). Each large square (5 mm) represents 0.2 seconds.

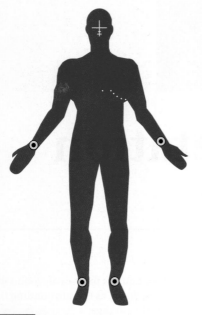

FIGURE 26–2

Limb leads are made up of 4 leads placed on the extremities: left and right wrist; left and right ankle.

ECG Interference and Quality

The ECG machine is designed to pick up electrical activity within the heart but it will pick up electrical activity from nearby machinery, such as pumps, TVs, drills, or machinery. The ECG should be repeated and modifiable problems corrected. Also check that all the electrodes are connected and have good contact with the skin (Figure 26-3).

Muscle tremor is something that can occur for a number of reasons, such as shivering due to cold, rigor, or Parkinson disease (see Figure 26-4).

Electrical Activity of the Heart

The electrical impulse usually originates in the sinoatrial node, high in the right atrium, traveling through the atria to the atrioventricular node and then down the bundle of His, bundle branches, and fascicular pathways to the ventricles. Purkinje fibers then conduct the electrical impulse from the inner surface known as the endocardium to the outer surface of the heart called the epicardium (Figure 26-5).

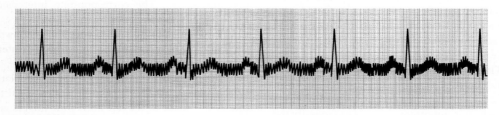

FIGURE 26–3

Electrical Interference.

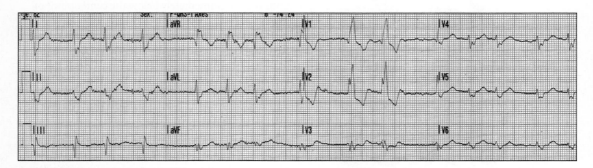

FIGURE 26–4

Atrial Fibrillation with Muscle Tremor. Irregularly-irregular rhythm of atrial fibrillation with baseline demonstrating underlying muscle tremor of the patient. Tall R waves in V_1 and V_2, and deep S wave in Lead I indicate RBBB. Axis-74° represents left axis deviation. Courtesy of Orange County (NC) EMS.

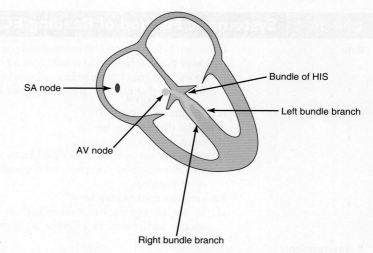

FIGURE 26–5

Origination of electrical activity.

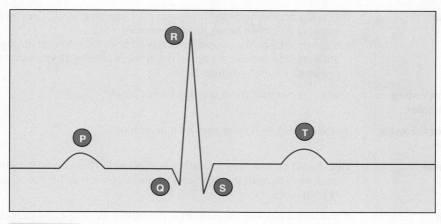

FIGURE 26–6

Parts of the ECG. P = P wave, atrial contraction; Q = Q wave, first negative deflection of the QRS complex; R = R wave, first upward deflection, ventricular contraction; ST = ST segment and T wave, repolarization.

Parts of the ECG

Atrial contraction is associated with the P wave of the ECG. Ventricular contraction is associated with the QRS complex (Figure 26-6).

Parts of the QRS

If the first deflection is downward, it is called a Q wave. Pathologic Q waves are greater than two small squares in depth. They are often followed by a reduced R wave and are indicators of myocardial tissue death. An upward deflection is called an R wave, even if not preceded by a Q wave. Any deflection below the baseline also called the isoelectric line following an R wave is referred to as the S wave.

Develop a systematic method of reading ECGs that is applied in every case (Table 26-1 and Figure 26-7).

1. **Is there a P wave?**
2. **Is each P wave the same shape?**
3. **Is each P wave followed by a QRS complex?**
4. **Is the P-R interval between three to five small squares?**
5. **Is the rhythm regular?**

Checking for Regularity

Place the edge of a piece of paper along the line of the rhythm strip and mark the center of two consecutive R waves. Compare this measurement with the next

Table 26–1	**Systematic Method of Reading ECG's**
Rate	If the rate is faster than 100 beats/minute, a tachycardia is present. A rate slower than 60 beats/min means that a bradycardia is present. To calculate the rate count the number of large boxes between successive R waves and divide that number into 300 (**Figure 26-7**)
Rhythm	Is it Regular or Irregular? A regular rhythm may be (1) sinus rhythm (2) sinus rhythm with extra (ectopic) beats such as atrial premature beats which are narrow complex or ventricular premature beats which are wide complex An irregular rhythm may be (1) an entirely ectopic mechanism such as atrial fibrillation or flutter, ventricular tachycardia or a 2nd or 3rd degree heart block
P wave present?	Yes or No
PR interval	This is the beginning of the p wave to the beginning of the QRS and should measure 3-5 small boxes (0.12-2 seconds) It is the time taken for excitation to spread from the SA node through the atrial muscle and the AV node, down the bundle of His and into the ventricular muscle (**Figure 26-5**)
P waves preceding QRS complex	Yes/No - If No then there may be a heart block
QRS waves following p waves	Yes/No - If No then there may be a heart block
QRS interval	This should be less than 3 small boxes and or 0.12 seconds. It represents excitation through the ventricles. If prolonged it may be due to a bundle branch block
QT length	If prolonged (>0.440 seconds) may predispose to ventricular tachycardia
Cardiac Axis	See text
ST segments	Look for elevation or depression

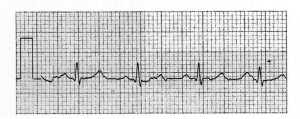

$$\text{Heart Rate} = \frac{300}{3} = 100 \text{ beats/minute}$$

FIGURE 26–7

Calculating the rate.

two R waves. If the measurements are the same, then the rhythm is regular.

Cardiac Axis

A simple method of working out the axis is to look at limb leads I, II, and III. In general if lead I is negative and lead III is positive and lead II is in the same direction as lead III, then this is right axis deviation (right on) (Figure 26-8). If lead I is positive and lead III negative and lead II and III are in the same direction, then this is left axis deviation (left outside) (Figure 26-9). Left axis deviation may suggest left ventricular hypertrophy. Right axis deviation may suggest right-sided heart strain such as found in pulmonary embolus (PE).

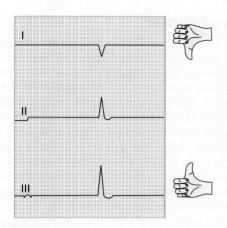

FIGURE 26–8

Right Axis Deviation – 'right on'.

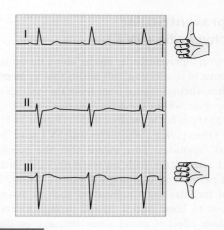

FIGURE 26–9

Left Axis Deviation – 'left outside'.

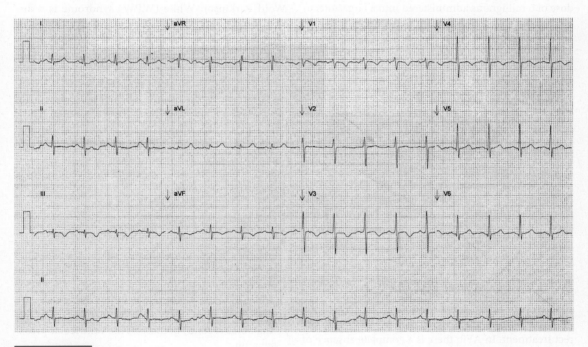

FIGURE 26–10

Sinus Tachycardia. Sinus tachycardia, rate=103. Narrow QRS complex, with each QRS preceded by a P wave. Also note T wave inversion in Lead III, T wave flattening in V_2 and T inversion in V_3. Courtesy of UNC Hospitals, Chapel Hill, NC.

Sinus Tachycardia

- R-R intervals constant and regular (Figure 26-10).
- One P wave per QRS complex.
- Rate is >100 bpm, but not usually >130 bpm at rest.

- Occurs normally during exercise/stress/pain. The patient is usually asymptomatic.
- Other causes may be hypovolemia/underlying medical problems such as hyperthyroidism or a result of sympathomimetic intake (ecstasy or cocaine).

Supraventricular Tachycardia (SVT)

The term supraventricular means "above the ventricles." In terms of conduction, this means that the abnormal rhythm is being initiated from above the ventricles from somewhere within the atria. The rate in SVT can be 100-250 bpm but is usually 140-200 (Figure 26-11).

Often patients who suffer with SVT have "paroxysmal" episodes. This means that the accelerated heart rate occurs with no warning, often lasting a brief period and stopping without treatment. Treatment includes vagal maneuvers such as asking the patient to blow into a 10-mL syringe to create a Valsalva effect. Carotid sinus massage or dipping the patient's head abruptly into a bucket of ice water are other vagal maneuvers that are often effective. If these actions are ineffective adenosine at an initial dose of 6 milligrams administered into a large antecubital vessel followed by an immediate flush may be used. Patients should be warned that they will feel a gripping sensation in their chest if adenosine is used. If it is ineffective, repeat after a few minutes using 12 milligrams again as a rapid push. Beta-blockers or synchronized cardioversion are used with specialist advice.

If patients are very tachycardic, hypotensive with evidence of hypoperfusion, with chest pain or severe pulmonary edema, primary synchronized cardioversion should be the first-line treatment.

There are a number of rhythms that fall into the category of SVT. These are atrial tachycardia, atrial flutter, atrial fibrillation, re-entry tachycardia (with accessory pathway), AV nodal re-entry, and Wolff-Parkinson-White syndrome (WPW) (AV bypass tract).

Atrial Fibrillation (AFib)

AFib (Figure 26-12) is the most common arrhythmia in most countries and is easily managed with the correct treatment. In AFib there is a complete absence of a sinoatrial stimulus, which would result in a P wave. In AFib the atria are fibrillating, or quivering, and that final 'atrial kick' that delivers the final 30% of blood from atria to the ventricles does not occur. AFib is an abnormality that exists above the ventricles at the sinoatrial node and, as a consequence of this, when a stimulus does get conducted through the AV node into the ventricles, the ventricles depolarize as they would do normally and therefore AFib will have a normal QRS complex (width less than three small squares).

Atrial Flutter

There are many similarities between atrial fibrillation and atrial flutter. Atrial flutter is an abnormality of conduction within the atria and, as with AFib, the ventricles work normally. The sequence of electrical impulses tends to be more regular than in AFib. The AV node (as in AFib), still acts as a "gatekeeper" and only conducts every second or third impulse due to the refractory period. The atria tends to flutter at around 300 bpm. As in AFib, these flutter waves bombard the AV node but in a much more organized and regular fashion. The flutter waves are also better defined than fibrillatory waves and tend to look like the teeth of a saw (for cutting wood); the ECG is often said to have a "saw-tooth" pattern (Figure 26-13).

Wolff-Parkinson-White Syndrome

Wolff-Parkinson-White (WPW) syndrome is a distinctive and important ECG abnormality caused by *preexcitation* of the ventricles. The WPW abnormality predisposes patients to paroxysmal SVT because of the presence of an extra conduction pathway. Patients may carry a pill in their pockets prescribed by their cardiologist for when this occurs. The acute treatment for WPW is ibutilide, procainamide, or flecainide. These drugs are capable of slowing the conduction through the accessory pathway. Adenosine should be used with caution if used at all. Digoxin, β-blockers and calcium-channel blockers are dangerous if given to these patients (Figure 26-14).

ECG features of WPW

■ The QRS is widened, giving the superficial appearance of a bundle branch block pattern. The wide QRS is caused not by a delay in ventricular depolarization but by early stimulation of the ventricles. The QRS is widened to the degree that the PR is shortened.

■ The PR is shortened (often but not always to less than 0.12 second) because of the ventricular preexcitation.

■ The upstroke of the QRS complex is slurred or notched. This is called a delta wave (see arrow) (Figure 26-15).

Heart Block

The time taken for the spread of depolarization from the SA node to the ventricular muscle is shown by the PR interval (0.12–0.2 or three to five small boxes). Heart block occurs when this pathway is delayed or interfered with.

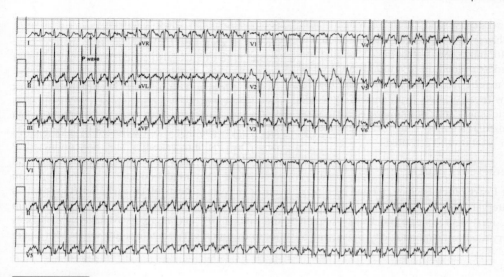

FIGURE 26–11

Supraventricular Tachycardia. Rate=195, narrow complex QRS (60 milliseconds) and prominent P wave (put in arrow) with PR interval 90 milliseconds. Courtesy of UNC Hospitals, Chapel Hill, NC.

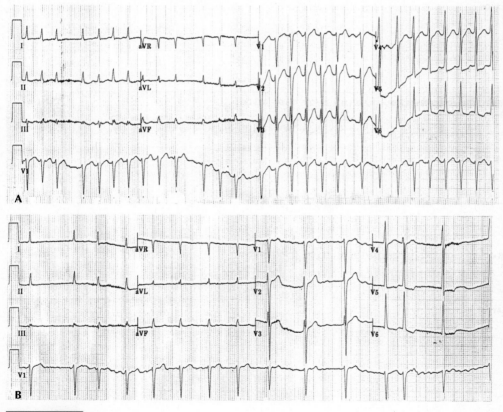

FIGURE 26–12

A and **B**, Atrial Fibrillation. A, narrow QRS complex with an irregularly irregular R-R interval, and no identifiable P waves. Ventricular rate is 163. B, After IV Diltiazem, the ventricular rate decreases to 88. The rhythm remains atrial fibrillation. Courtesy of UNC Hospitals, Chapel Hill, NC.

Heart blocks cause bradycardia (slow heart rate). If the patient has *symptomatic* bradycardia with a rate of less than 40, intravenous atropine (0.5 milligram doses repeated as needed up to a total limit dose of 3 milligrams) may be used to increase the heart rate. In bradycardia with associated hypotension, syncope, altered consciousness, and pulmonary edema, atropine may be used as a temporizing measure while the external pacer is set up and activated.

First Degree Heart Block

First- degree heart block is characterized by a prolonged PR interval (greater than 0.2 seconds or five small boxes). First degree heart block may suggest coronary artery disease, digoxin toxicity, or electrolyte disturbance.

Second Degree Heart Block

Second-degree heart block has two major types: Mobitz type I block (also called Wenckebach block) and Mobitz type II block.

In **Mobitz I block or Wenckebach block** there is progressive lengthening of the PR interval from beat to beat until a beat is "dropped." The dropped beat is a P wave that is not followed by a QRS complex. The PR interval after the nonconducted P wave is shorter than the PR interval of the beat just before the nonconducted P wave. Common causes of Wenckebach block include drugs such as β-blockers, calcium-channel blockers (diltiazem and verapamil), and digoxin. Wenckebach block is not uncommon with acute inferior wall AMI (Figure 26-16).

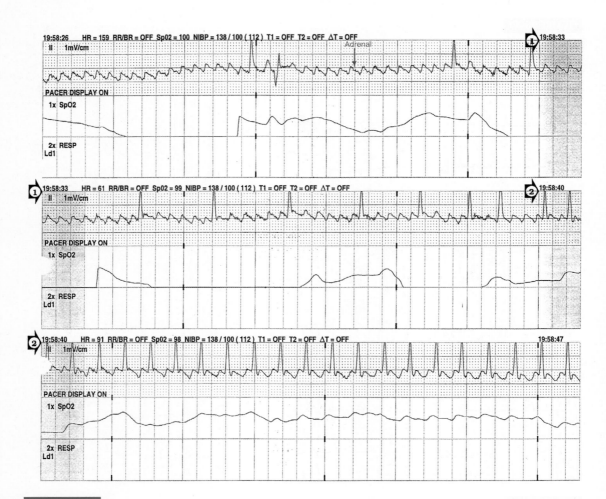

FIGURE 26–13

Atrial Flutter. Note the "sawtooth" atrial waves at a rate of about 300 per minute. Top rhythm strip: ventricular response rate is about 20 per minute. Middle rhythm strip: ventricular response rate is about 60 per minute. Bottom rhythm strip: ventricular response rate is about 160 per minute. Courtesy of UNC Hospitals, Chapel Hill, NC.

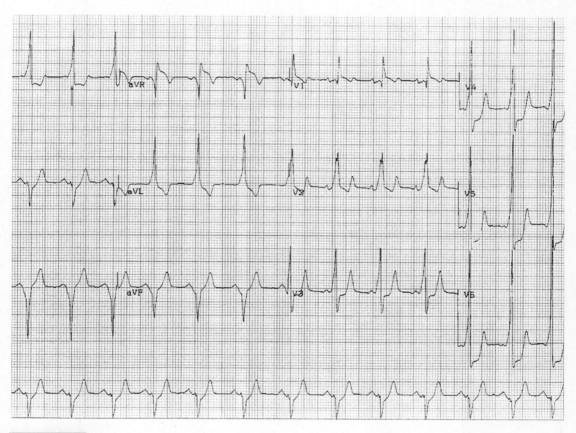

WPW. The arrow points to the delta wave. Courtesy of NC Baptist Hospital, Winston-Salem, NC.

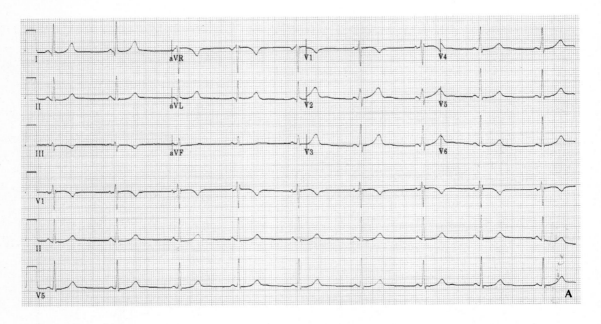

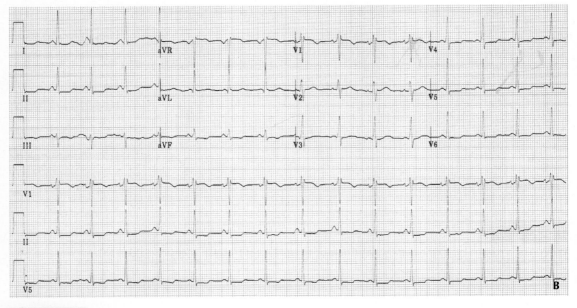

FIGURE 26–15

WPW with delta waves. Note short PR interval of 112 milliseconds (about 3 small squares) and the gentle upward slope of the beginning of the R wave. The gentle sloping is especially prominent in Lead V$_4$. Courtesy of UNC Hospitals, Chapel Hill, NC.

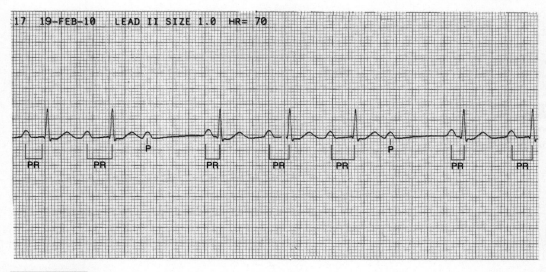

FIGURE 26–16

Second Degree Block, Mobitz I Wenckebach. Courtesy of UNC School of Medicine Human Simulator Lab, Jim Barrick, EMT-P.

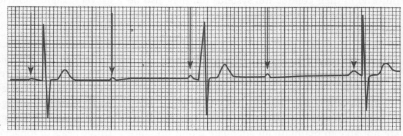

FIGURE 26–17

Second Degree Block, Mobitz II.

Mobitz II block AV block is a rarer and more serious form of second-degree heart block. Its characteristic feature is the sudden appearance of a single, nonconducted sinus P wave without the progressive prolongation of PR intervals seen in classic Mobitz type I (Wenckebach) AV block and shortening of the PR interval in the beat after the nonconducted P wave as seen with type I block (Figure 26-17). Mobitz type II block may be seen with anterior wall AMI, and can progress into complete heart block.

Therefore cardiologists generally treat patients with anterior wall AMI and Mobitz type II AV block by inserting a pacemaker.

The term ***advanced second-degree AV block*** refers to the distinct ECG finding of two or more consecutive nonconducted sinus P waves (Figure 26-18). For example, with sinus rhythm and 3:1 block, every third P wave is conducted; with 4:1 block, every fourth P wave is conducted, and so forth. This type of advanced block does not necessarily indicate a

Mobitz II mechanism. However, unless advanced second-degree AV block has a reversible cause (e.g., drug toxicity or hyperkalemia), a permanent pacemaker is usually required.

Third Degree Heart Block

Third-degree block, also called complete heart block, is a serious and potentially life-threatening arrhythmia. In third-degree heart block atrial contraction is normal but no beats are conducted to the ventricles. The ventricles are instead paced by an escape pacemaker located somewhere below the point of block in the AV junction.

The P waves bear no relation to the QRS complexes, and the PR intervals are completely variable because the atria and ventricles are electrically disconnected (Figure 26-19).

It is most commonly seen in older patients who have chronic degenerative changes (sclerosis or

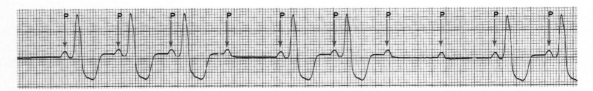

FIGURE 26–18

Second Degree Block, Mobitz II Advanced. Courtesy of UNC School of Medicine Human Simulator Lab, Jim Barrick, EMT-P.

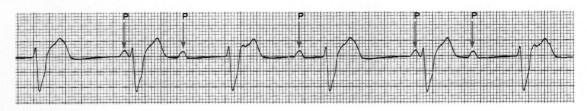

FIGURE 26–19

Third Degree Block. Courtesy of UNC School of Medicine Human Simulator Lab, Jim Barrick, EMT-P.

fibrosis) in their conduction systems but may also be seen in digitalis toxicity, Lyme disease, or acute anterior wall AMI.

Ventricular Tachycardia and Ventricular Fibrillation

Sustained ventricular tachycardia (VT) (Figure 26-20) is a life-threatening arrhythmia as many patients are not able to maintain an adequate blood pressure

at very rapid ventricular rates and the condition may degenerate into ventricular fibrillation, causing cardiac arrest.

Pulseless ventricular tachycardia is an indication for immediate defibrillation.

Sustained VT refers to an episode that lasts at least 30 seconds and generally requires termination by antiarrhythmia drugs or electrical cardioversion. Nonsustained VT suggests that the episodes are short (three beats or longer) and terminate spontaneously.

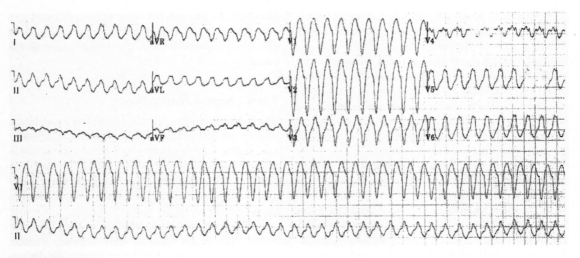

FIGURE 26–20

12-Lead ECG Ventricular Tachycardia. Courtesy of UNC School of Medicine Dept of Anaesthesiology, Frances W. Smith EMT-P.

VT is usually associated with coronary artery disease. Patients who have VT in the absence of coronary artery disease may have other cardiac abnormalities, including cardiomyopathy, mitral valve prolapse, valvular heart disease, QT interval prolongation or, in an otherwise normal heart, an abnormality described as primary electrical instability.

Summary of ECG Criteria for VT

- There are no normal-looking QRS complexes.
- Rate: Greater than 100 beats/minute and usually not faster than 200 beats/minute.
- Rhythm: Usually regular but may be irregular.
- P waves: In rapid VT the P waves are usually not recognizable. At slower ventricular rates, P waves may be seen after the QRS, and may represent normal atrial depolarization from the sinus node at a rate slower than VT, but the electrical activities do not affect one another.
- The width of the QRS is 0.12 second or greater.
- The QRS shape is often bizarre (Figure 26-21).

A distinct type of VT is called **torsades de pointes** and is characterized by a continuously changing axis of polymorphic QRS morphologies (Figure 26-22).

Causes

- Drugs, particularly antiarrhythmic agents, psychotropic agents, tricyclic antidepressants, and other noncardiac drugs such as methadone, cisapride, and erythromycin and related antibiotics.
- Electrolyte imbalances, especially hypokalemia, hypomagnesemia, and hypocalcemia, which prolong repolarization can also cause this lethal arrhythmia.
- Hereditary long QT syndromes.

Ventricular Fibrillation

In ventricular fibrillation (VF) the ventricle quivers asynchronously and ineffectively. (**Figure 26-23** and **Figure 26-24**) The heart cannot pump any blood

and the patient becomes unconscious immediately in 'cardiac arrest'. VF requires immediate defibrillation with an unsynchronized shock (2). (**Figure 26-25**)

Bundle branch block

If there is abnormal conduction through either the right or left bundle branches there will be a delay in the depolarisation of part of the ventricular muscle causing a widening of the QRS complex. The QRS should be less than 3 small boxes in width (0.12 seconds). If it

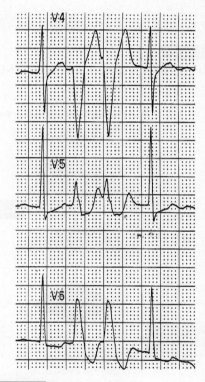

FIGURE 26–21

ECG showing Ventricular Tachycardia, Monomorphic. Two beats of non-sustained Ventricular Tachycardia. Courtesy of UNC Hospitals, Chapel Hill, NC.

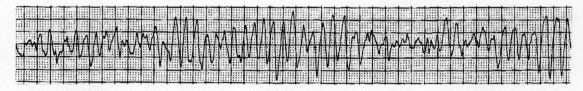

FIGURE 26–22

Torsades de Pointe. Courtesy of UNC Heart Center, Chapel Hill, NC Paula Miller, MD.

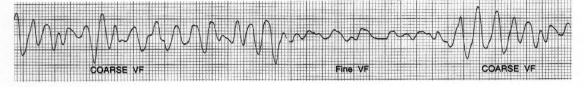

FIGURE 26–23

Ventricular Fibrillation. Courtesy of UNC School of Medicine Human Simulator Lab, Jim Barrick, EMT-P.

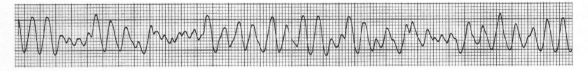

FIGURE 26–24

Ventricular Fibrillation (coarse). Courtesy of UNC School of Medicine Human Simulator Lab, Jim Barrick, EMT-P.

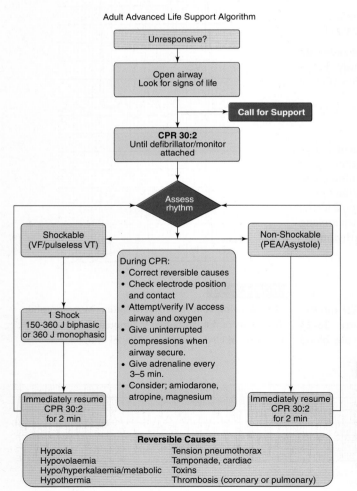

FIGURE 26–25

Algorithm for Unconscious Patient[2]. Adapted from the 2005 American Heart Association Guidelines for Cardiopulmonary Resuscitation and Emergency Cardiovascular Care: Pt 1 Introduction: Circulation. 2005;112 [Suppl I]:IV-1-IV-5; Nov 28 2005.

is greater than this then abnormal conduction through the ventricles via a slower pathway has occurred. Right bundle branch block (RBBB) may suggest a problem in the right side of the heart. Left bundle branch block (LBBB) is always an indication of heart disease usually of the left side of heart. When LBBB or RBBB are present it makes it challenging to further interpret the ECG.

Right bundle branch block is best seen in Lead V_1 where an RSR^1 pattern is seen. (**Figure 26-26**)

Left bundle branch block is best seen in V_6, where there is a broad complex resembling the letter 'M' known as an M pattern. (**Figure 26-27**)

The mnemonic 'WILLIAM MORROW' is helpful in recalling the patterns associated with LBBB and RBBB. An M type pattern is seen in V_6 in Left bundle branch block with a W type pattern seen in V_1. An M type pattern is seen in V_1 in right bundle branch block with a W type pattern in V_6 in right bundle branch block. (**Figure 26-28**)

Left Bundle Branch Block with Atrial Fibrillation and Rapid Ventricular Response

The broad QRS complex in Lead I identifies this as a LBBB. The irregular-irregular rhythm means this is NOT Ventricular Tachycardia, because VT has a regular rhythm. There are no P waves visible, and the irregularly irregular rhythm identifies this as atrial fibrillation. (see **Figure 26-29**)

Acute Myocardial Infarction

When myocardial blood supply is abruptly reduced or cut off to a region of the heart the ECG changes that occur concern the ST segment. ST elevation indicates acute myocardial injury, either infarction or pericarditis. The leads in which the elevation occurs indicate the region of the heart involved. Anterior heart wall damage shows in the chest leads and inferior heart wall damage in Leads II, III, and aVL.

Tall broad T waves may be seen (also called hyperacute T waves) in advance of the ST changes. ST elevation (**Figure 26-30**) indicates the need for reperfusion with thrombolysis or angioplasty. Subsequently Q waves appear, and the T waves become inverted. The ST segments return to baseline within 24-48 hours usually unless pericarditis or a heart wall aneurysm has developed. (**Figure 26-31 and Figure 26-32**).

T wave inversion

T waves are normally inverted in Leads aVR and V_1. Sometimes, T wave inversion occurs in Lead III, V_2 and V_3 (in some African-Americans). T wave inversion may indicate ischaemia, ventricular hypertrophy, bundle branch block, digoxin treatment or may be a normal variant. (**Figure 26-33** and **Figure 26-34**)

If an infarct is not involving the full thickness of the heart wall then there will be T wave inversion but no pathological Q waves (Non STEMI).

Location of Infarct

AMIs are generally localized to a specific portion of the left ventricle, affecting either the anterior or the inferior wall.

1. **Anterior Infarction:** ST elevation in Leads V_3-V_4, but often also in Leads V_2 and V_5. (**Figure 26-35**)
2. **Inferior Infarction:** ST elevation in Leads II and III and aVF. (**Figure 26-36**)
3. **Lateral Infarction:** changes in Leads I, aVL V_5-V_6. (**Figure 26-37**)
4. **Posterior Infarction:** tall R waves and ST depressions may occur in Leads V_1 and V_2. In most cases of posterior AMI, the infarct extends either to the lateral wall of the left ventricle, producing characteristic changes in Lead V_6, or to the inferior wall of that ventricle, producing characteristic changes in Leads II, III, and aVL (see **Figure 26-38**).
5. **AMI in presence of LBBB:** An indicator of myocardial infarction in the presence of left bundle-branch block is ST change— that is, ST deviation in the same (concordant) direction as the QRS complex. Concordant ST changes in the presence of left bundle-branch block include ST-segment depression of at least 1 mm in Lead V_1, V_2, or V_3 or in Lead II, III, or aVF and elevation of at least 1 mm in Lead V_5. Extremely discordant ST deviation (>5 mm) is also suggestive of myocardial infarction in the presence of left bundle-branch block. (see **Figure 26-39**)

ECG indicating pacemaker spikes

Note the small positive deflection before the wide QRS complexes seen in Leads V_3 through V_6. The positive deflection represents the electrical discharge of the pacemaker wire which is in the right ventricular cavity. There are no P waves evident. The QRS complex is broad because the electrical impulse is propagated by muscle-to-muscle activation in the ventricles, and not through the right or left bundle branches. **Figure 26-40** and **Figure 26-41** show pacer spikes.

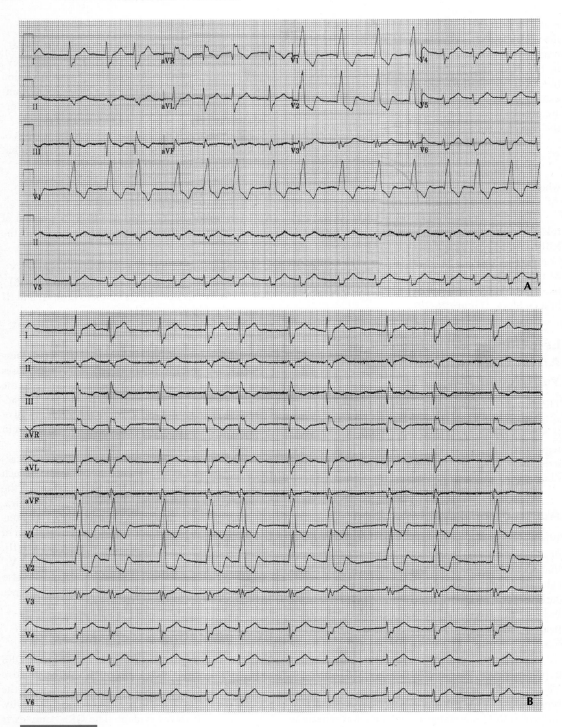

FIGURE 26–26

Right Bundle Branch Block. Tall R waves in V_1 and deep S waves in Lead V_6 indicate Right Bundle Branch Block. ST changes associated with RBBB are generally opposite the direction of the QRS complex. Courtesy of UNC Hospitals.

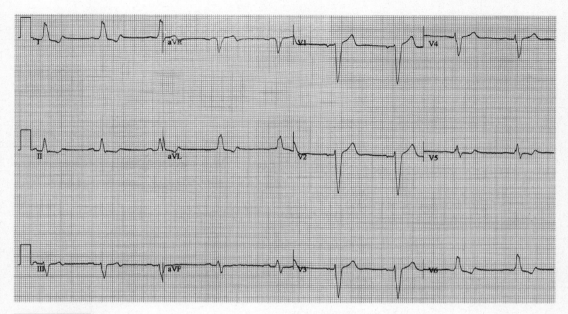

FIGURE 26–27

Left Bundle Branch Block with Sinus Bradycardia. Courtesy of UNC Heart Center, Chapel Hill, NC, Paula Miller, MD.

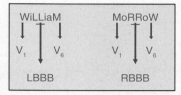

FIGURE 26–28

WILLIAM MORROW pneumonic.

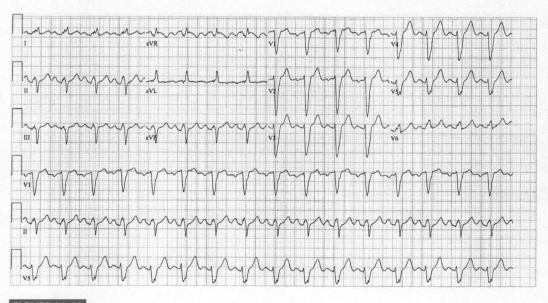

FIGURE 26–29

Left Bundle Branch Block. LBBB is characterized by a QRS duration >120 milliseconds. The wide QRS is most evident in Leads I and V$_6$. Courtesy of UNC Hospitals.

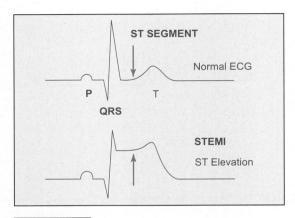

FIGURE 26–30

Acute ST segment elevation.

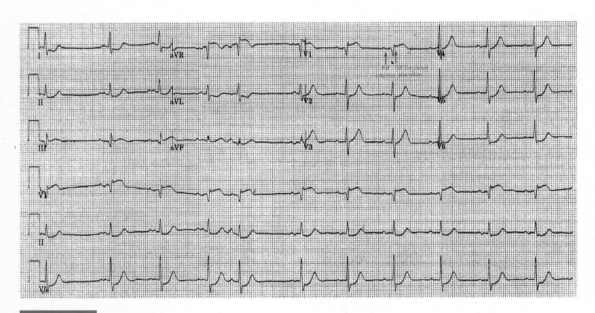

FIGURE 26–31

ST Elevation. Prominent ST elevation in Lead V_1. To detect ST elevation, compare the ST segment with the previous PR interval. Make sure the ECG lead is recorded in a straight line. Courtesy of UNC Hospitals and Alamance Co (NC) EMS.

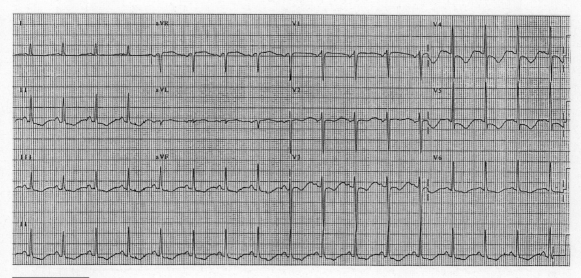

FIGURE 26–32

ST Depression. ST depression is evident in Leads V_4, V_5, and V_6. The ST is depressed when compared to the preceding PR interval of the QRS segments in V_4, V_5, and V_6. Courtesy of UNC Hospitals.

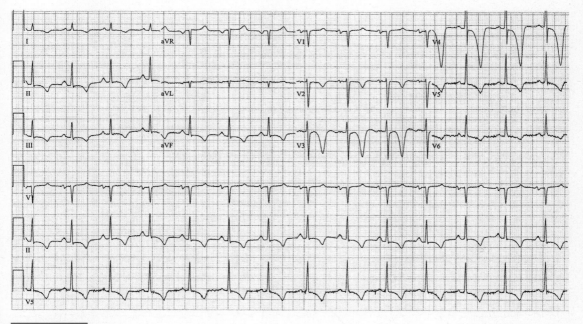

FIGURE 26–33

T-wave inversion. T wave inversion is noted in Leads I, II, III, aVF, and V_2-V_6. The T wave inversion is very deep in leads V_3-V_4 suggesting lateral endocardial ischemia. Courtesy of UNC Hospitals.

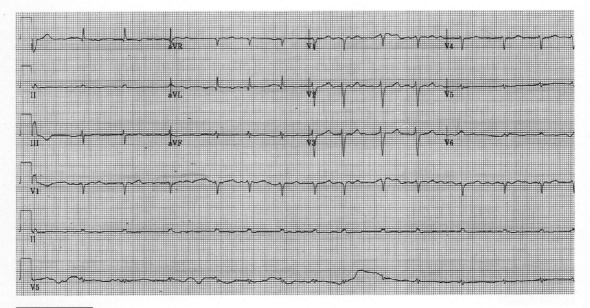

FIGURE 26–34

Flattened T-wave. Note flattened T waves in Leads II, aVF, and V₅. The underlying rhythm is atrial fibrillation. Courtesy of UNC Hospitals.

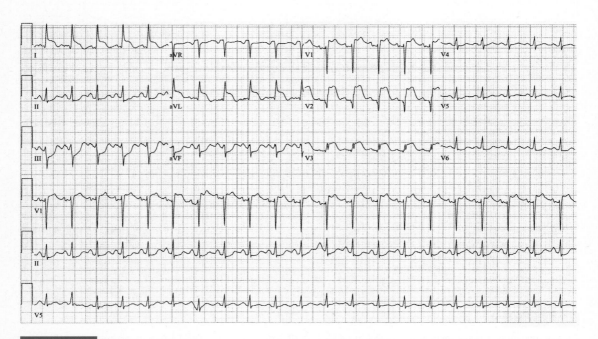

FIGURE 26–35

Anterior AMI. Marked ST elevation in Leads I, aVL, V₂, V₃, and V₄ with reciprocal ST depression in Leads II, III, and aVF. Courtesy of UNC Hospitals.

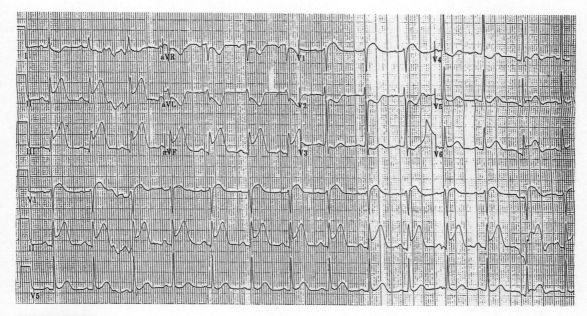

FIGURE 26–36

Acute Inferior Infarction. Note marked ST elevation in Leads II, III, and aVF, with reciprocal changes of ST depression most marked in Lead aVL. Courtesy of UNC Hospitals.

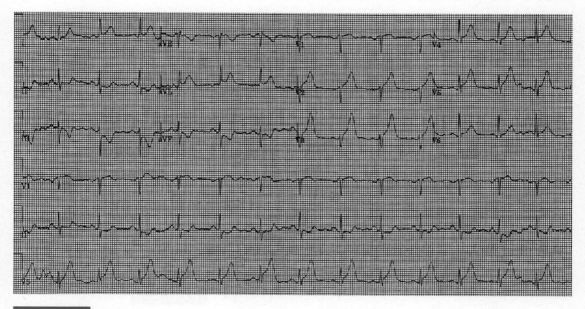

FIGURE 26–37

Lateral Infarction: see changes in Leads I, aVL, V_4, and V_6. Courtesy of UNC School of Medicine Dept of Anaesthesiology, Frances W. Smith, EMT-P.

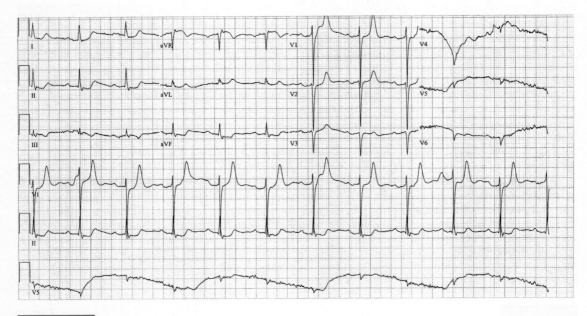

FIGURE 26–38

Posterior Infarction. Note very small R waves in V_2-V_5 and no R wave in V_6. In a normal ECG, the R waves increase in prominence from V_1-V_6. The reciprocal changes of ST segment depression evident in I, II, and aVF indicate an acute MI responsible for the lack of R waves in the lateral precordial leads. Courtesy of UNC Hospitals.

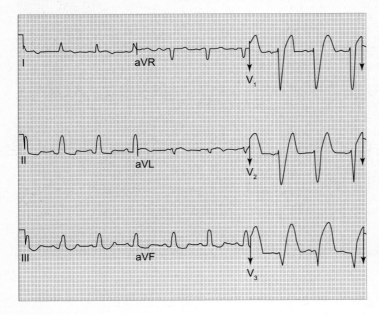

FIGURE 26–39

AMI in the presence of LBBB – Sgarbossa criteria.

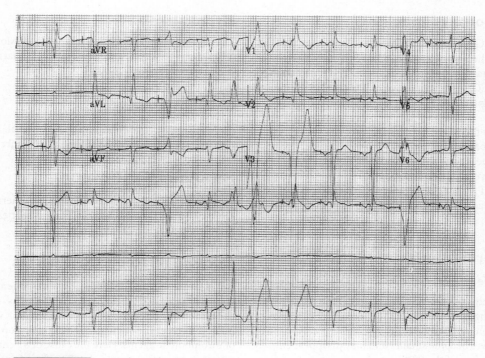

FIGURE 26–40

Atrial Pacemaker. Courtesy of NC Baptist Hospital, Winston-Salem, NC, David Cline, MD.

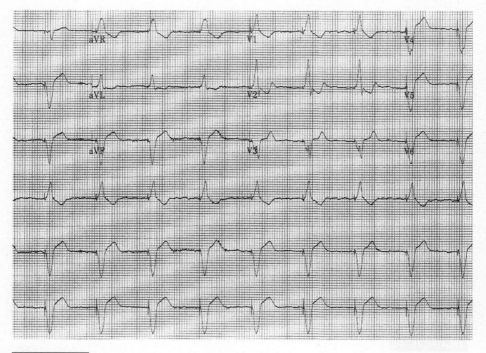

FIGURE 26–41

Ventricular Pacemaker. Courtesy of NC Baptist Hospital, Winston-Salem, NC, David Cline, MD.

Pulmonary Embolism

The ECG features of Pulmonary Embolism are those of right heart strain as the right heart struggles to overcome the blockage in the pulmonary circulation.

ECG signs suggestive of Pulmonary Embolism are: (**Figure 26-42**)

■ Sinus tachycardia.
■ Right axis deviation.
■ Tall peaked P waves, especially in Lead II.
■ T wave inversion in Leads V_1-V_4.
■ $S_1Q_3T_3$ changes: S wave in Lead I, a Q wave in Lead III and an inverted T wave in Lead III are seen.

Hyperkalaemia

ECG features: (Figure 26-43)

■ Initially tall tented T waves meaning there is narrowing and peaking of the T waves.
■ Prolonged PR intervals.
■ P waves become smaller and may disappear entirely.
■ Widening of the QRS complexes.
■ Sine wave pattern.

Hypokalemia

The most common pattern seen is ST depressions with prominent U waves and prolonged repolarization. (**Figure 26-44**)

Calcium levels

Hypocalcemia causes prolonged QT interval. Hypercalcemia causes shortened QT interval. (**Figure 26-45**)

Hypothermia

Prominent J waves (see arrows) with hypothermia are referred to as Osborn waves. They disappear with rewarming. (**Figure 26-46**)

Cocaine related ECG changes

ECGs are abnormal in 56 to 84% of patients with cocaine-associated chest pain; as many as 43% of cocaine-using patients with chest pain but without infarction meet the standard ECG criteria for the use of thrombolytic agents. Here the cause of ST changes is artery spasm rather than a clot. The treatment is generally medical management rather than thrombolysis.

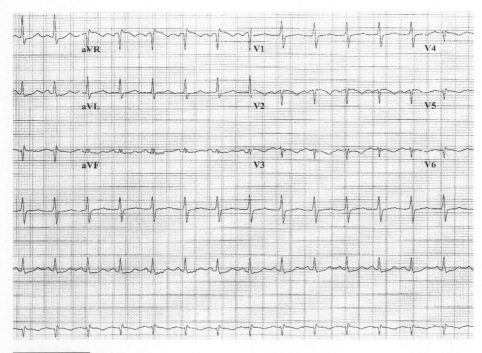

FIGURE 26–42

ECG Pulmonary Embolism S1Q3T3. Courtesy of NC Baptist Hospital, Winston-Salem, NC, David Cline, MD.

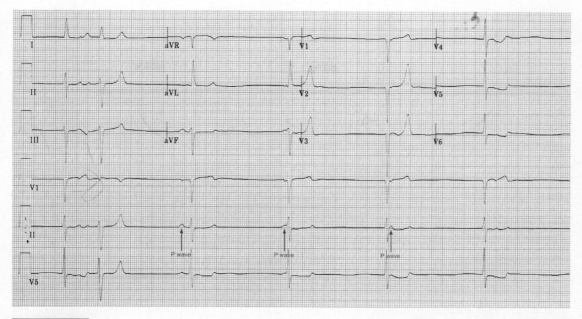

FIGURE 26–43

Hyperkalemia. Tall peaked T waves of hyperkalemia are seen in Leads V_2 and V_3. The narrow and regular QRS complex (104 milliseconds) (rate=38) without a preceding P wave indicates a junctional rhythm. P waves are seen without any relationship to the QRS complexes *(arrows)*. The patient's serum potassium was 6.9 meq/L at the time this ECG was performed. The ECG changes of AV dissociation and marked bradycardia indicate severe hyperkalemia. Courtesy of UNC Hospitals.

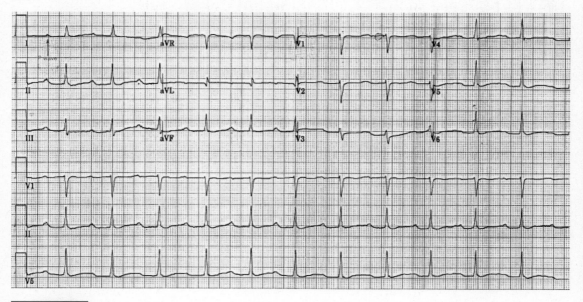

FIGURE 26–44

Hypokalemia. Hypokalemia: Potassium 2.09 meq/L. Note prolonged PR, QT and QTc intervals. Courtesy of UNC Hospitals.

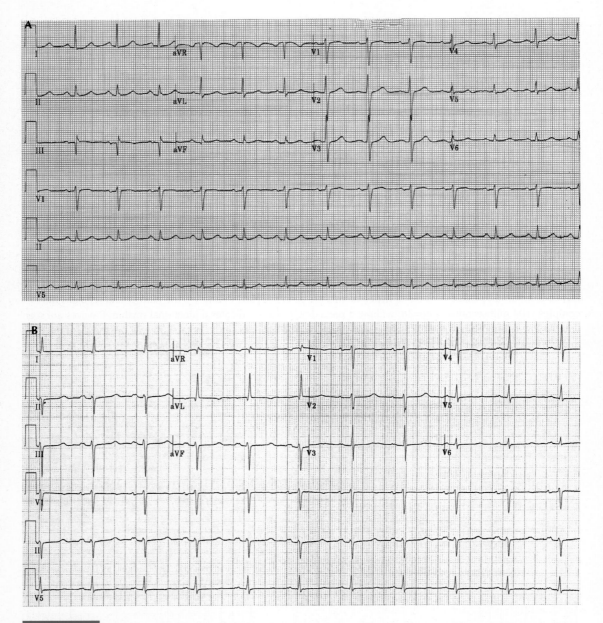

FIGURE 26–45

ECG's comparing Normal Calcium and Hypocalemia. **A**, Normal calcium, QT 414 milliseconds. **B**, Hypocalcemia, calcium 3.9 meq/L total calcium, QT 598 milliseconds and QTc 607 milliseconds. Courtesy of UNC Hospitals.

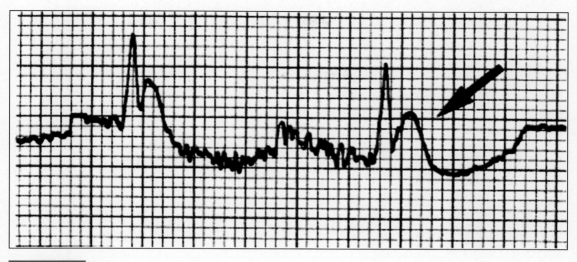

FIGURE 26–46

Hypothermia. Rhythm strip from patient with temperature of 25°C (77°F) showing atrial fibrillation with a slow ventricular response, muscle tremor artifact, and Osborn (J) wave *(arrow)*. Reprinted with permission, Figure 192-1, 6th ed. Tintinalli's Emergency Medicine Study Guide.

References

1. Gitter MJ, Goldsmith SR, Dunbar DN, Sharkey SW. Cocaine and chest pain: clinical features and outcome of patients hospitalized to rule out myocardial infarction. *Ann Intern Med*. 1991 Aug 15;115(4): 277-82. PMID: 1854111

2. American Heart Association Guidelines for Cardiopulmonary Resuscitation and Emergency Cardiovascular Care: Part 1 Introduction: *Circulation*. 2005;112 [Suppl I]:IV-1-IV-5; Nov 2005, (doi:10.1161/*CIRCULATION AHA*.105.166550 http://circ.ahajournals.org/content/vol112/24_suppl/)

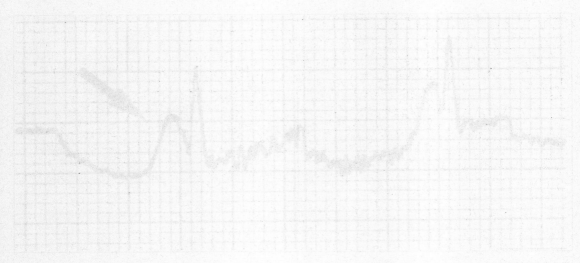

CHAPTER 27

Prehospital Fibrinolysis

Conor Deasy

KEY LEARNING POINTS

- "Time is heart".
- PCI wins if prehospital fibrinolysis saves less than 1 hour of time.
- Fibrinolysis checklists improve patient safety.

- Established protocols with a PCI facility are needed to avoid confusion, indecision, and time delays.

INTRODUCTION

Fibrinolysis is dissolution of an arterial clot by drugs or mechanically with a variety of intraarterial catheters. Fibrinolysis during cardiac catheterization is termed percutaneous coronary intervention [PCI]. Fibrinolysis is also used for acute ischemic stroke. **In this chapter, the term "prehospital fibrinolysis" means the administration of fibrinolytic agents for coronary artery clot dissolution.**

Out-of-hospital administration of fibrinolysis by paramedics, nurses, or physicians using an established protocol is safe and feasible for patients with ST elevation myocardial infarction (STEMI) with no contraindications to the treatment.[17] However, prehospital fibrinolysis requires adequate training and provisions for the diagnosis and treatment of STEMI and its complications, including strict treatment protocols, a prehospital fibrinolysis checklist, ECG acquisition and interpretation skills,

experience with defibrillators and in ACLS protocols, and the ability to communicate with medical control. In this chapter, the evidence surrounding prehospital fibrinolysis is described. Some recent controversies are also discussed. The treatment pathway for patients with STEMI is described from dispatch, to paramedic assessment, through prehospital treatment, including prehospital fibrinolysis.

PURPOSE OF PREHOSPITAL FIBRINOLYSIS

The benefits of fibrinolysis in patients with acute myocardial infarction (AMI) are time-dependent: **"Time is heart." When patients are treated within an hour of onset of symptoms, mortality is reduced up to 48%.[1,2]**

Percutaneous coronary intervention (PCI) is preferred over prehospital fibrinolysis IF a

skilled facility is available and the time to PCI from onset of symptoms is less than 1 hour.[4,17]

However, *if the time period of 1 hour to PCI cannot be met*, prehospital fibrinolysis for STEMI significantly *decreases* the time to coronary artery clot dissolution and *decreases* hospital mortality.[3] The CAPTIM (Comparison of Primary Angioplasty and Pre-hospital fibrinolysis In acute Myocardial infarction) compared 30-day and 5-year outcomes between prehospital fibrinolysis and primary angioplasty for acute STEMI. It found outcomes equivalent for acute STEMI (onset of symptoms within 6 hours), for prehospital fibrinolysis with transport to an interventional facility, and primary angioplasty (percutaneous coronary intervention or PCI).[4,5]

Prehospital fibrinolysis and subsequent PCI, also called "facilitated percutaneous coronary intervention (PCI)," increases the risk of intracranial bleeding and reinfarction.[6,7] **Therefore key prehospital decisions depend upon the accurate diagnosis of STEMI and a determination of how rapidly PCI can be accomplished** (see **Table 27-1, Table 27-2, and Table 27-3**).

Rapidly identify patients with STEMI and quickly screen them for indications and contraindications to fibrinolytic therapy or PCI.

Hospitals with capabilities for PCI should have a clear protocol directing EMS and ED triage in initial management. Confusion about the method of reperfusion, e.g., prehospital or ED fibrinolysis or PCI, delays definitive therapy.

Patients with extensive ECG changes (consistent with a large acute MI) and a low risk of intracranial

Table 27–1	**STEMI: Indications for Fibrinolysis or PCI**[17]

Chest pain lasting >15 minutes and less than 12 hours **with:**

- ST-segment elevation of >2 mm in two or more contiguous precordial leads or >1 mm in two or more adjacent limb leads
  or
- Presumed new left bundle branch block (LBBB) but discuss this with medical support
  or
- Reciprocal ST segment depression (V_2–V_3) due to posterior wall damage but discuss this with medical support

bleeding receive benefit from fibrinolysis.[18] Patients with symptoms highly suggestive of acute myocardial infarction and ECG findings consistent with left bundle branch block (LBBB) are also appropriate candidates for intervention because they have the highest mortality rate when LBBB is caused by an extensive myocardial infarction. However, indications for fibrinolysis therapy in new LBBB require complex decision-making that is best discussed first with medical support from the specialist center.

The benefits of fibrinolysis are less impressive in inferior wall infarction except when it is associated with RV infarction (ST-segment elevation in lead V_4 or anterior ST-segment depression).[18]

Table 27–2	**History Taking in the Patient with Possible Acute Myocardial Infarction**[8]
Commenced when?	What time did the pain start?
History/risk factors	History of ischemic heart disease (IHD), smoking, diabetes, high cholesterol, high blood pressure, family history of IHD
Extra Symptoms	Symptoms such as back pain, shortness of breath, nausea, sweating, palpitations, dizzy, weak, feelings of impending doom
Stays or radiates	Does the pain travel anywhere?
Timing	Is it there continuously or does it come and go; how long does it last?
Place	Where is the pain?
Alleviates/aggravates	Does anything improve or worsen the pain?
Intensity	Rate the pain on a scale from 1–10
Nature	Describe the pain – listen without suggesting descriptors such as dull, crushing, sharp, or vise-like pain

Adapted from Newberry L, Barnett GK, Ballard N. A new mnemonic for chest pain assessment. *J Emerg Nurs* Feb;31(1): 84, 2005.

Table 27–3	Comparison of Indications for Fibrinolysis and PCI	
Prehospital or ED Fibrinolysis Is Generally Preferred if:	**An Invasive Strategy (PCI) Is Generally preferred if:**	
Early presentation (≤3 hours from symptom onset)	Late presentation (symptom onset >3 hours ago)	
Invasive strategy is not an option (e.g., lack of access to skilled PCI facility or difficult vascular access) or procedure would be delayed	Skilled PCI facility available with surgical backup	
Medical contact to balloon or door to balloon is expected to be >90 minutes	Medical contact to balloon or door to balloon <90 minutes	
(Door to balloon) minus (door to needle) is >1 hour	(Door to balloon) minus (door to needle) is <1 hour.	
No contraindications to fibrinolysis	Contraindications to fibrinolysis, including increased risk of bleeding and ICH	
	High risk from STEMI (CHF, cardiogenic shock).	
	Diagnosis of STEMI is in doubt	

CHF = congestive heart failure; ICH = intracranial hemorrhage; PCI = percutaneous coronary intervention; STEMI = ST-elevation acute myocardial infarction.

PATIENT SELECTION: HISTORY TAKING

"CHEST PAIN" is a helpful mnemonic to ensure that a focused yet complete chest pain history has been taken from the patient[8] (**Table 27-2**).

The following are justifications of the various equipment and drugs that are listed in Table 27-4:

Table 27–4	Equipment and Drugs Needed for Prehospital Fibrinolysis

- ■ Monitor ECG/BP/oxygen saturation
- ■ 12-lead ECG +/– transmission capability
- ■ 100% oxygen
- ■ Chewable Aspirin 325 milligrams PO if not allergic
- ■ NTG/GTN 2 puffs if no contraindications
- ■ Fibrinolytic checklist
- ■ Intravenous cannula
- ■ Morphine 2.5 milligrams to 10 milligrams IV for pain
- ■ Enoxaparin 30 milligrams IV
- ■ IV bolus fibrinolytic agent (ie reteplase or tenecteplase)
- ■ Defibrillator

ECG = electrocardiogram; BP = blood pressure; GTN = ; NTG = nitroglycerin.

ECG

Routine use of the 12-lead out-of-hospital ECG with advance ED notification reduces the time interval to fibrinolysis. Advance ED notification may be achieved with direct transmission of the ECG itself or verbal report (via telephone) of the ECG interpretation by out-of-hospital personnel. Where transmission of the ECG to the ED is not feasible, the ability of paramedics to accurately read 12-lead ECGs is crucial to the success of both safe prehospital fibrinolysis and/or prehospital activation of the PCI facility. **Paramedics can diagnose STEMI and identify appropriate PCI activations with a high degree of accuracy.**[16]

Aspirin

Ideally, dispatchers should advise the patient with suspected acute coronary syndrome (ACS) to chew a single dose (325 milligrams) of aspirin (ASA) after making sure the patient is not allergic to aspirin. **Aspirin is safe and the earlier it is given, the greater the reduction in risk of mortality.**[9] If the patient has not already taken an aspirin, give him or her *chewable* aspirin (325 milligrams) not coated, swallowed aspirin tablets.[10–13] **Low-dose aspirin (75 or 81 milligrams) is not an adequate dose. Chewable or soluble aspirin is absorbed more quickly than swallowed tablets.**[14,15] **If the patient is allergic to aspirin, give clopidogrel, 300 milligrams PO instead.**

The cause of an acute myocardial infarction is usually an occlusion of blood platelets in a coronary artery, which then leads to a blood clot formed by a network of fibrin and other blood clotting factors. The clot stops blood flow in the coronary artery, and if obstruction is prolonged, cardiac muscle served by the occluded artery dies. Aspirin prevents platelet clumping and reduces the degree of coronary artery blockage. Once aspirin is given, it has an effect on platelets for the entire life of a platelet, which is about 10 days.

Fibrinolytic Agents

Fibrinolytic agents are compounds that dissolve the fibrin network of a blood clot. Second-generation fibrin-specific agents that are available as a single dose or bolus (i.e., reteplase, tenecteplase) are the fibrinolytics of choice. Bolus doses of fibrinolytic agents are easier to administer, have a lower chance of medication errors (and the associated increase in mortality when such medication errors occur), and less internal bleeding than fibrinolytics that have to be administered as an infusion.[21,22]

Low Molecular Weight Heparin

In those patients less than 75 years of age and receiving fibrinolytic therapy for STEMI, low molecular weight heparin (LMWH) is also administered. Enoxaparin is given as an intravenous bolus of 30 milligrams. **Do not give enoxaparin to patients over 75 years old because they could experience more bleeding complications.**[24] Give heparin with fibrinolytics when treating acute myocardial infarction, but **NEVER give heparin when fibrinolytics are given for stroke.** If heparin is given along with fibrinolytics in a patient with acute stroke, there is a great risk of intracerebral bleeding.

Advanced Considerations: Antiplatelet Agents and Fibrinolytics

Acute myocardial infarction (AMI) is generally caused by platelet aggregation and thrombus formation at the site of a ruptured atherosclerotic plaque. If obstruction to blood flow is prolonged, AMI occurs.

Platelets cause obstruction by platelet adhesion, aggregation, and activation. *Platelet adhesion* is the sticking of platelets to an area of damaged endothelium. *Platelet aggregation* is progressive accumulation of platelets at the site of injury. *Platelet activation* is the release of substances by the aggregated platelets, which further enhances aggregation. Activated platelets

become cross-linked with fibrinogen molecules, and a stronger clot is formed.

Aspirin inhibits platelet aggregation by a very specific mechanism - that of preventing the formation of thromboxane A_2 through the arachidonic acid pathway. This effect is immediate and requires an aspirin dose >160 milligrams. Aspirin alone reduces the relative mortality rate from AMI by about 25%.

Clopidogrel irreversibly inhibits the platelet adenosine diphosphate receptor, resulting in a reduction in platelet aggregation through a different mechanism than aspirin. It has an immediate effect. Clopidogrel (300 milligrams PO) should be given for AMI if the patient is allergic to aspirin. Patients up to 75 years of age with STEMI receiving fibrinolysis, aspirin, and heparin are generally also given a 300-milligram oral loading dose of clopidogrel.[25]

Glycoprotein (GP) IIb/IIIa antagonists are stronger antiplatelet agents than aspirin because they interrupt platelet activation regardless of agonist. GP IIb/IIIa inhibitors are not currently recommended in patients receiving prehospital fibrinolysis for STEMI. In patients treated with PCI without fibrinolysis, it may be helpful in reducing mortality rates and short-term reinfarction. There is no evidence documenting a better outcome by giving GP IIb/IIIa inhibitors out of hospital or early in the ED.

Fibrinolytic agents lyse the acute thrombosis directly or indirectly as plasminogen activators. Plasminogen is a proteolytic enzyme, which binds directly to fibrin during clot formation to form a plasminogen-fibrin complex. Fibrinolytic agents activate plasminogen in the plasminogen-fibrin complex and cause fibrin lysis.

Any patient factors that increase the risk of hemorrhage from fibrinolytic therapy are relative or absolute contraindications to the use of fibrinolytic agents (see **Fibrinolysis Checklist in Box 27-1**). Intracranial hemorrhage is more common with tissue plasminogen activator (tPA) than with streptokinase. The benefits of therapy should always be balanced against the risks.

Only about half of patients have early and substantial restoration of coronary blood flow from fibrinolytic agents. When fibrin is lysed, thrombin is exposed. The exposed thrombin activates platelets, instituting a cycle of thrombus formation. This is why heparin and antiplatelet therapy are given with fibrinolytics.

Nitroglycerin (NTG or GTN)

Nitroglycerin relieves ischemic chest pain. It also dilates the coronary arteries (particularly in the region of plaque disruption) and decreases preload (venous return). To administer GTN spray one to two doses under the tongue. If giving the GTN tablet, place 500 micrograms (1 tablet) under the tongue and instruct the patient to allow it dissolve.

Do not give nitrates to patients with hypotension (SBP <90 mm Hg or >30 mm Hg below baseline), bradycardia (<50 beats/minute), or tachycardia (>100 beats/minute). Administer nitrates with extreme caution if at all to patients with suspected inferior wall MI with possible right ventricular (RV) involvement because blood pressure in these patients is volume-dependent and nitroglycerin will cause severe hypotension. Do not administer nitrates to patients who have received a phosphodiesterase inhibitor for erectile dysfunction within the last 24 hours (longer for some preparations).

Morphine

Morphine sulfate is the analgesic of choice for continuing pain unresponsive to nitrates. Morphine is a venodilator that reduces ventricular preload and oxygen requirements. If hypotension develops, elevate the patient's legs, administer volume, and monitor for signs of worsening pulmonary vascular congestion. Start with a 2- to 4-milligram IV dose, and give additional doses of 2 to 4 milligrams IV at 5- to 15-minute intervals.

Beta-blockers (β-blockers)

β-Blockers can cause delayed hypotension and heart block, especially in the elderly; therefore they are generally not part of prehospital ED and treatment guidelines for STEMI.

Most deaths associated with ST elevation MI happen in the first hour and are caused by ventricular fibrillation (VF) or pulseless ventricular tachycardia (VT).[27-29] IV administration of β-blockers to patients without hemodynamic or electrical contraindications can reduce the incidence of VF and PVCs,[33,34] reduce the size of the infarct, reduce the incidence of cardiac rupture, and reduce mortality in patients who do not receive fibrinolytic therapy.[30-32] In patients who do receive fibrinolytic agents, IV β-blockers decrease post-infarction ischemia and nonfatal AMI. A small but significant decrease in death and nonfatal infarction has been observed in patients treated with β-blockers soon after infarction.[35]

General contraindications to β-blockers are moderate to severe heart failure and pulmonary edema,

bradycardia (<60 beats/minute), hypotension (SBP <100 mm Hg), signs of poor peripheral perfusion, second-degree or third-degree heart block, or reactive airway disease.

PROCEDURE FOR PREHOSPITAL FIBRINOLYSIS

Patient Positioning

Position the patient sitting in a comfortable position at 45 degrees on 100% oxygen, attach an ECG monitor, and place an IV access in the antecubital fossa. Perform a 12-lead ECG. Inform the patient about the benefits of fibrinolysis as well as of the risk of bleeding and hemorrhagic stroke, if this is the proposed treatment (Figure 27-1).

Complications and Complicating Factors

Hypertension

The presence of high blood pressure (Systolic BP >175 mm Hg) on presentation increases the risk of hemorrhagic stroke after fibrinolytic therapy. Even if blood pressure is lowered with β-blockers or nitrates before administration of fibrinolytic agents, the risk of stroke may not be reduced. Fibrinolytic treatment of STEMI patients who present with an Systolic BP >180 mm Hg or a diastolic blood pressure >110 mm Hg is contraindicated in the prehospital setting.[20]

Stroke

The incidence of stroke increases with advancing age, reducing the relative benefit of fibrinolytic therapy.[19] **Factors that increase the risk of stroke are age (≥65 years), low body weight (<70 kg), initial hypertension (≥180/110 mm Hg), and use of** fibrinolytic **agents.** The risk of hemorrhagic stroke ranges from 0.25% with no risk factors to 2.5% with three risk factors.[23]

Cardiogenic shock

Infarction of ≥40% of the left ventricular (LV) myocardium usually results in cardiogenic shock and carries a high mortality rate. **Cardiogenic shock and congestive heart failure are not contraindications to fibrinolysis, but PCI is the preferred treatment.**

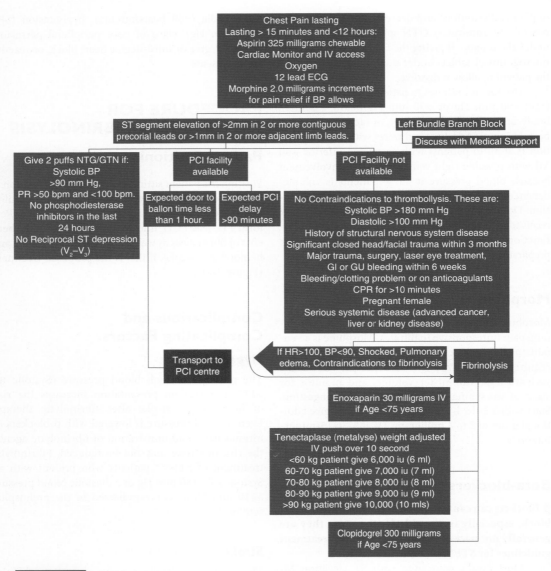

FIGURE 27–1

Suggested Prehospital fibrinolysis treatment algorithm.

Right Ventricular (RV) Infarction

RV infarction or ischemia may occur in up to 50% of patients with inferior wall MI. Suspect RV infarction in patients with inferior wall infarction, hypotension, and clear lung fields. If infarction is suspected, nitrates, diuretics, or any vasodilators should be avoided because severe hypotension may result. This hypotension is often easily treated with an IV fluid bolus.

Web Resources

American Heart Association 2005 Guidelines for CPR and ECC (update expected December 2010) http://www.americanheart.org/presenter.jhtml?identifier=3035517. accessed December 2009, verified April 2010.

BOX 27-1   Fibrinolysis Checklist[17]

Chest pain for longer than 15 minutes and less than 12 hours?
ECG showing ST elevation of >2 mm in 2 or more contiguous precordial leads or >1 mm in 2 or more adjacent limb leads or new presumed new LBBB?
Are there any contraindications to prehospital fibrinolysis?

Contraindications to Prehospital Fibrinolysis	Yes	No
Systolic BP greater than 180 mm Hg		
Diastolic BP greater than 100 mm Hg		
History of structural central nervous system disease		
Significant closed head/facial trauma within previous 3 months		
Recent (within 6 weeks) major trauma, surgery (including laser eye surgery), GI/GU bleed		
Bleeding or clotting problem or client on blood thinners		
CPR for longer than 10 minutes		
Pregnant female		
Serious systemic disease (e.g., advanced/terminal cancer, severe liver or kidney disease)		

Consider for Direct Transfer to a PCI Facility	Yes	No
Heart rate greater than or equal to 100 beats per minute AND systolic BP less than 100 mm Hg		
Pulmonary edema		
Signs of shock (cold/clammy)		
Contraindications to fibrinolytic therapy		

References

1. Boersma E, Mercado N, Poldermans D, et al. Acute myocardial infarction. *Lancet* 2003 Mar 8;361(9360): 847–58. Review. PMID: 12642064

2. Keeling P, Hughes D, Price L, et al. Safety and feasibility of prehospital thrombolysis carried out by paramedics. *BMJ.* 2003 Jul 5;327(7405):27–8. PMID: 12842952 *(British Medical Journal)*

3. Morrison LJ, Verbeek PR, McDonald AC, et al. Mortality and prehospital thrombolysis for acute myocardial infarction: A meta-analysis. *JAMA.* 2000 May 24–31;283(20):2686–92. PMID: 10819952

4. Bonnefoy E, Lapostolle F, Leizorovicz A, et al, for the CAPTIM study group. Primary angioplasty versus prehospital fibrinolysis in acute myocardial infarction: a randomised study. *Lancet* 2002 Sep 14; 360(9336):825–9. PMID: 12243916

5. Bonnefoy E, Steg PG, Boutitie F, et al; CAPTIM Investigators, Mercier C, McFadden EP, Touboul P. Comparison of primary angioplasty and pre-hospital **fibrinolysis** in acute myocardial infarction (CAP-TIM) trial: a 5-year follow-up. *Eur Heart J.* 2009 Jul; 30(13):1598–606. Epub 2009 May 8.

6. Afilalo J, Roy AM, Eisenberg MJ. Systematic review of **fibrinolytic**-facilitated percutaneous coronary intervention: potential benefits and future chal-lenges. *Can J Cardiol.* 2009 Mar;25(3):141–8. Review. PMID: 19279981

7. Ellis SG, Tendera M, de Belder MA, et al; FINESSE Investigators. Facilitated PCI in patients with ST-elevation myocardial infarction. *N Engl J Med.* 2008 May 22;358(21):2205–17. PMID: 18499565

8. Newberry L, Barnett GK, Ballard N. A new mnemo-nic for chest pain assessment. *J Emerg Nurs.* 2005 Feb;31(1):84–5. PMID: 15682135

9. Acute Coronary Syndromes. ECC Committee, Sub-committees and Task Forces of the American Heart Association. 2005 American Heart Association Guidelines for Cardiopulmonary Resuscitation and Emergency Cardiovascular Care. *Circulation.* 2005 Dec 13;112(24 Suppl):IV1–203. Epub 2005 Nov 28.

10. Haynes BE, Pritting J. A rural emergency medical tech-nician with selected advanced skills. *Prehosp Emerg Care.* 1999 Oct-Dec;3(4):343–6. PMID: 10534037

11. Funk D, Groat C, Verdile VP. Education of parame-dics regarding aspirin use. *Prehosp Emerg Care* 2000 Jan-Mar;4(1):62–4. PMID: 10634286

12. Freimark D, Matetzky S, Leor J, Boyko V, et al. Tim-ing of aspirin administration as a determinant of sur-vival of patients with acute myocardial infarction treated with thrombolysis. *Am J Cardiol.* 2002 Feb 15;89(4):381–5. PMID: 11835915

13. Verheugt FW, van der Laarse A, Funke-Kupper AJ, et al. Effects of early intervention with low-dose aspirin (100 mg) on infarct size, reinfarction and mortality in anterior wall acute myocardial infarction. *Am J Cardiol*. 1990 Aug 1;66(3):267–70. PMID: 2195861

14. Feldman M, Cryer B. Aspirin absorption rates and platelet inhibition times with 325-mg buffered aspirin tablets (chewed or swallowed intact) and with buffered aspirin solution. *Am J Cardiol*. 1999 Aug 15;84(4):404–9. PMID: 10468077

15. Sagar KA, Smyth MR. A comparative bioavailability study of different aspirin formulations using on-line multidimensional chromatography. *J Pharm Biomed Anal*. 1999 Nov;21(2):383–92. PMID: 10703994

16. Trivedi K, Schuur JD, Cone DC. Can paramedics read ST-segment elevation myocardial infarction on pre-hospital 12-lead electrocardiograms? *Prehosp Emerg Care*. 2009 Apr-Jun;13(2):207–14. PMID: 19291559

17. ECC Committee, Subcommittees and Task Forces of the American Heart Association. 2005 American Heart Association Guidelines for Cardiopulmonary Resuscitation and Emergency Cardiovascular Care. *Circulation*. 2005 Dec 13;112(24 Suppl):IV1–203. Epub 2005 Nov 28. (available at: http://circ.aha journals.org/cgi/content/full/112/24_suppl/IV-89

18. Indications for **fibrinolytic** therapy in suspected acute myocardial infarction: collaborative overview of early mortality and major morbidity results from all randomised trials of more than 1000 patients. **Fibrinolytic** Therapy Trialists' (FTT) Collaborative Group *Lancet*. 1994 Feb 5;343(8893):311–22. Review. Erratum in: Lancet 1994 Mar 19;343(8899):742. PMID: 7905143

19. Mahaffey KW, Granger CB, Sloan MA, et al. Risk factors for in-hospital nonhemorrhagic stroke in patients with acute myocardial infarction treated with thrombolysis: results from GUSTO-I. *Circulation*. 1998 Mar 3;97(8):757–64. PMID: 9498539

20. Aylward PE, Wilcox RG, Horgan JH, et al. Relation of increased arterial blood pressure to mortality and stroke in the context of contemporary thrombolytic therapy for acute myocardial infarction: a random-ized trial. GUSTO-I Investigators. *Ann Intern Med*. 1996 Dec 1;125(11):891–900. PMID: 8967669

21. Van de Werf F, Barron HV, Armstrong PW, et al; ASSENT-2 Investigators. Assessment of the Safety and Efficacy of a New Thrombolytic. Incidence and predictors of bleeding events after **fibrinolytic** therapy with fibrin-specific agents: a comparison of TNK-tPA and rt-PA. *Eur Heart J*. 2001 Dec;22(24): 2253–61. PMID: 11728145

22. Giugliano RP, Antman EM; Caeteris paribus—all things being equal. *Eur Heart J* 2001 Dec;22(24): 2221–3 PMID: 11728139

23. Simoons ML, Maggioni AP, Knatterud G, et al. Indi-vidual risk assessment for intracranial haemorrhage during thrombolytic therapy. *Lancet*. 1993 Dec 18–25;342(8886–8887):1523–8. PMID: 7902905

24. Wallentin L, Goldstein P, Armstrong PW, et al; Effi-cacy and safety of tenecteplase in combination with the low-molecular-weight heparin enoxaparin or un-fractionated heparin in the prehospital setting: the Assessment of the Safety and Efficacy of a New Thrombolytic Regimen (ASSENT)-3 PLUS random-ized trial in acute myocardial infarction. *Circulation*. 2003 Jul 15;108(2):135–42. Epub 2003 Jul 7. PMID: 12847070

25. Sabatine MS, Cannon CP, Gibson CM, et al; Addition of clopidogrel to aspirin and **fibrinolytic** therapy for myocardial infarction with ST-segment elevation. *N Engl J Med*. 2005 Mar 24;352(12):1179–89. Epub 2005 Mar 9. PMID: 15758000

26. ISIS-4 (Fourth International Study of Infarct Survival) Collaborative Group. ISIS-4: a randomised factorial trial assessing early oral captopril, oral mononitrate, and intravenous magnesium sulphate in 58,050 patients with suspected acute myocardial infarction. *Lancet*. 1995 Mar 18;345(8951):669–85. PMID: 7661937

27. Pantridge JF, Geddes JS. A mobile intensive-care unit in the management of myocardial infarction. *Lancet*. 1967 Aug 5;2(7510):271–3 PMID: 4165912

28. Cohen MC, Rohtla KM, Lavery CE, et al. Meta-analysis of the morning excess of acute myocardial infarction and sudden cardiac death *Am J Cardiol*. 1997 Jun 1;79(11):1512–6. Erratum in: *Am J Cardiol* 1998 Jan 15;81(2):260. PMID: 9185643

29. Colquhoun MC, Julien DG. Sudden death in the community: the arrhythmia causing cardiac arrest and results of immediate resuscitation. *Resuscitation*. 1992; 24: 177A.

30. Hjalmarson A, Herlitz J, Holmberg S, et al. The Goteborg metoprolol trial: Effects on mortality and morbidity in acute myocardial infarction: limita-tion of infarct size by beta blockers and its potential role for prognosis. *Circulation*. 1983;67 (Supp I): 126–132.

31. Metoprolol in acute myocardial infarction (MIAMI). A randomised placebo-controlled international trial. The MIAMI Trial Research Group. *Eur Heart J*. 1985 Mar;6(3):199–226. PMID: 2863148

32. Randomised trial of intravenous atenolol among 16 027 cases of suspected acute myocardial infarction: ISIS-1. First International Study of Infarct Survival Collaborative Group. *Lancet*. 1986 Jul 12;2(8498): 57–66. PMID: 2873379

33. Rehnqvist N, Olsson G, Erhardt L, Ekman AM. Metoprolol in acute myocardial infarction reduces ventricular arrhythmias both in the early stage and after the acute event. *Int J Cardiol*. 1987 Jun;15(3): 301–8. PMID: 3298080

34. Herlitz J, Edvardsson N, Holmberg S, et al; Göteborg Metoprolol Trial: effects on arrhythmias. *Am J Cardiol*. 1984 Jun 25;53(13):27D–31D. PMID: 6731325

35. Roberts R, Rogers WJ, Mueller HS, Lambrew CT, et al. Immediate versus deferred beta-blockade following thrombolytic therapy in patients with acute myocardial infarction: Results of the Throm-bolysis in Myocardial Infarction (TIMI) II-B Study. *Circulation* 1991 Feb;83(2):422–37. PMID: 1671346

CHAPTER 28

Prehospital Stroke Assessment

Judith Tintinalli

PURPOSE OF PROCEDURE

EMS providers need to be proficient in assessing possible signs of stroke. Stroke is a neurologic emergency, and improvement of stroke care is a worldwide concern.[1-5] **EMS is a key link in the chain of modern EMS care.** Patients who call EMS for stroke reach emergency care at least one hour earlier than patients who do not use EMS.[6] One hour makes a difference for those patients and institutions that administer thrombolytics for acute ischemic stroke. And one of the most important factors affecting stroke recovery is treatment in a stroke unit[1-6]; therefore EMS units play the leading role in transporting a stroke patient to the most appropriate hospital. Several validated stroke assessment scales are presented below. Use your local protocols for stroke assessment.

If you think the patient has a possible stroke, notify the most appropriate ED immediately. **Carefully document the last time the patient was seen to be normal and document the source of this information.** Obtain the names and phone numbers of family and observers so that if the time of onset of symptoms needs to be verified in the ED, time will not be wasted trying to find out the best sources of information.

None of these scales have been used or validated in transient ischemic attack (TIA). **In patients with TIA, symptoms may have resolved by the time of EMS assessment.** Patients (or their family members) who describe features of stroke that have resolved still require ED transport and assessment.

PREHOSPITAL STROKE ASSESSMENT

Cincinnati Prehospital Stroke Scale[7]

The **Cincinnati Prehospital Stroke Scale**[7] is a simple three-part test that can help identify the presence of an acute stroke or TIA. **If any one sign is positive**, immediately transport the patient to an ED, preferably an ED in a hospital with a stroke unit.

1. *Facial droop*: Ask the patient to smile, show the teeth or pucker the lips. Compare movement of both sides of the face.
   - Normal: Both sides of face move equally.
   - Abnormal: One side of face does not move as well as the other (or at all).
2. *Arm drift*: Ask the patient to close the eyes and hold the arms straight out in front while you count to 10. If one arm does not move, or one arm winds up drifting down more than the other, that could be a sign of a stroke.
   - Normal: Both arms stay steadily elevated.
   - Abnormal: One arm cannot be raised, or one arm drifts down compared with the other.

Table 28–1	ABCD and ABCD² score			
Letter	**Element**	**Definition**	**ABCD**	**ABCD²**
A	Age	≥60	1	1
B	Blood Pressure	>140/≥90 mm Hg	1	1
C	Clinical Features	Unilateral weakness	2	2
		Speech problem (no weakness)	1	1
D	Duration	≥60 minutes	2	2
		10-59 minutes	1	1
		< 10 minutes	0	0
D²	Diabetes		n/a	1
Total			6	7

3. **Speech:** Have the person say a phrase like, "You can't teach an old dog new tricks," or some other simple, familiar saying. If the person slurs the words, gets some words wrong, or is unable to speak, that could be sign of stroke.
   ■ Normal: Patient repeats phrase correctly and with no slurring of speech.
   ■ Abnormal: Slurred or inappropriate words or cannot speak or does not understand what you are asking.

Ambulance Victoria® Stroke Assessment[8]

1. **Facial Droop**: Patient shows teeth or smiles.
2. **Speech**: Patient says "You can't teach an old dog new tricks".
3. **Hand Grip.**
4. **Blood Glucose Level**: If point of care testing demonstrates hypoglycemia, treat with glucose and reassess.

The Los Angeles Prehospital Stroke Screen (LAPSS)[9]

{Criteria state that patient may still be having a stroke if criteria are not met.}

   Screening criteria: all should be "yes" or can be "unknown."

   Age > 45 years old.
   History of seizure disorder or epilepsy *absent*.
   Symptoms began < 24 hours ago.

Patient not wheelchair-bound or bedridden at baseline.
Blood glucose level is between 60 and 100 mg/dL.

Examination

Facial smile or grimace: one side droops compared to the other side.
Hand grip: weak or unable to grip.
Arm weakness: arm drifts down from horizontal position.

Advanced Considerations: the ABCD and ABCD² Score

Stroke is often preceded by a transient ischemic attack (TIA), which is "a transient episode of neurologic dysfunction caused by focal brain, spinal cord, or retinal ischemia without acute infarction."[10] TIA symptoms resolve in 24 hours or less. The ABCD system is a tool that helps quantify the risk of stroke (within hours or a few days) after a TIA. A score of ≥3 indicates a high risk of stroke.[11,12] Scores <3 can still be associated with stroke but the risk is lower (Table 28-1).[13]

References

1. De Lecinana-Cases MA, Gil-Nunez A, Diez-Tejedor E 'Relevance of stroke code, stroke unit and stroke networks in organization of acute stroke care – the Madrid acute stroke care program' Cerebrovasc Dis 2009; 27 Suppl 1:140–7 PMID 19342844.
2. Teasell R, Meyer MJ, McClure A et al 'Stroke rehabilitation: an international perspective' Top Stroke Rehabil 2009 Jan-Feb; 16(1):44–56.

3. Kusuma Y, Venketasubramanian N, Kiemas LS et al 'Burden of stroke in Indonesia' Int J Stroke 2009 Oct; 4(5):379–80.

4. Kuptniratsaikul V, Kovindha A, Massakulpa P, Permsirivanich W et al 'Inpatient rehabilitation services for patients after stroke in Thailand: a multi-centre study' J Rehabil Med 2009 Jul; 41(8):684–6.

5. Putman K, De Wit L, Schupp W et al 'Variations in follow-up services after inpatient stroke rehabilitation: a multicentre study' J Rehabil Med 2009 Jul; 41(8): 646–53.

6. George MG, Tong X, McGruder H, Yoon P, Rosamond W, Winquist A, Hinchey J, Wall HK, Pandey DK; Centers for Disease Control and Prevention (CDC) MMWR Surveill Summ. 2009 Nov 6;58(7):1–23.

7. Kothari RU, Pancioli A, Liu T, Brott T, Broderick J (April 1999). "Cincinnati Prehospital Stroke Scale: reproducibility and validity". *Ann Emerg Med* 33 (4): 373–8. PMID 10092713.

8. http://www.ambulance.vic.gov.au/Paramedics/Qualified-Paramedic-Training/Clinical-Practice-Guidelines.html, accessed 2/10. verified 3/26/10.

9. Kidwell CS, Starkman S, Eckstein M, Weems K, Saver JL. "Identifying stroke in the field. Prospective validation of the Los Angeles prehospital stroke screen (LAPSS)." Stroke 2000 Jan;31(1):71–6.

10. Easton JD, Saver JL, Albers GW et al 'Definition and evaluation of transient ischemic attack: a scientific statement for healthcare professionals from the American Heart Association/American Stroke Association Stroke Council; Council on Cardiovascular Surgery and Anesthesia; Council on Cardiovascular Radiology and Intervention Council on Cardiovascular Nursing; and the Interdisciplinary Council on Peripheral Vascular Disease' Stroke 2009 Jun;40(6): 2276–93 PMID 19423857.

11. Giles MF, Rothwell PM 'Risk prediction after TIA: the ABCD system and other methods' Geriatrics Oct 2008, 63:10, 10–16.

12. Fothergill A, Christianson TJH, Brown RD, et al 'Validation and Refinement of the ABCD2 Score: A Population-Based Analysis' Stroke 2009; 40; 2669–2673.

13. Ong MEH, Chan YH, Lin WP et al 'Validating the ABCD2 Score for Predicting Sroke risk after transient ischemic attack in the ED' Am J Emerg Med Jan 2010 28:44–48.

CHAPTER 29

Helmet Removal

Gürkan Özel

KEY LEARNING POINTS

- EMS providers should be knowledgeable about different types of helmets and proper techniques to safely remove them.
- Two individuals are needed for proper helmet removal. One individual must always focus on neck stabilization and prevention of neck flexion.

- Common indications for helmet removal are management of the patient's airway and detection and control of any hidden bleeding into the posterior helmet. A major contraindication for helmet removal is the presence of penetrating injury to the head involving helmet fragments or other foreign objects.

When helmet users experience injury, the helmet may interfere with the care rendered by the EMS providers, and it may be necessary to remove the helmet in the field. There are many different types of helmets, all with unique features. Some examples are motorcycle helmets, athletic helmets used for sporting events, safety helmets for workplace use, and military type helmets. EMS providers should be able to assess the indications and contrindications for helmet removal and should know helmet removal techniques. **Motorcycle helmets are the focus of this chapter.** However, the principles of motorcycle helmet removal apply to most other types of helmets. An exception are the helmets worn during American football games. Such helmets have different characteristics and require specialized techniques to be removed properly.

INDICATIONS AND CONTRAINDICATIONS FOR HELMET REMOVAL

Helmets are mainly designed to protect the integrity of the skull. They do not necessarily protect the wearer from spinal injuries.

There are four basic types of motorcycle helmets: full face, flip-up, open face, and off-road (Figure 29-1).

Full-face helmets fit the head snugly, can prevent the assessment of a patient's airway and breathing, and also limit access to the airway. Helmets can make it very difficult to provide supplemental oxygen and to immobilize the neck properly. Large-sized helmets also flex the neck when the patient is lying supine on the ground. **For these reasons, full-face helmets need to be**

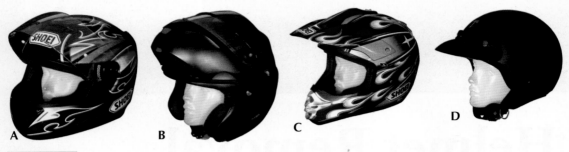

FIGURE 29–1

Types of common motorcycle helmets. **A**, Full face **B**, modular flip-up **C**, off-road **D**, open face. Photo courtesy of Gürkan Özel.

removed early in patient assessment.[1-2] By removing the helmet, the EMS provider can also assess for any bleeding on the scalp, or for hidden bleeding into the back of the helmet.

Procedure

Helmet removal requires *two individuals*. One individual must concentrate on maintaining manual immobilization of the head and neck while the helmet is still in place.

Step 1

Open the face shield to allow the second EMS provider to assess the patient's airway.

Once the decision is made to remove the helmet, explain the procedure to the patient. Then, the first EMS provider, who is already stabilizing the head and neck, holds the helmet with palms pressed on both sides of the helmet and fingertips curled over the lower magrin of the helmet. The second EMS provider kneels at the side of the patient and unfastens (or cuts if necessary) the chin strap (Figure 29-2).

Step 2

Once the chin strap is released, the second EMS provider then places one hand on the neck, as far under the head as possible on the occiput. The other hand of the second EMS provider grasps the mandible of the patient with the thumb and the first two fingers supporting the angle of the mandible on both sides (Figure 29-3).

Step 3

The first EMS provider holding the helmet pulls the sides of the helmet apart, just to clear the patient's face,

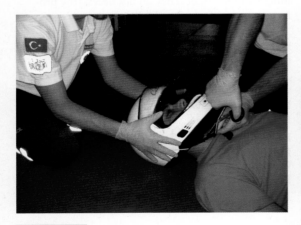

FIGURE 29–2

Step 1: Stabilization. Photo courtesy of Gürkan Özel.

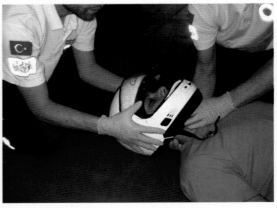

FIGURE 29–3

Step 2: First EMS with hand on neck while second EMS supports the mandible. Photo courtesy of Gürkan Özel.

and gently pulls the helmet in a straight line while rotating its lower end to clear the patient's nose. Keep the back of the helmet (helmet's posterior surface) in contact with the ground to prevent neck flexion during helmet removal (Figure 29-4).

Step 4

The first EMS provider stops when the helmet is nearly halfway off the patient's head. The second EMS provider now repositions his or her hands and supports the occipital area of the patient's head, preventing it from falling on the ground freely once the helmet is completely removed (Figure 29-5).

Step 5

The first EMS provider holding the helmet continues to pull the sides of the helmet apart, gently slipping it off the patient's head (Figure 29-6).

Step 6

Once the helmet is completely removed, the first EMS provider takes hold of the patient's head and provides manual immobilization (Figure 26-7).

Step 7

The second EMS provider may place a padding under the patient's head to maintain the neck in a

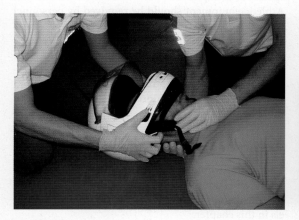

FIGURE 29–4

Step 3: Removal of helmet. Photo courtesy of Gürkan Özel.

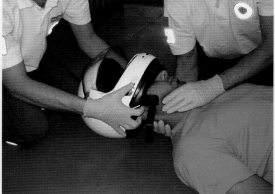

FIGURE 29–5

Step 4: Pause removal; second EMS repositions hands to support occiput. Photo courtesy of Gürkan Özel.

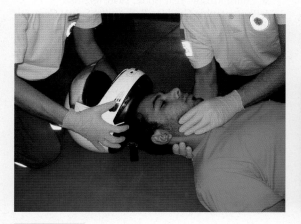

FIGURE 29–6

Step 5: Continue helmet removal. Photo courtesy of Gürkan Özel.

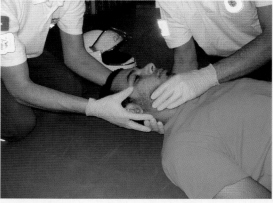

FIGURE 29–7

Step 6: First EMS takes over manual stabilization of the head. Photo courtesy of Gürkan Özel.

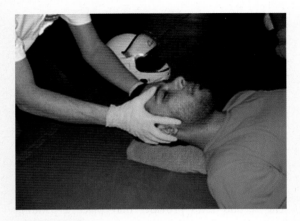

FIGURE 29–8

Step 7: Place padding under head, continue patient assessment. Photo courtesy of Gürkan Özel.

neutral in-line position. Then, patient assessment is continued, a cervical collar is applied, and the patient is placed on a backboard or another device to complete full spinal immobilization if needed (Figure 29-8).

Keep a few things in mind when the helmet is removed from the patient.

- At no time during the process should both of the EMS providers be moving their hands simultaneously.[1] Instead, one EMS provider should always be maintaining neck immobilization.
- **Clearing the patient's nose** is one of the most difficult movements during the removal of a full-face helmet. The EMS provider pulling the helmet off should be slowly rotating the helmet with up-and-down rocking motions. **Stop if the patient's nose is caught, move the helmet toward the patient's torso a little, and retry.**
- If the helmet is broken following the crash but is on the patient's head, helmet fragments could be impaled in the scalp or skull. If this is the case, do not remove the helmet. Instead, just remove the face shield to allow access to the patient's mouth

and nose. Helmets should also be left in place when an object impales the helmet and goes through to the scalp or the skull.

The procedure for the removal of other types of helmets is similar. Most other helmets are easier to remove compared to full-face helmets. Front panels of flip-up helmets should be flipped up by pressing the release mechanisms located on both sides of the helmet. This turns the helmet into an open-face model and allows for easy access to the patient's airway. One exception in helmet removal technique would be the helmets worn during American football games. Those helmets have different characteristics and when combined with protective shoulder pads, they require special techniques and considerations to remove. Athletic equipment should be removed by personnel trained and experienced in the removal of sports equipment.[3] Regular EMS providers are encouraged to attend special training sessions in order to learn how to remove this type of helmet. Guidelines developed by professional organizations should be followed when approaching the injured athlete wearing one of those helmets.

Acknowledgments

The author would like to thank Tolga Kanik (EMT), Memduh Haldun Ülkenli (EMT), and Aytaç Alaydin from Ankara, Turkey, for their participation as models in this chapter.

References

1. Butman AM, Martin SW, Womacka RW, McSwain NE. Comprehensive Guide to Pre-Hospital Skills. St. Louis: Mosby-Year Book, 1996; 682-684.
2. A Photographic Guide to Prehospital Spinal Care. 5th ed. Copyright © Emergency Technologies, Ellimintyt,Victoria, Australia; 20 August 2004, pp. 64-69. http://emergencytechnologies.com.au/psm.htm. (Accessed September 17, 2009.)
3. Salomone JP, Pons PT: PHTLS: Prehospital Trauma Life Support, 6th Edition. Mosby EMS. St. Louis, Mo., 2007; p. 268.

CHAPTER 30

Spinal Immobilization

Devin T. Price, Gürkan Özel

There are few skills used by EMS providers that offer such a variety of techniques, approaches, and equipment choices as those skills involving cervical and spinal immobilization. These skills are commonly used but frequently applied incorrectly. All too often EMS providers focus a great portion of their time on the cervical spine but fail to give the same degree of concern and attention to detail when stabilizing the lower portions of the spine.

The spine is composed of 33 vertebrae. The cervical region has seven vertebrae (C1 through C7), the thoracic region has 12 vertebrae (T1 through T12), and the lumbar region has five vertebrae (L1 through L5). The sacral region consists of five vertebrae, all fused together to form one continuous bone mass known as the sacrum. The coccygeal region consists of four vertebrae, all fused together to form the coccyx or tailbone. (Figure 30-1).

The vertebrae provide vertical structural support, house the spinal cord, and protect the spinal cord from injury (Figure 30-2).

Different forces applied to the spine can result in a number of different types of injures; therefore the EMT must give special consideration to the mechanism of injury. This is particularly important when evaluating spinal injuries and making decisions regarding extrication, packaging, and transport. In some cases the rescuer may decide not to utilize any spinal precautions, but this decision must be based on a careful review of the mechanism of injury, patient complaint, obvious injuries, and any comorbid factors that may exist. The graph below shows data from the United Kingdom breaking down the various causes of spinal cord injury and is fairly representative of most urban populations (Figure 30-3).

Blunt or penetrating trauma can cause spinal injury by compression, distraction, rotational, and lateral forces. Deceleration forces can result in hyperextension and hyperflexion. **Compression** injuries, also known as **axial loading**, result from force being applied to the spine from above such as from diving injuries and falls on the head. Compression impacts vertebral bodies together and can result in "burst" fractures. With **distraction** injuries of the spine, unusual forces are applied to the spine that may result in its lengthening, tearing of the spinal ligaments, and even the separation of the vertebral bodies from one another. Distraction injures are frequently severe and result in grave or permanent disabling injuries to the patient. Mechanisms associated with distraction injuries include hanging and clothesline injuries.

Rotational injures are commonly seen in motor vehicle accidents and sports-related injuries. In this case the force of energy causes a twisting of the spinal column and can result in not only vertebral and spinal cord injury but serious soft-tissue

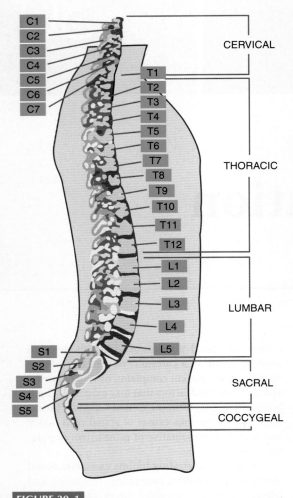

FIGURE 30–1

Spinal vertebrae.

injury to the surrounding site. **Lateral** forces can lead to vertebral fractures, soft-tissue injury, and in severe cases, distraction of the spinal cord.

Hyperextension and **hyperflexion** spine injuries can stretch and tear spinal ligaments and spinal nerve roots. The disks between the vertebrae can bulge, tear, or rupture, and vertebrae can be forced out of their normal position, resulting in spinal cord injury (Figure 30-4).

STEPS IN PATIENT EVALUATION

As you approach an incident or receive information about an injury, consider the **mechanism of injury** to assess the possibility of spinal injury. If the mechanism suggests possible spine injury, assume this is valid. Is there head injury? Head and spine injuries are frequently associated. Always treat for spine injury in the head-injured patient. Does the mechanism of injury suggest multisystem trauma (e.g., high-speed accident)? Spine injuries are associated with multisystem trauma.

Next, consider the **patient complaint and ask focused questions**. If the patient complains of neck or back pain or discomfort, assume possible spine injury. Ask if numbness or changes in feeling have occurred in a capelike distribution or in the shoulders, arms, or legs. These complaints suggest spine injury. If the patient complains of a lightning-shock in the neck or back, assume spine injury.

Next perform a **physical examination**. Are there any obvious injuries present, including "step-offs," bruising, and obvious blunt or penetrating trauma? Is there paralysis or weakness of the arms or legs? Is there head injury?

Finally, **comorbid factors** must be considered when debating whether the risk of serious spinal injury exists. The elderly and those with preexisting spinal injury are more likely to injure the spine. Other signs and symptoms that require concern for spine injury are competing pain or injuries (joint dislocations, large painful lacerations or abrasions, injuries above the level of the shoulder), altered mental status, and patient impairment from alcohol or drugs.

Mechanism of Injury

According to Sir Isaac Newton's First Law of Motion *"every object in a state of uniform motion tends to remain in that state of motion unless an external force is applied to it."* In other words, "a body in motion stays in motion until acted on by an outside force." For example, when a patient falls off a ladder to the ground, he or she acquires energy in the form of motion. When the patient actually strikes the ground, several things occur. Depending on the nature of the surface (grass, water, concrete), some of the energy associated with the fall will be transmitted to the surface. We see this in the form of a splash when an object hits a body of water. The patient's body also distributes and absorbs the energy of impact. Bone and soft tissues are pushed, compressed, and stretched, resulting in abrasions, lacerations, avulsions, or fractures.

As EMS providers, we can learn a lot about the mechanism of injury based upon our initial assessment of the scene. Look at the energy transfer that occurs in a car crash, for example. Examine the car

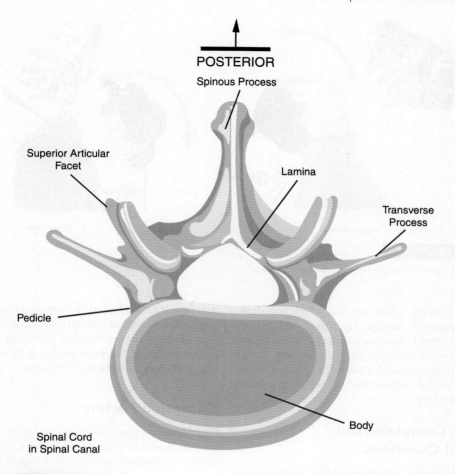

POSTERIOR

Spinous Process

Superior Articular
Facet

Lamina

Transverse
Process

Pedicle

Body

Spinal Cord
in Spinal Canal

FIGURE 30–2

Components of a typical vertebra.

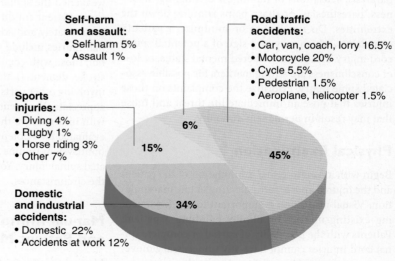

**Self-harm
and assault:**
• Self-harm 5%
• Assault 1%

**Road traffic
accidents:**
• Car, van, coach, lorry 16.5%
• Motorcycle 20%
• Cycle 5.5%
• Pedestrian 1.5%
• Aeroplane, helicopter 1.5%

**Sports
injuries:**
• Diving 4%
• Rugby 1%
• Horse riding 3%
• Other 7%

6%

15%

45%

**Domestic
and industrial
accidents:**
• Domestic 22%
• Accidents at work 12%

34%

FIGURE 30–3

Typical activities associated with
spinal injury.

*Data taken from a survey of 126 new patient admissions to
Duke of Cornwall Spinal Treatment Centre, 1997–1999*

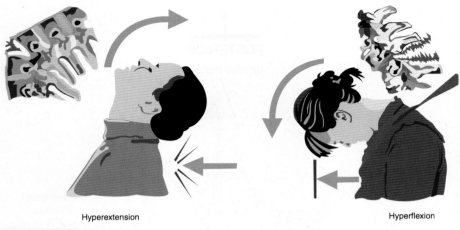

Hyperextension

Hyperflexion

FIGURE 30–4

Hyperextension and hyperflexion injuries.

bumpers, crumple zones, steering wheel, and dashboard for potential damage. Significant vehicle body damage, passenger space intrusion, and fully deployed restraint devices create a picture of severe energy transfer. We can use such evidence as a predictor for the potential for serious injury, including possible spinal cord injury.

Patient Complaint and Focused Questions

This will be information provided by patients regarding their specific complaint of pain or discomfort. Complaints may range from neck or back pain to paralysis, sensations of numbness or tingling, weakness, paresthesias, or sharp pains running down the extremities. Do not ignore or minimize a patient's complaints, which may be a sign of a potential spinal cord injury. Head injury, altered mental status, or loss of consciousness are strong markers for possible associated spine injury. Prioritize the complaints on those injuries that pose an immediate life threat and those that may result in permanent disability.

Physical Examination

Begin with a careful visual examination of the patient and the injured area before palpating or any manipulation. Visual inspection is important to avoid worsening existing injuries by blindly handling a patient. Patients with the possibility of partial or complete spinal cord injuries cannot have any unnecessary movement or manipulation of the spine, as this may cause permanent disability. Examine for signs of blunt or

penetrating trauma along the spinal column. Do not forget to consider that injures that occur anteriorly can also result in deeper injuries, including the spine. Without moving the spine, palpate it for abnormalities, displacement, or bony protrusions.

Comorbid Factors

Certain patient populations or preexisting conditions can predispose to serious spinal injury. For example, patients with osteoporosis (the thinning of bone tissue and loss of bone density over time) can have severe injury even from seemingly minor mechanisms of injury. Preexisting spinal injuries may have already weakened the spinal column or its supporting structures. Patient conditions that might make it difficult to accurately and adequately assess for potential spinal injuries include those impaired by drugs or alcohol, those with cognitive dysfunction (e.g., caused by stroke, dementia), those with painful or large injuries involving other parts of the body, and those who fail to appreciate the potential for serious injury. Any patient with injury above the level of the shoulder should be evaluated for a potential spinal injury. Head injury and multisystem trauma are major risk factors for associated spinal injury. Your index of suspicion must match the circumstances.

Manual Immobilization and Patient Movement

Manual movement techniques (log roll, lifting) and immobilization devices (for example, the long spine board, the scoop, vacuum mattress, cervical immobilization devices, and the Kendrick Extrication Device (K.E.D.®) stabilize body position and restrict movement in situations with the potential for spinal injury. Different devices are used in different regions and by different EMS systems. Two methods for manual patient movement are the log roll and the two or three person lift.

MANUAL PATIENT MOVEMENT

Patients found in a prone position or in a lateral recumbent position will require repositioning into a supine position for spinal immobilization and for further treatment and transport. Concerns about crew safety and ergonomics are the first priority. For patient care, the ABC's are paramount, and in most cases assessing and maintaining a patent airway requires the patient to be on his or her back (supine). Before moving the patient, first consider the safest and most effective means to accomplish this task. Then the process of repositioning and moving the patient can begin.

The **log roll** is the method for repositioning the patient from a prone or lateral position onto the back (supine). The supine position is needed for airway control, intravenous access, and transport.

Indications

1. Patients found in a prone or lateral recumbent position who are unable to move themselves into a supine position or more appropriate position for treatment and transport.
2. Patients found in a prone or lateral recumbent position who require ongoing in-line spinal immobilization.
3. When movement of a patient is necessary to complete a full head-to-toe physical exam, including visualization and palpation of the posterior body.

Advantages

1. Proper log roll technique reduces the risk of causing or worsening existing injury to the patient.
2. A well-coordinated log roll maintains in-line spinal immobilization.
3. The rescuers reduce the risk of injury to themselves by using proper ergonomics and by distributing the workload associated with rolling a patient.

Disadvantages

1. A minimum of two people are needed to safely move the patient and reduce the risk of injury to rescuers.
2. Some patients may not cooperate or allow the rescuers complete control over positioning.

Procedure

1. Gather at least two EMTs to safely move the patient.
2. Before moving the patient, complete the visual inspection and the physical examination. Once the patient is supine, the posterior chest and upper and lower back cannot be inspected or examined. If the patient is turned before the back is checked, the log roll will have to be repeated.
3. Next, place the long board alongside the patient to allow easy transfer onto the board.
4. EMT #1 is positioned at the patient's head and manually stabilizes the head and neck. EMT #1 is responsible for directing all movement in an organized and coordinated manner and never releases the patient's head until he or she is completely secured with the spinal immobilization equipment (Figure 30-5).
5. EMT #2 is positioned alongside the patient so he or she has access to the patient's shoulders and hips. If a *third* EMS provider is available, he or she is positioned next to EMT #2 by the patient's hips and legs (Figure 30-6).
6. EMT #1 coordinates turning of the patient. One way this can be done is once EMT #1 has control of the head and neck, on the count of 3 all EMTs turn the patient simultaneously. If the patient is on his or her face (prone), this may require two steps, with the patient moved from the face-down position the side and then onto the back (Figures 30-7 and 30-8).
7. Finally, proceed with the remaining portions of the patient assessment or treatment necessary prior to transport.

Movement of a patient from a bed or the ground to the gurney can be difficult. The **stretcher lift** is an effective and safe technique. This maneuver needs at least two people, and it is best to have three. Use the stretcher lift in situations of confined space, narrow hallways, and frequent turns where fixed length transport devices (i.e., long board, scoop, gurney) will not work.

Indications

1. Patients who are unable to walk or where the medical situation prevents walking.
2. Unable to utilize conventional patient movement devices (e.g., long board, scoop).

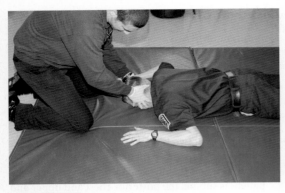

FIGURE 30–5

Log roll procedure Step 4.

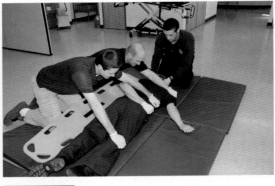

FIGURE 30–6

Log roll procedure Step 5.

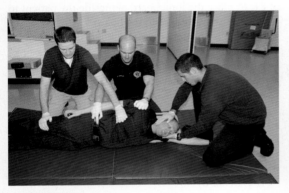

FIGURE 30–7

Log roll procedure Step 6A.

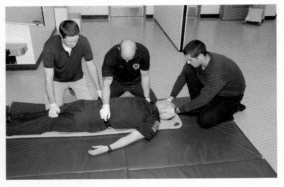

FIGURE 30–8

Log roll procedure Step 6B.

3. Confined space, narrow access, or multiple turns involved with patient removal.

Contraindications

1. Do not attempt the stretcher lift under conditions unsafe for the patient or EMTs. For example, if the patient is too large or heavy, or if multiple EMS personnel are unavailable, do not try the stretcher lift.
2. Do not use the stretcher lift for violent or uncooperative patients who might pose harm to the EMTs.

Advantages

1. Patients can easily be moved without any additional equipment required.
2. Patients are easily moved from confined spaces, around corners, and into different confined spaces as necessary.
3. Any level of provider or rescuer can perform this maneuver.

Disadvantages

1. Patients are held closely, putting EMTs at risk for biohazard or infectious exposure.
2. If incorrectly applied or if an inadequate number of personnel are involved, there is great risk of injury to the EMS providers and or unsafe handling of the patient.
3. Cannot be used with uncooperative or combative patients.

TWO OR THREE PERSON LIFT

Procedure

1. If the patient is on the floor, then each EMS provider kneels next to the patient. If the patient is in a bed, then each EMS provider lines up alongside the patient. If two rescuers are available, one is responsible for the patient's head (airway) and

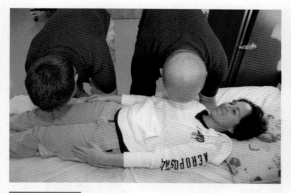

FIGURE 30–9

Bed or Ground to Stretcher Lift Step 2.

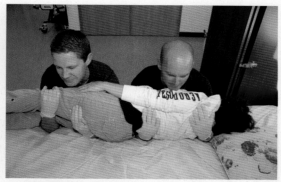

FIGURE 30–10

Bed or Ground to Stretcher Lift Step 4.

5. The EMS provider at the head is the designated team leader, and upon his or her direction each EMT side-steps with the patient from the pick-up point to the destination (gurney, bed) (Figure 30-11).
6. Reverse the steps outlined in step #2 to 4 to place the patient onto the gurney or bed.

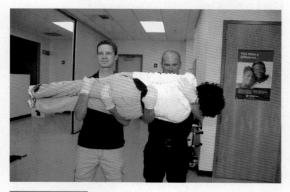

FIGURE 30–11

Bed or Ground to Stretcher Lift Step 5.

upper torso and the second is responsible for the lower torso, pelvis, and thighs. If three rescuers are available, the second rescuer takes control of the torso and the third EMS provider is responsible for the pelvis and legs.

2. Ideally, log roll the patient onto his or her side so the EMTs can slide their hands underneath the patient. If this is not possible, then each EMT slides his or her hands underneath the patient, ensuring that the critical regions (head/shoulders, shoulder/pelvis, pelvis/lower extremities) are under the EMS provider's hands (Figure 30-9).

3. Interlace one arm with the other EMT's arm, so that the two arms are criss-crossed. This will provide mutual support and a locking mechanism to prevent the patient from slipping and to minimize strain on the EMTs.

4. Once both EMTs have a firm and secure grip, rotate the patient so that the patient is facing the EMS providers, resting against the EMS provider's chest (Figure 30-10).

SPINAL IMMOBILIZATION

Spinal immobilization is a relatively easy task that requires knowledge of the immobilization options and comfort with the correct use of equipment.

Cervical Collars

1. After identifying the need for spinal immobilization, assemble the necessary equipment (Figure 30-12).

2. The EMT #1 applies and maintains cervical immobilization. Do not release the hand hold until the patient is either fully secured to all of the spinal equipment or until one is relieved by another EMS provider (Figure 30-13).

3. EMT #2 assesses the patient's circulation, sensation, and motion in all four extremities *before* any movement or equipment application and *after* securing the patient to spinal immobilization equipment (Figures 30-14 and 30-15).

4. EMT #2 then measures the patient for proper size selection of a cervical collar. If an adjustable collar is used, adjust it accordingly. First measure the distance from the bottom of the patient's mandible to the top of the patient's clavicle. Measure the same distance on the premarked cervical collar (Figures 30-16 and 30-17) and either select the appropriate size or adjust the collar to the

appropriate size. **Although the collar will help** *limit* **movement of the patient's head and neck, it will not truly immobilize the head and neck, so EMT #1 must maintain continuous in-line stabilization.**

5. Apply the cervical collar according to the manufacturer's directions. Some collars allow for a frontal application and some require that the back of the collar be put into place before positioning the front (Figure 30-18).

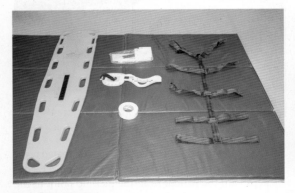

FIGURE 30–12
Cervical collar equipment.

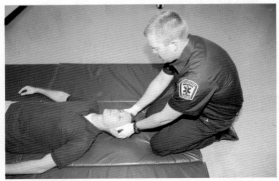

FIGURE 30–13
Cervical collar procedure Step 2.

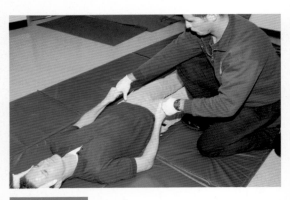

FIGURE 30–14
Cervical collar procedure Step 3A.

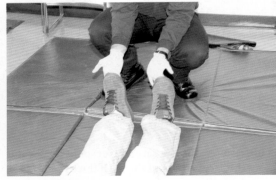

FIGURE 30–15
Cervical collar procedure Step 3B.

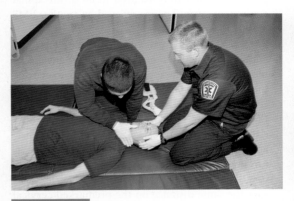

FIGURE 30–16
Cervical collar procedure Step 4A.

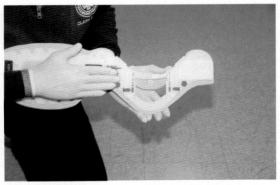

FIGURE 30–17
Cervical collar procedure Step 4B.

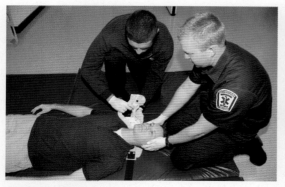

FIGURE 30–18

Cervical collar procedure Step 5.

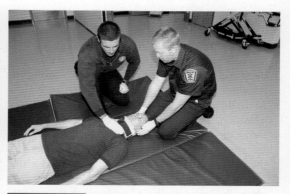

FIGURE 30–19

Cervical collar procedure Step 6.

6. Ensure that the collar is properly sized and firmly in position. (Figure 30-19). Improperly sized or positioned cervical collars may allow movement of the patient's head and cervical spine. Improperly sized collars can actually displace the patient's head anteriorly or posteriorly, negating the benefits of the collar. Collars that are too tight or too small can restrict the patient's ability to breathe, cough, or swallow.

LONG SPINE BOARD (BACKBOARD)

Long spine boards (also known as backboards) are used by EMS systems around the world for patient extrication and spinal immobilization. They are typically made out of plastic composites (fiberglass, carbon fiber) or wood (plywood). Holes are cut on the sides of the board for grasping the board and for passing straps to secure the patient to the board. Most backboards are X-ray translucent, so transfer to other devices is not needed when obtaining radiographs in the ED.

Indications

1. Patients with potential spinal injuries.
2. Patients with potential spinal injuries who need extrication from a vehicle.
3. Can also be used as full-body splint in multitrauma patients.

Contraindications

1. In patients with chronically deformed spines (such as kyphosis or scoliosis) in whom the head and neck cannot be placed in a neutral line, long spine boards

are contraindicated and an alternative method (such as full-body vacuum splints) for spinal immobilization is needed.

Advantages

1. Fairly rapid application makes it a favorable device for most EMS systems.
2. Allows easy extrication from a variety of patient positions.

Disadvantages

1. Is a poor device for supporting body contour in patients with spinal injuries.
2. Patients experience pain in pressure points during long transports unless the board is well padded.

Procedure

Once a cervical collar has been properly placed on a patient, the next step in fully securing the spine is placement of the patient on a long spine board. To secure the patient to a long spine board, use either wide adhesive tape, straps, or other commercially available securing devices. Also use a securing mechanism specifically designed to stabilize the head and neck onto the backboard. See Figure 30-25, in step #5 which demonstrates one example of head and neck stabilization onto the backboard.

1. With EMT #1 stabilizing the patient's head and neck (Figure 30-20), additional EMS providers place themselves alongside the patient. EMT #1 at the patient's head is responsible for coordinating all patient movement until the patient is fully secured onto the backboard.

2. The additional EMS providers assure equal distribution of the patient's body weight by interlacing their arms as they prepare the patient for a log roll. (Figure 30-21). This provides safe patient movement and minimizes the risk to the EMS providers responsible for moving the patient.

3. At the direction of EMT #1 who maintains neck stabilization, the patient is rolled onto his or her side facing the two assistant rescuers (Figure 30-22). Do not over-roll the patient, and if possible, do not roll the patient onto an injured body part. Once the patient is on his or her side, an additional assistant places the long spine board underneath the patient. If possible, leave several inches of the board at the patient's head exposed so that if he or she needs to be centered onto the board, it can be done in one single move.

4. Once the patient is properly aligned onto the board, EMT #1, who is holding the patient's head,

calls for a slow and coordinated movement of the patient back onto the long spine board (Figure 30-23). If the patient needs to be centered on the board, or if the patient's head needs to be aligned along the upper portion of the board, EMT #1 holding the head will continue to coordinate the patient's movement.

5. Utilizing a restraint device, secure the head and cervical spine and the rest of the body to the spineboard. Place one strap over the upper torso (at or above the nipple line), another over the pelvic wings, one over the midthigh, and another over the midcalf region. Do not place straps over any known or suspect fracture sites. Make sure the straps are not so tight that they interfere with patient breathing, CPR, or other critical patient care treatment (Figures 30-24 and 30-25).

6. EMT #1 may now release his or her hold on the patient's head. Prior to moving the patient, reassess

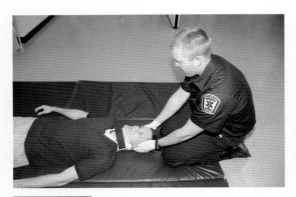
FIGURE 30–20
Long spine board procedure Step 1.

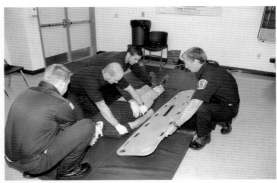
FIGURE 30–21
Long spine board procedure Step 2.

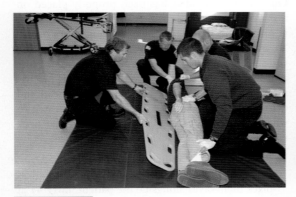
FIGURE 30–22
Long spine board procedure Step 3.

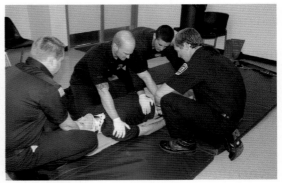
FIGURE 30–23
Long spine board procedure Step 4.

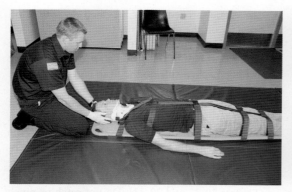

FIGURE 30–24

Long spine board procedure Step 5A.

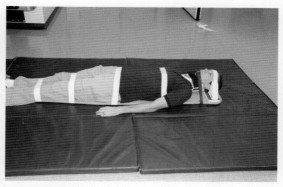

FIGURE 30–25

Long spine board procedure Step 5B.

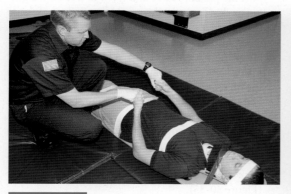

FIGURE 30–26

Long spine board procedure Step 6.

circulation, sensation, and movement. Document any changes that may have occurred (Figure 30-26).
7. Pregnant women in the third trimester can be placed on a backboard, with a wedge or rolled blankets under the board to angle the woman onto her left side in order to avoid hypotension from pressure on the inferior vena cava.

SCOOP STRETCHER

The scoop stretcher is a device that splits into two long halves, so patients can be picked up with minimal body movement. Scoop stretchers are made of lightweight metal alloys, usually aluminum, and can be folded in the middle for easy storage. Some models are made out of plastic components and combine features of a long backboard and a scoop stretcher (Figure 30-27).

Most scoop stretchers are x-ray lucent and allow easy patient handling and transfer in the ED.

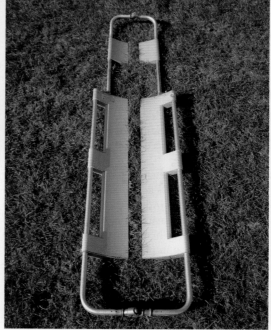

FIGURE 30–27

Example of a Scoop Stretcher.

Indications

1. Patients with hip and pelvic injuries.
2. Patients with spinal injuries who need to be lifted and transferred to another stretcher (a backboard or a full-body vacuum splint).

Contraindications

1. Unstable patients.

Advantages

1. Allows picking up the supine patient in the position found without causing much movement.
2. Fits narrow spaces where other stretchers cannot be used.
3. Provides good body support by design.

Disadvantages

1. Best for patients already in the supine (face-up) position.
2. Does not allow efficient strapping of the patient. This becomes problematic if the patient vomits and needs to be tilted to one side or when the patient has to be carried up or down steep areas.
3. The patient's weight tends to bend it in the middle; therefore it does not provide full spinal immobilization (if available two other rescuers can support the stretcher on either side to overcome this difficulty).
4. The locking mechanism of the latches is critical, and the stretcher may unlatch with improper use or handling, causing the patient to tumble to the ground.

Procedure

1. If a spinal injury is suspected, EMT #1 maintains manual immobilization of the head and neck throughout the procedure. Place a cervical collar if not already done.
2. Place the scoop stretcher on the ground next to the patient. Align the head curve of the stretcher with the patient's head. Adjust the length of the scoop stretcher by releasing the length-locking pins (Figure 30-28). When adjusting the length, keep the head portion in place while sliding the bottom half of both pieces down past the bottom of the patient's feet by about 20 cm. Most devices have autolock properties at predetermined points. Simply slide the adjustable part of the device until it clicks and locks into position. Repeat for the other half of the device. Pay close attention to both halves of the scoop stretcher so both halves are adjusted and locked at the same length.
3. Once the proper length is determined and the device is locked, split the device in two and place both halves on either side of the patient (Figure 30-29). Do not lift the stretcher's halves over the patient.
4. Maintain spinal immobilization. One provider kneels down on one side of the patient and slightly elevates the patient's torso toward them, while the other EMS provider on the opposite side slides one long half of the scoop stretcher under the patient (Figure 30-30). This half should reach the midline of the patient's back.

5. The same procedure is repeated by the EMS provider on the opposite site (Figure 30-31). Use a sea-saw or gentle rocking movement to place the second half of the scoop stretcher so that the locking mechanisms on the head end and the foot end will face each other for easy locking.
6. Assemble the device together once both halves of the scoop stretcher are properly placed on both sides of the patient. Start with the head end of the device and gently lock the mechanism while keeping the head and neck immobilized. Now, move down to the foot end and lock the mechanism there (Figures 30-32 and 30-33). Do not catch or pinch the patient's skin, hair or clothing when locking the halves together. If anything gets caught, gently support the patient's head and torso to free hair, clothing or skin from the device. At this point make sure the device is properly locked so it will not give way when lifting the patient.
7. Strap the patient onto the scoop stretcher before lifting. Use three straps, one on the chest, one on the hips, and the last one on the legs (Figure 30-34). Pad underneath the head and strap the head to the stretcher in the final step.
8. When using a scoop stretcher to lift a patient with a potential hip fracture with no likelihood of spinal trauma, pick up the patient without head and neck immobilization and without a cervical collar (Figure 30-35).

It is possible to place the patient and the scoop stretcher onto a moving stretcher for transport. A patient with suspected spinal injury can also be put onto a full body vacuum splint or a backboard by using the scoop stretcher.

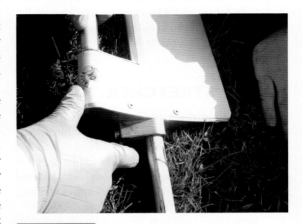

FIGURE 30–28

Scoop stretcher procedure Step 2.

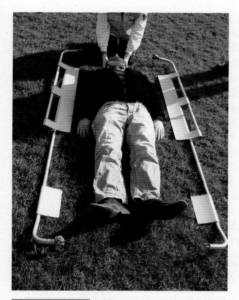

FIGURE 30–29

Scoop stretcher procedure Step 3.

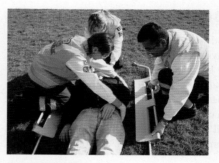

FIGURE 30–30

Scoop stretcher procedure Step 4.

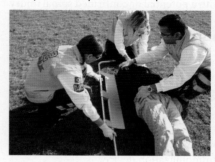

FIGURE 30–31

Scoop stretcher procedure Step 5.

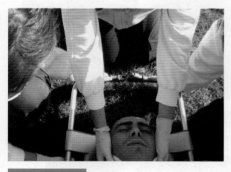

FIGURE 30–32

Scoop stretcher procedure Step 6A.

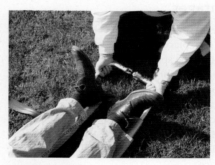

FIGURE 30–33

Scoop stretcher procedure Step 6B.

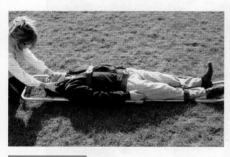

FIGURE 30–34

Scoop stretcher procedure Step 7.

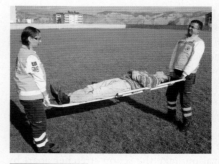

FIGURE 30–35

Scoop stretcher procedure Step 8.

FULL-BODY VACUUM SPLINT

The full-body vacuum splint is typically a 90 cm × 180 cm vinyl or nylon bag filled with thousands of polystyrene beads. Once the patient is placed on the splint, the air is evacuated by using a hand pump through one or more valves placed on the mattress. The splint conforms perfectly to body contour, provides a rigid support, relieves pressure on dependent areas, and provides insulation.

Indications

1. Patients with a potential or confirmed spinal injury.

Contraindications

1. None.

Advantages

1. Provides superior conformity to patient's body contour.
2. Relieves pressure points and eliminates pain resulting from immobilization device.
3. Provides insulation from cold.

Disadvantages

1. Physical examination of the back is difficult once the splint is in place (perform examination prior to placement on the splint).
2. Cannot be used for extrication as it is not rigid enough to support extrication maneuvers.
3. If the vacuum splint is punctured, the splint may loose function, with potential injury to the patient. Place tape over the puncture site to fix the problem temporarily. The vacuum inside will help hold the tape in place.

Procedure

1. Place the patient on a scoop stretcher following the steps above.
2. Place the full-body vacuum splint on the ground next to the patient. Gently pat the mattress's inner surface to evenly distribute the beads inside (Figure 30-36).
3. Lift the scoop stretcher with the patient on it, and place it on the full-body vacuum splint. (Figure 30-37).
4. With one EMS provider providing head and spine immobilization, take the scoop stretcher apart by using the pins on the head-end and foot-end. Gently pull the halves of the scoop from under the patient, one piece at a time (Figures 30-38 and 30-39).

5. While maintaining manual immobilization of the head and neck, the second and third EMS providers place the straps so that the splint wraps the patient's body (Figure 30-40).
6. Place the pump on the valve and begin evacuating air. Other EMS providers help to shape the splint by folding the edges as the splint takes shape. Fold the head-end of the mattress and let the EMS provider at the head immobilize by placing hands over the folded sections against both sides of the patient's head (Figure 30-41). Make sure to leave adequate room to reach the patient's arms for procedures such as IV access and blood pressure measurement.
7. Once the splint is completely rigid, close the valve and check to make sure there is no air release (Figure 30-42).

Now the patient can be moved onto the main stretcher (Figure 30-43).

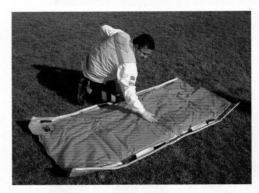

FIGURE 30–36

Full body vacuum splint Step 2.

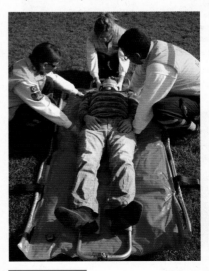

FIGURE 30–37

Full body vacuum splint Step 3.

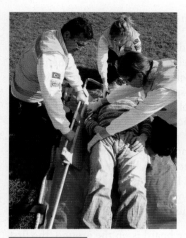

FIGURE 30–38
Full body vacuum splint Step 4A.

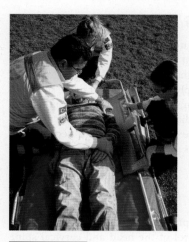

FIGURE 30–39
Full body vacuum splint Step 4B.

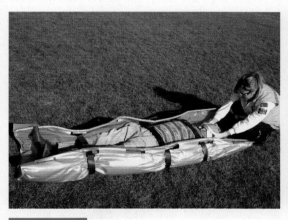

FIGURE 30–40
Full body vacuum splint Step 5.

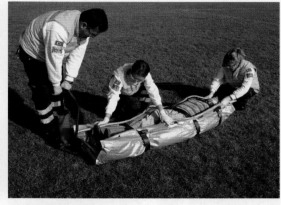

FIGURE 30–41
Full body vacuum splint Step 6.

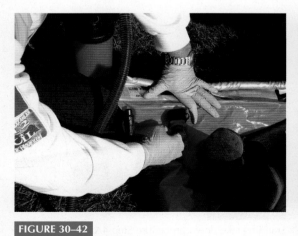

FIGURE 30–42
Full body vacuum splint Step 7A.

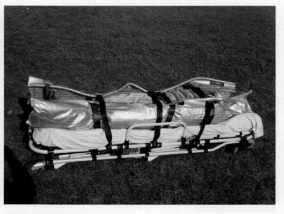

FIGURE 30–43
Full body vacuum splint Step 7B.

STANDING TAKE-DOWN

During an initial patient encounter it may become evident that a patient needs spinal precautions. Don't allow a patient with possible spinal injuries to ambulate, even if it's simply just walking over to the stretcher. In such a situation, a standing take-down is recommended to immediately secure the patient's spine. A minimum of three EMS providers are necessary to safely complete this maneuver.

Procedure

1. The first EMS provider stands behind the patient and takes control of the head and cervical spine (Figure 30-44).
2. A second EMS provider sizes and applies a cervical collar while the first rescuer maintains continuous control of the patient's head (Figure 30-45). Position a long spine board behind the patient.
3. The second and third EMS providers will then position themselves on either side of the patient. Facing the patient, the two EMS providers each grab hold of the spine board with the provider's arm nearest to the patient (Figure 30-46).
4. Using their opposite hands, the second and third EMS providers place their hands alongside the patient's head and assume responsibility for ensuring head and neck immobilization. This maneuver frees up the first EMS provider to assume responsibility for the spine board and control its descent to the ground (Figure 30-47).

Once the spine board is on the ground, the first EMS provider reassumes responsibility for maintaining in-line stabilization, and the two remaining EMS providers align and secure the patient onto the spine board (Figure 30-48).

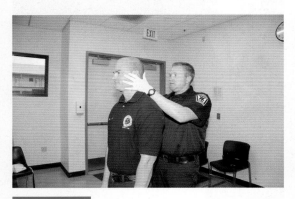

FIGURE 30–44

Standing take down procedure Step 1.

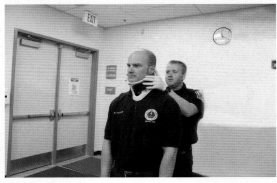

FIGURE 30–45

Standing take down procedure Step 2.

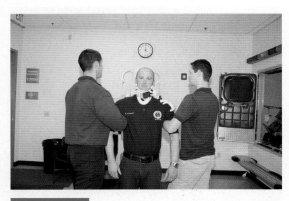

FIGURE 30–46

Standing take down procedure Step 3.

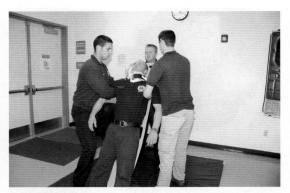

FIGURE 30–47

Standing take down procedure Step 4A.

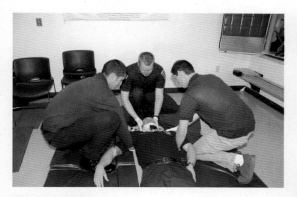

FIGURE 30–48

Standing take down procedure Step 4B.

SEATED PATIENTS

Patients in seated positions may warrant spinal precautions. Whether a patient is found at home seated after a fall or seated inside the car after a motor-vehicle crash, precautions must be taken to ensure that injury is not worsened during extrication or transport. Removing a patient from a chair can be done simply with three EMS providers.

Removal from a Chair

Procedure

1. The first EMS provider assumes responsibility for maintaining in-line cervical stabilization and coordinates all subsequent patient movement. A second EMS provider sizes and places a cervical collar (Figures 30-49 and 30-50).
2. The second and third EMS providers are responsible for the movement and manipulation of the patient's seat. In some cases a "chair lift" may be done, or if the chair lift maneuver is unsafe for the rescuers, the chair itself can be moved. With the first EMS provider coordinating the patient movement, the remaining two EMS providers reposition the chair in a slow and controlled manner until the patient is supine (Figures 30-51 and 30-52).
3. At the direction of the first EMS provider, position the patient onto a long spine board for securing and subsequent transport (Figures 30-53 and 30-54).

Removal from a Car

Procedure

1. The first EMS provider assumes responsibility for maintaining in-line cervical stabilization and coor-

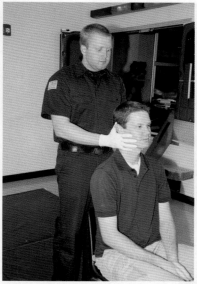

FIGURE 30–49

Removal from a chair procedure Step 1A.

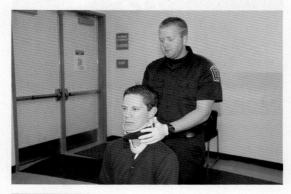

FIGURE 30–50

Removal from a chair procedure Step 1B.

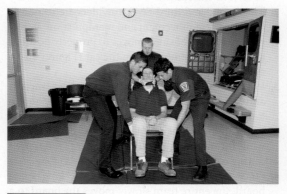

FIGURE 30–51

Removal from a chair procedure Step 2A.

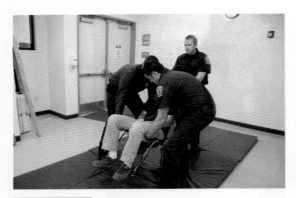

FIGURE 30–52

Removal from a chair procedure Step 2B.

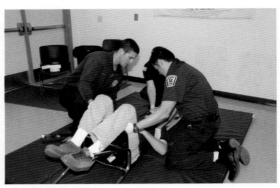

FIGURE 30–53

Removal from a chair procedure Step 3A.

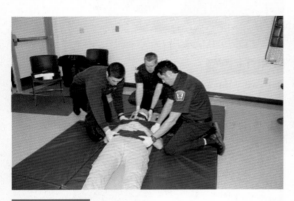

FIGURE 30–54

Removal from a chair procedure Step 3B.

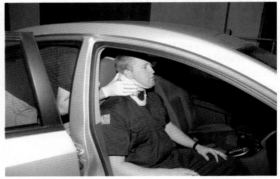

FIGURE 30–55

Removal from a car procedure Step 1.

dinates all subsequent patient movement. A second EMS provider sizes and places a cervical collar (Figure 30-55). Before movement of the patient, check his or her circulation, sensation, and motion in all four extremities.

2. The second and third EMS providers are responsible for patient movement and manipulation. It may require a series of small moves to properly position the patient for removal from the car (Figures 30-56 and 30-57).

3. With an EMS provider maintaining in-line traction and stabilization, slowly lower the patient onto a long spine board (Figure 30-58). Make sure that adequate personnel are available to ensure safety while lifting and supporting the patient's full weight during extrication.

4. Once the patient is centered on the long spine board, the entire team slowly moves the board to a safe working area to secure the patient onto the board. An EMS provider should always maintain in-line stabilization (Figure 30-59).

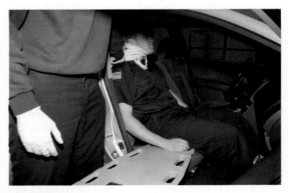

FIGURE 30–56

Removal from a car procedure Step 2A.

5. Once the patient is secured to the long spine board and prepared for transport, reassess, complete, and document the patient's CSM (Figure 30-60).

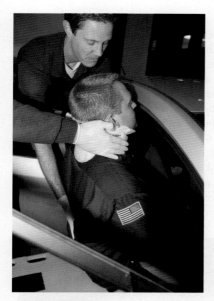

FIGURE 30–57

Removal from a car procedure Step 2B.

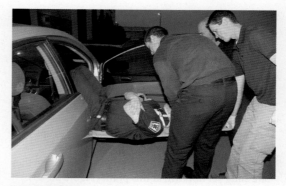

FIGURE 30–58

Removal from a car procedure Step 3.

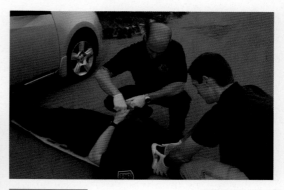

FIGURE 30–60

Removal from a car procedure Step 5.

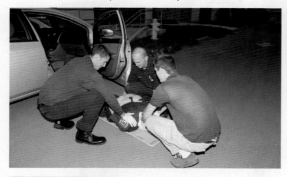

FIGURE 30–59

Removal from a car procedure Step 4.

SEATED PATIENT WITH KENDRICK EXTRICATION DEVICE (K.E.D.®)

The Kendrick Extrication Device (KED®) is a device used to secure sitting patients when spinal precautions are required. The K.E.D.® is most often used in motor vehicle crashes on stable patients, as it takes a few minutes for proper application and extrication. For unstable patients, use long spine boards whenever rapid extrication is needed. The K.E.D.® device is x-ray translucent so it can remain in place during ED evaluation.

Indications

1. Sitting patients with a potential or confirmed spinal injury.

2. Extrication of patients from confined spaces while maintaining spinal precautions.

Contraindications

1. Unstable patients.

Advantages

1. Prevents or minimizes spinal movement effectively during the extrication.
2. Can be used in confined spaces where other devices will not fit.
3. Can be used as a pediatric spinal immobilization device.

Disadvantages

1. It takes a few minutes to properly apply the device, lengthening the scene time.

Procedure

1. Prior to any patient movement, check the patient's circulation, sensation, and motion in all four extremities.

2. The first EMS provider has responsibility for maintaining in-line cervical stabilization and coordinates all subsequent patient movement. A second EMS provider sizes and places a cervical collar.
3. Place the K.E.D.® behind the patient and make sure it is centered. Place the wings or sides of the device in the patient's axillae (Figure 30-61).
4. Attach the leg straps, ensuring they are well placed in the inguinal fold (Figure 30-62). Leg straps may be snug, but do not fully tighten them yet.
5. Attach each of the colored chest straps, ensuring they are snug yet not firm at this point (Figure 30-63).
6. Beginning with the leg straps and working up, firmly tighten the straps by feeding the loose end

into the D-rings. Ask the patient to take a deep breath prior to securing the top chest strap, which will allow the patient to breathe freely without the constriction of the K.E.D.®
7. If available and utilized in your EMS system, place the chin strap on, followed by the head strap of the K.E.D.® The chin strap should not restrict the patient's ability to breathe or obstruct vomiting (Figure 30-64).
8. The patient can now be lifted or moved to a long spine board for transport. If the patient is placed flat on the ground or a board, loosen the two leg straps as needed for patient comfort.
9. Reassess circulation, sensation, and mobility.

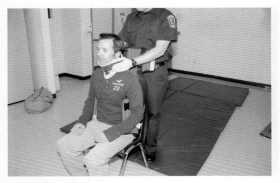

FIGURE 30–61
Seated patient KED procedure Step 3.

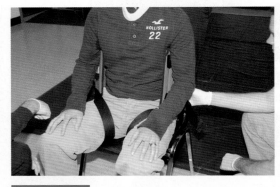

FIGURE 30–62
Seated patient KED procedure Step 4.

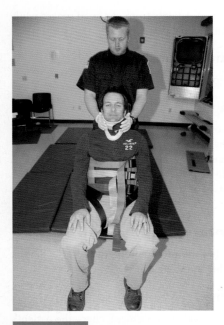

FIGURE 30–63
Seated patient KED procedure Step 5.

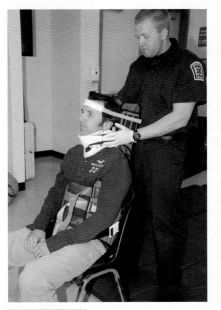

FIGURE 30–64
Seated patient KED procedure Step 7.

CHAPTER 31

Stabilization of Pelvic Fractures

Gürkan Özel

Pelvic fractures can cause life-threatening blood loss. Bleeding results from the sacral venous plexus, the hypogastric artery, fracture surfaces, and surrounding soft tissue. Stabilizing the pelvis in the field, especially during patient rescue and transport, is an important skill that can save a patient's life.[1-3]

Motor vehicle crashes, pedestrians struck by cars, motorcycle accidents, and falls from heights are associated with pelvic fractures. Assessing the risk of a pelvic fracture in the field is difficult. **The most important factors suggesting pelvic fracture are mechanism of injury and patient complaint of pelvic pain.**[1] Other signs associated with pelvic fracture are ecchymoses around the pelvis, perineum, or scrotum, open wounds over the pelvis, or rectal or vaginal bleeding. In the trauma patient with a mechanism of injury suggestive of pelvic fracture, do not compress or manipulate the pelvis. Pain on pelvic compression or possible pelvic instability on pelvic compression are insensitive signs of pelvic fracture, and pelvic compression may worsen bleeding and pelvic injury.[1]

Pelvic stabilization may reduce bleeding by reducing movement of bone ends and preventing further bony and vascular injury and clot disruption.

Several commercial pelvic binders, such as Pelvic Binder™ (Pelvic Binder, Inc., Dallas, Texas, US), Sam Sling (SAM Medical Products®, Newport, Oregon US), T-POD® (Pyng Medical Corporation, Richmond, BC, Canada), or PelviGrip™ (YMS, Cape Town, South Africa) are available. These devices provide mechanical stabilization of the pelvis, are easy to use in the field, and have auto-stop buckles that prevent harmful over-compression (see Figure 31-1).

Wrapping the pelvis with a bed sheet is a good improvisation. However, it is difficult to determine how tightly the sheet should be tied, and the sheet can loosen or unwrap during transport (see Figure 31-2).

Place the bed sheet or the pelvic binder over the lower pelvis, over the greater trochanters of the hips. This location provides the best mechanical stability of the pelvic ring. Once a pelvic stabilizer is placed, do not remove it in the field.

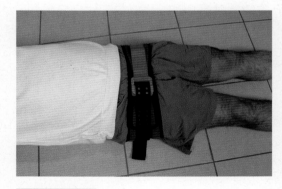

FIGURE 31–1

Application of a SAM Sling. Photo courtesy of SAM Medical Products®, Newport, Oregon.

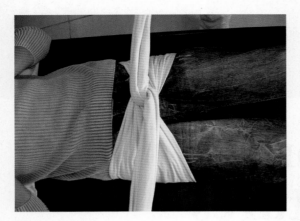

FIGURE 31–2

Application of a bed sheet wrap.

Even the smallest manipulation of the pelvic girdle can increase hemorrhage. Lift the patient with a scoop stretcher whenever possible. Place a bed sheet or a commercial pelvic binder on the backboard prior to patient placement. Then, place the patient on the backboard and secure the pelvis with the sheet or device already laid on the backboard. Full-body vacuum splints can also help stabilize unstable pelvic injuries. An additional EMS provider should *preform* the vacuum splint in order to accommodate the patient's body and injuries and to provide rigid support to the pelvis during the removal of air.

Acknowledgments

The author wishes to thank the staff of Tunceli 112 ASH, Turkey (Turkish EMS) for their contribution to the photographs.

References

1. Lee C, Porter K. The prehospital management of pelvic fractures. *Emerg Med J* 24(2): 130, 2007. Review PMID: 17251627
2. Melamed E, Blumenfeld A, Kalmovich B, et al. Prehospital care of orthopedic injuries. Israel Defense Forces Medical Corps Consensus Group on Prehospital Care of Orthopedic Injuries. *Prehospital Disaster Med* 22(1): 22, 2007.
3. Salomone JP, Pons PT, *PHTLS Prehospital Trauma Life Support*, 6th ed. St. Louis: Mosby; 2007.

CHAPTER 32

Extremity Splinting and Care of Open Fractures

Devin T. Price, Gürkan Özel

EXTREMITY SPLINTING

General Principles

Extremity immobilization is indicated for suspected extremity fractures, for extremities with possible neurovascular compromise, or to prevent dislodgement of an intravenous or intraosseous line. Proper immobilization prevents further limb injury and decreases patient pain during movement and transport. Immobilization is done by applying commercial or improvised (Figure 32-1) splints to the injured extremity.

Specific examination and splinting principles are applicable to all splinting techniques: (1) assess neurovascular function before and after splinting; (2) check the joints above and below the injury; (3) include the joints above and below the injury when immobilizing; and (4) provide pain relief according to local EMS protocols.

Assess circulation by palpating the pulse distal to the injury or by determining distal capillary blood flow. To assess capillary blood flow, gently press the tip of the nail until the nailbed blanches; then release pressure. Color should rapidly return to the nailbed. Normal capillary refill time is ≤2 seconds. However, many factors besides

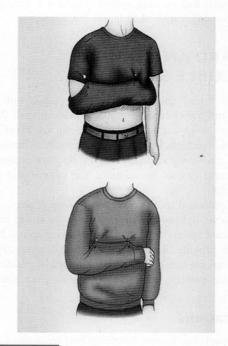

FIGURE 32–1

Improvised splint for the forearm, using safety pins and the patient's own clothing. Photo courtesy of Ricardo Ong, MD, US Army.

vascular injury can cause delayed capillary fill: shock, dehydration, cold, compartment syndrome (swelling of an injured muscle to such an extent that it cuts off arterial blood flow), or peripheral vascular disease.

Examine the joints below and above the suspected injury for associated injuries. For example, a fall onto an outstretched hand can transmit the energy of the fall not only to the wrist but also to the forearm, elbow, or shoulder.

Immobilize the joint above and below the area of injury to prevent movement of the injured part. To properly immobilize the forearm, make sure the splint extends to the elbow and wrist. **Maintain the wrist in a natural position at about 15 degrees of extension, like holding a soda can. Maintain the elbow at 90 degrees, the knee at 5 to 15 degrees' flexion, and the ankle at 90 degrees.**

Treat pain according to local EMS protocols. It may be necessary to provide pain relief before splinting. Do not give anything by mouth.

Immobilization is done by applying commercially made or improvised splints and by making sure there is sufficient padding on the splint for patient comfort. Some of the basic types of splints are padded cardboard or wooden splints, flexible splints, inflatable air splints, and vacuum splints. Traction splints are used to stabilize mid–shaft femur fractures.

BOARD AND FLEXIBLE SPLINTS

Padded board splints are typically made out of wood and are encased in a foam padding shell that provides good support for long bone fractures or multiple fractures of the same extremity. Although splints may come in different sizes, they are nonmalleable and cannot be adjusted for patient size or condition.

Cardboard splints come in a variety of sizes, are disposable, lightweight, and can even be cut to size. Cardboard splints are not as firm as wood splints but they do provide basic support. Although most cardboard splints come with some lightweight padding, additional padding is often needed for patient comfort.

Indications

1. Suspected or known extremity fracture.
2. Major trauma or crush injury to an extremity.
3. Suspected vascular compromise.
4. Immobilization for an intravenous or intraosseous line.

Advantages

1. Most of these splints are easily applied and relatively inexpensive.

Disadvantages

1. Application may extend on-scene time when rapid transport is required.
2. Improperly applied immobilization devices can result in further soft-tissue damage and accelerate bone fragmentation.

Procedure

1. If an extremity fracture is suspected, first apply manual immobilization, keeping the extremity in as normal an anatomic position as possible, and maintain this position until the immobilization device has been applied (Figure 32-2).
2. Before moving or splinting the extremity, check distal circulation, sensation, and motion (Figure 32-3). If these are not intact, see discussion below on Pulseless Extremity.
3. Select the best immobilization device for securing the extremity. Immobilize the bones and joints above and below the suspected fracture site in order to prevent movement of the injured part. When using a simple cardboard or wooden board, pad the splint for patient comfort. Wrap the splint with a soft gauze or elastic bandage (Figure 32-4).
4. **Remove all jewelry and watches from the injured limb before splinting.** Remove rings with a ring cutter if the limb or digits are already swollen. Whenever possible, place a gauze pad in the patient's hand in order to maintain normal anatomic position of the wrist (Figure 32-5). If EMS protocols allow, treat pain before splinting.
5. Start from the distal end of the extremity, and moving proximally, wrap the splint snugly with gauze or an elastic bandage (Figure 32-6).
6. Once the splint is properly secured, it is imperative that the patient's distal circulation, sensation, and motion (CSM) are once again affirmed as being intact and unchanged from the earlier assessment (Figure 32-7).
7. Sling and swathe the upper extremity in the final step, using two pieces of triangular bandage (Figure 32-8).

Flexible splints, such as Sam® Splints, have an inner layer of aluminum alloy encased in closed cell foam. The splint is malleable and comfortable. Once properly positioned, it provides a rigid support for the

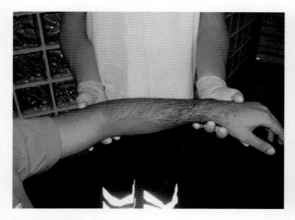

FIGURE 32–2

Manually immobilize the forearm. Photo courtesy of Devin Price and Gürkan Özel.

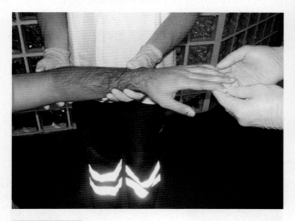

FIGURE 32–3

Check circulation, sensation and motion. If the forearm is injured, assess distal circulation by checking the radial pulse or by checking capillary refill in the nailbeds. Have the patient move his or her fingers or make a fist to check distal motor function. Lightly touch the fingers to make sure sensation is intact. These maneuvers can be done without causing any pain or movement of the injured forearm. Photo courtesy of Devin Price and Gürkan Özel.

FIGURE 32–5

Gauze pad in hand. To immobilize the forearm, make sure the splint extends below the wrist and above the elbow. Note the gauze pad in the patient's hand to maintain normal wrist position. Photo courtesy of Devin Price and Gürkan Özel.

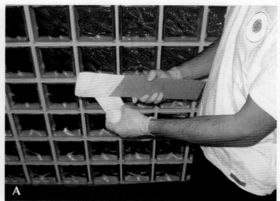

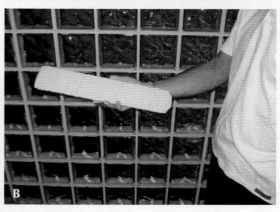

FIGURE 32–4

A and **B**. Wrap the splint with gauze or other padding for patient comfort. Photos courtesy of Devin Price and Gürkan Özel.

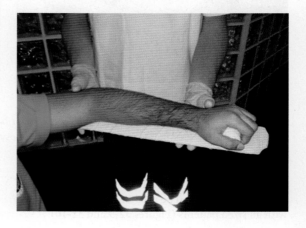

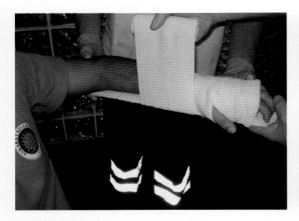

FIGURE 32–6

Wrap the splint and arm with gauze or an elastic bandage, moving from distal to proximal. Check pulse or capillary refill, sensation, and motor function again. Photo courtesy of Devin Price and Gürkan Özel.

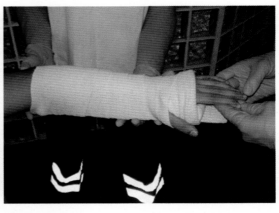

FIGURE 32–7

Check pulse or capillary refill, sensation, and motor function again. Have the patient move his or her fingers. Photo courtesy of Devin Price and Gürkan Özel.

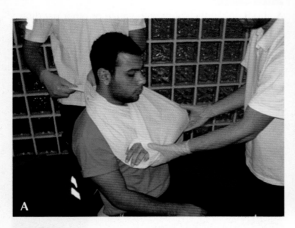

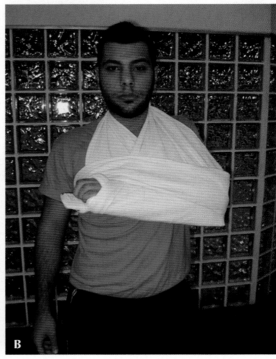

FIGURE 32–8

A and **B** Applying triangular bandage. Apply a triangular bandage to keep the arm steady and immobile and at the level of the heart o minimize swelling. Photos courtesy of Devin Price and Gürkan Özel.

extremity above and below the fracture site. The splint is radiolucent and can be used in all temperatures and with all sized patients (Figures 32-9 and 32-10).

The Fracture-Pak® is a tubular or cylindrical splint that is easy to apply and is available for upper and lower extremities (Figure 32-11).

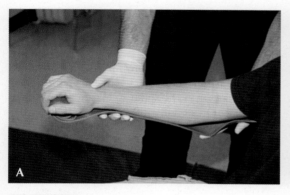
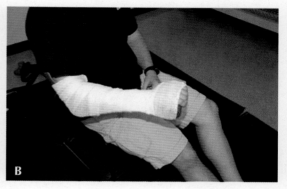

FIGURE 32–9

Sam® splint. **A**, A flexible splint applied to the forearm. The splint extends from above the elbow to below the wrist. **B**, Apply gauze or an elastic bandage to secure the splint. Photos courtesy of Devin Price and Gürkan Özel.

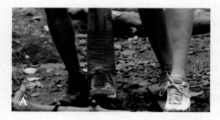

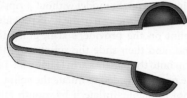

SAN SPLINT FOLDED IN HALF
AND EDGES BENT

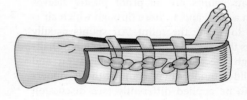

SAN SPLINT APPLIED TO A FRACTURED
LEG OR ANKLE

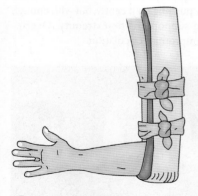

SAN SPLINT APPLIED TO A FRACTURED HUMERUS

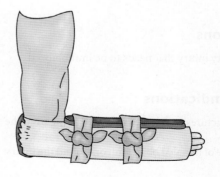

SAN SPLINT APPLIED TO A FRACTURED FOREARM

FIGURE 32–10

A, Sam® splint; flexible splint applied to the lower extremity; **B**, Different applications of flexible splints. Photos courtesy of Devin Price and Gürkan Özel.

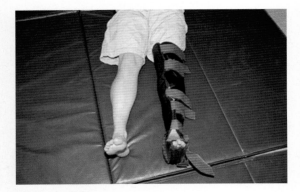

FIGURE 32–11

Putting Fracture-Pak® on leg. Tubular or cylindrical splint applied to the lower extremity and fastened with velcro strips. The splint immobilizes the thigh, knee, leg, ankle, and foot. Photo courtesy of Devin Price and Gürkan Özel.

INFLATABLE AIR SPLINTS

Inflatable air splints are air-proof plastic sleeves that contain a valve and air hose through which air is introduced to inflate the splint. Air splints usually have zippers that extend either the full length or halfway through the splint for easy application and removal. Older models may come without zippers and need to be applied differently (see discussion below).

Inflatable air splints come in variety of sizes and shapes. Some adult sizes can also accommodate children (e.g., adult half arm for child full arm, or adult half leg for child full leg).

Indications

1. Extremity injury that needs to be immobilized.

Contraindications

1. Open fractures with bone ends protruding from the injury.
2. Presence of impaled objects on or around the injury site.

Advantages

1. Provides compression to help to control active bleeding and swelling while providing immobilization.

Disadvantages

1. May not be shaped to conform to angulated fractures.
2. Changing atmospheric pressures (either air transport or extreme environmental temperatures) may cause the air in the splint to expand or contract, causing over- or underinflation.
3. Can compromise circulation if overinflated for long period of time.
4. Can easily be ruptured by foreign objects and sharp materials.

Procedure

1. With one EMS provider applying manual support to the injured site, assess circulation, sensation, and motion (CSM) distal to the injury site on the extremity before placing the air splint.
2. Choose an appropriately sized splint. Remove the patient's watch, rings, and other jewelry so that nothing remains under the splint. Unzip the splint and place it around the area before zipping it closed (Figure 32-12). Once the splint is properly located, zip it closed. **Do not catch the patient's skin in the zipper.**
3. If the air splint is a straight model without a zipper, first place the splint on the arm of the EMS provider. With the splint on the provider's arm, grasp the patient's hand, and then slide the splint from the provider's arm onto the patient's arm (Figure 32-13).
4. Next, use the pump provided to inflate the splint. If a pump is not available, inflate it by mouth after wiping the mouthpiece clean with an alcohol swab (Figure 32-14).
5. Inflate the air splint just enough to make a small indentation by pushing on it gently, but with enough air to provide support to the extremity. Overinflation may compromise circulation.

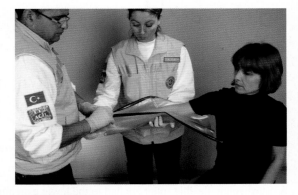

FIGURE 32–12

Applying an inflatable splint with a zipper.

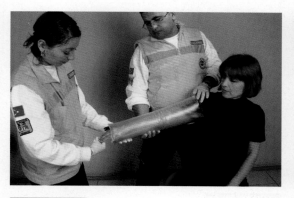

FIGURE 32–13

Putting on an unzippered inflatable arm splint. Slip the inflatable splint from the provider's arm onto the patient's arm.

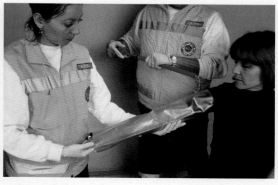

FIGURE 32–14

Use the pump to fill the splint with air. Photo courtesy of Devin Price and Gürkan Özel.

6. After inflating, shut the valve off and reassess CSM distal to the injury site. If there is compromise, deflate the splint a little and reassess. If neurovascular function is still compromised, remove the splint completely and reapply. Once inflation is complete and the valve is shut off, you should assess the circulation, sensation, and motion distal to the injury site. If CSM is compromised, deflate the splint a little and reassess. If CSM is still compromised, you should take off the splint completely and again resplint.

7. Sling and swathe as needed to relieve pressure on the extremity.

8. Inflated air splints may leak air over time, resulting in loss of extremity support. Therefore periodically check air splints during patient transport. If the splint is punctured, remove it and apply another splint.

9. Inflatable air splints are reusable devices, so clean and disinfect them after each use, following your local EMS protocols for cleaning.

VACUUM SPLINTS

Vacuum splints are rectangular bags filled with polystyrene beads. When air is vacuumed from the splint, the beads are tightly pressed against each other and the splint takes the shape of the body region and comfortably supports the injured extremity or spinal column.

Vacuum splints typically have one or more valves through which air is evacuated by special hand pumps. Those pumps may work one-way or can evacuate air both when the pump is pushed in and pulled out.

Vacuum splints come in variety of sizes. The full-body vacuum splint can also be used for spinal immobilization in adults. **Vacuum splints can provide good splinting for extremities in any situation, including splinting for angulated and open fractures.** An adult leg splint can be used as a full-body splint for children. All vacuum splints are x-ray translucent and can be left on when radiographs are taken. However, if the splint is punctured or if the valve is mistakenly opened to allow air to enter the splint, the splint will no longer provide immobilization. Vacuum splints are reusable, so they should be cleaned and disinfected after use.

Procedure

1. While one EMS provider provides manual support to the injured site, assess CMS distal to the injury site on the extremity before placing the vacuum splint.

2. Choose the appropriate splint for the region to be immobilized. Lay the splint on the ground and pat the beads to disribute them evenly through the splint (Figure 32-15).

3. Attach the pump to the valve and evacuate some air out of the splint, making sure it is hardening. Evacuate enough air so that the splint becomes gently stiff but still shapeable. Close the valve and make sure there is no air movement in or out of the splint. This step will let you make sure that the splint is properly functioning (Figure 32-16).

4. Apply the splint to the extremity. One EMS provider stabilizes the extremity, holds the vacuum splint in place, and fastens the velcro straps or buckles. **Make sure not to encircle the entire extremity.** Overlapping edges can be folded out. The second EMS provider uses the hand pump to evacuate the remaining air from the splint. Both EMS providers continually shape the vacuum splint as it stiffens to

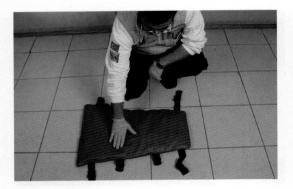

FIGURE 32–15

Patting the beads. Lay the splint open and distribute the beads throughout the splint. Photo courtesy of Devin Price and Gürkan Özel.

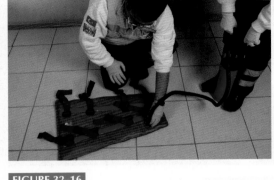

FIGURE 32–16

Attach the pump and inflate. Attach the valve and evacuate air so the splint stiffens. Photo courtesy of Devin Price and Gürkan Özel.

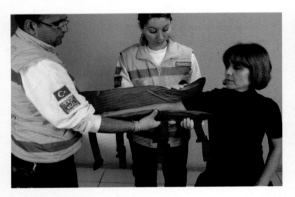

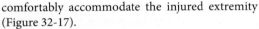

FIGURE 32–17

Shaping the vacuum splint as it stiffens. Photo courtesy of Devin Price and Gürkan Özel.

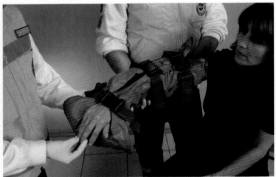

FIGURE 32–18

Attach buckles or velcro straps and recheck CSM. Photo courtesy of Devin Price and Gürkan Özel.

comfortably accommodate the injured extremity (Figure 32-17).

5. Once the splint is rigid and fully supporting the extremity, carefully close the valve without letting air in and then remove the pump. Fasten the velcro straps or buckles. Assess the circulation, sensation, and motion distal to the injury. If compromised, let some air in in order to soften the splint. If circulation still doesn't return, remove the vacuum splint completely and repeat the entire procedure (Figure 32-18).

6. Sling and swathe as needed to support the extremity.

7. If a vacuum splint is used for splinting a lower extremity, fold the distal end of the splint onto the bottom of the foot and bend the patient's knee slightly while supporting the splint underneath until enough air is removed to make the splint rigid (Figure 32-19).

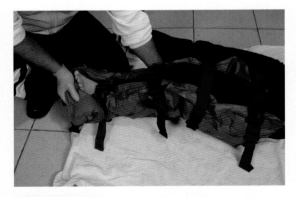

FIGURE 32–19

Fold the splint so it braces the bottom of the foot, and bend the knee slightly. Photo courtesy of Devin Price and Gürkan Özel.

TRACTION SPLINTS

If one suspects a proximal or mid–shaft femur fracture, consider the application of a traction splint. **Traction splints should not be applied in the case of certain types of injuries** (see discussion below). Traction splints pull the injured extremity to realign the ends of the fractured bone. Gentle traction reduces the risk of vascular, nerve, and soft-issue injury. Traction reduces spasm of the thigh muscle of the thigh and corrects shortening and or rotation of the leg. Traction splints come in adult and pediatric sizes, and there are several different designs. The application of a traction splint usually requires at least two rescuers, and it takes several minutes to safely apply.

Indication

Known or suspected mid–shaft femur fractures.

Contraindications

1. Injury at the pelvis, hip, knee, lower leg, or ankle.
2. Multiple extremity fractures.
3. Partial amputation of the extremity.
4. Open fractures: bone ends protruding or visible.
5. Lack of training in traction splint application.

Equipment

1. The Hare traction splint® (Figure 32-20) was invented in the early 1960s as a modification of the Thomas half-ring device, which had been in existence throughout the 20ᵗʰ century. Secured to the pelvis and the ankle, it uses telescoping rods to adjust its length. Once traction is applied to the device, built-in elastic bands secure the limb to the splint for stabilization.

2. The Sager splint® (Figure 32-21) also uses a telescoping rod to adjust the length of the splint, but instead of being placed underneath the patient's ischial tuberosity, the splint is placed medially between the patient's legs. Using the lateral perineal area, the ischial pad is placed and the ankle is used to provide support for the lower strap from which traction is applied. The Sager splint® can be used on bilateral femur fractures and in some cases may facilitate transport with aeromedical transport services.

3. The Reel traction splint® (Figure 32-22) is an articulating splint that folds in half and can articulate at the knee or hip. It can be applied anteriorly or posteriorly and can also be applied to angulated injuries where the principle "immobilize in the position found" should be followed. It is often used in the military.

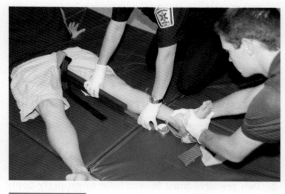

FIGURE 32–21

Sager splint.® Photo courtesy of Devin Price and Gürkan Özel.

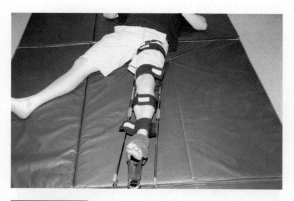

FIGURE 32–20

Hare traction splint.® Photo courtesy of Devin Price and Gürkan Özel.

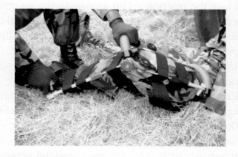

FIGURE 32–22

Reel traction splint.® Photo courtesy of Ricardo Ong, MD, US Army.

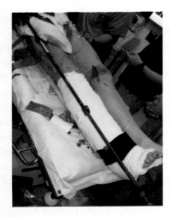

FIGURE 32–23

Slishman splint.® Note the metal part of the splint is a ski pole. There are two red straps, one at the groin and the other at the ankle. Photo courtesy of Ricardo Ong, MD, US Army.

4. The Slishman splint® (Figure 32-23) was originally improvised with a collapsable ski pole and a pulley system. It is light and portable, places traction on the thigh but not the foot, and has only two straps. It can also be used for the upper arm/shoulder.

Procedure (Hare Traction Splint®)

1. Properly identify a possible *closed* fracture of the *proximal or midshaft femur*. Ensure that no contraindications to traction splinting exist, and if they do, consider alternative means of immobilization.
2. Two rescuers must be available to properly apply the traction device.
3. Assess and document distal circulation, sensation, and motion. Clearly mark the pulse location sites on the skin so that you can easily reassess them after application of the traction splint (Figure 32-24).
4. Place the traction splint alongside the *unaffected* extremity to size the length properly. The goal is to have both legs of equal length when the splint is properly applied (see Figure 32-25).
5. Undo the velcro straps before placing the splint underneath the injured leg.
6. Place the padded bar or seat under the injured leg against the patient's ischial tuberosity and make sure the splint is completely underneath the patient's femur. **Do not let the pad slide above the ischial tuberosity or** it can compress the sacral nerve and cause nerve damage (i.e., inability to flex the foot).
7. Firmly secure the groin strap. Make sure the strap does not go over the suspected fracture site (Figure 32-26).

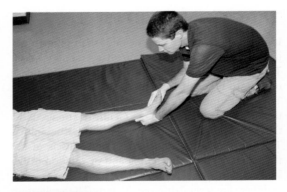

FIGURE 32–24

Check pulse of foot and put an "X." Check the dorsalis pedis pulse and place an "x" on the skin where you feel the pulse. Photo courtesy of Devin Price and Gürkan Özel.

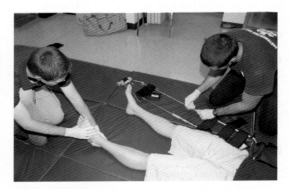

FIGURE 32–25

Place the Hare traction splint® alongside the unaffected extremity to determine proper leg length. Another rescuer checks circulation and provides gentle manual traction to the injured leg. Photo courtesy of Devin Price and Gürkan Özel.

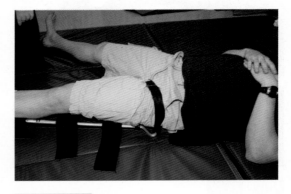

FIGURE 32–26

Secure the groin strap. Photo courtesy of Devin Price and Gürkan Özel.

8. Attach the ankle hitch and hook it to the traction strap (Figure 32-27).

9. Slowly tighten the traction strap until pain or muscle spasm decreases in intensity. Make sure both leg lengths are equal. The first rescuer does not release manual traction until the splint has been fully secured to the patient. If the patient's pain does not decrease, continue to apply traction but do not stretch the injured leg past the length of the unaffected leg.

10. The first rescuer can release the hold on the patient's injured leg. Secure all of the velcro straps around the patient's leg, ensuring that no strap is placed over the suspected fracture site (Figure 32-28).

11. Reassess the patient's pulse, sensation, and motor function. Check pulse at the premarked skin site on the top of the patient's foot. Check sensation with a gentle touch, and check motion by having the patient wiggle his or her toes.

12. Make sure the traction splint is firmly secured before moving the patient.

Procedure (Sager Splint®)

1. Follow steps 1 to 3 as listed above for the Hare traction splint.

2. Position the Sager splint® between the patient's legs, resting the ischial perineal cushion (the saddle) against the ischial tuberosity (Figure 32-29). The pulley wheel should be on the inside of the leg, and the wheel should be facing the injured leg.

3. One rescuer applies manual traction to the injured leg.

4. The second rescuer firmly secures the thigh strap, ensuring that it goes high up on the thigh but not over the suspected fracture site (Figure 32-30).

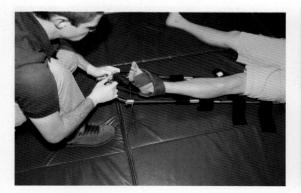

FIGURE 32–27

Ankle hitch. Attach the ankle hitch and hook it to the traction strap. Photo courtesy of Devin Price and Gürkan Özel.

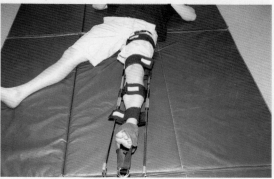

FIGURE 32–28

Hare traction splint® in place with all straps secured. Photo courtesy of Devin Price and Gürkan Özel.

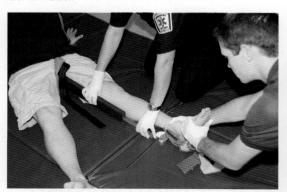

FIGURE 32–29

Place the Sager splint® between the patient's legs. Note the location of the pulley wheel. The arrow points to the pulley wheel (next to the left hand of the top rescuer). Photo courtesy of Devin Price and Gürkan Özel.

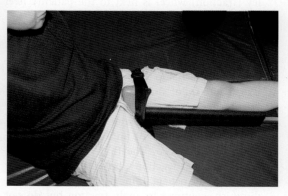

FIGURE 32–30

Thigh strap is secured. Apply thigh straps of Sager splint.® Photo courtesy of Devin Price and Gürkan Özel.

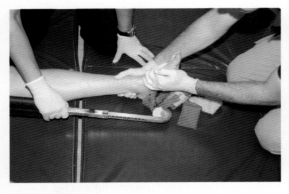

FIGURE 32–31

Spring clip pulley at heels. Extend the shaft until the pulley wheel is at the patient's heel. Photo courtesy of Devin Price and Gürkan Özel.

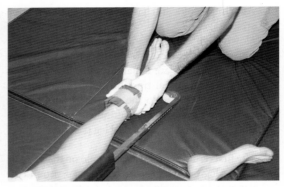

FIGURE 32–32

Secure the ankle harness around the ankle. Photo courtesy of Devin Price and Gürkan Özel.

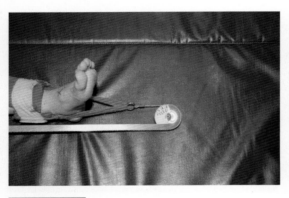

FIGURE 32–33

Hitch and pulley with traction applied. Make sure the two leg lengths are the same. Photo courtesy of Devin Price and Gürkan Özel.

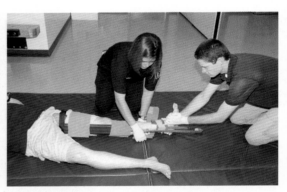

FIGURE 32–34

Secure all straps. Photo courtesy of Devin Price and Gürkan Özel.

5. Lift the spring clip to extend the shaft until the pulley (traction) wheel is next to the patient's heel (Figure 32-31).
6. Position the ankle harness beneath the heel and just above the ankle. Using the attached hook and loop straps, wrap the ankle harness snugly around the ankle and attach it to the pulley (Figure 32-32).
7. Extend the splint shaft to achieve the amount of traction desired while checking the traction amount registered on the traction scale. Go up to 10% of the patient's body weight, or until the pain or muscle spasms are reduced. The first rescuer does not release manual traction until the splint is fully secured to the patient. If the patient's pain does not diminish, continue to apply traction but do not extend the injured leg past the length as the unaffected leg (Figure 32-33).

8. Adjust the thigh strap at the upper thigh, making sure it is snug and secure; then firmly secure the elastic leg straps. Ensure that none of the leg straps are over the suspected fracture site. The first rescuer can release the hold on the injured leg once the traction splint is properly secured (Figure 32-34).
9. Reassess CSM.
10. Make sure the traction splint is firmly secured before moving the patient.

CARE OF OPEN FRACTURES

Purpose of Procedure

To properly manage an open fracture in a prehospital environment.

Patient Selection

Any patient with a suspected or obvious open fracture. Obvious open fractures have protruding bone or bone visible through the injury site. **Suspicion for open fracture is high if there is a break in the skin near a suspected fracture. Immobilize the limb in the position found.** If an open fracture is not severely angulated or displaced and patient transport is expected within 6 to 8 hours, treat the injury with a standard compression dressing and splint, pad the splint with a cotton sheet, and ensure that bony prominences are protected. Administer antibiotics if transport time to definitive care is prolonged. If the open fracture is severely angulated or displaced or transport is not expected within 6 to 8 hours, follow the procedure described below.

Risks and Precautions

Improper management of open fractures leads to the risk of osteomyelitis, which is a significant factor in morbidity. **In general, do not reduce an open fracture with exposed bone unless the extremity is pulseless, extremely angulated, or if time to transport to definitive care exceeds 6 to 8 hours.** Reduction of an open fracture introduces bacteria into the soft tissue and bone, increasing the chance of osteomyelitis.

Equipment

- Sterile gauze pads and gauze roll.
- Povidone-iodine solution.
- 3-Inch medical tape.
- Elastic wrap.
- Splinting device.
- Cotton sheet.
- Traction device or limb immobilizer.
- Sterile saline or tap water.
- Antibiotics.
- Analgesia and sedation.

Anesthesia and Procedural Monitoring

It is best to administer an IV narcotic. Dose according to your local EMS protocol. Benzodiazepines may be given in addition to a narcotic, as they relax muscles. Ensure that you have IV access and have naloxone available. Monitor oxygen saturation and apply a cardiac monitor.

Step-by-Step Technique

Non–traction splinting:

1. Assess and document neurovascular status.
2. Remove any particulate matter from wound.
3. Irrigate with copious sterile saline (at least 1L); non-sterile tap water or other potable water is acceptable.
   - Use at least 1 L.
   - Non–sterile tap water or other potable water is acceptable.
4. There is little evidence to identify the optimal irrigation solution for bone segments: saline, povidone-iodine, soap; chlorhexidine, or others.[1,2] Follow local protocols.
5. **Do not apply traction device if there are injuries *at* the hip or *at* the knee for fear of causing neurovascular injury.**
6. Apply sterile dressing to wound.
7. Splint injury (there are many commercially available options; refer to Figure 32-10B.
   - Pad splint with a cotton sheet, if available.
   - Immobilize from the joint above to the joint below.
     Keep wrist in natural position at 15 degrees of extension – like holding a can.
     Elbow at 90 degrees.
     Knee at 5 to 15 degrees flexion.
     Ankle at 90 degrees.
   - Wrap with elastic bandage to secure in place.
   - Do not splint circumferentially or too tightly so that circulation is compromised (allow space to accommodate for swelling). Reassess neurovascular status to ensure it is unchanged.
8. Relieve stress on injured limb with sling support. Administer antibiotics (IV ceftriaxone or cefazolin).
9. Continue to manage analgesia and sedation.
10. Evacuate immediately to definitive orthopedic care.

Do

- Splint the injury to the joints above and below.
- Remove any particulate matter and irrigate the wound with at least 1 L NS (more if evacuation is delayed and reduction is required in the field).
- **Reduce a fracture with exposed bone if severely displaced, pulseless, and/or time to transport is expected to exceed 6 to 8 hours.**
- Administer a dose of IV antibiotics as early as possible.

Do Not

- Splint circumferentially.
- Forget to continuously reassess neurovascular status.
- Reduce a fracture with exposed bone if transport to definitive care is expected within 6 to 8 hours.
- Apply traction splints to injuries directly *at* the hip or *at* the knee for fear of causing neurovascular injury.

References

1. van Winkle BA, Neustein J "Management of open fractures with sterilization of large, contaminated, extruded cortical fragments' *Clin Orthop Relat Res* 1987 Oct; 223; 275-81.
2. Flow Investigators. 'Fluid Lavage of Open Wounds (FLOW): design and rationale for a large, ulticenter collaborative 2 × 3 factorial trial of irrigating pressures and solutions in patients with open fractures' *BMC Musculoskelet Disord.* 2010 May 6; 11(1):85 [Epub ahead of print PMID 20459600].

CHAPTER 33

Pulseless Extremity

Gürkan Özel

KEY LEARNING POINTS

- Injured extremities are usually splinted in the position found.

- Attempt to realign an extremity should be made only after the life threats have been addressed and if there is a circulatory compromise, sensory deficit or if the extremity cannot be splinted in the position found.

- Attempts to realign an extremity in the field should never delay the rapid transport of critically injured patient to the hospital.

- Pulseless extremities can be left in place when transport time to hospital is short.

- Gentle traction on longitudinal axis is usually all it takes to realign an angulated extremity.

- Dislocated joints should be best left in place unless there is circulatory compromise distal to the injury site. Gentle rotation can be attempted to restore circulation. Rapid transport is required if unsuccessful.

- If an extremity is grossly angulated and pulseless after an open fracture, realigning the extremity by gentle traction on bone ends can be attempted. Bleeding control and general wound care should preceed the splinting of open fractures.

Sometimes injured extremities are found to be grossly angulated. In general, EMS providers can attempt to realign an injured and angulated extremity, *only* after life threathening injuries are addressed and *if* there is:

- Compromised circulation distal to the injury.
- Presence of sensory deficit distal to the injury.
- An extremity that cannot be effectively immobilized in the position found, risking further damage to the underlying structures and increasing pain during movement and transport.

> **Caution: Attempts to realign an extremity in the field should never delay the rapid transport of a critically injured patient to the hospital.**

The decision to reduce or not to reduce the fracture or realign the extremity also requires good judgement, a complete physical exam, careful consideration of all other factors involved, and sufficient skill in the technique of reduction and realignment[1].

In urban or suburban areas, where transport times are short, attempts to realign a pulseless extremity should be left to skilled hands in the ED. EMS providers should focus on safe and rapid transport to an appropriate medical facility. If, however, the patient with the pulseless extremity is located in a rural area or in any remote or wilderness environment, long transport times may result in a hypoxic and necrotic extremity. An attempt to realign a pulseless extremity is more reasonable, even warranted, where transport times to definitive medical care are prolonged (many hours to days).

When realigning an injured extremity, do not worry about a perfect solution. Instead, do your best to realign the extremity as close to normal anatomical position as possible, in order to restore circulation and facilitate proper and effective immobilization by splinting or other means. EMS providers attempting to realign injured extremities are encouraged to seek online medical direction to discuss risks and benefits of the procedure, even if clinical protocols do not require such communications.

Realigning an injured extremity is done by grasping the joints immediately distal and immediately proximal to the injured site, and applying *gentle* longitudinal traction followed by *gentle* positioning of the extremity, trying to approximate a straight line[2]. The key here is to use the least amount of force for traction when realigning extremities. **Excessive traction can further injure underlying structures.** (See **Figure 33-1**)

While small bones can be realigned by a single provider, angulated long bones (such as humerus) require at least two EMS providers to safely and effectively achieve realignment. One EMS provider immobilizes the proximal end of the injured extremity while the second EMS provider immobilizes and applies gentle traction on the distal end of the injured site, followed by realigning into an approximately straight position. Once the extremity is realigned, continue gentle traction and support of the extremity until splinting is completed. (See **Figure 33-2**)

If an injured extremity results in several broken bones and multiple angulations, try to reposition the misaligned pieces one at a time, starting from the most

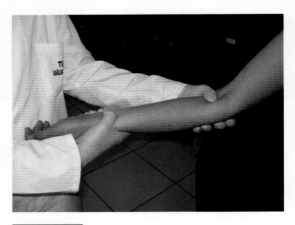

FIGURE 33–1

Gentle traction to reduce pulseless extremity (arm). Photo courtesy of Gürkan Özel.

distal end and moving towards the proximal sites while supporting the already realigned sections. The second EMS provider should anchor the proximal end of the injured segments throughout the procedure.[2]

Dislocation of a moving joint is another concern for EMS providers if there is a circulatory compromise. Reducing dislocations in the field, without X-ray capability, is generally not a modern EMS procedure. Attempts to realign a dislocated limb can convert a pure dislocation to a fracture-dislocation and result in further damage to underlying structures[3]. If there is no circulatory compromise, gently support the extremity and splint it in a comfortable position for the patient prior to transport.

If, however, there is no pulse and no capillary fill, gently straighten or rotate the joint a little to see if the circulation returns. If gentle manipulation does not restore the pulse, immobilize the joint, support the extremity to avoid traction stress, and rapidly transport to the nearest appropriate medical facility.

Immediately stop attempts to realign a deformed extremity if:

- Patient complains of increasing pain.
- EMS provider encounters mechanical resistance.
- Circulatory compromise or sensory or motor deficit worsen.
- The attempt causes further visible damage in the extremity.

If the EMS provider has to stop the realigning attempt for the reasons mentioned above, support the extremity in most comfortable position for the patient and splint it *as is*. Rapid transport to an appropriate medical facility is once again warranted.

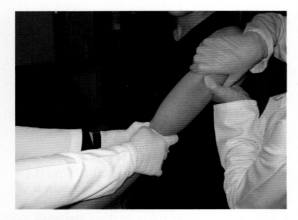

FIGURE 33–2

Gentle traction to reduce pulseless extremity (forearm). Photo courtesy of Gürkan Özel.

References

1. Critical care paramedic: Bryan Bledsoe, Randall W. Benner, Prentice Hall, Inc. Upper Saddle River, NJ pp: 537–538, January 2006.
2. *Comprehensive Guide To Pre-Hospital Skills: A Skills Manual For —EMT-BASIC, EMT-INTERMEDIATE, EMT-PARAMEDIC* **by Alexander M. Butman, BA, D.Sc., REMT-P, Scott W. Martin, BS, REMT-P, Richard W. Vomacka, BA, REMT-P, Norman E. McSwain, Jr., FACS, REMT-P ©1995 Emergency Training, Akron, OH ISBN Number:0-940432-09-9**.
3. Judith E. Tintinalli, Gabor D. Kelen, J. Stephan Stapczynski, eds, Emergency Medicine, A Comprehensive Study Guide, 6e © 2004, McGraw-Hill, New York, Chapter 267, Injuries to the Bones, Joints & Soft Tisse, pp 1653. 2004.

Other suggested readings

1. Quinn RH, Macias DJ: The Management of Open Fractures. Wilderness and Environmental Medicine: Vol. 17, No. 1, pp. 41–48. 2006.
2. PHTLS Prehospital Trauma Life Support, 6th Ed. National Association of Emergency Medical Technicians @2007, MosbyEMS, St. Louis, MO, pp 320.

CHAPTER 34

Impaled Objects

Gürkan Özel

KEY LEARNING POINTS

- Impaled objects should be left in place and stabilized with bulky dressings to prevent movement.
- If an impaled object interferes with the patient's airway, or if a patient cannot be loaded into the ambulance with the object, try to shorten the object into a managable size.

- Any time an impaled object is removed, either by accident or selectively, control bleeding with direct pressure, and quickly transport to an appropriate hospital.

Removal of an impaled object may worsen the injury or may result in uncontrolled internal bleeding. For these reasons, **removal of impaled objects is contraindicated in the prehospital environment.** Instead, stabilize impaled objects in place. For many objects, a bulky dressing can be placed and secured around the object for stabilization (Figure 34-1). Sometimes creativity is needed when managing impaled objects in the field.[1,2]

For objects impaled in the eye, have the patient close both eyes as much as possible and place a paper cup with the bottom removed or a hole punched in the bottom to accommodate the impaled object. Apply adequate padding to stabilize the impaled object. Try to have the patient keep both eyes closed once the impaled object is stabilized in place in order to prevent movement of the injured globe during transport.

The only times to consider removal of impaled objects in the prehospital environment would be

- **If they interfere with the patient's airway.**
- **If the patient cannot be transported with the object in place.**

Every attempt should be made to cut the impaled object into a managable size so that the patient can safely be loaded into an ambulance and transported to the hospital. Fire departments and civil defense units are usually equipped with cutting tools and will assist the EMS providers when requested. The skin is the pivot point for impaled objects, and any movement *outside* the skin will cause significant movement of the object end *inside the body*. If the object cannot be shortened or removed for transport, request a physician, preferably a surgeon, to come to the scene to provide assistance in removal.

Impaled objects in the soft tissue of the cheek of the face can usually be safely removed. Bleeding can be controlled by placing gauze pads inside on the mucosal surface and outside against the skin of the cheek and applying pressure.

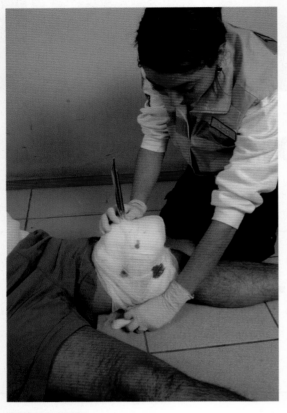

FIGURE 34–1

Impaled object; bulky dressing to stablilize impaled object. Photo courtesy of Gürkan Özel.

If impaled objects are accidentaly removed, aggressively control bleeding with direct pressure and rapidly transport the patient to an appropriate medical facility. Notify the ED beforehand if at all possible, so that the appropriate specialists will be ready to provide care.

Bring removed impaled objects to the hospital with the patient whenever possible. Be prepared to provide a detailed report of the incident, including the type and size of the object, its location on the body, and the angle of the object's entry.

References

1. *PHTLS Prehospital Trauma Life Support.* 6th ed., St. Louis: Mosby, 2007; 306.
2. Bledsoe B, Benner RW, eds. *Critical Care Paramedic,* ©Prentice Hall, Inc., A Pearson Education Company, Upper Saddle River, New Jersey; 2006;481.

CHAPTER 35

Hemorrhage Control

Ricardo Ong

PURPOSE OF PROCEDURE

To preserve a victim's blood by controlling life-threatening compressible hemorrhage at the wound site.

PATIENT SELECTION

Any patient who has sustained an injury resulting in continued hemorrhage without intervention. This can be arterial (brisk, pulsating, bright red blood) or venous (low flow, oozing, darker red blood) in nature, resulting from penetrating (high-velocity or low-velocity missile, stab wound) or blunt trauma (open fracture).

RISKS AND PRECAUTIONS

The most significant risk is the inability to properly control potentially life-threatening hemorrhage. Applying a tourniquet or a pressure dressing too tightly risks the viability of the circulation to the injured limb. The EMT should be careful when applying a tourniquet and pressure dressing and understand the indications and potential complications, but not hesitate to use a tourniquet if the situation calls for it. Very proximal wounds may be difficult to apply a pressure dressing or tourniquet to; do your best to control the hemorrhage.

EQUIPMENT

- Gauze roll.
- 4 × 4 Gauze pads.
- Self-adhering, multipurpose, elastic wrap
- Tourniquet
- Hemostatic agent

PATIENT POSITIONING

Patient positioning largely depends on the location of the wound (e.g., arm, leg, upper, lower portion). Place the patient in a relatively comfortable position, typically lying supine on the ground. Position the patient so as to allow easy access to the wound. Do not compromise ventilation by leaning on the patient's chest or over the airway.

ANESTHESIA AND PROCEDURAL MONITORING

No anesthesia is typically required. In fact, if you are spending time preparing an anesthetic or pain medication, you are wasting the most precious resource this patient has - his or her own blood.

If the patient is conscious and the airway is unobstructed, continuous verbal communication is the best way to monitor the patient. If the patient is unconscious and unable to communicate, you will not have time to place the patient on a cardiac monitor before attempting to control the hemorrhage if you are alone.

If you have a partner, one person can attend to the hemorrhage while the other sets up the monitor. If no monitor is available, use a portable, battery-operated finger pulse-oximeter, which will provide an auditory pulse indicator as well as a visual pulse-oximetry (oxygen saturation) reading.

PRESSURE DRESSING

Step-by-Step Technique

1. Apply direct pressure to the wound with gauze pads or a roll. If gauze is not immediately available, use your fingers and hand to control the point of hemorrhage (see Figure 35-1).

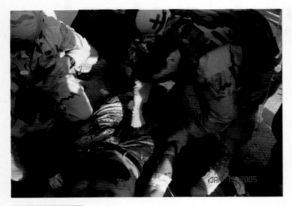

FIGURE 35–1

Direct pressure to control compressible hemorrhage. Photo courtesy of US Army.

2. Prepare the pressure dressing. Extend the gauze roll while keeping it off the ground and as clean and sterile as possible.
3. Pack the wound with the gauze roll. Use as many gauze rolls as needed to fill the wound.
4. Place another rolled or wadded-up gauze roll over the packed wound to serve as a focal pressure point.
5. Stabilize the gauze packing with several 4 × 4 gauze pads.
6. Wrap the dressing firmly with the self-adhering elastic wrap. Do not constrict the wound so tightly that you cut off arterial circulation if the artery is intact.
7. Assess the neurovascular status of the limb. If you did not observe brisk, pulsating, bright red bleeding and do not suspect arterial hemorrhage, then make sure you can still palpate a distal pulse. If you can no longer palpate the distal pulse, then lessen the tension of the pressure dressing.

Outcomes Assessment

You have effectively and correctly applied the pressure dressing if you observed the following steps:

1. Neurovascular status intact: In the absence of an arterial injury and/or a significant nerve injury, the patient should have a palpable distal pulse and intact motor and sensory function.
2. Hemorrhage control: Dressing remains dry and is not soaked with blood. If dressing soaks through with blood, consider reapplying the pressure dressing, applying a tourniquet, and/or applying a hemostatic agent.

Tourniquet Application

If the wound continues to bleed, consider use of a tourniquet. Given the concerns over inappropriate use of tourniquets and potential complications of prolonged limb ischemia, only use a tourniquet when indicated and apply the correct technique. Consider tourniquet use as a temporary hemorrhage control technique, but do not hesitate to apply it if the patient is in danger of fatal hemorrhage. The patient is better off risking potential loss of a limb (even though the risk is low if the tourniquet is applied correctly in the appropriate situation) rather than losing his or her life.

There are many effective tourniquets commercially available today. Ensure that the tourniquet you use is relatively wide (at least 2 inches or 5 cm) and has a windlass device that allows you to tighten it. Figure 35-2 illustrates an improvised tourniquet and Figure 35-3 is an example of a commercial tourniquet.

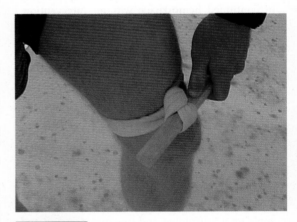

FIGURE 35–2

Improvised tourniquet. Improvised tourniquet with windlass. Photo courtesy of US Army.

Step-by-Step Technique

1. Place the tourniquet approximately 2 inches (5 cm) above the wound (Figure 35-4).
2. Secure the tourniquet in place as indicated by the type of tourniquet (Figure 35-5).

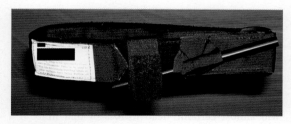

FIGURE 35–3

Commercial tourniquet. Example of a new type of commercially available tourniquet. Photo courtesy of US Army.

3. Tighten the windlass until the bleeding stops (Figure 35-6).
4. Secure the windlass so the tourniquet will not loosen (Figure 35-7).
5. Undress the wound; clean it of excess, clotted blood.
6. Reapply the pressure dressing as described above.
7. After several minutes, slowly release the tourniquet over a one-minute period.
8. If the wound continues to bleed, retighten the tourniquet and leave it in place.
9. Prepare to evacuate the patient or consider using a hemostatic agent.

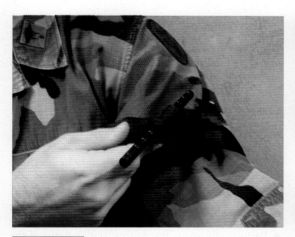

FIGURE 35–4

Tourniquet Placement. Photo courtesy of US Army.

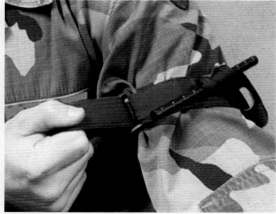

FIGURE 35–5

Secure tourniquet. Photo courtesy of US Army.

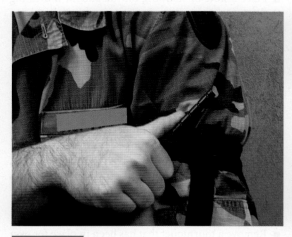

FIGURE 35–6

Tighten windlass. Tighten the windlass until bleeding stops. Photo courtesy of US Army.

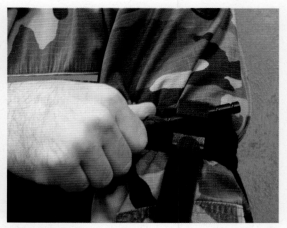

FIGURE 35–7

Secure windlass. Photo courtesy of US Army.

Outcomes Assessment

1. Neurovascular assessment. If the tourniquet is applied correctly, no pulse should be palpated.
2. Hemorrhage control. Dressing remains dry and is not soaked with blood. If dressing soaks through with blood, consider either reapplying the tourniquet or applying a hemostatic agent.

HEMOSTATIC AGENT APPLICATION

If the wound continues to bleed, consider use of a topical hemostatic agent. There are numerous different and effective hemostatic agents commercially available today - products made with collagens , zeolites , chitosans , or polysaccharides . Some current products are Heme-Con™, QuikClot™, Celox™, D-Stat™. Some are available in granule form, others in dressing form. Ensure you are familiar with the both the indications, contraindications, and specific application technique for the product you choose to use. Most of these agents have a relatively similar application technique as described below.

Step-by-Step Technique

1. Control hemorrhage proximal to the wound, preferably with a tourniquet.
2. Undress the wound and evacuate it of excess, clotted blood.
3. Apply the hemostatic agent in granule, dressing, or gauze form.
4. Apply pressure dressing over the hemostatic agent, as described above.
5. Maintain pressure over the wound for 10 to 15 minutes before releasing the tourniquet.
6. Slowly release the tourniquet over a one-minute period.
7. If the wound continues to bleed, retighten the tourniquet and reapply the hemostatic agent.
8. If the wound still continues to bleed, retighten the tourniquet and leave in place.

Outcomes Assessment

1. Neurovascular assessment. If the hemostatic agent is effective in controlling the hemorrhage, sensation and a pulse should return (assuming the artery is intact).
2. Hemorrhage control. Dressing remains dry and is not soaked with blood. If dressing soaks through with blood, consider either reapplying the hemostatic agent or attempt to control the bleeding through direct pressure; prepare to evacuate the patient immediately.

Complications

The main complication is limb ischemia and neurovascular compromise. A tourniquet left on indefinitely will almost certainly lead to loss of that limb. If a tourniquet is kept on for more than 6 hours, when it is released, metabolic toxins from the injured extremity will flood the circulation and cause shock and metabolic acidosis. Therefore, if a tourniquet has been in place for more than 6 hours, it is best to leave it there to preserve the life of the patient at risk of losing the limb.

Follow-up and Patient Instructions

Transport the patient immediately to the nearest appropriate medical facility. Instruct the patient not to modify the dressing or tourniquet in any way.

Do

- Obtain immediate control of hemorrhage through direct pressure.
- Consider a tourniquet as a temporary hemorrhage control device.
- Use a tourniquet that has a windlass, which provides the mechanical advantage required for it to be effective.
- Periodically assess the neurovascular status of the limb.
- Periodically reassess the wound to make sure the dressing, tourniquet, or hemostatic agent is effective.
- Place a note or marking on the patient indicating that a tourniquet or hemostatic agent has been applied.

Do not

- Use a tourniquet or hemostatic agent on a hemorrhage that is easily controlled with a basic pressure dressing.
- Hesitate to use a tourniquet to gain control of potentially life-threatening hemorrhage uncontrolled by a conventional pressure dressing.
- Use a tourniquet less than 2 inches (5 cm) wide, such as rope or cord, unless nothing else is available (narrow tourniquets create more tissue damage).
- Remove a tourniquet that has been in place for over 6 hours.
- Attempt to clamp a vessel with forceps (very difficult to do in a field environment).

CHAPTER 36

Eye Injuries

Ricardo Ong

PURPOSE OF PROCEDURE

To properly manage a patient with a potentially ruptured globe in order to protect it from further damage.

PATIENT SELECTION

Any patient with suspected globe rupture or penetrating eye injury (Table 36-1).

Table 36–1	Signs and Symptoms of Eye Injury

History
- Vision Change
- Explosion, hammering, or metal grinding
- Known or suspected foreign body in the eye
- Eye protection is shattered

Symptoms
- Loss of, or decreased vision
- Eye pain or foreign body sensation
- Photophobia or double vision
- Eye discharge

Signs
- Decreased visual acuity. Test with visual acuity card if available; count fingers at 1 meter (3 feet); test light perception
- Normal vision makes significant injury less likely but does not rule it out
- Large subconjunctival hemorrhage
- Non-circular, irregular, or tear-dropped shaped pupil (Fig 36-1)
- Dark brown tissue at junction of sclera and cornea (Fig 36-1)

RISKS AND PRECAUTIONS

The aqueous fluid within the eye cannot be replaced. It is critical that you act to preserve the fluid remaining in a ruptured globe. Do not palpate any globe that is potentially ruptured. Do not attempt to remove any foreign bodies. Do not apply a pressure patch to a potentially ruptured globe.

EQUIPMENT

- Rigid, sterile metal eye shield.
- Cravat.
- Medical tape.
- Oral or IV fluoroquinolone.

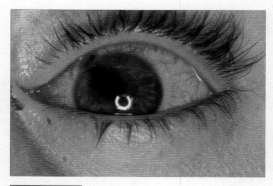

FIGURE 36–1

Tear-drop shaped pupil with dark brown tissue at junction of sclera and cornea. Photo courtesy US Army.

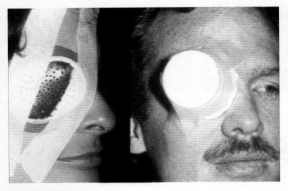

FIGURE 36–2

Rigid metal eye shield. Photo courtesy US Army.

ANESTHESIA AND PROCEDURAL MONITORING

Does not apply to eye injuries.

Step-by-Step Technique

Globe rupture suspected or obvious.

1. Apply sterile rigid metal shield to eye. (Figure 36-2).
2. Secure with tape.
3. Ensure that no pressure is applied to the globe itself.
4. Administer antibiotic (oral or IV fluoroquinolone).

   If no premade rigid eye shield is available, use a padded cup or fashion a doughnut-shaped bandage from a cravat (see Figures 36-3).

Outcomes Assessment

Visual acuity does not worsen and infection is prevented by application of the eye shield.

Complications

Permanent visual impairment and/or infection. To avoid introducing air into the globe, minimize barometric changes if possible (this consideration is always secondary to expeditious transport to obtain ophthalmologic evaluation).

Follow-up and Patient Instructions

Transport for immediate ophthalmologic evaluation. Do not remove the eye shield. Do not palpate, irrigate, or allow any pressure on the globe.

Do

- Protect a ruptured globe from further loss of aqueous fluid.
- Give an initial dose of antibiotics if available.
- Assume the globe is ruptured if history, signs, and symptoms are consistent with rupture, even if perforation is not obvious.

Do not

- Palpate a potentially ruptured globe!
- Irrigate a potentially ruptured globe!
- Attempt to remove any foreign bodies!
- Assume the globe is not ruptured just because visual acuity is normal!
- Apply any topical ointment to a ruptured globe!
- Apply a pressure patch to a potentially ruptured globe!

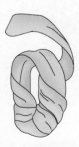
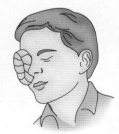
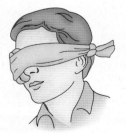
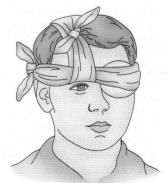

FIGURE 36–3

Doughnut-shaped bandages.

CHAPTER 37

Burns

Ricardo Ong

PURPOSE OF PROCEDURE

To protect burn wounds from unnecessary contamination and infection.

PATIENT SELECTION

Any patient with second- (partial-thickness) or third-degree burns (see Table 37-1).

RISKS AND PRECAUTIONS

For small burns, focus on wound management. For burns >20% total body surface area (TBSA) or >10% of TBSA in the very old, very young, and those with significant chronic medical disease, consider other potentially life-threatening factors; look for inhalation injury and airway compromise, signs of carbon monoxide poisoning, cervical spine injury in an accident, and signs of shock. Address each issue accordingly if concerned. See Figure 37-1 for estimating percentage of total body surface area.

If the burn patient will be evaluated by trained medical personnel within the first 24 hours, then generally initial field treatment with ointment will not be needed; however, if evacuation is delayed beyond 24 hours or the patient is expected to manage his or her own wounds at home, be prepared to engage in aggressive wound management, dressing changes, and antibiotic ointment application.

EQUIPMENT

- Sterile burn dressing
- Gauze roll
- 4×4 gauze pads
- Medical tape
- Elastic wrap
- Antibiotic cream or ointment (bacitracin, silver-based ointment)
- Antibiotic dressings (silver-based)
- Analgesia and sedation (narcotic, benzodiazepine).

Table 37–1	Depth of Burn
Depth	**Description**
First Degree	Erythema of top skin layer, no blisters
Second Degree	Blistering, top layer of skin (epidermis) injured, showing deeper layer (dermis). For partial second-degree burns, the dermis will blanch. For deep second-degree burns, the dermis does not blanch when compressed
Third Degree	Skin is pale, charred, and leathery. All skin layers are involved

ANESTHESIA AND PROCEDURAL MONITORING

Managing burns wounds can be very painful for the patient. Initial wound management can typically be performed without analgesia or sedation; however, expect that the patient will eventually require analgesia if evacuation is delayed and you expect to manage this patient in a prehospital setting for longer than 24 hours or if the patient is managing his or her own wounds at home.

BURN WOUND DRESSING

Step-by-Step Technique

1. Stop the burning process.
   a. Thermal burns: remove smoldering or hot clothing.
   b. Electrical burns: turn off the current (do not directly touch casualty or step on any wires).
   c. Chemical burns: remove particulate matter, decontaminate as described below, and treat as a thermal burn after decontamination.
   Acid/bases: flush with water immediately for at least 30 minutes (hours for alkali burns, which penetrate more deeply).
   White phosphorus (WP): deprive of air, submerge in water.
   Hydrofluoric acid (HF): topical application of 2.5% calgonate gel (Calgonate®).

   Or

   ■ 7 grams of calcium gluconate per 5 ounces Surgilube gives you a 5% solution/gel. (These come in tubes identified in ounces rather than cc's.)

   Or

   ■ The easiest way to remember is to use one large Surgilube tube which is 4.25 ounces + 10 vials calcium gluconate (each vial has 10 cc), = 5 to 10% calcium gluconate.
   Tar/asphalt: cool in water, then apply petroleum jelly, mineral oil, or vegetable oil to dissolve the hardened material.
2. Expose wounds by removing clothing.
3. Do not débride small (<2 cm) unruptured blisters (but unroof them if they rupture, lie across a joint, or are >2 cm).
4. Apply sterile burn dressing.
   a. Several premade burn dressings are commercially available.

   b. If no sterile burn dressing is available, improvise using plastic wrap or a plastic bag (something that will prevent fluid loss from the wound).
   c. Cover extensive burns with a sterile sheet, if available, or clean linen.
5. Secure burn dressing with gauze pads and tape or wrap in gauze roll or elastic bandage if possible (limbs).

PROLONGED EVACUATION

If you expect to remain in a prehospital setting for >24 hours, change dressings at least once daily, preferably twice. You may need to administer a narcotic or sedative agent to the patient, either orally or IV, to facilitate dressing changes. For adults, provide IV fluids at a rate of 4 cc × weight in kilograms × % TBSA in the first 24 hours. For children, the rate is 3 cc × weight in kg × % TBSA.

> **FORMULA–1.** Formulas for first 24 hours of IV fluid administration for second- and third-degree burns.

Adults: 4cc × weight in kg × % TBSA.*
Children: 3cc × weight in kg × % TBSA.*
*TBSA = total body surface area

Step-by-Step Technique

1. Thoroughly clean the wound, preferably with a surgical detergent, but soap and water are fine.
2. Apply silver-based ointment to wounds but never to the face (bacitracin to face). Consider use of commercially available silver-based dressings (note that these must be kept moist with water, not saline).
3. Dress wound with sterile gauze.
4. Secure with gauze roll or elastic wrap.

Outcomes Assessment

Prevention of infection is the main goal of emergency care.

Complications

Wound infection and cellulitis. Infection can progress systemically to sepsis. Use of silver-based ointments on the face can lead to gray-colored staining of skin.

Follow-up and Patient Instructions

Wound care: silver-impregnated dressings need to be changed every 2 to 5 days; keep the dressings moist. Change cream or ointment applications at least once a day, preferably twice. Wet the dressing before removing to prevent disruption of the healing process, wash with soap and water, reapply topical cream or ointment, reapply sterile dressing, and keep the dressings clean and dry.

If wounds are <10% body surface area (Figure 37-1) and the patient is reliable, the patient may perform wound care at home and receive follow-up twice a week. If the patient is unreliable or wounds are >10% body surface area, expect daily follow-up or possible hospitalization.

Do

- Always stop the burning process first.
- Always assess for inhalation injury, Carbon monoxide (CO) poisoning, cervical spine injury, and shock.
- Unroof blisters if they rupture, lie across a joint, or are larger than >2 cm. (1 inch)
- Use bacitracin for facial burns, silver-based ointment for all others.
- Change dressings at least once daily, preferably twice, if remaining in a prehospital environment for >24 hours or if the patient plans to manage the wounds at home.

Do not

- Remove clothing stuck to the burn area.
- Directly touch a patient receiving a shock.
- Delay flushing a chemical burn to remove clothing.
- Use a silver-based antibiotic ointment on the face (may cause skin or corneal staining).
- Débride small (<2 cm) (<1 inch) unruptured blisters.
- Use prophylactic IV or oral antibiotics for prehospital burn wound management.

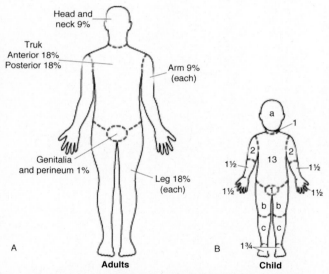

Relative percentage of body surface area (% BSA) affected by growth

Body Part	Age				
	0 yr	1yr	5 yr	10 yr	15 yr
a = 1/2 of head	9 1/2	8 1/2	6 1/2	5 1/2	4 1/2
b = 1/2 of 1 thigh	2 3/4	3 1/4	4	4 1/4	4 1/2
c = 1/2 of 1 lower leg	2 1/2	2 1/2	2 3/4	3	3 1/4

FIGURE 37–1

Lund-Browder chart. Estimating percentage of total body surface area. (*Exclude area of the degree burn erythema when estimating*) The Lund-Browder chart is the most accurate method for estimating burn extent and must be used in the evaluation of all pediatric patients.

CHAPTER 38

Snake Bites

Ricardo Ong

PURPOSE OF PROCEDURE

To properly manage a venomous snake bite injury.

PATIENT SELECTION

Any patient with suspected or obvious snake bite from a potentially venomous snake.

RISKS AND PRECAUTIONS

Ensure that the site is safe and that further exposure to the offending snake is eliminated. A venomous snake bite causes neurologic or cardiovascular compromise to the victim, possibly resulting in death. However, the most important considerations remain rapid transport, intensive care, and administration of antivenom; expeditious transport should be arranged as soon as possible. Recommended treatment for a snake bite from the Crotalidae family (North American rattlesnake, copperheads, and water moccasins) is to immobilize the bitten limb with a standard splint. Venom sequestration techniques such as the pressure immobilization technique can be used for snakes in the Elapidae family (coral snakes). The prehospital provider needs to make an informed decision on which techniques to use based on factors such as the type of snake, potential severity of the bite, size of the victim, and time to transport. **Note that pressure immobilization is not recommended in Crotalidae bites because few people die from these bites, and there is a greater risk of worsening the local necrotizing effects of the toxin.**

EQUIPMENT

- Sterile gauze pads or gauze roll
- Elastic wrap
- Arm or leg immobilizer
- Splinting material and device

ANESTHESIA AND PROCEDURAL MONITORING

No analgesia or sedation should be required for this procedure. However, the toxin can create a very painful local reaction that may require narcotic analgesia for ongoing management.

PRESSURE IMMOBILIZATION DRESSING

Step-by-Step Technique

1. Assess and document neurovascular status of injured limb.
2. Clean the wound with soap and water.
3. Apply sterile dressing to wound to protect from secondary infection.
4. Wrap the entire limb with an elastic ACE™ bandage (Figure 38-1).
   a. Wrap the elastic bandage firmly enough to compress the lymphatics and smaller superficial veins, generally as firmly as you would wrap a sprained joint.
   b. Do **not** wrap the bandage so tightly that the arterial or larger venous circulation is compromised.

Fang marks

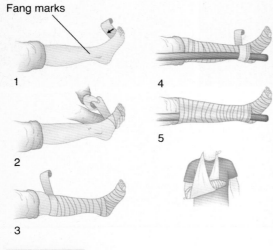

1

2

3

FIGURE 38–1

Pressure immobilization for snake bite.

4

5

5. Immobilize the injured limb with an immobilizer, splint, or sling.
6. Ensure that the patient minimizes use of the limb. If the limb cannot be immobilized (i.e., the patient needs to walk from a remote area), the attempt to sequester the venom will be futile. If this is the case, do not bother with a pressure immobilization dressing.
7. Manage pain as needed.
8. Evacuate patient immediately to a definitive care center.

Note: use standard splinting techniques (as if you were splinting and injured limb) for Crotalidae bites, not the pressure immobilization technique.

Outcomes Assessment

Remember that the pressure immobilization technique is intended to sequester the venom, thereby preventing systemic absorption. If it has been applied effectively, systemic absorption and toxicity should be avoided or mitigated through delayed absorption.

Complications

Applying the pressure immobilization technique to a Crotalidae bite can result in increasing local pain and necrosis.

Follow-up and Patient Instructions

Ensure that the patient understands that immobilization is critical and that he or she must make the best effort possible to minimize use and movement of the injured limb. If the patient needs to walk or use the bitten limb, immobilization is likely to be ineffective. Make all practical efforts and suggestions to minimize use. Immediate attention at an appropriate medical facility is required.

Do

- Immobilize the injured limb to minimize use if applying the pressure immobilization technique.
- Arrange for immediate transport of the patient.

Do not

- Attempt to incise the bite site or suck out the poison with your mouth.
- Apply commercial suction devices.
- Apply a tourniquet.
- Forget to continuously reassess neurovascular status.
- Apply any technique that will impede immediate transport of the patient.
- Apply a pressure immobilization dressing to a limb bitten by a Crotalidae (North American rattlesnake, copperhead, or water moccasin).

Web Resources

1. World Health Organization Snake Antivenom Immunoglobulins: http://bit.ly/afzgEF.

CHAPTER 39

Prehospital Pain Management

Gürkan Özel

KEY LEARNING POINTS

- Pain is the most common reason patients seek help from EMS providers. EMS providers tend to underestimate patients' perception of pain, resulting in undertreatment of pain.

- Before managing pain, assess pain level properly.

- Patient's self-reporting is the most reliable indicator of the existence of pain.

- "Numeric Pain Intensity Scale," "Simple Descriptive Pain Intensity Scale," "Visual Analog Scale," and "Wong-Baker FACES Pain Rating Scale" are some of the tools used when assessing patients' pain.

- Pain management can be accomplished by nonpharmacologic interventions and pharmacologic interventions.

- Reassess pain after interventions to document pain improvement.

- Education progams designed especially for EMS providers that address prehospital pain management strategies are valuable.

Pain is an unpleasant sensory and emotional experience associated with actual or potential tissue damage or described in terms of such damage. It is one of the most common patient complaints encountered by EMS personnel. The management of pain is a vital aspect of patient care. In order to provide optimal patient care, pain should be correctly assessed and treatment options for pain relief should be considered and then applied. EMS providers are the first in the line of proper pain management for patients. However, historically, EMS providers tend to underestimate and undertreat the pain in the field.[1-4]

PAIN ASSESSMENT

Pain is a subjective finding and has physical, psychological, mental, cultural, and gender-related properties. Since EMS providers can underestimate the patient's perception of pain, they should approach the patient *without bias* when assessing pain. **Patient self-reporting is the most reliable indicator of the existence and intensity of pain.**[5]

Proper history taking and questioning of the patient with regard to his or her own perception of pain is an important step. EMS providers can use various tools to assess pain. Pain rating scales are

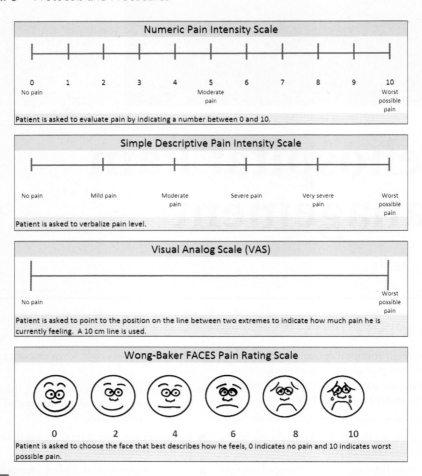

FIGURE 39–1

Wong-Baker FACES Pain Rating Scale. Reprinted with permission from Hockenberry MJ, Wilson D. *Wong's Essentials of Pediatric Nursing*. ed. 8, St. Louis: Mosby, 2009.

useful tools for pain assessment. See Figure 39–1 for commonly used pain rating scales.

For adults or children who cannot verbally express themselves, look for pain clues. including facial expressions (frowning, grimace), vocalization (moaning, groaning, or crying), or physical actions (guarding, limited or lost mobility, restlessness). EMS providers should carefully evaluate these clues and develop an appropriate pain management strategy based on all available information.

PAIN MANAGEMENT

Once all life threats have been addressed, pain management can be started. Interventions for pain management can be divided into two sections: non-

pharmacologic interventions and pharmacologic interventions.

Nonpharmacologic Interventions

Nonpharmacologic interventions include therapeutic communication with the patient such as recognition, empathy, talking and reassurance, and relieving anxiety. Some nonpharmacologic interventions such as acupuncture, massage, transcutaneous electrical nerve stimulation (TENS), and hypnosis suit the management of chronic pain but are of little use in the prehospital environment.

Other important techniques EMS providers can use for pain management are splinting fractures, applying cold packs to the injured parts, padding pressure points in spinal immobilization, and otherwise providing comfort the for the patient before and during transport. These techniques may reduce pain and make the overall prehospital experience more comfortable.

Pharmacologic Interventions

Pharmacologic agents used for pain management should be carefully selected for their primary indications, contraindications, possible adverse effects, the patient's overall hemodynamic status, and other related factors. Some of the selected agents are discussed below. Depending on local availability, patients' specific needs, and the medical director's approval, other pharmacologic agents can be used when treating pain. Avoid narcotic analgesia in patients with head injuries because narcotics can interfere with subsequent neurologic examination. Analgesics may need to be combined with hypnotics and sedatives when managing severe pain caused by movement and manipulation.[9]

Morphine

Morphine is a potent opiate analgesic and is the most commonly used agent for pain management. In the prehospital setting, it should be used whenever long-lasting pain relief is desired. Patients experiencing myocardial infarction whose pain is not relieved by nitrates and burn patients are good candidates for morphine administration unless there is no other contraindication, such as sensitivity to drug or hypotension. Morphine can cause histamine release, resulting in itching and skin flushing. Morphine can be administered IV, IM, or SC. Morphine's onset of action is 5 minutes when given by the IV route, with peak effects occuring in 20 minutes. The duration of action is up to 6 hours. The typical adult dose for morphine is 2.0 to 10 milligrams administered slowly and titrated to effect.

Fentanyl

Fentanyl is a synthetic opiate and is 100 times more potent than morphine. Its short onset and relatively short duration of action make it a favorable prehospital medication for controlling acute pain. Another advantage of fentanyl is that it seems to result in less nausea and vomiting than morphine, and it does not release histamine. Fentanyl can be used safely as an effective pain medication by EMS providers in the field for the multisystem trauma patient as well as for acute abdominal pain.[6,7] Peak effect is reached within 3 to 5 minutes, and the duration of action is 30 to 60 minutes. The typical adult dose is 50 to 100 micrograms IV. Do not give fentanyl by rapid IV push, as it can cause severe muscle rigidity, bronchospasm, or laryngospasm. Give fentanyl IV slowly, over 20 to 30 seconds or more.

Meperidine

Another synthetic opiate, meperidine, has about one tenth the potency of that of morphine sulfate. It can be used for moderate to severe pain, but it can cause respiratory depression and does cause histamine release. The onset of action for meperidine is 5 minutes when given IV. Peak effect is reached within 30 minutes, and duration of action is 2 hours. The typical adult dose is 25 to 100 milligrams.

Tramadol (Contramal®)

Tramadol is a non–narcotic opiate agonist that has an effect comparable to that of morphine for acute pain.[8] The IV form of the drug is available in Europe and Turkey. The dose is 1 to 2 milligrams/kg/IV, and it is typically given in a dose of 100 milligrams IV. The onset of action after IV administration is within minutes. Peak effect is reached in 15 to 30 minutes and duration of action is 4 hours.

Nitrous Oxide

Nitrous oxide is an inhaled agent that is mixed with oxygen (typically 50:50) and can be self- administered by patients using a tight sealing mask. At low doses it has analgesic effects, whereas at higher doses it shows anesthetic properties. It has immediate onset and its effect is relieved almost immediately after discontinuation of the medication.

Ketorolac

Nonsteroidal anti-inflammatory drugs (NSAIDs) are one of the options that are used by various EMS systems for managing pain in the prehospital arena. Ketorolac is a NSAID that is particularly useful for renal and biliary colic pain. It can be administered IV or IM. The time of onset is 10 to 15 minutes, with peak effects occurring in 60 minutes. Duration of action is 6 hours. The typical adult dose is 15 to 30 milligrams IV or 30 to 60 milligrams IM.

REASSESSMENT AND DOCUMENTATION

Reassess and document interventions for pain management and the patient's response to treatment.

Check vital signs, mental status, cardiac rhythm, and oxygen saturation values before and after the interventions. Most pharmacologic agents are titrated to effect in order to minimize side effects and provide necessary pain relief. Treatment strategies can be modified after reassessing the pain of the patient.

EDUCATION

Proper educational programs should be planned and delivered to address pain management issues in the prehospital setting. Education can increase understanding of pain principles and the use of appropriate pharmacologic pain treatment, and can result in improved documentation.[10,11]

References

1. Merskey H, Bogduk N, eds. *Classification of Chronic Pain.* 2nd ed. Seattle: IASP Press, 1994; pp 209–214.
2. Bryan E. Bledsoe, JM. Pain and comfort: pathophysiology of pain and prehospital treatment options. *J Emerg Med Services* June 2003;28(6):50–67.
3. Jones GE, Machen I. Pre-hospital pain management: the paramedics' perspective. *Accid Emerg Nursing* 2003 Jul;11(3):166–72.PMID: 12804613.
4. Ho K, Spence J, Murphy MF. "Review of pain measurement tools." *Ann Emerg Med,* 1996 Apr;27(4):427–32. Review. PMID: 8604852.
5. Alonso-Serra HM, Wesley K. Prehospital pain management. *Prehosp Emerg Care* 2003 Oct-Dec;7(4):482–8. PMID: 14582104.
6. *PHTLS Prehospital Trauma Life Support.* 6th ed. St. Louis: Mosby, 2007; 325–326.
7. Kanowitz A, Dunn TM, Kanowitz EM, et al. Safety and effectiveness of fentanyl administration for prehospital pain management. *Prehosp Emerg Care* 2006 Jan-Mar;10(1):1–7. PMID: 16418084.
8. Vergnion M, Desgesves S, Garcey L, et al. Tramadol, an alternative to morphine for treating posttraumatic pain in the prehospital situation. *Anesth Anal* 2001 Jun;92(6):1543–6.PMID: 11375843.
9. Tintinalli JE, Gabor D, Kelen, J. Stapczynski S, eds. *Emergency Medicine: A Comprehensive Study Guide.* 6th ed. © *2004, McGraw-Hill, New York* **p 1657.**
10. Lord B. Pain management: can education make a difference? *J Emerg Primary Health Care* 2003; Vol 1 : Issue 3-4 Article Number: 990056–12.
11. French SC, Salama NP, Baqai S, et al. Effects of an educational intervention on prehospital pain management. *Prehosp Emerg Care* 10 (1): 71, 2006.

CHAPTER 40

Obstetrics and Gynecology

Kim Hinshaw, Helen Simpson, Malcolm Woollard

INTRODUCTION

In this section we will describe practical approaches for managing the common and important EMS situations in obstetrics and gynecology. The approaches described can be adapted to local circumstances (e.g., dependent on equipment, facilities, local drug regimens, degree of training, geography).

There are an estimated 4 million neonatal deaths and 500,000 maternal deaths worldwide each year. Most deaths occur in developing countries, where 43% of births are attended by relatively unskilled, traditional birth attendants. This is particularly the case in rural areas.[1]

EMS practitioners may be the first line of skilled help in these circumstances, and simple interventions can be lifesaving. The specific approaches described for both maternal and neonatal resuscitation are based on the UK experience of the authors, and it is accepted that specific elements may vary from country to country.

Procedures and protocols for the management of emergencies in pregnancy depend upon the gestational age of the fetus and the trimester of pregnancy. If the patient does not know her expected date of confinement or the exact gestational age, the gestational age can be calculated by adding 9 months and 7 days to the first day of the last menstrual period. At 20 weeks of gestation, it should be possible to palpate the uterus at the umbilicus. **A delivery of ≥24 weeks' gestation is compatible with fetal survival outside the uterus.** Because it can be difficult or impossible to determine the exact gestational age in the prehospital setting, 20 weeks of gestation is generally used as the cut-off point for potential fetal viability. For this reason, pregnancy is often divided into early (<20 weeks) and late (≥20 weeks) when managing problems of pregnancy.

LIST OF TERMS AND DEFINITIONS

Here we define terms relating to obstetric and gynecologic management used specifically in this section. Other terms used are in accord with the definitions set in the first chapter – Standard EMS Terms and Definitions.

1. Antepartum hemorrhage – bleeding from the genital tract after 20 weeks of gestation and before delivery of the baby (see sections on Placental Abruption and Placenta Previa).
2. Birth Attendant.
   a. Skilled birth attendant – WHO defines a skilled attendant as "an accredited health professional – such as a midwife, doctor, or nurse – who has been educated and trained to proficiency in the skills needed to manage normal (uncomplicated) pregnancies,

childbirth and the immediate postnatal period, and in the identification, management and referral of complications in women and newborns."

  b. Traditional birth attendant — traditional birth attendants are generally untrained although this is an aim of the WHO Safer Motherhood initiative. They are an integral part of many rural societies in developing countries and may be the only help available to women in labor.

3. Breech presentation — when the baby's buttocks or legs are presenting during late pregnancy or labor.

4. Cervix — the neck of the womb.

5. Cord prolapse — when the umbilical cord appears during labor before delivery of the baby has occurred.

6. Eclampsia — the onset of generalized grand mal seizures, often (but not exclusively) associated with pre-existing pre-eclampsia.

7. Ectopic pregnancy — a pregnancy sited outside of the uterine cavity, most commonly in the fallopian tube.

8. Midwife (see birth attendant - skilled).

9. Miscarriage — spontaneous loss of a pregnancy before 20 to 24 weeks (depends on country definition) and most commonly in the first 12 weeks.

10. Placental abruption — separation of a normally sited placenta that may be to a minor or major degree, often associated with abdominal pain (see Antepartum Hemorrhage).

11. Placenta previa — a situation in which the placenta lies in front of the baby, attached to the uterine wall close to or covering the cervix in late pregnancy; it usually occurs with painless vaginal bleeding after 24 weeks (see Antepartum Hemorrhage).

12. Postpartum hemorrhage (PPH) — bleeding from the genital tract after delivery of the baby (often defined as >500 mL). Primary PPH occurs within 24 hours of delivery. Secondary PPH occurs after 24 hours and may be associated with infection.

13. Pre-eclampsia — high blood pressure in pregnancy (almost exclusively beyond 20 weeks) associated with generalized edema and proteinuria. May range from mild to severe. The latter may be life-threatening.

14. Pregnancy-induced hypertension — a significant and persistent rise in blood pressure above non-pregnant levels.

15. Shoulder dystocia — an acute labor emergency in which the baby's shoulders impact against the pubic bone after delivery of the head. This requires specific maneuvers to allow prompt delivery of the baby before hypoxic brain damage ensues and to prevent damage to nerve plexuses.

16. Trimester — pregnancy is divided into thirds, each lasting approximately 13 weeks (i.e. first, second, and third trimesters).

17. Vasa previa — a rare cause of bleeding in late pregnancy or labor. Bleeding is from a ruptured fetal vessel in the membranes and perinatal mortality is very high (see Antepartum Hemorrhage).

COLLAPSE AND TRAUMA IN PREGNANCY

KEY LEARNING POINTS

For Material Cardiac Arrest or Trauma in Pregnancy ≥20 Weeks' Gestation

■ Manage pregnant women ≥20 weeks of pregnancy with 15 to 30 degrees of left lateral tilt.

■ Use large-bore cannulas to secure intravenous access; provide 50% more IV fluid volume.

■ In cardiac arrest, perform CPR with the patient in the left lateral tilt position and follow standard ACLS algorithms.

■ In maternal cardiac arrest, perimortem cesarean section should be undertaken as soon as possible if the fetus is potentially viable. Perimortem cesarean section is most effective if performed within 5 minutes of maternal cardiac arrest. Alert the receiving unit of the potential need for urgent delivery on arrival.

Cardiac Arrest

Purpose of Procedure

This procedure aims to provide a structured approach to the management of the pregnant patient in cardiac arrest, regardless of cause. **Maternal resuscitation is the best fetal resuscitation, so maternal resuscitation is always the priority. Specific maneuvers for fetal viability are generally directed to gestations' ≥20 weeks of pregnancy.**

Patient Selection

This procedure is appropriate for all pregnant patients in cardiac arrest regardless of cause, but particularly those in the second and third trimesters. Although the incidence of cardiac arrest is low in this group of patients, more common causes include pre-existing cardiovascular disease; road traffic accidents; suicide secondary to psychiatric illness; domestic violence; substance abuse; thromboembolic conditions, and hemorrhage.[2,3] More than half of the women who die during pregnancy are obese, and many have not attended prenatal care clinics.

Risks and Precautions

There are two major risks or performance errors to the pregnant patient in cardiac arrest. **The first is the failure to position the patient in the left-lateral tilt position,** resulting in compression by the gravid uterus of the inferior vena cava, significantly reduced venous return to the heart, reduced cardiac filling pressures, and consequently coronary perfusion pressures that are too low to support perfusion of the myocardium. Chest compressions only produce blood flow of approximately 15 to 30% of normal under ideal circumstances: if a patient in the third trimester is left lying on her back, cardiac blood flow may be reduced to virtually nothing and resuscitation will be futile. **The second is failure to transport the patient immediately to definitive care, simultaneous with performing CPR. It is inappropriate for EMS personnel to stay on the scene and treat the patient in accordance with "normal" resuscitation protocols, since the definitive treatment of maternal cardiac arrest after 24 weeks is an emergency cesarean section. If this can be performed within five minutes of the onset of arrest, the probability of the survival of the mother and fetus is maximized.**

Equipment

- Spine board and straps.
- Blankets and pillows (for padding).
- Intubation kit (ideally including capnograph [waveform end-tidal CO_2 monitor] and esophageal detector device; tracheal tube introducer or stylet; and surgical cricothyroidotomy kit).
- Ventilator (preferably automated volume-cycled, self-inflating bag as an alternative).
- Defibrillator/ECG monitor.
- Venous and adult intraosseous access kit.
- Adrenaline, atropine, amiodarone, magnesium.
- Radio or mobile phone to prealert the receiving ED.

Patient Positioning

All pregnant women in cardiac arrest should be strapped on a spine board tilted to the left at an angle of 15 to 30 degrees as soon as possible (see Figure 40-1). In the interim, until sufficient health-care

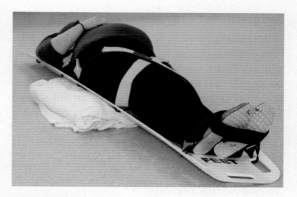

FIGURE 40–1

Use of spine board to maintain a 15- to 30-degree left lateral tilt. Photo courtesy of Jason Poposki, School of Biomedical Sciences, Charles Sturt University, New South Wales, Australia.

providers are available, the EMT who is providing chest compressions kneels at the patient's right side and places his or her thighs under the right side of the patient's chest, hip, and buttock to facilitate a tilt (Figure 40-2). **Failure to tilt the patient will mean that chest compressions are ineffective and resuscitation will fail.**

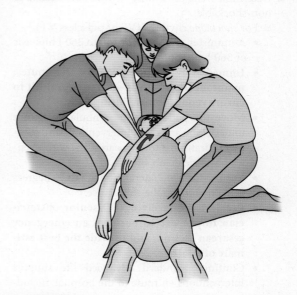

FIGURE 40–2

Manual displacement of the uterus to the patient's left. Photo courtesy of Woollard M, Simpson H, Hinshaw K, Wieteska S. *Pre-hospital Obstetric Emergency Training.* Oxford: Wiley-Blackwell, 2010, reprinted with permission.

Sedation and Procedural Monitoring

If the patient recovers spontaneous circulation *after* intubation, sedation is needed to allow controlled ventilation to normalize blood gases. **It is most important that ventilation is strictly controlled (and therefore is ideally delivered using an automated ventilator) to ensure normocapnia**: both elevated and reduced levels of CO_2 will result in reduced blood flow to the patient's brain and will exacerbate any hypoxic damage that has already occurred.

Step-by-Step Technique

■ **Position the patient in a 15- to 30-degree lateral tilt,** ideally by strapping her to a spine board with padding under the right side.

■ Confirm the occurrence of cardiac arrest.

■ Commence uninterrupted chest compressions (for a minimum of 2 minutes if the patient is in non–witnessed ventricular fibrillation/tachycardia arrest).

■ Intubate the patient with a cuffed tracheal tube or, if unavailable, a cuffed supraglottic airway device such as a laryngeal mask airway.

■ Confirm airway device placement with waveform capnography **and** an esophageal detector device.

■ Begin ventilations at ten per minute.

■ Determine if the presenting rhythm is shockable or non-shockable.

  ■ For *shockable* rhythms (VF or pulseless VT).

    • Administer **one** shock at 150 to 360 J biphasic or 360 J monophasic.

    • **Immediately resume CPR for 2 minutes; maintain the 15- to 30-degree lateral tilt to ensure venous return during CPR.**

    • Move the patient to the ambulance **before** undertaking any other interventions and commence transport to the nearest ED with a senior obstetrician on site.

    • Ensure that a left lateral tilt of 15 to 30 degrees is maintained in the ambulance.

    • **Prealert the receiving ED/senior obstetrician to prepare to perform an emergency cesarean section, and provide the best estimate of fetal age.**

    • Continue standard advanced life support interventions en route to the hospital, including obtaining intravenous or intraosseous access, administering drug therapy, and treating reversible causes, but stop for **nothing.**

  ■ For *non-shockable* rhythms.

    • Immediately resume CPR for 2 minutes.

    • Obtain IV or intraosseous (IO) access.

    • Give epinephrine 1 milligram IV or IO.

• Move the patient to the ambulance **before** undertaking any other interventions and commence transport to the nearest ED with a senior obstetrician on site.

• Ensure that a left-lateral tilt of 15 to 30 degrees is maintained in the ambulance.

• **Prealert the receiving ED/senior obstetrician to prepare to perform an emergency cesarean section on arrival.**

• Continue standard advanced life support interventions en route to hospital, including administering drug therapy and treating reversible causes, but stop for **nothing.**

Figure 40-3 charts the appropriate steps for the management of out-of-hospital maternal cardiac arrest.

Outcomes Assessment

The most valid measure of outcome from cardiac arrest is survival of the mother and fetus to discharge with normal neurologic function. **However, an important measure of the success of prehospital treatment is the on-scene time: this must be as short as possible to facilitate the minimum interval to performing emergency cesarean section in the receiving ED.**

Complications

In maternal cardiac arrest, early intubation with a cuffed endotracheal tube is recommended to protect against regurgitation, aspiration, and Mendelson syndrome (aspiration pneumonia, itself often fatal). If tracheal intubation is not available or possible, a cuffed supraglottic airway device such as a laryngeal mask airway (LMA) offers a less reliable alternative. Avoid ventilation with non-cuffed devices because they do not protect against gastric insufflation and regurgitation.

TRAUMA IN PREGNANCY

Purpose of Procedure

Road traffic accidents and domestic violence are leading causes of death during pregnancy. The anatomic and physiologic changes of pregnancy and the associated increased metabolic requirements exhaust many maternal compensatory mechanisms or result in injury specific to pregnancy, such as placental abruption. Consequently, a severely injured pregnant woman may appear to compensate adequately initially but will then decompensate rapidly. Since **maternal blood volume at term is increased up to 50%, fluid**

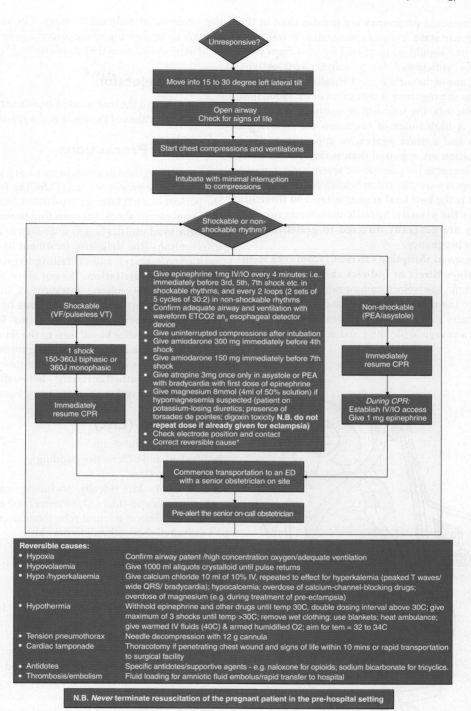

Unresponsive?

Move into 15 to 30 degree left lateral tilt

Open airway
Check for signs of life

Start chest compressions and ventilations

Intubate with minimal interruption to compressions

Shockable or non-shockable rhythm?

Shockable
(VF/pulseless VT)

1 shock
150-360J biphasic *or*
360J monophasic

Immediately resume CPR

- Give epinephrine 1mg IV/IO every 4 minutes: i.e.. immediately before 3rd, 5th, 7th shock etc. in shockable rhythms, and every 2 loops (2 sets of 5 cycles of 30:2) in non-shockable rhythms
- Confirm adequate airway and ventilation with waveform ETCO2 an$_d$ esophageal detector device
- Give uninterrupted compressions after intubation
- Give amiodarone 300 mg immediately before 4th shock
- Give amiodarone 150 mg immediately before 7th shock
- Give atropine 3mg once only in asystole or PEA with bradycardia with first dose of epinephrine
- Give magnesium 8mmol (4ml of 50% solution) if hypomagnesemia suspected (patient on potassium-losing diuretics; presence of torsades de pointes; digoxin toxicity **N.B. do not repeat dose if already given for eclampsia)**
- Check electrode position and contact
- Correct reversible cause*

Non-shockable
(PEA/asystole)

Immediately resume CPR

During CPR:
Establish IV/IO access
Give 1 mg epinephrine

Commence transportation to an ED with a senior obstetrician on site

Pre-alert the senior on-call obstetrician

Reversible causes:

• Hypoxia	Confirm airway patent /high concentration oxygen/adequate ventilation
• Hypovolaemia	Give 1000 ml aliquots crystalloid until pulse returns
• Hypo /hyperkalaemia	Give calcium chloride 10 ml of 10% IV, repeated to effect for hyperkalemia (peaked T waves/ wide QRS/ bradycardia); hypocalcemia; overdose of calcium-channel-blocking drugs; overdose of magnesium (e.g. during treatment of pre-eclampsia)
• Hypothermia	Withhold epinephrine and other drugs until temp 30C, double dosing interval above 30C; give maximum of 3 shocks until temp >30C; remove wet clothing: use blankets; heat ambulance; give warmed IV fluids (40C) & armed humidified O2; aim for tem = 32 to 34C
• Tension pneumothorax	Needle decompression with 12 g cannula
• Cardiac tamponade	Thoracotomy if penetrating chest wound and signs of life within 10 mins or rapid transportation to surgical facility
• Antidotes	Specific antidotes/supportive agents - e.g. naloxone for opioids; sodium bicarbonate for tricyclics.
• Thrombosis/embolism	Fluid loading for amniotic fluid embolus/rapid transfer to hospital

N.B. *Never* terminate resuscitation of the pregnant patient in the pre-hospital setting

---

FIGURE 40–3

Management of cardiac arrest in the pregnant patient. Modified, and reprinted with permission of Woollard M, Simpson H, Hinshaw K, Wieteska S. *Pre-hospital Obstetric Emergency Training*. Oxford: Wiley-Blackwell, 2010. *Adapted from*: Resuscitation Council (UK). Adult Advanced Life Support Algorithm. Available at: <http://www.resus.org.uk/pages/gl5algos.htm> Accessed 29th December 2009.

requirements in pregnancy are greater than in the nonpregnant state. Volume resuscitation in multisystem trauma should be increased by 50% from what would be anticipated for a nonpregnant patient. Further, one of the earliest compensatory mechanisms in trauma in pregnancy is restriction of the blood flow to the placenta: *the fetus will be sacrificed to save the mother.* **A high index of suspicion for significant injuries and a more aggressive approach to fluid resuscitation are required than is the case for most adults** (except in the presence of severe pre-eclampsia or eclampsia – see discussion below). **Maternal resuscitation is the best fetal resuscitation and therefore is always the priority. Specific maneuvers for fetal viability are generally directed to gestations ≥20 weeks of pregnancy.**

Placental abruption can result from even seemingly minor direct or indirect abdominal trauma. For example, low-velocity motor vehicle accidents and falls onto the abdomen from the standing position or down stairs can result in placental abruption even without any vaginal bleeding, abdominal pain, or clin-ical evidence of abdominal injury. The mechanism appears to be shearing of the placenta from the more rigid uterine wall caused by deceleration.[4,5]

Patient Selection

The approach to the treatment of significant trauma is the same regardless of the cause of the injuries.

Risks and Precautions

The three main risks or errors in managing significant trauma during pregnancy are (1) **failing to position the patient in a left lateral tilt position**, thus worsening hypovolemic shock; (2) **spending too much time on scene** to administer largely unproven or ineffective interventions (the definitive treatment of trauma is most often surgery); and (3) **failing to provide adequate fluid resuscitation.** Do not allow permissive hypotension/low volume intravenous infusion in pregnant women. **Remember that one of the main maternal compensatory mechanisms in hypovolemia is to sacrifice blood flow to the fetus.**

An important step in reducing injuries to the mother and fetus in road accidents is instruction on **how to wear a seatbelt correctly – below the "bump" of the abdomen rather than on it** (see Figure 40-4).

Equipment (List)

- Spine board and straps.
- Blankets and pillows (for padding).
- Cervical collars.
- Intubation kit (ideally including capnograph [waveform end-tidal CO_2 monitor] and esophageal detector device; tracheal tube introducer or stylet; and surgical cricothyroidotomy kit).
- High-concentration oxygen masks.
- Ventilator (preferably automated volume-cycled, self-inflating bag as an alternative).
- Needle thoracocentesis kit.
- Wound dressings, tourniquets, and hemostatic dressings.
- Splints (including traction splints).
- Venous and adult intraosseous access kit.
- Defibrillator/ECG/noninvasive blood pressure reader/oxygen saturation monitor.
- Opiate analgesics, ketamine, succinylcholine, Ringer's lactate, or NS for infusion.
- Radio or mobile phone to prealert the receiving ED.

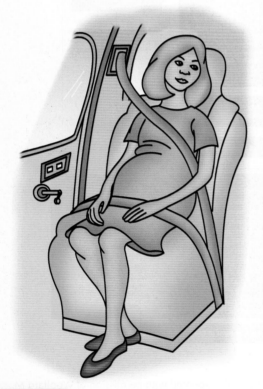

FIGURE 40–4

Proper position for shoulder harness and lap belt in pregnancy.

Patient Positioning

Secure the patient on a spine board tilted to the left at an angle of 15 to 30 degrees as soon as possible (refer to Figure 40-1). In the interim, until sufficient healthcare providers are available, one EMT kneels at the patient's left side and manually displaces the uterus to the left (refer to Figure 40-2). **Failure to tilt the patient will reduce maternal cardiac output, cause hypotension, and decrease blood flow to the fetus.**

Anesthesia and Procedural Monitoring

Any pregnant patient with a Glasgow Coma Score (GCS) of eight or less requires early intubation to minimize the risk of regurgitation and aspiration. An obtunded patient who is still breathing spontaneously needs rapid sequence intubation. Succinylcholine is widely used as a short-term paralytic, and ketamine has been extensively used as an induction agent in pregnancy. Ketamine has dose-dependent toxic effects, such as transient increases in maternal blood pressure, increased uterine tone, increased muscle tone in neonates, and neurologic and respiratory depression in neonates. Therefore **low doses should be used to minimize these effects – for example 1 milligram/kg IV of ketamine.** Once anesthesia has been induced, it can be maintained with repeated low doses of ketamine and morphine, and if needed, paralysis may be maintained with an intermediate duration paralyzing agent such as rocuronium. **Remember that this combination of drugs will cause neonatal neurologic and respiratory depression.**

Control maternal ventilation (ideally with an automated ventilator) to ensure normocapnia. Both elevated and reduced levels of CO_2 will result in reduced blood flow to the brain of both mother and fetus and will exacerbate any damage that has already occurred following a primary traumatic brain injury or a hypoxic episode.

Step-by-Step Technique

- Control any external visible catastrophic hemorrhage, using direct and indirect pressure and tourniquets and hemostatic dressings where indicated.
- Manually displace the uterus to the left until the patient can be secured to a spine board and tilted.
- While manually stabilizing the mother's cervical spine, open, maintain, and protect the airway as needed and perform early tracheal intubation if the Glasgow Coma Score is eight or less.
- Deliver high-concentration oxygen. Provide ventilatory assistance if oxygen saturation or tidal volume is inadequate.
- If the patient has a thoracic injury, management and intervention are the same as for a nonpregnant

patient (for example, needle thoracocentesis for tension pneumothorax). **Make sure the spine board straps are not fastened so tightly that they prevent chest excursion when the patient breathes.**
- Disposition.
  - Any significant airway, breathing, or circulation problem is time-critical and requires immediate transfer to the *nearest* ED (not necessarily one with an obstetric unit).
  - Non–time-critical pregnant women ≥20 weeks of pregnancy who are injured should be taken to an ED with an associated obstetric unit for immediate assessment and cardiotocographic monitoring.
- Non–time-critical pregnant women ≥ 20 weeks of pregnancy who are *apparently* uninjured after a motor vehicle crash or abdominal trauma should be taken to an ED or directly to an appropriate obstetric unit for immediate assessment and cardiotocographic monitoring.
- Secure the patient onto a spine board and place a pad under the right side of the board to produce a 15- to 30-degree tilt to the left.
- Insert one or two large-bore (14-gauge) cannulas en route (do NOT delay on scene to do this). If it is not possible to gain IV access, use intraosseous access.
- Administer crystalloids **to maintain a systolic BP (SBP) of >100 mm Hg.**
- Administer analgesia for pain. If the patient is hypotensive, replace intravascular volume with NS and use morphine cautiously. Morphine will cause respiratory depression in the neonate.
- Apply splints to pelvic and long bone fractures.
- If time permits, perform a 12-lead ECG and blood glucose monitoring en route.
- Give nothing by mouth, as the patient is likely to require anesthesia and surgery.
- If the patient has been burned, assess, treat, and manage burns in exactly the same manner as for a nonpregnant patient. If burns are estimated to be more than 25% of body surface area (BSA) give 1 L of crystalloid IV or intraosseously.
- If the patient has a non–time-critical problem, perform a full secondary survey.

Figure 40-5 provides an algorithm for the management of the hypovolemic pregnant patient.

Outcomes Assessment

The most useful measures of prehospital activity are *on-scene time,* which should be as short as possible (10 minutes in the non-trapped patient is a reasonable target), and whether or not a pre*alert message* has been passed to the receiving hospital. These key

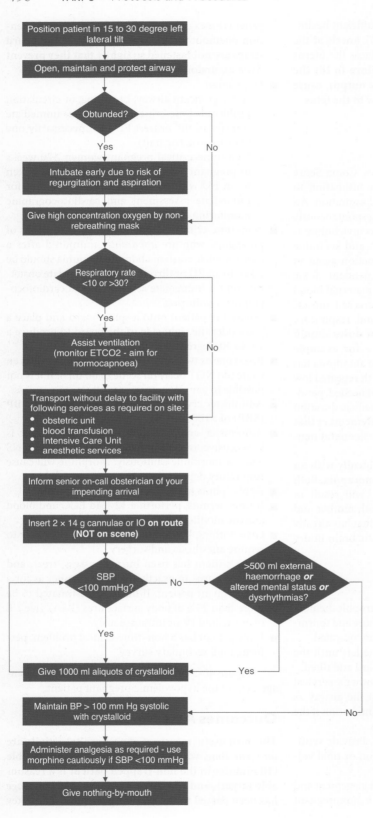

FIGURE 40–5

Universal hypovolemia in pregnancy algorithm. Reprinted with permission of Woollard M, Simpson H, Hinshaw K, Wieteska S. *Pre-hospital Obstetric Emergency Training.* Oxford: Wiley-Blackwell, 2010.

interventions have been empirically shown to positively impact on outcome, whereas this is not the case for other clinical interventions in trauma.

Complications

Early intubation with a cuffed tracheal tube is ideal in unconscious pregnant trauma victims because of the high probability of regurgitation and aspiration. Inadequate fluid resuscitation remains a risk because of to the failure to anticipate fluid losses and the inappropriate use of restricted fluid resuscitation algorithms. Inadequate fluid replacement risks fetal death.

Placental abruption is a complication of even seemingly minor direct or indirect abdominal trauma in pregnancy and is a leading of cause of fetal death in major maternal trauma. Therefore, in women in the last trimester of pregnancy, any direct or indirect abdominal trauma or multisystem trauma requires rapid transport of the patient to the ED or obstetric unit, and **immediate maternal resuscitation and monitoring of fetal heart rate and uterine contractions** to identify possible placental abruption. **Delays in the instituting such monitoring can result in fetal death from placental abruption.**

Follow-up and Patient Instructions

Any pregnant woman involved in a road traffic accident or other cause of *potential* abdominal trauma (even following a minor road traffic accident involving deceleration) should be urgently seen in the ED and evaluated by an obstetrician to identify silent placental abruption.

VAGINAL BLEEDING IN EARLY PREGNANCY (≤20 WEEKS OF PREGNANCY) (MISCARRIAGE AND ECTOPIC PREGNANCY)

KEY LEARNING POINTS

For Vaginal Bleeding ≤20 Weeks of Pregnancy

- Use the term miscarriage rather than spontaneous abortion.

- Shoulder tip pain or severe abdominal pain may imply significant intra-abdominal bleeding associated with a ruptured ectopic pregnancy.

- If shock is out of proportion to the amount of visible bleeding, consider cervical shock miscarriage or ruptured ectopic pregnancy.

Purpose of Procedure

To allow the EMT to manage the common complications of miscarriage and ectopic pregnancy in the prehospital setting.

Patient Selection

Miscarriage means spontaneous loss of the pregnancy. The upper limit of gestation varies from country to country but is usually between 20 to 24 weeks. Miscarriage is more common in the first 12 weeks of pregnancy, and overall almost 20% of pregnant women will miscarry. Most patients have varying amounts of vaginal bleeding and may have associated abdominal pain or cramping. It is sometimes better to use the term miscarriage than spontaneous abortion because some may read negative connotations into the word abortion. In all cases a final diagnosis cannot be made without a formal ultrasound assessment to determine fetal viability. The commonly used terms used to describe a miscarriage follow.

Threatened miscarriage: usually just light bleeding and no pain. Most result in ongoing pregnancies.

Inevitable miscarriage: heavier bleeding, the cervix is open, but no tissue has been passed as yet.

Incomplete miscarriage: the cervix is open but some fetal/placental tissue is retained in the uterine cavity.

Complete miscarriage: all the placental/fetal tissue has passed, the cervix has closed, and bleeding has stopped.

Missed miscarriage: usually little bleeding but on ultrasound assessment the pregnancy is found to be nonviable.

Septic miscarriage: infection following any miscarriage but usually after an incomplete miscarriage or following surgical evacuation of the uterus. Look for signs of sepsis such as headache, nausea, flushes, sweating, shivering, and rise in pulse and temperature.

In the acute situation, management depends on the clinical situation rather than the absolute diagnosis.

Ectopic pregnancy is increasing in incidence and affects between 1 to 2% of pregnancies. Risk factors include previous pelvic inflammatory disease, sterilization, and previous ectopic pregnancy. Presentation is often with unilateral lower abdominal pain and slight bleeding, usually at around 6 to 8 weeks of pregnancy. Most ectopic pregnancies are located in the fallopian tube but can be in other sites (e.g., the ovary or cervix). Acute presentation with hypovolemic shock is associated with tubal rupture. **There may be shoulder tip pain and signs of peritonitis (severe abdominal pain and a rigid, tender abdomen).**

Risks and Precautions

Most patients are stable and transfer is not 'time-critical.' However EMTs should be aware of the following acute emergencies that require urgent intervention:

- Shock (cervical): in incomplete miscarriage, tissue may lodge in the open cervix, with profuse vaginal bleeding. The patient's blood pressure is low, and there may be *bradycardia* rather than tachycardia.
- Shock (hypovolemic).
  - Miscarriage: may manifest with very heavy vaginal bleeding leading to circulatory collapse.
  - Ectopic pregnancy: erosion of an ectopic pregnancy into the vasculature of the fallopian tube may lead to catastrophic intra-abdominal bleeding and collapse. **The only definitive treatment is urgent surgery.**
- Shock (septic): may be a rare presentation associated with miscarriage. Look for cardiovascular instability, fever, "air hunger," and a bounding pulse.
- In all cases, manage these situations as time critical-and transfer patients urgently after initial stabilization.

Equipment (List)

- High-concentration oxygen masks.
- Venous and adult intraosseous access kit.
- Opiate analgesics, Ringer's lactate, or NS for infusion.
- Radio or mobile phone to prealert the receiving ED.

Patient Positioning

- **Not critical in pregnancies under 20 weeks of pregnancy.** *After 20 weeks*, position the patient in a 15- to 30-degree left lateral tilt, ideally by strapping her to a spine board with padding under the right side.

Anesthesia and Procedural Monitoring

- Blood pressure, pulse, respiratory rate (note temperature).

Step-by-Step Technique

To be used when the patient is cardiovascularly unstable or in the presence of heavy bleeding or severe pain.

- Fully assess the ABC's: document respiratory rate, pulse rate and quality, and blood pressure.
- Provide high-flow oxygen via a non–rebreather mask; aim for oxygen saturations of 94 to 98%.
- Insert one or two large-bore (14-gauge) cannulas (but DO NOT delay transfer to receiving unit). If it is not possible to gain IV access, use an intraosseous cannula.
- Administer crystalloids **to maintain a systolic BP (SBP) of 100 mm Hg.**
- Take a brief patient history regarding gestation, degree of bleeding, and quantity of pain. Review any ultrasound information that may be available in patient-held records.
- Arrange rapid transfer to the nearest ED if bleeding continues or the patient is hemodynamically unstable.
- Inform the receiving unit of the patient's condition. Confirm if a ruptured ectopic pregnancy is suspected or if there is significant vaginal bleeding, as surgery will be required.
- Administer analgesia as appropriate.
- Do not administer anything by mouth.
- Bradycardia secondary to cervical shock can be treated with atropine and IV fluids.

Outcomes Assessment

- On-scene time in time-critical situations.
- Appropriate prealert message sent to receiving unit.

Complications

Continuing hemorrhage (vaginally or intra-abdominally) may lead to cardiac arrest. Manage as per local protocols. Local standing orders or directions from medical control may allow the use of an oxytocic injection IV or IM in cases of very heavy vaginal bleeding associated with miscarriage. In the ED or obstetric unit or by specially trained providers, any pregnancy tissue lodged in the cervical os can be removed during pelvic examination as part of the resuscitation process.

VAGINAL BLEEDING IN LATE PREGNANCY (>20 WEEKS OF PREGNANCY) (PLACENTA PREVIA, PLACENTAL ABRUPTION, VASA PREVIA)

KEY LEARNING POINTS

For Vaginal Bleeding >20 Weeks of Pregnancy

- Do not attempt vaginal or pelvic examination in case the placenta is low-lying (i.e., previa), as this might provoke catastrophic hemorrhage.

- In placental abruption, the amount of external revealed bleeding may not reflect the true amount of bleeding, which may be concealed under the placenta or within the uterus.

- A hard, woody, tender uterus suggests a major placental abruption.

- Pregnant patients may lose large amounts of circulating blood volume before showing any changes in blood pressure or heart rate — gain IV access as early as possible.

Purpose of Procedure

To allow the EMS practitioner to manage bleeding complications in later pregnancy (antepartum hemorrhage or hemorrhage before delivery).

Patient Selection

Antepartum hemorrhage is similar to any bleeding from the genital tract after 20 to 24 weeks' gestation (this time frame varies from country to country). It usually is due to bleeding from within the uterus. Although deaths from antepartum hemorrhage are rare, bleeding prior to delivery may weaken the patient's ability to cope with a subsequent postpartum hemorrhage. **The amount of vaginal bleeding may not reflect the true amount of bleeding, which may be concealed within the uterus.**

Bleeding from the following types of conditions is identified:

Placenta Previa

The placenta is sited completely or partially in the lower part of the uterus and can overlie the cervix. Bleeding is usually painless, and the patient may have several small episodes before a major hemorrhage occurs. Bleeding usually starts after 24 weeks and is often bright red. The patient may know that she has placenta previa from previous ultrasound scans. If the placenta remains low and lies in front of the fetus in late pregnancy, delivery by planned cesarean section is required and is usually done around 37 weeks' gestation. **Vaginal examination should never be performed in cases of bleeding in late pregnancy until placenta previa has been excluded by ultrasound scan.** Vaginal examination in the presence of placenta previa can cause catastrophic bleeding.

Placental Abruption

This occurs when a *normally sited* placenta separates from the uterine wall during late pregnancy or in labor. It is usually an unpredictable event, although it can be associated with blunt abdominal trauma (e.g., seat belt injury). It may occur at the time of the trauma or may be delayed by 3 to 4 days. Abruption is also associated with cocaine use, hypertension, and pre-eclampsia. **Hemorrhage is commonly entirely or partially concealed** (no vaginal bleeding) in the uterus, often under the placenta. Bleeding can cause abdominal pain as blood tracks into the muscle wall of the uterus. Most abruptions are minor, but occasionally total blood loss can be significant and can result in immediate fetal death and major maternal complications, including cardiovascular collapse, disseminated intravascular coagulopathy (DIC), and renal failure. Maternal deaths are still reported associated with major abruption.[2,3]

Vasa Previa

Vasa previa is an extremely rare condition that usually leads to fetal death but does not cause the mother specific harm. It occurs when a fetal vessel in the membranes ruptures. The fetus has a low blood volume and quickly exsanguinates. This diagnosis cannot be made in the prehospital situation and presents in a similar way to that of placenta previa.

Risks and Precautions

Most patients will be stable. However, pregnant women may lose a great deal of circulating blood volume before showing any changes in blood pressure or heart rate. Therefore any bleeding in late pregnancy has the potential to be extremely serious for both mother and fetus and can occasionally lead to unpredictable and profound maternal collapse. Gaining early IV access is recommended, even if the patient appears to be stable.

Overall major abruption is more unpredictable than placenta previa. In severe cases, the mother may lose two thirds or more of her circulating volume, which sequesters under the placenta. Be wary if there is minimal vaginal bleeding in a patient who has severe and continuous uterine pain. **The uterus will be tender and may feel "woody" (or "hard as wood"), and** the mother may have noticed that fetal movements have ceased. Abruption is time-critical and the patient should be transferred urgently to an appropriate obstetric unit after initial stabilization.

Equipment (List)

- Spine board and straps.
- Blankets and pillows (for padding).
- High-concentration oxygen masks.
- Venous and adult intraosseous access kit.
- Opiate analgesics, Ringer's lactate, or NS for infusion.
- Radio or mobile phone to prealert the receiving ED.

Patient Positioning

- Place the patient at a 15- to 30-degree left lateral tilt to maintain optimum maternal circulation (ideally by strapping her to a spine board with padding under the right side).

Anesthesia and Procedural Monitoring

- Blood pressure, pulse, respiratory rate.
- If equipment and time allow, check fetal heart rate; this should be between 120 and 160 beats per minute. Absence of the fetal heart tones may imply fetal death in association with severe hemorrhage (revealed or concealed).

Step-by-Step Technique

To be used when the patient is cardiovascularly unstable or when there is heavy bleeding or severe pain.

- Fully assess ABC's: document respiratory rate, pulse rate and quality, and blood pressure.
- Provide high-flow oxygen via a non–rebreathed mask; aim for oxygen saturations of 98%.
- Insert one or two large-bore (14-gauge) cannulas en route to the receiving unit (but DO NOT delay transfer). If it is not possible to gain IV access, consider using an intraosseous cannula.
- If the patient is hypotensive, administer crystalloids **to maintain a systolic BP (SBP) >100 mm Hg.**

- Ask to see the patient's maternity records (if available). Briefly review the history of the gestation, degree of bleeding/pain, fetal movements, and any high blood pressure during pregnancy. Review any available ultrasound information.
- Arrange rapid transfer to the nearest maternity unit staffed with an obstetrician and operating room facilities.
- Inform the receiving unit of the woman's condition. Confirm if there is significant vaginal bleeding, as surgery will be required.
- Administer analgesia as appropriate.
- Do not administer anything by mouth.

Outcomes Assessment

- On-scene in-time critical situations.
- Appropriate prealert message sent to receiving unit.

Complications

Continuing major antepartum hemorrhage may lead to cardiac arrest (see section on Cardiac Arrest in Pregnancy). Remember to inform the receiving unit if CPR is required. The patient will probably require urgent perimortem cesarean section on arrival.

SEVERE PRE-ECLAMPSIA AND ECLAMPSIA

KEY LEARNING POINTS

For Pre-Eclampsia and Eclampsia

- Hypertension and edema of the fingers and face can represent pre-eclampsia.
- Severe pre-eclampsia is often associated with some of the following symptoms: headache, visual disturbances (flashing lights), and/or pain in epigastrium or right upper quadrant.
- Avoid excessive IV fluid input, which may precipitate pulmonary edema and adult respiratory distress syndrome (ARDS).
- Maintain IV fluid input at 85 mL/hour or less.
- Eclamptic seizures can occur in late labor or immediately post partum.

Purpose of Procedure

To allow the EMT to identify and manage severe pre-eclampsia and eclampsia.

Patient Selection

Pregnancy-Induced Hypertension

This is a significant rise in blood pressure occurring after 20 weeks' gestation **in the absence of proteinuria or other features of pre-eclampsia**. Most cases are mild, with blood pressure levels of around 140/90 mm Hg. Fifteen percent of women who present with pregnancy-induced hypertension will develop pre-eclampsia.

Pre-eclampsia

Pre-eclampsia is hypertension associated with proteinuria, usually developing after 20 weeks of pregnancy. It may be associated with excessive peripheral edema. Some edema of the legs is common in almost all pregnant women. However, *edema of the fingers and face* is more likely to represent pre-eclampsia. Risk factors for pre-eclampsia include pre-existing hypertension, multiple pregnancies, obesity, age <16 and >40 years, and a history of renal disease or diabetes. While only a minority of cases advance to severe disease, pre-eclampsia accounts for 13.6% of maternal deaths related to direct pregnancy causes.[2]

Severe Pre-eclampsia

In severe pre-eclampsia **the blood pressure is significantly raised (≥160/110 mm Hg) with proteinuria and one or more of the following symptoms and signs: headache, visual disturbances (flashing lights, blurred vision), and pain in epigastrium or right upper quadrant.** Severe pre-eclampsia may develop with acute symptoms and little prior warning or may progress from mild pre-eclampsia. There is a risk of intracranial hemorrhage and eclamptic grand mal seizures.

Eclampsia

Eclampsia is the development of acute seizures in pregnancy or immediately post partum, without the pre-existence of any primary neurologic disorder such as epilepsy.

Risks and Precautions

- Always keep the mother in the left lateral decubitus position in order to maintain cardiac output and avoid hypotension.
- **Because excessive IV fluid administration can precipitate pulmonary edema and adult respiratory distress syndrome, only provide IV fluid at a rate to keep the IV line open (NS, 85 mL/hour or less).**
- Complications of eclampsia include multiorgan failure, disseminated intravascular coagulopathy, recurrent seizures or status epilepticus, intracranial hemorrhage, aspiration of gastric contents from repeated seizure activity, and hypoxia.

Equipment (List)

- Spine board and straps.
- Blankets and pillows (for padding).
- High-concentration oxygen masks.
- Venous and adult intraosseous access kit.
- Ringer's lactate (LR) or NS for infusion.
- Radio or mobile phone to prealert the receiving ED.

Patient Positioning

- If the patient is ≥20 weeks of gestation, place her in a 15- to 30-degree left lateral tilt.

Monitoring

- Monitor maternal blood pressure and heart rate.
- If equipment allows, check fetal heart rate; this should be between 120 and 160 beats per minute. Absence of the fetal heart tones may imply fetal death, particularly in cases of eclampsia with recurrent seizures.

Step-by-Step Technique

- Fully assess ABC's: document respiratory rate, pulse rate and quality, and blood pressure. Blood pressure assessment is critical in cases of severe pre-eclampsia and eclampsia.
- In cases of eclampsia, provide high-flow oxygen via a non–rebreathed mask in the postictal phase. Aim for oxygen saturations of 94 to 98%.
- Insert one or two large-bore (14-gauge) cannulas en route to the receiving unit (but DO NOT delay transfer). If it is not possible to gain IV access, consider using an intraosseous cannula.
- Ensure intravenous fluid is restricted to less than 85 mL/hour to avoid development of pulmonary edema.
- Give magnesium sulfate, 2 grams IV, over 15 minutes if transport time to the ED is less than a few minutes. Follow the bolus with 2 grams magnesium IV over 1 hour.
- For status epilepticus, treat according to standard protocol after magnesium sulfate has been administered.
- For diastolic blood pressure >110 mm Hg: if magnesium has not lowered the blood pressure, give

hydralazine in a 10 milligrams IV bolus if transport time to the ED or obstetric unit is prolonged.

- Ask the patient's family to provide any available maternity records with the history such as gestation, degree of bleeding/pain, fetal movements, or high blood pressure during pregnancy. Review any available ultrasound information.
- Arrange *rapid transfer* to the nearest maternity unit staffed with an obstetrician.
- Do not administer anything by mouth in case cesarean delivery is required.

Outcomes Assessment

- On-scene time in time-critical situations.
- Appropriate prealert message sent to receiving unit.

LABOR AND NORMAL VAGINAL DELIVERY

Purpose of Procedure

To allow the prehospital practitioner to identify labor and conduct a normal vaginal delivery. **A delivery of ≥24 weeks is compatible with fetal survival outside the uterus.**

Patient Selection

The patients are pregnant women whose delivery is imminent, and there is insufficient time to transfer them to an ED or maternity unit. **An imminent delivery is a head that is crowning.**

Risks and Precautions

Avoid transport with a patient with an imminent delivery, and instead assist in delivery at the scene. Judging whether there is sufficient time to reach the hospital for an in-hospital delivery can be difficult. **A head that is obviously crowning is clear evidence that delivery is imminent.**

In established labor three to four contractions occur every ten minutes, each contraction lasting for about one minute. More than five contractions in ten minutes can suggest a placental abruption. Membranes can rupture at any point before or during labor.

Equipment (List)

- Blankets and towels.

- Delivery pack.
- Sterile gloves and personal protective equipment.
- Neonatal resuscitation equipment: rubber suction bulb, hemostats, cord clamps, sterile towels, and drapes.

Patient Positioning

The typical delivery position is with the woman on her back because this allows the best visualization and control of the delivery. If the patient prefers another position, such as the knee-chest position, all delivery maneuvers must be done in the opposite direction of the illustrated positions (Figure 40-6).

Anesthesia and Procedural Monitoring

- Imminent delivery does not allow for anesthesia.

Step-by-Step Technique

- Ask permission to check the perineal area.
- Gaping of the vaginal opening with an obvious presenting fetal part visible confirms that delivery is imminent. There may be gaping of the anus as well.
- Note the color of any vaginal liquid.
- Prepare for delivery.

Normal Vaginal Delivery (Figure 40-6)

- Open delivery pack and ensure there are cord clamps, scissors, and dry towels/blankets in which to wrap the baby.
- Ensure that the neonatal resuscitation equipment is at hand — bag and mask.
- Allow the mother to push with her contractions.
- When the head crowns, it will no longer recede between the contractions and will stay, distending the perineum. At this stage ask the woman to pant rather than push to try and control the delivery.
- The head will deliver by extension so that the forehead delivers first, followed by the face and then the chin.
- It is not necessary to check for the umbilical cord as usually the body will deliver the fetus through any loops of cord.
- After the head delivers, it will rotate slightly to look sideways.
- Place one hand on each side of the baby's head, gently, so they cup the baby's ears.

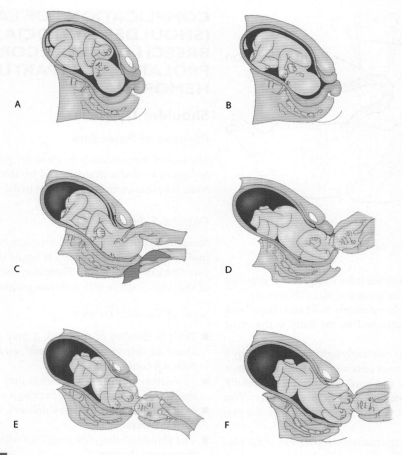

FIGURE 40–6

Normal vertex delivery (occiput anterior position). Maneuvers of normal delivery for vertex presentations. **A**, Engagement, flexion, and descent. **B**, Internal rotation. **C**, Extension and delivery of the head. After delivery of the head, suction the infant's nose and mouth and make sure the umbilical cord is not wrapped around the infant's neck. **D**, Rotate to bringing the infant's chest into an anteroposterior direction in the pelvis. **E**, Anterior shoulder delivery. **F**, Posterior shoulder delivery. After delivery, support the infant's head and gently deliver the shoulder. Do not pull.

■ The anterior shoulder should deliver as the woman pushes. Guide the head gently downward as she pushes until the shoulder delivers.

■ Do NOT pull vigorously, as this can cause injury to the infant's nerves of the arm and shoulder (brachial plexus injury).

■ Once the anterior shoulder has delivered, guide the baby upward with gentle traction to deliver the posterior shoulder followed by the rest of the body. The infant will be very slippery. ***Do not DROP the infant.***

■ Place the baby on the mother's abdomen to allow the skin to skin contact and to help keep the baby warm.

■ **Document the date and time of delivery of the baby.**

■ Dry the infant with a towel and then cover with a fresh dry blanket/towel.

■ If the baby does not take a gasp and commence breathing within the first minute or remains blue or white, assess as per newborn life support guidelines.

■ Wait for the cord to stop pulsating before cutting and dividing, unless the baby needs resuscitation.

■ To clamp the cord place a cord clamp 1 to 2 cm from the baby's abdomen and a second cord clamp 2 to 3 cm distally to the first. Ensure that the clamps are firmly closed and cut BETWEEN the two

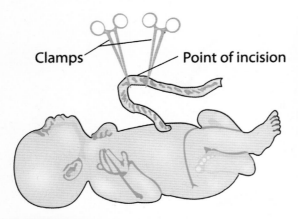

FIGURE 40–7

Clamping and cutting the umbilical cord.

clamps. Check that the baby's fingers and genitalia are clear of the clamps and scissors (Figure 40-7).

- If the cord snaps immediately, hold and clamp both ends. The end attached to the baby is the most important.
- Rarely, the cord is extremely tight around the baby's neck and you cannot remove it, or the baby cannot deliver through the cord. In this case carefully clamp and divide the cord before delivery. You must ensure that you cut the cord between the two clamps.
- Otherwise await spontaneous separation of the placenta before cutting the umbilical cord.
- Signs of separation are.
  - Cord lengthens.
  - Uterus rises up and is easier to palpate.
  - Often a small gush of blood.
- The placenta should deliver spontaneously normally within the first 30 minutes following delivery. Ask the mother to give little pushes to expel it. **Do not pull the placenta.** Too much traction can cause uterine inversion (uterus turns inside-out), tearing of the umbilical cord, or tearing of the placenta and severe bleeding.
- **Note the time of delivery of the placenta and the total blood loss. Place the placenta in a clean container or placental basin and take it to the hospital.**

Outcomes Assessment

Check maternal blood pressure and pulse following delivery.

Transport patient and infant to the nearest appropriate hospital.

COMPLICATIONS OF LABOR (SHOULDER DYSTOCIA, BREECH DELIVERY, CORD PROLAPSE, POSTPARTUM HEMORRHAGE)

Shoulder Dystocia

Purpose of Procedure

The aim of this section is to allow the practitioner to recognize shoulder dystocia and be able to perform some simple maneuvers to attempt to deliver the baby.

Patient Selection

Shoulder dystocia can occur during any delivery but is more common when the baby is big or the mother is very obese or has diabetes. There may also be a history of shoulder dystocia with previous pregnancies.

Signs of Shoulder Dystocia

- Prior to delivery of the head, it may appear to be about to deliver and then "bob" away or retract between contractions.
- At delivery of the head, the chin may appear tight against the perineum (turtle neck sign or turtle sign).
- When the head of the baby delivers, it will fail to turn sideways.
- The shoulders then fail to deliver with the normal downward traction.

Risks and Precautions

- Pulling vigorously downward on the baby's head can cause brachial plexus injury (this paralyzes the arm). By following the procedures described below and using only a normal level of downward traction, the risk of brachial plexus injury can be minimized.
- Most babies are likely to deliver with the maneuvers described below, but some babies will not; if this occurs, immediate transfer to a maternity unit should be undertaken. Warn the admitting unit of the situation. DO NOT wait any longer to begin transport to an obstetric unit or ED.
- Anticipate the need for neonatal resuscitation.
- A postpartum hemorrhage can follow shoulder dystocia.

Equipment (List)

- Delivery equipment.
- Blankets and towels.
- Neonatal resuscitation equipment.

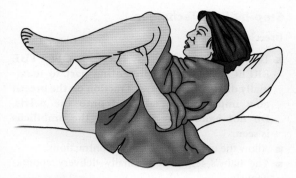

FIGURE 40–8

McRoberts maneuver, knee-chest position with the patient on her back. This opens up the pelvis for easier delivery.

Patient Positioning

■ If shoulder dystocia is anticipated or occurs, place the woman in the **McRoberts position** (Figure 40-8).

■ Have the mother lie flat with only one pillow below her head.

■ Bring the knees up toward her chest and move the knees apart.

■ You can ask the mother or her partner to hold the legs in this position.

■ This maneuver alone can lead to delivery in 60 to 70% of cases.

Step-by-Step Technique

Identification of Shoulder Dystocia

■ At delivery of the head, with a contraction attempt to deliver the anterior shoulder with gentle downward traction as described in the normal delivery section.

■ If the shoulders no not deliver, you have diagnosed **shoulder dystocia.**

■ Ask the patient to assume the McRoberts position as described above.

■ Attempt to deliver the shoulders.

■ Ask the patient to push and use gentle downward traction to attempt to deliver the shoulders again.

■ Try this for 1 to 2 minutes.

Assistant's Use of Constant Pressure

■ If you fail to achieve delivery, identify where the fetal back lies. This will often be the opposite side to the direction in which the baby is facing.

■ Ask whomever is assisting you to stand on the side of the baby's back (e.g., if the baby is facing left, stand on the mother's right side).

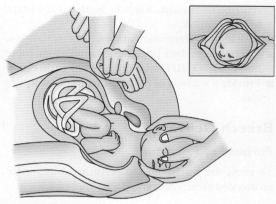

FIGURE 40–9

Compression two finger-breadths above the mother's pubic symphysis to release the impacted shoulder.

■ Ask the assistant to use his or her hands in a CPR grip, and place the heel of the hand two finger breadths above the symphysis pubis (see Figure 40-9).

■ Ask the assistant to apply **moderate downward pressure for 1 to 2 minutes** to move the baby's shoulder.

■ Attempt to deliver the baby while the assistant applies the pressure for 1 to 2 minutes.

Assistant Rocking Pressure

■ After 2 minutes ask your assistant to apply intermittent pressure.

■ Continue to try to deliver the baby while the assistant applies **rocking pressure** two finger breadths above the symphysis pubis.

■ Try this maneuver for 1 to 2 minutes.

All Fours Position

■ If delivery still does not occur, ask the mother to move into the all fours position.

■ Ensure that the mother's hips are well flexed.

■ The mother's bottom should be elevated.

■ The mother's head should be as low as possible.

■ Continue to attempt delivery for 1 to 2 minutes in this position.

■ It may be easier to deliver the posterior shoulder first in this position.

Transfer

■ If the baby still does not deliver, scoop mother and baby and move without further delay to the nearest staffed obstetric unit. Keep the mother in the lateral left tilt position.

- Give high-concentration oxygen.
- Insert one or two large-bore cannulas en route; however, DO NOT delay on the scene to do this.
- Provide a warning of the situation to the accepting unit.

Breech Delivery

Purpose of Procedure

To allow the practitioner to perform an imminent, unattended breech delivery.

Patient Selection

The woman may know the baby is in a breech presentation.

There will be evidence of labor as described in the normal labor section.

On inspection of the perineum, the following may be visible:

- Buttocks.
- Feet or soles of feet.
- Swollen or bruised genitalia.
- Meconium (it will look like black toothpaste).

Risks and Precautions

The more preterm the delivery, the more likely the baby is to present in the breech position.

- At term only 3% of babies present in the breech position.
- At 28 weeks 20% of babies present in the breech position.

Ask the mother if she knows whether the baby is in the breech position.

Equipment (List)

- Delivery equipment.
- Blankets and towels.
- Neonatal resuscitation equipment.

Patient Positioning

- Semirecumbent.
- Buttocks at the edge of the bed.
- Support feet on chairs if available.
- The mother may be able to support her own legs.

OR

- Squatting: remember that in this position you will be behind the mother, so be aware that the fetal back will appear reversed.

Step-by-Step Technique

Breech Delivery

- The basic principle is **HANDS OFF THE BREECH. Allow the presenting part to maximally dilate the introitus. Traction on the breech may impact the fetal head onto the pelvis. Do not handle the fetus until the umbilicus is seen.**
- Allow the mother to push with contractions.
- The baby's legs will normally delivery spontaneously.
- If the legs do not deliver, place your hand on the back of the fetal thigh, and gently flex the baby's knee. The breech should then rotate so that the baby's sacrum is anterior (facing upward). Grasp the baby so that your fingers are on the baby's thighs.
- Keep the baby's body parallel with the floor as it delivers to avoid hyperextension of the neck.
- The arms usually deliver spontaneously.

Figure 40-10 shows for maneuvers for imminent breech delivery.

- If the above fails to work, perform the Løvset maneuver[6] (see Figure 40-11).
  - Hold the baby over the pelvic girdle.
  - Lift slightly toward the maternal symphysis.
  - Rotate until one of the shoulders is in the anterior position.
  - The arm may spontaneously deliver.
  - If delivery does not occur, run a finger over the shoulder and down to the elbow.
  - Sweep the arm across the front of the baby's chest to deliver.
  - Rotate the baby back to the sacroanterior position.
  - Repeat in the opposite direction if the second arm fails to deliver.
- Wrap a towel around the baby during the delivery to keep it warm.
- Keep the baby's body parallel with the floor until the nape of the neck is visible.
- The head may delivery spontaneously – aim to control the delivery – ask the mother to pant.
- ***Do not drop the infant.***
- Should delivery still not occur, place the mother in the McRoberts position (see Shoulder Dystocia).
- Ask an assistant to give suprapubic pressure – downward towards the pelvis.
- Should delivery still not occur, transfer mother and baby to the nearest maternity unit.
- Inform the maternity unit of the situation.

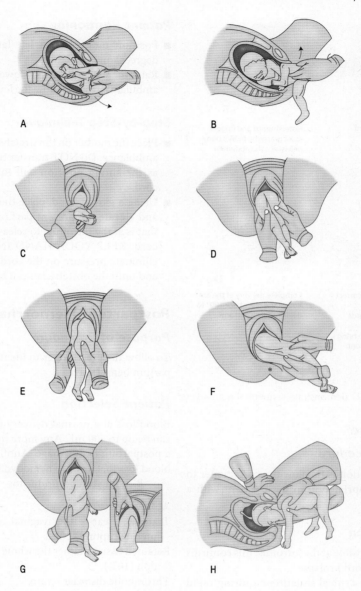

FIGURE 40–10

Maneuvers for imminent breech delivery. Management of the vaginal frank breech delivery. **A,** The operator's hand is placed behind the fetal thigh, putting gentle pressure at the knee and allowing delivery of the leg. **B,** A similar maneuver of the opposite leg. **C,** The feet are grasped with the thumb and third finger over the lateral malleolus and the second finger is placed between the two ankles. **D,** With maternal expulsive efforts, the breech is delivered to the level of the umbilicus. The sacrum should be kept anterior. **E,** Again, with maternal expulsive efforts, the infant is delivered to the level of the clavicles, keeping the sacrum anterior. **F,** The fetus is rotated 90 degrees allowing visualization of the now anterior right arm. **G,** The arm is well visualized and a single digit is used to deliver it. Delivery of the opposite arm is accomplished by rotating the fetus 180 degrees in a clockwise direction and repeating the maneuver. **H,** Delivery of the fetal vertex is accomplished by placing the operator's fingers over the maxillary processes of the fetus, keeping the body parallel to the floor. The body should never be lifted above the parallel position to prevent hyperextension of the neck. An assistant applies suprapubic pressure, aiding flexion of the fetal head and accomplishing delivery.

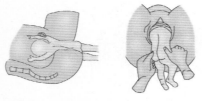

A

Here the arms are extended and cannot be delivered

B

Note: thumbs and fingers must grasp the baby's bony pelvis, not the abdomen

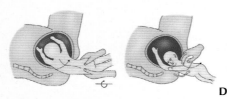

C

Grasp baby's pelvis using correct 'pelvic grip'
Gently flex the baby upwards ('sideways')
Finally rotate baby 180° to bring the posterior arm to the front where it can be delivered

D

Complete delivery of the arm
Rotate the baby back 180° to deliver the second arm

FIGURE 40–11

Løvset maneuver, A-D demonstrate sequential maneuvers.

Cord Prolapse

Purpose of Procedure

The aim of this section is to allow the practitioner to identify and appropriately transfer a patient with a prolapsed cord.

Patient Selection

If a loop of cord is visible at the introitus, this confirms the diagnosis of a cord prolapse.

This is a time-critical situation requiring rapid transfer to the nearest obstetric unit.

Risks and Precautions

Cord prolapse is more common with transverse lie or breech presentation.

If delivery appears to be imminent, that is, head/breech is seen at the introitus along with the cord – proceed with delivery and be prepared to deal with a neonatal resuscitation.

Equipment List

- Delivery pack and neonatal resuscitation equipment if delivery is imminent.
- Gloves.

Patient Positioning

- Position mother on a left lateral tilt (15 to 30 degrees) on a stretcher.
- Raise the patient's hips by lowering the head of the ambulance trolley below the level of the pelvis.

Step-by-Step Technique

- Place the mother on the stretcher and transfer to the ambulance. Do NOT transfer the patient in a chair, as the sitting position will further compress the cord.
- Using a gloved hand, place the hand in the vagina and elevate the present part of the baby (the part that is at the introitus) to release pressure from the cord. KEEP YOUR HAND IN THE VAGINA to eliminate pressure on the cord during the transfer and until the obstetrician can take over.

Postpartum Hemorrhage

Purpose of Procedure

To allow the practitioner to identify and treat a postpartum hemorrhage.

Patient Selection

Blood loss at a normal delivery (or breech delivery) can be up to 500 mL. Any more than this is defined as a postpartum hemorrhage. Another definition is any blood loss that leads to hemodynamic instability.

Bleeding can occur due to:

Atonic uterus 70%.
Trauma – tears either vaginal or cervical or rarely uterine rupture (20%).
Retained tissue – either the whole placenta or a cotyledon (10%).
Thrombotic disorder – rare.

Risks and Precautions

Ask the mother and check for a history in the maternity notes of

- Previous postpartum hemorrhage.
- Enlarged uterus – polyhydramnios, large baby.
- Grandmultiparity – five deliveries or more.
- Known uterine fibroids.
- Maternal age over 40.
- Maternal obesity.

There is also an increased risk of postpartum hemorrhage in the presence of antepartum hemorrhage or shoulder dystocia.

- If any of these factors are identified and time allows, place a **large-bore canula** (14 gauge).

Equipment (List)

- Intravenous cannulas – large-bore (14 gauge).
- Intravenous crystalloid.
- Gloves.
- Sanitary pads or similar protection.

Step-by-Step Technique

- Fully assess ABC's.
- Obtain intravenous access via large-bore cannula (14 gauge).
- Give intravenous crystalloids to maintain a systolic BP of 100 mm Hg.
- Check for perineal and obvious vaginal tears – local compression with a sanitary towel may reduce the bleeding.
- Arrange rapid transfer to a staffed obstetric unit.
- Inform the accepting unit of the patient's condition.

Web Resources

1. Resuscitation Council (UK). *Adult Advanced Life Support Algorithm.* Available at: http://www.resus. org.uk/pages/gl5algos.htm Accessed 29th December 2009.
2. Royal College of Obstetricians and Gynaecologists. *Clinical greentop guidelines.* Available at: http://www. rcog.org.uk/womens-health/guidelines Accessed 29th December 2009.
3. Advanced Life Support in Pregnancy (ALSO) available at: http://www.aafp.org/online/en/home/cme/ aafpcourses/clinicalcourses/also.html and http:// www.aafpfoundation.org/online/foundation/home/ programs/humanitarian/internationalfund/also.html.

Selected Readings

1. Howell C, Grady K, Cox C, eds. *Managing Obstetric Emergencies and Trauma – the MOET Course Manual.* 2nd ed. London: RCOG Press, 2007; p 380.
2. Woollard M, Simpson H, Hinshaw K, Wieteska S, eds. *Pre-hospital Obstetric Emergency Training.* Oxford: Wiley-Blackwell, 2010; p 211.

References

1. Davis JB, Jokhio AH, Winter HR, Cheng KK. An intervention involving traditional birth attendants in Pakistan. *N Engl J Med* 353: 1417, 2005.
2. Confidential Enquiry into Maternal and Child Health. Why Mothers Die 2000-2002. Report on Confidential Enquiries into Maternal Deaths in the United Kingdom. London: *CEMACH;* 2004.
3. Lewis, G, ed. The Confidential Enquiry into Maternal and Child Health (CEMACH). Saving Mothers' Lives: reviewing maternal deaths to make motherhood safer - 2003–2005. The Seventh Report on Confidential Enquiries into Maternal Deaths in the United Kingdom. London: *CEMACH*; 2007.
4. Pearlman MD, Tintinalli JE, Lorenz RP. Blunt trauma during pregnancy. *New Engl J Med* 323 (23): 1609, 1990.
5. Crosby WM, Snyder KG, Snow C, et al. Impact injuries in pregnancy. 1. experimental studies. *Am J Obstet Gynecol* 101: 100; 1968.
6. Løvset J. Shoulder delivery by breech presentation. *J Obstet Gynaecol Brit Emp* 44: 696, 1937.

CHAPTER 41

Pediatric Procedures

Nadeemuddin Qureshi, Mohammed Al-Mogbil, Khalid Abu Haimed

Prehospital care is an integral component of emergency services in which initiated treatment protocols have a significant impact on long-term outcomes for patients. The ability of EMS personnel to perform lifesaving procedures on children takes priority over other aspects of treatment. For example, inability to establish a patent airway in a child in respiratory distress will lead to significant morbidity and mortality. This chapter describes the most common lifesaving pediatric procedures that EMS personnel need to have proficiency in when taking care of sick children in a prehospital setting.

AIRWAY

Respiratory distress is a common problem in pediatric patients. In the field or in the ED, management of the pediatric airway is always a challenge due to multiple differences between the pediatric and adult airway. The variation in equipment sizes and medication doses adds additional difficulty. Table 41-1 outlines the major differences between the pediatric and the adult airway and suggests solutions for overcoming these difficulties.[1,2]

Indications for Airway Management

1. Respiratory failure or impending respiratory failure.[3]
2. Respiratory rates <12 or >60 bpm plus nonpurposeful or unresponsive to painful stimuli.
3. Cardiopulmonary failure.
4. Shock: helps decrease the work of breathing.
5. Neurologic resuscitation: pediatric Glasgow Coma Score (GCS) < 8 or consider in anyone with GCS <12 and decreasing mental status; hyperventilation to P_{CO_2} of 30 to 35 mm Hg.
6. To protect airway during transport.

Opening the Airway

The initial step in airway management is opening the airway using the chin lift and/or jaw thrust maneuver.

Chin Lift Maneuver

Indications   Children with a decreased level of consciousness with upper airway obstruction except trauma victims.

Contraindications   Trauma victims even if radiographs do not show spinal injury.

Procedure

1. Identify unresponsiveness.
2. Place the right hand on the patient's forehead and the other hand on the mandible just lateral to the chin.
3. Gently depress the forehead with one hand and extend the neck while lifting the chin with the other hand (Figure 41-1).

Table 41–1	Pediatric Airway Differences from Adults and Possible Measures to Overcome These Difficulties	
Anatomic Considerations	**Management**	
Prominent occiput can cause airway obstruction	Use 1-inch towel roll below shoulders	
Relatively larger tongue can cause airway obstruction	Use oropharyngeal or nasopharyngeal airway	
Larynx is anterior and cephalad	Need to get lower and look up to see cords	
Epiglottis is U-shaped and floppy	Use a straight laryngoscope blade to lift the epiglottis directly	
Short tracheal length (newborn 4–5 cm and 18-month old 7–8 cm); ET tubes dislodged easily	Reassess tube position frequently	
Cricoid area of child is smallest area of the airway	Avoid cuffed tubes in children <8 years	
Large amounts of adenoidal tissue can make nasotracheal intubations difficult, causing laceration and bleeding	Avoid nasal airways in children less than 1 year old	
Diaphragmatic breathers	Decompress stomach with nasogastric tube to ventilate more easily	

4. Sometimes the chin needs to be lifted up firmly by using the lips or teeth. Be careful of loose teeth.
5. Confirm adequate ventilation by observing the chest wall rise and performing auscultation.

Complications   The chin lift maneuver can exacerbate spinal cord injury and therefore should not be applied to trauma victims.

Hyperextension in neonates and young children can cause obstruction rather than relieving it.

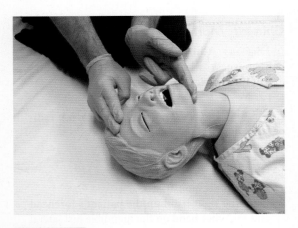

Use the chin lift maneuver to open the airway and place the airway in a neutral position. Photo courtesy of Dr. Nadeemuddin Quereshi.

Jaw-Thrust Maneuver

This maneuver allows opening the airway in patients with suspected spinal cord injury.

Indications   Patient's neck needs immobilization.

Contraindications   No absolute contraindications, however, may be difficult to apply in children with maxillofacial injuries.

Procedure

1. Place both hands at the mandibular angles and push the mandible anteriorly without moving the neck (Figure 41-2).
2. Confirm ventilation by observation and auscultation.

Complications   Spinal cord injury may occur if the spine is not adequately secured.

Airway Stents

The next step in airway management after applying appropriate positioning maneuvers is the use of airway stents. Nasopharyngeal and oropharyngeal airways provide a stent to protect obstruction of the airway caused by soft tissue. These airways can be used to facilitate effective ventilation in intubated and non-intubated patients.

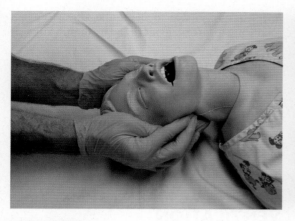

FIGURE 41–2

Jaw-thrust maneuver. Photo courtesy of
Dr. Nadeemuddin Quereshi.

Oropharyngeal Airways

Oropharyngeal airways are semicircular tubes available in various sizes to provide an adequate stent for overcoming soft-tissue obstruction mainly caused by a large tongue. These can be used in both intubated and nonintubated patients. Figure 41-3 shows the different sizes of oropharyngeal airways.

Indications

To relieve upper airway obstruction.
Bite block for endotracheal (ET) tube.
To facilitate oral and pharyngeal suctioning.

Contraindications In conscious patients or patients with intact airway reflexes, the use of an oropharyngeal airway may trigger laryngospasm or bronchospasm.

Do not use if foreign body aspiration is suspected.

Equipment Multiple sizes are available from 55 to 90 mm. Measure the distance from the lips to the angle of mandible to identify the appropriate size for the oral airway. To select the right size, place the airway on the patient's cheek extending up to the angle of the mandible.

Procedure

1. After identifying the appropriate size airway, open the patient's mouth and suction out secretions.
2. Place a tongue blade at the base of the tongue.
3. Pull the tongue forward with the blade.
4. Insert the airway with 1 to 2 cm protruding from the incisors.

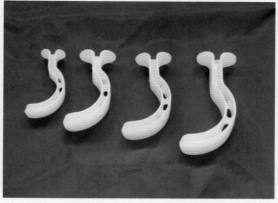

FIGURE 41–3

Different sizes of oropharyngeal airways. Photo courtesy of Dr. Nadeemuddin Quereshi.

5. Perform the jaw thrust with your fingers until the flange is even with the lips.
6. Remove the jaw thrust and check that the tongue and lips are not caught by the airway.

Complications Inappropriate sized airways can cause airway obstruction.

An airway that is too large will stimulate surrounding structures, triggering laryngospasm and or bronchospasm.

An airway that is too small will push the tongue posterior to cause airway obstruction.

Nasopharyngeal Airways

A soft rubber tube that provides a stent from the nares to the glottis.

Indications Upper airway obstruction in conscious patients. In children who have extensive adenoidal tissue and tonsils the obstruction may not be relieved with an oral airway. A nasopharyngeal airway in such patients may serve as a perfect conduit to relieve upper airway obstruction. The NP airway is also useful in patients in whom it is difficult to place an oral airway, e.g., those with trismus or in status epilepticus.

Contraindications

Midface, basilar, and nasal trauma or history of nasal facial surgery (cleft palate repair).
Coagulopathy (epistaxis).
Foreign body aspiration.

Equipment Nasopharyngeal airway sizes from 16 F to 34 F. Measure the right size from the tip of the nose to the tragus of the ear (Figure 41-4).

Procedure

1. Select the correct size (see Figures 41-5A, B).
2. Lubricate NP airway with jelly.
3. Hold the tube between the two fingers and pass it into the nostril with the bevel pointing away from the nasal septum.
4. If you meet resistance, gently rotate and advance the NP tube.

5. If you are unable to insert the airway, do not attempt to force it. Remove and try the other side or a smaller size.
6. Appropriate sized ET tubes can be used as nasopharyngeal airways.

Complications

Bleeding from adenoidal tissue, especially if you try to force an inappropriate size.
Ineffective in relieving the obstruction if airway is too long or too short.

BAG-VALVE MASK (BVM) VENTILATION

Respiratory failure is the commonest cause of cardiac arrest in children compared to adults. Factors responsible include higher baseline airway resistance and fewer muscle fatigue- resistant muscle fibers in the intercostals and the diaphragm. Small changes in airway diameter have a large impact on overall airway resistance in children compared to adults, as explained by Poiseuille's law that resistance is inversely proportional to the radius to the power of four. This predisposes children to rapid respiratory failure followed by cardiac arrest. For this reason BMV ventilation is a crucial skill in pediatric resuscitation. Early recognition of respiratory failure and intervention may potentially save the child from cardiopulmonary arrest.[4,5]

Indications

Respiratory failure due to any etiology in which assisted or controlled ventilation is required.

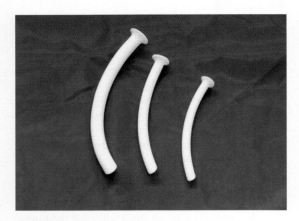

FIGURE 41–4

Nasopharyngeal airways of different sizes. Photo courtesy of Dr. Nadeemuddin Quereshi.

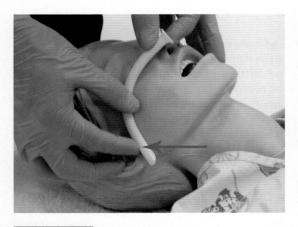

FIGURE 41–5A

Inappropriately sized nasopharyngeal airway. Photo courtesy of Dr. Nadeemuddin Quereshi.

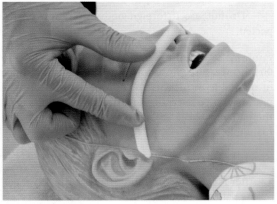

FIGURE 41–5B

Correct size nasopharygeal airway. Photo courtesy of Dr. Nadeemuddin Quereshi.

Contraindications

Absolute

Meconium aspiration in a newborn.
Diaphragmatic hernia.

Relative

Facial injury.
Pneumothorax.
Complete obstruction from a foreign body.

Equipment

- Self-inflating bags (neonate, child, and adult bags) (Figure 41-6).
- Appropriate sized bags.
  - 250-cc bags for neonates (3 to 6 months).
  - 450-cc bags for infant or child (<5 years).
  - 750-cc bag or adult bag for older children.
- Appropriate masks (Figure 41-7 B) covering base of nose up to chin cleft.
- (Figure 41-7A illustrates inappropriate size mask covering eyes).
- Oxygen supply.

Procedure

1. Select the appropriate sized bag and mask for the patient.
2. Apply chin lift or jaw thrust maneuver to open the airway.

3. Look for any chest wall movement; listen for air movement.
4. Stabilize the head and neck in a "sniffing" position to keep the upper airway open (Figure 41-8A & B).
5. Place the mask covering the nasal bridge to the chin cleft.
6. Hold mask using a "CE" grip: C = is thumb and index grip mask forming a "C"; E = third fourth, and fifth fingers on angle of jaw forming an "E"[4] (Figure 41-9).

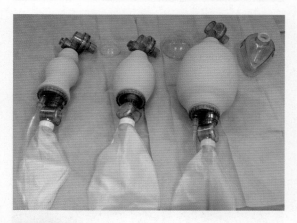

FIGURE 41–6

Self-inflating bags in neonatal, child, and adult sizes. Photo courtesy of Dr. Nadeemuddin Quereshi.

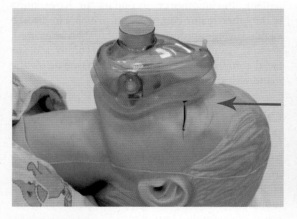

FIGURE 41–7A

Inappropriate mask size covering the eyes. Photo courtesy of Dr. Nadeemuddin Quereshi.

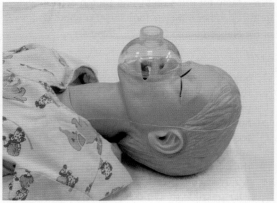

FIGURE 41–7B

Appropriate size mask covering base of nose up to chin cleft. Photo courtesy of Dr. Nadeemuddin Quereshi.

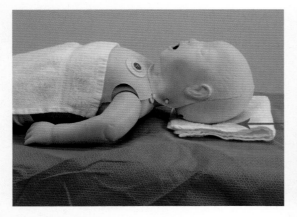

FIGURE 41–8A

Flexed neck. WRONG position. Photo courtesy of Dr. Nadeemuddin Quereshi.

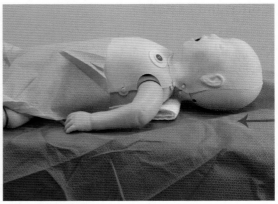

FIGURE 41–8B

Correct "SNIFFING" position. Photo courtesy of Dr. Nadeemuddin Quereshi.

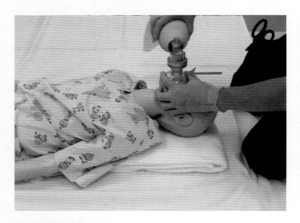

FIGURE 41–9

"CE" clamp for BVM ventilation Thumb & forefinger form "C", other 3 fingers form the "E". Photo courtesy of Dr. Nadeemuddin Quereshi.

7. Say "Squeeze/Release/Release" as you ventilate the child; this will slow you down and allow proper exhalation time.
8. Sometimes it is preferable to use a two-person technique in which one person using both hands applies the mask in the "CE" clamp position and the other person compresses the bag.
9. Apply cricoid pressure (Sellick maneuver) whenever possible to avoid aspiration of gastric contents.
10. Observe for chest rise and listen to breath sounds. Monitor the vital signs, especially the O_2 saturation monitor.

Special Considerations

Do not overventilate young children. The required tidal volume is 6 to 8 mL/kg. In addition 2 to 3 mL/kg is the dead space of the device.[6] Therefore attempt to deliver 10 mL/kg tidal volume with each breath. Monitor chest rise with each breath delivered, as this confirms delivery of an adequate tidal volume. Overventilation leads to gastric distention and vomiting.

Complications

The most common complication is aspiration pneumonitis. BVM ventilation does not protect against aspiration; however, the risk can be reduced by applying cricoid pressure and avoiding overventilating the patient. Pneumothorax secondary to barotrauma is the other major complication, which can also be avoided using appropriate tidal volumes. A large mask pressing against the eye can cause vagal bradycardia or facial compression. Pushing on soft tissue below the mandible can obstruct the airway.

ORAL INTUBATION PROCEDURE

Endotracheal (ET) intubation is perhaps the most important procedure in pediatric resuscitation. In children, respiratory failure precedes cardiopulmonary arrest. Establishing a patent functioning airway is of paramount importance.[3,7]

Two fundamental differences exist between BVM ventilation and tracheal intubation. A BVM delivers positive pressure to the entire upper airway, including the esophagus, thus increasing the risk of aspiration. The ET tube restricts the delivery of positive pressure to the lungs, prevents gastric aspiration, and provides access for tracheal suctioning. In meconium aspiration performing BVM ventilation will push the meconium particles farther down into the lungs, ET intubation will limit meconium deposits and provide access for pulmonary toilet. Similarly, in diaphragmatic hernia ventilation using a BVM will inflate the stomach, causing respiratory compromise, whereas ET intubation will limit the inflation to the lungs and protect the stomach from herniating into the thoracic cavity and causing respiratory distress.

Indications

Respiratory failure due to any etiology.
Tracheal suctioning for meconium staining.
Diaphragmatic hernia.

Contraindications

Epiglottitis.

Equipment

- Use length-based color-coded resuscitation tape whenever possible.
- Battery-powered laryngoscope handle, extra batteries and bulbs.
- Laryngoscope blades: curved (MacIntosh) size 1–3, straight (Miller) size 0–3.
- Cuffed and uncuffed ET tubes (one size smaller and one larger than anticipated).[8]
- Lubricating jelly.

- Disposable pediatric stylets.
- Suction.
- Pulse oximetry.
- Pediatric end-tidal CO_2 detector.
- MSOAP (monitors, suction, oxygen supply, airway equipment, pharmacy).

Drug Regimens for Emergent Intubation

Tables 41-2 through 41-6 provide the most commonly available and used drugs for performing intubations. Based on availability, any drug regimen which includes a sedative or atropine, with or without a neuromuscular agent, will be able to accomplish intubation safely.

Procedure

1. Open airway and ventilate with a BVM for 1 to 3 minutes with 100% O_2.
2. Select proper ET tube (Figure 41-10).
3. Insert stylet in ET tube.
4. Select proper sized blade and visualize the larynx (Figure 41-11).
5. Suction as needed.
6. Apply cricoid pressure to prevent regurgitation.
7. Under direct visualization, insert ET tube 2 to 3 cm past the cords (Figure 41-12 and Figure 41-13).
8. Each attempt should not exceed 30 seconds; hyperventilate between attempts.
9. Remove stylet and ventilate with a BVM.
10. Confirm placement with the following methods:
    a. Bilateral chest and epigastric auscultation or
    b. Capnography (or a capnometer if capnography is not available) (Figure 41-14).

Table 41–2	**Sedative Dosing Guidelines**			
Medication	**Route**	**Dose (milligram/kg)**	**Onset/Duration**	**Side Effects**
Midazolam	IV	0.05–0.15	2–3 minutes/ 30–60 minute 4–6 minutes/ 6–12 hours	Respiratory depression, hypotension, dependence, tolerance
Thiopental	IV	2–5	10–20 seconds/ 5–8 minutes	Respiratory depression, hypotension, dependence, tolerance
Ketamine	IV	0.5–2	1–2 minutes/ 60 minutes	Tachycardia, increased blood pressure, bronchodilation, apnea, hypoxia, laryngospasm
Etomidate	IV	0.1–0.3	<1 minute/ 3–5 minutes	Limited data on use in neonates for sedation. Few side effects in children and adults— emesis, myoclonic jerks

Table 41–3	**Neuromuscular Blocking Agents**			
Medication	**Route**	**Dose (milligram/kg)**	**Onset/Duration**	**Side Effects**
Succinylcholine	IV	1–2 mg/kg	30–60 seconds	Hyperkalemia Increased ICP, IOP Bradyarrhythmias
Rocuronium	IV	1 mg/kg	60–90 seconds	Tachycardia
Atracurium	IV	0.5 mg/kg	90 seconds	Hypotension Histamine release

ICP = intracranial pressure; IOP = intraocular pressure.

Table 41–4	**Adjunctive Medications**			
Drugs	**Routes**	**Dose**	**Onset of Action**	**Effects**
Atropine	IV	0.01–0.02 mg/kg	30 seconds	Prevents bradycardia, reduces secretions
Lidocaine	IV	1–2 mg/kg	60 seconds	May prevent ICP increase

ICP = intracranial pressure.

Table 41–5	**ET Tube Sizes, Preferred Laryngoscope Blades and Placement by age.**					
Age	**Premature and Up to 6 Months**	**<1 Year**	**1–2 Years**	**3–5 Years**	**5–8 Years**	**>10 Years**
ETT size (mm)	3.0–3.5	4.0	4.0–4.5	5.0	5.5–6.0	6.5–7.0
Laryngoscope blade size	0	0–1	1	2	2	3
Placement at the lip (cm)*	9	12	13	14	15	20

*Rule of thumb: ETT placement at the lip in cm = size × 3.

Table 41–6	**Airway Equipment by Weight (Premature Infants)**			
Weight (grams)	**ET Size (mm)**	**Suction Catheter (F)**	**Oral Airway size**	**Laryngoscope Straight Blade size**
<1000	2.5	5	000	0
1000–1250	2.5, 3.0	5, 6	000	0
1250–2500	3.0	6	00	0 or 1
2500–3000	3.0, 3.5	6, 8	0	1
>3000	3.0, 3.5, 4	8	0	1

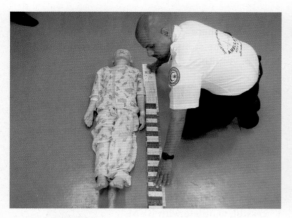

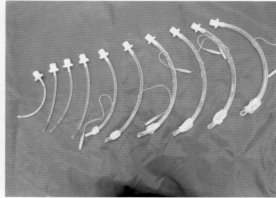

FIGURE 41–10

Endotracheal tubes cuffed, uncuffed, and in various sizes. Photo courtesy of Dr. Nadeemuddin Quereshi.

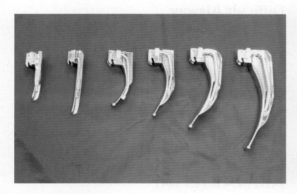

FIGURE 41–11

Straight and curved laryngoscope blades. Photo courtesy of Dr. Nadeemuddin Quereshi.

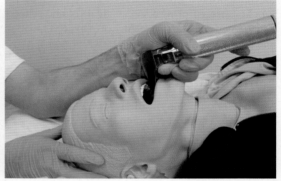

FIGURE 41–12

Vocal cord visualization. Photo courtesy of Dr. Nadeemuddin Quereshi.

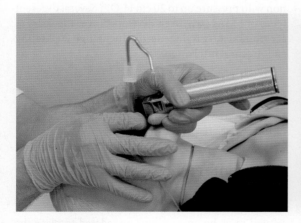

FIGURE 41–13

ETT with stylet inserted. Photo courtesy of Dr. Nadeemuddin Quereshi.

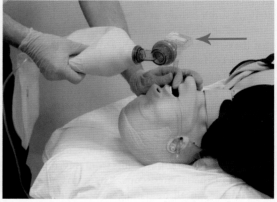

FIGURE 41–14

CO_2 detector confirms ETT placement. Photo courtesy of Dr. Nadeemuddin Quereshi.

- Direct visualization of tube passing through vocal cords.
11. Secure the tube.
12. Consider spinal immobilization to prevent extubation.
13. Reassess tube placement after each patient movement. If any doubt about placement exists, confirm by capnography or direct visualization.

Postprocedure Care

After successful intubation the biggest challenge is to maintain and secure the airway for transport. Children have smaller tracheal lengths (newborns = 4 to 5 cm and 18-month-old children = 7 to 8 cm); making dislodgement a common occurrence.[6,8] It cannot be overemphasized that the patient must be immobilized for transport, using paralytic agents if needed. Observe for chest rise, ensuring adequate tidal volume delivery and thereby reducing the incidence of hyperventilation and associated complications.

Complications

Several serious complications can develop during intubation. The most common include:

Failure to intubate.
Poor oxygenation.
Mechanical trauma.
Barotraumas.
Aspiration pneumonitis.

Inability to intubate should be addressed immediately with a rescue device to prevent hypoxic injury. Esophageal intubation is thought to be the most disastrous complication and should be recognized immediately. A sudden drop in O_2 saturation, drop in heart rate, and/or loss of measured exhaled CO_2 may mean that the ETT has become displaced or is in the esophagus. Direct visualization is the best method to determine the correct position of the ETT.

Barotrauma usually occurs secondary to large tidal volumes.[6] Utilizing the appropriate size bag while monitoring the delivered tidal volume and peak inspiratory pressure will enable the paramedic to identify any change in lung mechanics immediately.

Mechanical trauma results from improper manipulation of the laryngoscope. The gums, teeth, lips, and tongue can all be damaged, and bleed, leading to a more difficult intubation. The most important complication is permanent vocal cord damage secondary to improper insertion of the tube. ***Never force the tube through the vocal cord***. Aspiration pneu-

monitis can be minimized by applying the Sellick maneuver where cricoid pressure[9] reduces the air entry into the stomach, thereby lowering the likelihood of vomiting.

Special Considerations

Defibrillation should precede intubation in cardiac arrest situations. Limit intubation attempts in the following circumstances:

Cardiac arrest – one attempt with ETT; if unsuccessful, ventilate with a BVM.
Respiratory arrest – two attempts with ETT; if unsuccessful, ventilate with BVM.
Head trauma – one attempt with ETT; if unsuccessful, ventilate with a BVM.

Difficult Airway

The majority of children will respond to BVM ventilation and ET intubation. Inability to ventilate using a BVM and failure to intubate after three attempts classifies the procedure as a difficult airway, and rescue devices should be considered. For EMS the two most important rescue devices are the laryngeal mask airway[10] and Combitube™.[11]

LARYNGEAL MASK AIRWAY (LMA)

The LMA is an airway rescue device. It has three components: mask, airway tube, and inflation line. The LMA mask sits just above the laryngeal inlet and forms a seal. This seal allows positive-pressure ventilation with pressure up to 20 cm H_2O.[12] Several different types of LMAs have been developed over the years to accommodate varying needs, including facilitating endotracheal intubation.

Advantages

Easily placed without need of laryngoscopy.
Little cardiac effect while inserting.[10]

Disadvantages

No protection from vomiting or aspiration of gastric contents.[13]
Patient must be unconscious or sedated to place the LMA.
Not a definitive airway unless the intubation LMA is used and an ET tube can then be placed.

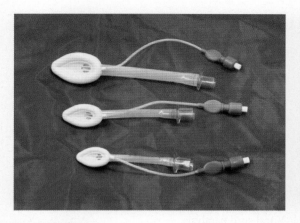

FIGURE 41–15

LMAs in different sizes. Photo courtesy of
Dr. Nadeemuddin Quereshi.

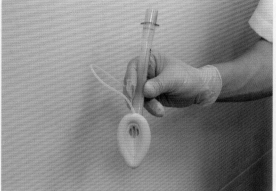

FIGURE 41–16

Checking cuff inflation. Photo courtesy of
Dr. Nadeemuddin Quereshi.

Equipment

Multiple sizes of LMA ranging from size 1 to size 7.
Usually at one end of the LMA the size and appro-
priate weight (kg) for which the given LMA can be
used are mentioned.
Lubricating gel.
Syringe 5 to 10 mL.

Placement of an LMA

1. Identify the correct size for the patient (Figure
   41-15 and Table 41-7).
2. Check cuff by inflating air (Figure 41-16).
3. Deflate the cuff and lubricate the posterior surface
   of the LMA with KY Jelly.
4. Preoxygenate the patient and place him or her in
   the "sniffing" position.
5. Hold the LMA like a pen grip, with the cuff deflated
   and the ventilating port facing down onto the
   tongue (Figure 41-17).

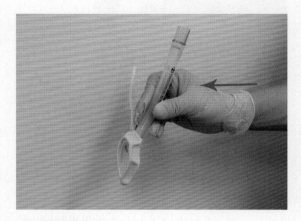

FIGURE 41–17

Cuff deflated and ready to insert using pen grip.
Photo courtesy of Dr. Nadeemuddin Quereshi.

Table 41–7	Laryngeal Mask Airway (LMA) Sizes		
LMA Size	**Age**	**Weight**	**Cuff Volume (cc)**
1	1 month	<5 kg	2–5 cc
1.5	<1 year	5–10 kg	2–5 cc
2.0	1–5 years	10–20 kg	7–10 cc
2.5	5–9 years	20–30 kg	10–14 cc
3.0	>10 years	30–50 kg	15–20 cc
4.0	>10 years	50–70 kg	25–30 cc
5.0	Adult	70–100 kg	25–30 cc
6.0	Adult	>100 kg	30 cc

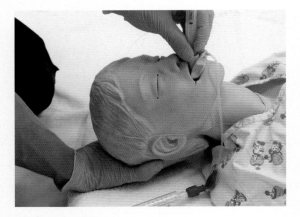

FIGURE 41–18

Using one to two fingers to guide the LMA into the oral cavity. Photo courtesy of Dr. Nadeemuddin Quereshi.

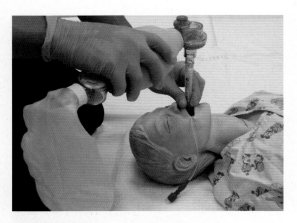

FIGURE 41–19

Postinsertion, inflate the cuff and attach to the ventilating bag. Photo courtesy of Dr. Nadeemuddin Quereshi.

6. Insert the LMA in the mouth with one or two fingers, guiding it against the palate (Figure 41-18).
7. Once you reach a point of resistance, inflate the cuff.
8. The LMA should seat itself on the glottis. Attach the end to a bag and start bagging the patient through the LMA (Figure 41-19).
9. Observe the chest rise and auscultate for breath sounds. Monitor heart rate and saturations.

Limitations

Contraindicated in an infant or child with an intact gag reflex.

Main disadvantage: not protective of the airway from regurgitated gastric contents.
Does not allow for administration of resuscitation medications.
May be more difficult than ETT to maintain during patient movement, and careful attention is required to make sure proper positioning is maintained.

Complications of LMA Placement

Coughing/bronchospasm.
Aspiration/regurgitation.
Trauma.
Lingual nerve palsy.
Vocal cord paralysis.
Hoarseness.
Stridor.
Pharyngeal or mouth ulcers.

COMBITUBE™

A Combitube™ is a combination of two tubes into one, as the name implies. It comes in two sizes and can be used in children who are at least 4 feet (120 cm) long. The large bulb is made of latex and therefore should not be used in patients with a latex allergy (Figure 41-20).

Indications

Patients with difficult airway problems and failed intubations.[14]
Patient must be >4 feet (120 cm), ≤7 feet (2 meters) in height.
Unconscious patient.

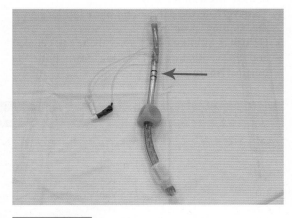

FIGURE 41–20

Combitube™. The black lines indicate the point of maximum tube insertion. Photo courtesy of Dr. Nadeemuddin Quereshi.

Contraindications

Esophageal varices.
Ingestion of caustic substances.

Procedure

1. Preoxygenate the patient.
2. Check both balloons.
3. Prepare and lubricate the tube.
4. Blindly insert the tube into the oropharynx till the incisors lie between the black marks on the proximal part of the tube (Figures 41-21, 41-22, and 41-23).
5. Inflate both balloons with the blue cuff with 100 cc of air, and the balloon with the white cuff with 15 cc of air (Figure 41-24A, 24B). (Helpful hint: "<u>B</u>lue = <u>b</u>ig tube").

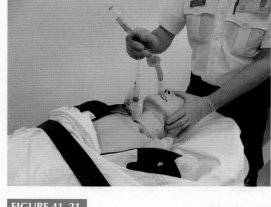

FIGURE 41–21

Insertion of the Combitube™. Photo courtesy of Dr. Nadeemuddin Quereshi.

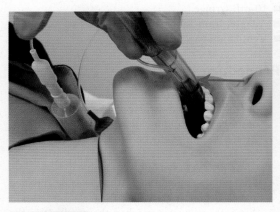

FIGURE 41–22

Black lines should be in between the central incisors. Photo courtesy of Dr. Nadeemuddin Quereshi.

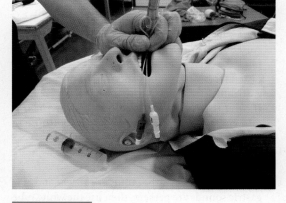

FIGURE 41–23

Combitube™ placed. Photo courtesy of Dr. Nadeemuddin Quereshi.

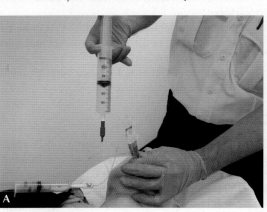

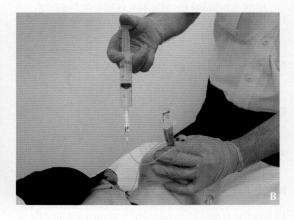

FIGURE 41–24

A, Blue balloon inflation, and **B**, white balloon inflation. Photos courtesy of Dr. Nadeemuddin Quereshi.

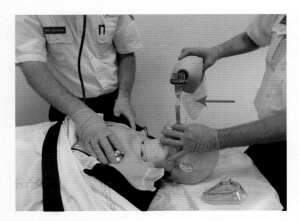

FIGURE 41–25

Ventilate through the blue tube and auscultate for breath sounds. Photo courtesy of Dr. Nadeemuddin Quereshi.

6. Start bagging using the blue tube (Figure 41-25). Auscultate for breath sounds.
7. Look for chest rise.
8. Listen for breath sounds and sounds over the epigastrium.
9. *If chest rise is positive, breath sounds are heard, and epigastric sounds are negative, continue to ventilate through the larger blue tube.*
10. In this case the white tube can be used to aspirate stomach contents.
11. If chest rise and breath sounds are absent and epigastric sounds are present, then use the white tube to ventilate the patient and assess for breath sounds and epigastric sounds. If breath sounds are present and epigastric sounds absent, you have intubated the trachea; continue bagging.
12. Confirm tube placement by using an end-tidal CO_2 detector.
13. Secure the tube.
14. Monitor vital signs, saturations, and capnograph reading.

Complications

Local damage to pharyngeal tissue due to mechanics of the device.

NEEDLE CRICOTHYROTOMY

This is the simplest surgical airway using a needle to enter the trachea and then ventilate the patient through the needle.[15]

Indications

Inability to intubate because of secondary trauma, foreign body, upper airway obstruction, or congenital deformity restricting endotracheal intubation.[16,17]

Use in children under 10 to 12 years of age in whom creating a surgical airway is technically difficult.

Contraindications

No absolute contraindications, as patient may die if this procedure is not accomplished. It may be difficult to perform in cases of neck injury.[18]

Equipment

- Gloves.
- 12- to 18-gauge Angiocath or intravenous catheter.
- 10-mL syringe.
- Adapter from 3.0 ET tube.
- Ventilation bag.

Procedure

1. Identify cricothyroid membrane; the inferior border of the thyroid cartilage is the superior border of the cricothyroid membrane.
2. Attach a syringe one half to three quarters filled with saline to a 12- to 14-gauge Angiocath.
3. Clean area with Betadine if possible.
4. Puncture the membrane with the needle, directed at a 45-degree angle toward the feet.
5. Aspirate as you enter; when the needle is in the trachea, bubbles should appear in the syringe.
6. Remove syringe.
7. Remove needle from Angiocath and advance the catheter.
8. Attach the adapter from the ET tube to the catheter.
9. Connect the bag to the ET tube adapter and start bagging the patient.
10. Have a team member hold the catheter to avoid kinking and dislodgement.

Complications

Complication rates are high (up to 40%).[17,18] Tracheal puncture can lead to subcutaneous emphysema. Puncture of vessels can lead to bleeding, and poor sterile technique will lead to infection.[18] The age limit is not clear; however, this procedure may be performed on children 8 years old and above.

Several case reports suggest that transtracheal jet ventilation, now *percutaneous translaryngeal ventila-*

tion (PTLV), may help in difficult or failed intubations. In patients in whom intubation has failed, PTLV was performed to obtain an airway. Once PTLV was introduced, intubating patients became easier. The high intratracheal pressure from PTLV seemed to lift the epiglottis and open the glottis, allowing visualization of the vocal cords and making intubation easier.[17,19]

TRACHEOSTOMY CHANGE

Tracheostomy tubes (TTs) are commonly used to support respiratory function in different primary and secondary respiratory disorders. TTs are available in different sizes. The most important characteristic is the inner and outer diameter of the TT, cuffed or uncuffed, and length, so that an equivalent can be identified and replaced if needed. Tracheostomy tubes can obstruct acutely and trigger sudden respiratory distress leading to arrest.[18]

Indications

Presence of a tracheostomy site.
Sudden onset of respiratory distress.
Tracheostomy tube dislodged.
Inability to oxygenate and/or ventilate.
Thick copious secretions.

Equipment

■ Tracheostomy tubes.
■ Multiple sizes. (When changing, confirm the outer diameter and inner diameter in addition to the tube size; Figure 41-26.).
■ Lubricant gel.

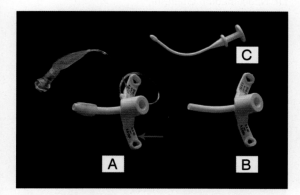

FIGURE 41–26

Tracheostomy tubes: **A**, Cuffed versus **B**, uncuffed. **C**, Obturator. Arrow points to writing indicating the size of the TT. Photo courtesy of Dr. Nadeemudin Quereshi.

Procedure

1. The most important thing is to have all airway equipment (including failed airway equipment) prepared to perform any intervention required during TT change.
2. Have available one smaller and one larger TT.
3. Lubricate the tube.
4. Extend the patient's neck to expose the TT.
5. Cut the TT straps.
6. Deflate the cuff if needed.
7. Remove the TT.
8. Insert the new TT.
9. Confirm placement by bagging and observing for chest rise.
10. If resistance is met, remove the tube and try with a smaller size. Alternatively, insert a small suction catheter into the stoma as a "stylet" and thread the ET tube over the catheter.
11. **Do not change a new TT if tube is <2 weeks old because false passage may result.**

Complications

Infections.
False track (especially if TT is <2 weeks old).
Cricoid stenosis.

CERVICAL SPINE IMMOBILIZATION

Cervical spine injuries are uncommon in children. Children with blunt trauma, accidents, or diving injuries are prone to have cervical spine injury.[20] These patients need to have their spine completely immobilized pending evaluation. Patients with an altered level of consciousness after injury also should have their spine immobilized.[21]

Indications

Any patient with a mechanism of cervical spine injury from blunt trauma, accidents, or diving (excluding isolated extremity injuries), should be evaluated for application of spinal immobilization.

Patients with an altered level of consciousness after injury should also be evaluated.

Equipment

■ Rigid backboard or other immobilization device.
■ Cervical collar (Figure 41-27).

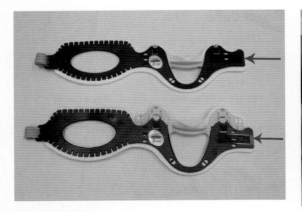

FIGURE 41–27

Cervical collar that is adjustable (arrows) to different pediatric sizes. Photo courtesy of Dr. Nadeemuddin Quereshi.

- Lateral cervical immobilization devices.
- Back board straps.
- Tape.

Procedure

1. Hold the patient's head and neck in a neutral position and maintain this throughout application of the collar (Figure 41-28).
2. Assess sensory and motor function of all extremities before and after collar application.
3. While one provider holds the patient in a neutral position, the second provider applies the collar (Figure 41-29, Figure 41-30, and Figure 41-31).
4. Place the patient on a spinal immobilization device with as little movement as possible (Figure 41-32).
5. Use towel rolls, foam head blocks, or equipment to immobilize the head so that no lateral movement occurs (Figures 41-33 and 41-34).
6. Secure the patient's head to the board at the forehead and chin (Figure 41-35).
7. Similarly immobilize the chest, hips, and knees to prevent any movement (Figures 41-36 and 41-37).
8. Recheck sensory and motor function of all extremities.
9. After complete body immobilization, the patient is ready for transport (Figure 41-38).

Complications

The major risk is damage to the spinal cord. Excessive neck movement can convert a subtle fracture into a

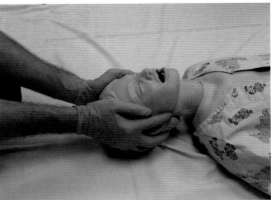

FIGURE 41–28

Head and neck in neutral position. Photo courtesy of Dr. Nadeemuddin Quereshi.

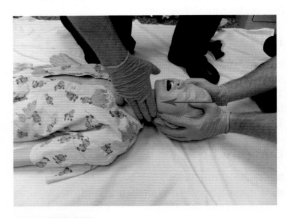

FIGURE 41–29

Measuring collar size. Photo courtesy of Dr. Nadeemuddin Quereshi.

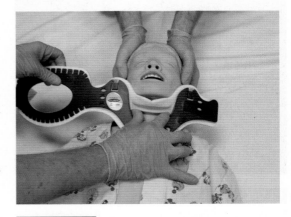

FIGURE 41–30

Collar application. Photo courtesy of Dr. Nadeemuddin Quereshi.

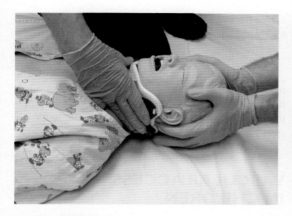

FIGURE 41–31

Collar application view 2. Photo courtesy of
Dr. Nadeemuddin Quereshi.

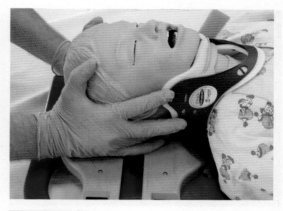

FIGURE 41–32

Placement on head board. Photo courtesy of
Dr. Nadeemuddin Quereshi.

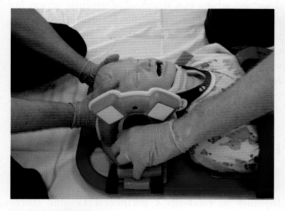

FIGURE 41–33

Head block applied to prevent lateral head movement.
Photo courtesy of Dr. Nadeemuddin Quereshi.

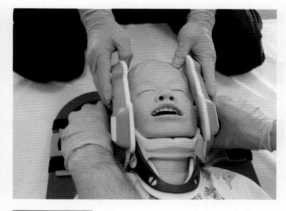

FIGURE 41–34

Head block to prevent head movement view 2. Photo
courtesy of Dr. Nadeemuddin Quereshi.

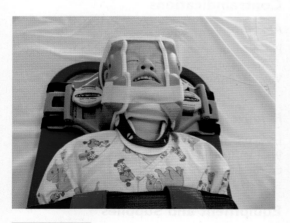

FIGURE 41–35

Securing forehead and chin. Photo courtesy of
Dr. Nadeemuddin Quereshi.

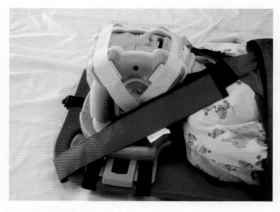

FIGURE 41–36

Shoulder strap applied to restrict any upper torso movement. Photo courtesy of Dr. Nadeemuddin Quereshi.

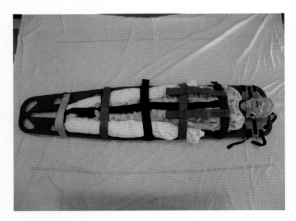

FIGURE 41–37

Immobilization of chest, hips, and legs. Photo courtesy of Dr. Nadeemuddin Quereshi.

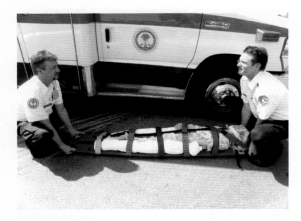

FIGURE 41–38

Ready for transport after complete body immobilization. Photo courtesy of Dr. Nadeemuddin Quereshi.

significant spinal cord injury with neurologic deficits. The other complication of immobilization is a circulatory or airway compromise. EMS providers should assess for these at frequent intervals. If patients vomit, logroll them on one side to prevent aspiration.

Special Considerations

Spinal immobilization can be omitted provided the following are documented:[20,22]

1. Mechanism of injury is not significant.
2. Neurologic examination is appropriate for age.
3. Patient is alert, oriented, and cooperative.
4. No neck, spinal, or upper back pain with active movement.

5. No neck or spinal tenderness elicited on palpation.
6. No distracting injuries or debilitating emotional conditions.

It is extremely important to document the neurologic examination before and after the application of immobilization, and in cases omitting immobilization, the reasons for this decision should be clearly stated.

VASCULAR ACCESS IN CHILDREN

Intraosseous (IO) Needle Placement

IO access has gained widespread acceptance in children and adults as a first line of vascular access for resuscitation.[23] Placing peripheral intravenous catheters may require time and present difficulty during circulatory shutdown.[24] Intraosseous administration of resuscitation medications and fluids in preterm and term neonates is an alternative when routine intravascular access is difficult.[25] For more detailed discussion of IO access, see Chapter 23, Parenteral Access.

Indications

A life-threatening event requiring fluid and medications immediately.
Inability to establish a peripheral IV line (three attempts or 90 seconds).
First-line approach for pediatric cardiac arrest.

Contraindications

Absolute

Potential insertion site with possible fracture (<6 weeks ago).
Vascular disruption to insertion site.

Relative

Local infection or burn over the site.
Prior IO attempt in the same bone.
Osteogenesis imperfecta.

Equipment and Supplies

■ IO needle (Figure 41-39).
■ Betadine swabs.

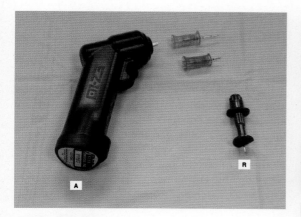

FIGURE 41–39

Commonly used intraosseous needles. A, = **EZ-10®** power operated; **B,** = Manual IO. Photo courtesy of Dr. Nadeemuddin Quereshi.

■ 5- to 10-mL syringe with saline flush.
■ IV tubing with three-way stopcock.
■ 4×4 gauze pads and tape.

Patient Preparation, Positioning, and Anatomic Landmarks

Place the patient in the supine position. Identify the IO site. The preferred sites are the proximal tibia, medial malleolus, or distal femur.

Procedure

1. Expose the lower leg.
2. Clean with Betadine.
3. Palpate the tibial tubercle (bony prominence below the kneecap) on the proximal tibia; 1 to 2 cm (two finger widths) below this is the insertion site (Figure 41-40).
4. Hold the IO needle perpendicular to the skin. Enter the skin gently until you reach the bony surface. Twist the needle handle with a grinding motion, applying a controlled downward force until a "pop" or "give" is felt indicating loss of resistance (Figure 41-41).
5. Remove the trochar, flush with saline, and aspirate the marrow (this may or may not be possible).
6. Attach the IV line tubing to the IO catheter (Figure 41-42).
7. Flush the line to make sure there is no resistance or fluid extravasation (Figure 41-43).
8. Secure the IO with 4×4 pads and tape.

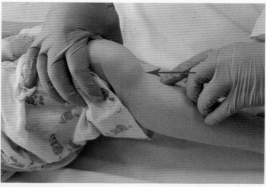

FIGURE 41–40

Identifying landmarks 2 cm below tibial tuberosity. Photo courtesy of Dr. Nadeemuddin Quereshi.

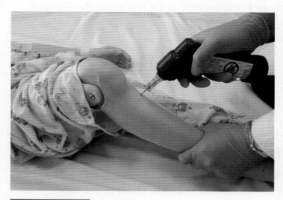

FIGURE 41–41

Under aseptic technique, hold the leg firmly and aim away from the growth plate. Photo courtesy of Dr. Nadeemuddin Quereshi.

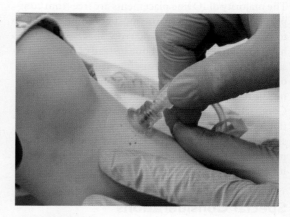

FIGURE 41–42

IV tubing attached. Photo courtesy of Dr. Nadeemuddin Quereshi.

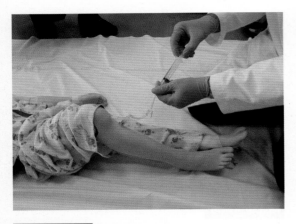

FIGURE 41–43

Bone marrow aspirate and flush using normal saline flush. Photo courtesy of Dr. Nadeemuddin Quereshi.

9. Placement is confirmed by the needle standing without support, bone marrow contents aspiration, and free flow of fluid.
10. Medications and fluids are delivered by either syringe push or via pressure bag.

Postprocedure Care

Secure the line well, as foot movement during transport can displace the IO line. Observe for subcutaneous fluid collection or the child crying when pushing fluids, indicating displacement or soft-tissue infiltration.

Complications

The majority of IO line placements are free from complications.[23,25] However, the most common is failure to place the needle in the marrow space. When this happens, move to another bone instead of trying in the same bone. Infections ranging from cellulitis to osteomyelitis can occur. The risk increases if the IO needle has been left in place for more than 24 hours.[25] Compartment syndrome can develop from extravasation of fluid into soft tissues. Therefore insertion sites should be examined periodically even hours after the procedure. Fracture of the bone has been reported in infants.

Special Considerations

Limit the IO attempts in each bone to two.
Gravity alone may not result in adequate flow of fluids through an IO device.

VENOUS ACCESS: EXTERNAL JUGULAR ACCESS

Intravenous access in children is one of the most challenging tasks.[26] To ensure blood sampling, drug delivery, and fluid resuscitation a reliable vascular access is needed. Most common sites used are antecubital, the dorsum of the hand, the scalp veins, the saphenous veins, and the external jugular vein. The external jugular vein has a low risk for pneumothorax or carotid injury and is safe in a child with coagulopathy. For more discussion of IV access, see Chapter 23, Parenteral Access.

Indications

In a critically ill patient requiring intravenous access for fluid or medication administration.
    Difficult IV access.

Equipment

- IV catheters 22 French.
- Saline flush.
- 5 cc syringe.

Procedure

1. Place the patient in a supine or Trendelenburg position. Tilt the patient's head toward the opposite (contralateral) side.
2. Identify the external jugular vein. It may dilate and be better seen with finger pressure on the upper surface of the clavicle or by pushing over the liver (hepato-jugular reflux).
3. Clean the area with Betadine.
4. Align the catheter with the vein and aim toward the clavicle.
5. Lightly place a finger just above the clavicle to produce a "tourniqueting" effect.
6. Puncture the vein midway between the angle of the jaw and the clavicle, and insert the cannula.
7. Remove the needle and check for blood flashback.
8. The vein tends to collapse easily. Do not attempt to withdraw a large amount of blood.
9. Secure the catheter and attach an IV line.
10. Flush the line to check for patency.

Postprocedure Care

Due to its anatomy, the external jugular vein is easily obstructed. Therefore maintaining a certain angle to ensure an uninterrupted flow is essential. Secure the line and immobilize the neck at an appropriate angle so the catheter does not kink.

Complications

Low incidence of pneumothorax and blood vessel damage.

AIRWAY FOREIGN BODY

A foreign body obstructing the airway is a life-threatening emergency. Utmost care is required when managing these patients. Management depends on the degree of obstruction and the clinical scenario associated with it.[27] A patient with a partial airway obstruction who is able to maintain ventilations and good O_2 saturation can be monitored and transferred to a nearby medical facility for foreign body removal in a more controlled environment. Patients with a complete obstruction need to have the foreign body removed immediately on site.

Equipment

1. Magill forceps (Figure 41-44).
2. Laryngoscopes.
3. Suction devices.
4. Airway supplies (bag, mask, tracheal tubes).
5. Surgical airway supplies (Angiocath with ETT adapter).

Procedure

1. Open the mouth and insert the laryngoscope.
2. Visualize the foreign body (Figure 41-45).
3. If the EMS provider is unable to see it, have an assistant give abdominal thrusts to bring the object into view.
4. After visualization, grasp it with the Magill forceps and remove it (Figure 41-46 and Figure 41-47).
5. If the object causing the obstruction is slippery, use suction or other tool.
6. If you are unable to visualize the foreign body, start BMV ventilation.
7. Pass the ET tube to establish the airway, and begin ventilation.
8. If you are unable to pass the ET tube, perform a surgical airway.
9. Establish the airway regardless of whether or not the foreign body removal is accomplished and before transferring the patient.

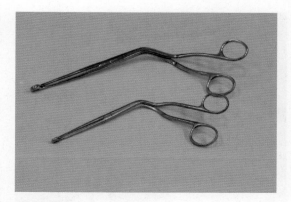

FIGURE 41–44

Magill forceps. Photo courtesy of Dr. Nadeemuddin Quereshi.

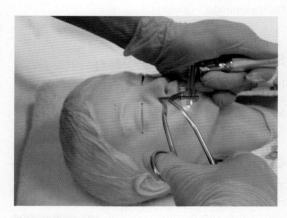

FIGURE 41–45

Laryngoscope visualization. Photo courtesy of Dr. Nadeemuddin Quereshi.

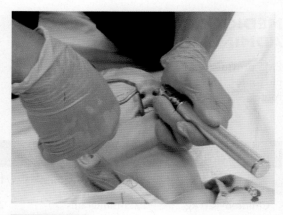

FIGURE 41–46

Insertion of Magill forceps. Photo courtesy of Dr. Nadeemuddin Quereshi.

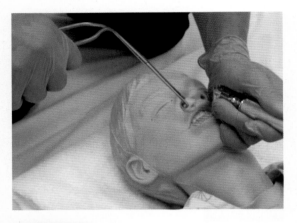

FIGURE 41–47

Removal of foreign body. Photo courtesy of Dr. Nadeemuddin Quereshi.

Special Considerations

In children with a foreign body obstruction first attempt BLS maneuvers (back blows & chest thrusts for a child <1-yr old or reverse Heimlich maneuver for a child >1-year old).

Complications

These methods should be reserved for unconscious patients with complete airway obstruction. Partial obstruction can become complete any time during transport or when attempting to remove a foreign body. Delay in diagnosis results in a significant increase in perioperative morbidity.[27]

MEDICATION ADMINISTRATION

EMS providers can deliver lifesaving drugs via multiple routes. These can be via IV, IO, ET, or nebulizer routes.

Nebulizer

The commonest nebulized medications used in children are bronchodilators. Multiple factors determine what amount of nebulized drug will reach the functional end point. These factors include minute ventilation (tidal volume X respiratory rate) of the patient, lung compliance, dose of the medication, duration of nebulization (time), and position of the apparatus delivering the drug. Therefore monitoring the therapeutic and side effects of the drugs is important, as administering the same dose may have a different range of effects in different children (Table 41-8). For more discussion, see Chapter 22, Airway and Respiratory Management.

Indications

Asthma exacerbation.
Croup.
Bronchospasm secondary to infections, drug side effects.

Contraindications

Children with poor respiratory effort.

Equipment

- Nebulizer machine.
- Face mask/mouthpiece with tubing.
- Nebulizing medication solutions.
- Reservoir for medication delivery.

Procedure

1. Prepare the nebulizing medication (correct dose per weight) and place it in the reservoir well of the nebulizer.
2. Connect the nebulizer to the O_2 source at 4 to 6 L per minute or adequate flow to produce a steady, visible mist.
3. Instruct the patient to inhale through the mouthpiece of the nebulizer. There needs to be a good seal around the mouthpiece. (Figure 41-48 and Figure 41-49).

Table 41–8	**Dosage Guidelines**		
	Albuterol (Ventolin™)	**Ipratropium (Atrovent™)**	**Racemic Epinephrine**
Children <20 kg	2.5 milligrams	250 micrograms	0.5 mL in 2 mL NS
Children >20 kg	5.0 milligrams	500 micrograms	1.0 mL in 2 mL NS

NS = Normal Saline.

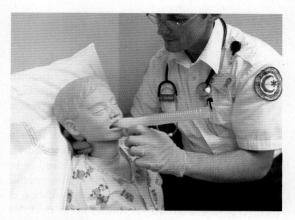

FIGURE 41–48

Nebulization using mouthpiece. Photo courtesy of
Dr. Nadeemuddin Quereshi.

4. The treatment should last until the solution is depleted.
5. Tapping the reservoir well near the end of the treatment will assist in utilizing all of the solution.
6. Monitor the patient for medication effects and change in condition.
7. Reassess the patient's vital signs, breath sounds, and presentation to determine the need for additional treatments.
8. Assess and document patient's respiratory effort before and after the treatment.
9. Document the treatment, dose, and route.

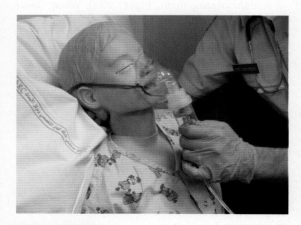

FIGURE 41–49

Nebulization via face mask. Photo courtesy of
Dr. Nadeemuddin Quereshi.

Complications

1. Medication overdose or underdose due to dosage error. Nebulizing time is essential to ensure adequate drug delivery, (e.g. Ventolin nebulization over 5 minutes will result in insufficient drug delivery.) Most nebulized medications need 15 to 20 minutes of nebulizing time for adequate dose delivery.
2. Profound side effects of given nebulized medications. This will limit the treatment options; (e.g. tachycardia due to albuterol may increase the work of breathing in a child with congenital heart disease).

Endotracheal Drug Delivery

The ET tube is an alternative route for four major resuscitation drugs.[26]

L: lidocaine.
A: atropine.
N: Narcan (naloxone).
E: Epinephrine.
ET dosages for L, A, and N are two to three times the IV or IO dosage.
The ET dosage of epinephrine is 10 times the IV or IO dosage.
Epinephrine 0.1 mg/kg of 1:1000 concentration (0.1 mL/kg) is given via ET tube.
Mix with 2 to 3 mL of normal saline to deliver at least 2 mL of liquid volume.

Indications

Administration of medications during resuscitation when vascular access is unavailable.

Contraindications

ET tube placement not confirmed.

Procedure

1. Confirm tube placement.
2. Prepare medication. Dosage needs to be 2 to 2.5 times the IV dose (excluding epinephrine).
3. Prepare a 10-mL normal saline flush to follow medication delivery administration.
4. Oxygenate and hyperventilate the patient.
5. Disconnect ventilation device from ET tube.
6. Inject the medication into the ET tube followed by the normal saline flush.
7. Reconnect the ventilation device.

8. Resume ventilation to circulate the given medication.
9. Monitor the patient for therapeutic and side effects.
10. Document the medication, dose, route, time, and patient response.

NASAL ACCESS

Recently greater interest has developed in this route, especially when treating status epilepticus patients. Intravenous access is difficult in a seizing patient and IO and ET tubes may not be required once the seizing stops. Multiple studies have shown intranasal midazolam (0.1 to 0.2 mg/kg dose) to effectively terminate seizures, and soon it may be considered as the first line of therapy in the prehospital setting. For more detailed discussion, see Chapter 23, Parenteral Access.

Indications

Status epilepticus.
Combative patients.
Difficult IV access.

Equipment

■ Medication dose.
■ Syringe.

Procedure

1. Prepare medication.
2. Explain the procedure to the patient.
3. Have the patient lie down supine with the head slightly extended.
4. Insert the medication into the nostril, aiming toward the septum.
5. Do not allow the patient to blow their nose after administration of the drug.
6. Keep the patient in the supine position for 15 to 20 minutes.
7. Monitor the patient for therapeutic and side effects.
8. Document the medication, dose, route, time, and patient's response.

Complication

Inadequate drug delivery and/or absorption resulting in suboptimal clinical effect.

PAIN MANAGEMENT IN CHILDREN

Pain is the leading cause for seeking emergency medical care services. Twenty percent of prehospital patients report moderate or severe pain. Pain has been termed "the fifth vital sign" after receiving increased attention from the Joint Commission on Accreditation of Health Care Organizations (JCAHO). In an attempt to improve pain management, protocols that address and treat pain in the prehospital setting need to be developed. These protocols should contain reliable assessment tools to measure pain, documentation of pain severity, and available medications to treat this pain, including side effects.[28].

Pain Assessment and Management

Indications

Children with pain.

Procedure

1. On initial patient assessment document pain severity along with a set of vital signs.
2. Document pain severity using a pain scale, such as.
   Visual analog scale (VAS): a 100-mm line with "no pain" at the beginning and "worst pain" at the end.
   Numeric rating scale (NRS): patients rate their pain with numbers, from no pain (0) to worst pain (10 or 100).
   Wong-Baker "faces" scale: this scale is used primarily in pediatric patients. The faces correspond to numeric values from 0 to 10. (see Chapter 39 Pain Management, Figure 39–1 Wong-Baker FACES Pain Rating Scale).
3. Treatment indications.
4. Select the appropriate drugs.
5. Measure vital signs pre- and postdrug delivery.
6. Document pre- and postdrug change in pain scale.
7. Monitor patient throughout the transport.

DRUG REGIMENS

Morphine

■ Analgesia.
■ Dose: 0.1 milligram/kg IV.
■ Onset: 5 to 10 minutes.
■ Duration: 3 to 4 hours.
■ Complications: respiratory depression, hypotension.
■ Acts synergistically with benzodiazepines.

Fentanyl

- Analgesia (more potent than morphine).
- Dose: 2 to 3 micrograms/kg IV, as slow IV bolus over 30-60 secs.
- Onset: 2 minutes.
- Duration: 30 minutes.
- Complications: respiratory depression, rigid chest, hypotension.
- Acts synergistically with benzodiazepines and together may cause significant respiratory compromise.

Nitrous Oxide

- Dissociative, euphoric, sedative; needs a specific scavenger for elimination.
- Onset: 1 to 2 minutes.
- Initial dose: 30 to 50% mixture with O_2.
- Administration: self-administered.
- Contraindications: pneumothorax, eye injuries, obstructed viscus.
- Complications: methemoglobinemia, hypoxia secondary to oxygen displacement, pulmonary toxicity due to nitrogen dioxide.

Ketamine

- Amnestic, analgesic, dissociative sedative, general anesthesia.
- Dose: 1 milligram/kg IV, IM 4 milligrams/kg, PO 6 to 8 milligrams/kg.
- Onset: 1 to 5 minutes IV/IM, 45 minutes PO.
- Duration: IV: 10 minutes; IM: 20 to 30 minutes.
- Complications: Laryngospasm, increased intracranial pressure (ICP) and intraocular pressure (IOP), hypertension, hallucinations/emergence reactions, increased salivation.
- Relative contraindications: Head injury, increased intraocular or intracerebral pressure, psychosis, age ≤3 months old

Nonsteroidal Antiinflammatory Drugs

Ketorolac can be administered IV (0.5 mg/kg up to 15 mg) or IM (1.0 mg/kg up to 30 mg).

Antagonist Agents

Naloxone (Narcan)

- Dose: .01–0.1 milligrams/kg.
- Indicated for reversal of narcotic agents.
- May result in agitation.

- Titrate reversal slowly to avoid tachycardia, hypertension, arrhythmias, and abrupt loss of sedation.

Special Considerations

1. Common painful ED procedures.
2. "Needlestick phobia" is an important consideration in the pediatric population. Every attempt should be made to minimize the pain associated with blood draws, intravenous line placement, lumbar puncture, and laceration repair. The following medications may help achieve this task.

Topical Analgesia

LET (lidocaine, epinephrine, and tetracaine):

- Lidocaine 4% gel, epinephrine 1:2000, tetracaine 0.5%.
- Good for superficial lacerations on face/scalp.
- Do not use on less vascular areas.

EMLA™ (eutectic mixture of lidocaine and prilocaine):

- 2.5% lidocaine.
- 2.5% prilocaine.
- Useful for painful procedures on intact skin.
- Must apply 60 minutes before procedure.

ELA-Max™ (similar to EMLA)

- 4% liposomal lidocaine.
- 30 minutes' application only.
- No occlusive dressing required.
- Useful in reducing venipuncture-related pain.

Infiltrative Analgesia

Lidocaine

- Maximum dose: 4 to 5 mg/kg without epinephrine; 7 mg/kg with epinephrine.
- Do not use epinephrine on distal extremity, nose, penis, or pinna of the ear.

Bupivacaine

- Maximum dose: 2 to 3 mg/kg.
- Four times more potent than lidocaine.
- Duration up to 7 hours with epinephrine.

NEWBORN PAIN MANAGEMENT

It was not too long ago that newborns were considered a "pain-free species". The concept of newborns possessing an immature neuroendocrine mechanism which fails to register painful stimuli has undergone a major transformation. Today various studies have demonstrated the need and benefit for adequate pain control in neonates undergoing painful procedures such as lumbar puncture, intravenous catheter placement, circumcision, and heelstick blood draws.

Pain scales for preterm and term neonates have been developed and use physiologic indicators (such as heart rate, respiratory rate, oxygen saturation, plasma cortisol or catecholamine levels, palmar sweating, and blood pressure) and behavioral changes (such as crying, body position, and facial expression).

- The Premature Infant Pain Profile (PIPP) uses physiologic indicators and facial expressions to evaluate pain.
- The Neonatal Infant Pain Scale (NIPS) uses crying, arm and leg movements, state of arousal, crying, and facial expressions.

- The CRIES scale specifically addresses **C**rying, **R**equirement for oxygen supplementation for Sa_{O_2} <95%, **I**ncreases in blood pressure and heart rate, facial **E**xpression, and **S**leeplessness. Other signs of pain include pallor, flushing, diaphoresis, dilated pupils, hyperglycemia, alterations in sleep and wakeful states, fussiness or listlessness, limb withdrawal, and arching or thrashing movements.

Table 41-9 provides an outline for therapies available to reduce pain in newborns.

Monitoring and Continued Assessment

Once the pain management strategy is decided, it is vital to continue frequent reassessment of the patient. The prehospital treatment form should document any change in patient status. Any clinical or technical problems encountered when administering the

Table 41–9	Pain Control Combination Therapies for Common Neonatal Procedures
Procedure	**Suggested therapy**
Heel lance	**Consider venipuncture** Sucrose pacifier Kangaroo care/swaddling
Percutaneous venous catheter	**Sucrose pacifier** Kangaroo care/swaddling EMLA™
Lumbar puncture	**Sucrose pacifier** EMLA™ Subcutaneous lidocaine infiltration
Subcutaneous or intramuscular injection	**Use IV medication if possible** Sucrose pacifier Kangaroo care/swaddling EMLA™
Umbilical catheter insertion	**Sucrose pacifier** Swaddling
Nasogastric or orogastric tube placement	**Sucrose pacifier** Kangaroo care/swaddling
Catheterization for urinalysis	**Sucrose pacifier** Swaddling

EMLA™ = eutectic mixture of lidocaine and prilocaine.

medication should be accurately documented. For patient safety it is important to monitor the level of sedation, pain control, and changes in vital signs. This is particularly important after drug administration as the majority of these agents can produce respiratory or hemodynamic changes.[29,30]

SPLINTING EXTREMITIES

An injured extremity needs to be immobilized so that secondary damage is prevented. Splints are created to immobilize extremities for this reason. Multiple different splints are available, although their function is the same. For more discussion, see Chapter 32, Extremity Splinting and Care of Open Fractures.

Indications

Immobilize injured extremity.

Equipment

- Cotton cast roll.
- Splint materials:
    - Fiberglass.
    - Traction splint (see lower extremities procedures).
    - Vacuum splint (see upper extremities procedures).
    - Preformed metal/plastic splint.
    - Bandage rolls.
    - Sling.

General Procedures

1. Expose the extremity: Expose the affected side and mark the potential site.
2. Assess for pulses, sensation, and motor function (neurovascular status).
3. If extremity is pulseless, perform gentle reduction prior to splinting.
4. Measure the splint size on the normal side and configure the splint to the same size.
5. Apply the splint proximal and distal to the area of injury. Do not secure the splinting device directly over the injury.
6. Secure the splint with Velcro or straps, depending on type of splint used.
7. Reassess neurovascular status of the extremity (pulse, sensory, motor), and if there is any worsening, remove the splint and reevaluate.

8. These procedures need to be followed for any extremity injury.

Procedure for Closed Femur Fracture using traction splint (Figure 41-50)

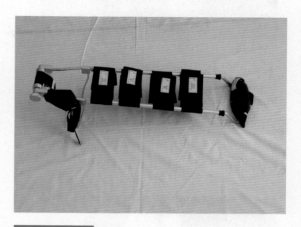

FIGURE 41–50

Traction splint. Photo courtesy of Dr. Nadeemuddin Quereshi.

1. Expose the extremity.
2. Mark the approximate fracture site (Figure 41-51).
3. Assess neurovascular status.
4. The EMS provider holds and applies manual traction in line until the patient feels some relief (Figure 41-52).
5. Place the ankle device and continue traction (Figure 41-53).
6. Measure the traction splint by using the uninjured leg and pull splint out approximately 4 to 6 inches past the foot and lock in place.
7. Place the proximal end of the traction splint under the patient's buttock on the injured side being careful to avoid any open wounds or placing too much pressure on the genitalia (Figure 41-54).
8. The extremity should rest on the support bands (Figure 41-55).
9. Secure the splint with the straps provided.
10. Attach the ankle device to the traction crank and slowly crank until resistance is met. Secure the support bands to the patient's leg, avoiding the injured area, knee, and ankle (Figure 41-56).
11. Reassess neurovascular status (pulses, sensation, and motor function). If there is any change of these parameters, release the traction and reevaluate.

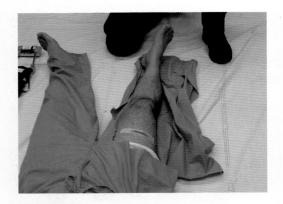

FIGURE 41–51

Expose the affected side and mark the potential site (leg). Photo courtesy of Dr. Nadeemuddin Quereshi.

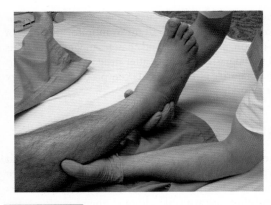

FIGURE 41–52

Apply manual traction before and after feeling the pulse. Photo courtesy of Dr. Nadeemuddin Quereshi.

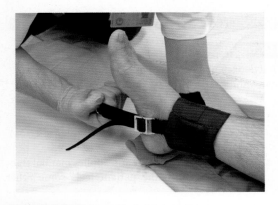

FIGURE 41–53

Using ankle hook, keep the traction on the extremity. Photo courtesy of Dr. Nadeemuddin Quereshi.

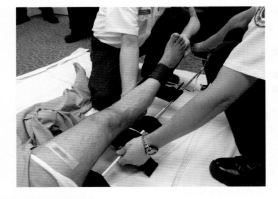

FIGURE 41–54

Application of the traction splint. Photo courtesy of Dr. Nadeemuddin Quereshi.

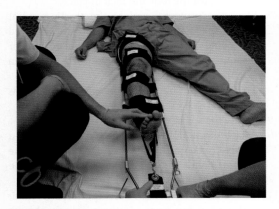

FIGURE 41–55

Limb immobilized and traction applied. Photo courtesy of Dr. Nadeemuddin Quereshi.

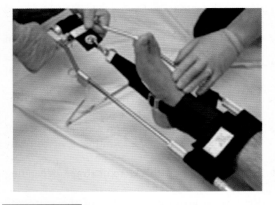

FIGURE 41–56

Pulley adjusted to deliver the right amount of traction. Photo courtesy of Dr. Nadeemuddin Quereshi.

Procedures for upper extremity using a vacuum splint.

1. A vacuum splint is one type of splint that may be used (Figure 41-57).
2. Expose the extremity.
3. Mark the approximate fracture site (Figure 41-58).
4. Assess neurovascular status.

5. Secure the splint with the straps provided. (Figure 41-59).
6. Air is pumped to ensure a rigid immobilization (Figure 41-60).
7. As in any splinting procedure, reassess neurovascular status of the extremity (pulse, sensory, motor), and if there is any worsening, remove the splint and reevaluate.

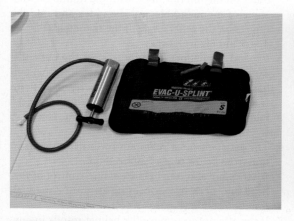

FIGURE 41–57

Vacuum splint. Photo courtesy of Dr. Nadeemuddin Quereshi.

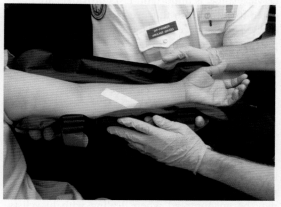

FIGURE 41–58

Expose the extremity and mark the affected site (forearm). Photo courtesy of Dr. Nadeemuddin Quereshi.

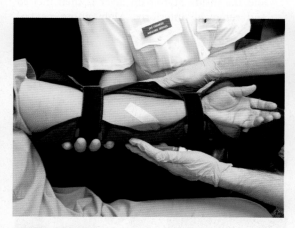

FIGURE 41–59

Splint applied. Photo courtesy of Dr. Nadeemuddin Quereshi.

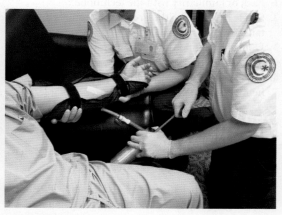

FIGURE 41–60

Air pumped to ensure a rigid immobilization. Photo courtesy of Dr. Nadeemuddin Quereshi.

HELMET REMOVAL

Helmets are being used today as a protective device in many sports and military activities. The objective is to protect an individual's head against high-velocity impact or injury. EMS providers might deal with those individuals during any stage of illness or injury where removal of the helmet is essential to complete their assessment and or management. Understanding the increased risk of injuries below the head in such high-velocity impact injuries, particularly injuries of the cervical spine, is important. EMS providers are mandated to accomplish this procedure safely and effectively. The objective is to remove the helmet safely and prevent the accidental slide of the patient's head, resulting in exacerbation of any possible cervical spine injuries. For more discussion, see Chapter 29, Helmet Removal.

Indications

The procedure is indicated for all patients wearing helmets who sustain an acute illness or injury. Helmets are being required more often in various athletic and recreational activities. For example, these situations may be encountered when dealing with bicyclists, motorcyclists, high-altitude climbers, skateboarders, skiers, American football players, Lacrosse players, parachuters, and occasionally baseball players.

Contraindications

1. Lack of familiarity with the technique.
2. Single provider, as the procedure requires an assistant to be present.
3. Damaged helmet that is penetrating the patient's head and/or neck.
4. Evidence of a possible cervical spine fracture and/or helmet deformity and no cast cutter available.

Equipment and Supplies

The following equipment and supplies are required to perform the helmet removal procedure.

1. EMS personnel protective equipment (PPE) including appropriate sized gloves and goggles.
2. Scissors and/or cast cutter.
3. Properly sized cervical collar.

Procedure Techniques

1. An EMS provider is positioned above or behind the patient and stabilizes the patient's head and neck by placing one hand on either side of the helmet with the fingers on the patient's mandible to prevent the helmet from slipping if the strap is loose (Figure 41-61).
2. Assess patient movement and sensation in the upper and lower limbs.
3. Direct an assistant to cut, loosen, or remove the helmet chin strap at the D-rings (Figure 41-62).
4. Direct the assistant to assume stabilization by placing one hand under the neck and occiput and the other on the interior neck, with the thumb on one angle of the mandible and the index and middle fingers on the other angle of the mandible (Figure 41-63 and Figure 41-64).
5. Expand the helmet laterally to clear the patient's ears and carefully remove the helmet. If the helmet has a face cover, this device must be removed first. If the helmet provides full facial cover, tilt the helmet backwards to clear to nose and then remove it (Figure 41-65).
6. The assistant must maintain in-line immobilization from below to prevent head tilt.
7. After removal of the helmet, assure control of the head and neck by performing an in-line manual immobilization (Figure 41-66).
8. If the attempt to remove the helmet results in any patient pain and or paresthesia, the helmet should be removed with a cast cutter. The head and neck must be stabilized during this procedure by dividing the helmet in the coronal plane through the ears. The outer rigid layer is removed first and the inside Styrofoam layer is then incised and removed anteriorly. Maintaining neutral

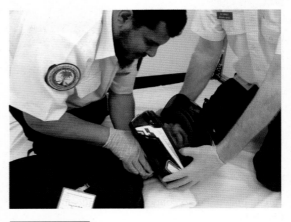

FIGURE 41–61

Secure the head and spine in a neutral position.
Photo courtesy of Dr. Nadeemuddin Quereshi.

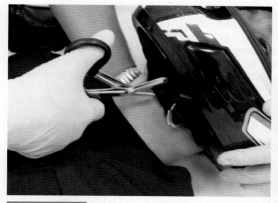

FIGURE 41–62

Cutting the chin straps. Photo courtesy of Dr. Nadeemuddin Quereshi.

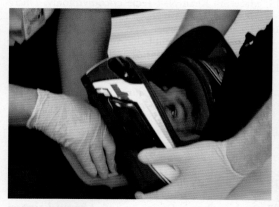

FIGURE 41–64

Stabilizing the mandible with the other hand. Photo courtesy of Dr. Nadeemuddin Quereshi.

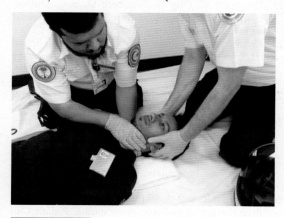

FIGURE 41–66

Post-helmet removal: align the head and neck before applying the cervical spine collar. Photo courtesy of Dr. Nadeemuddin Quereshi.

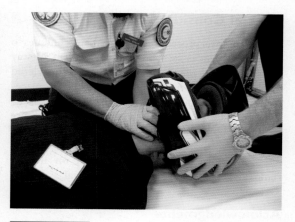

FIGURE 41–63

Stabilize the neck by placing one hand below the neck and occiput. Photo courtesy of Dr. Nadeemuddin Quereshi.

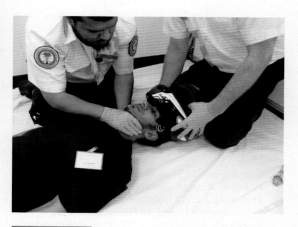

FIGURE 41–65

Helmet removed by the first EMS provider. Photo courtesy of Dr. Nadeemuddin Quereshi.

alignment of the head and neck, the posterior portion is then removed.

9. Direct the assistant to place and properly tighten the cervical collar while you maintain manual in-line stabilization of the patient's head and neck.
10. Reassess the patient response to the intervention.

Complications

The most common complication of the helmet removal procedure is the movement of the patient's neck and worsening of spine injury.

Special Considerations

Helmet removal procedures are essential techniques to complete patient assessment and management. Airway assessment and management are better considered during the in-line immobilization before the placement of the cervical collar. Coordination between the EMS provider and the assistant is essential to ensure minimal mobilization of the neck to prevent any complications.

For more detailed information on helmet removal, see Chapter 29 Helmet Removal.

Acknowledgments

The authors would like to thank the EMS services of King Faisal Specialist Hospital and Research Center for collaborating in producing the illustrations developed for this manuscript.

References

1. Santillanes G, Gausche-Hill M. Pediatric airway management. *Emerg Med Clin North Am* 26(4): 961, 2008.
2. Orenstein JB. Prehospital pediatric airway management. *CPEM* 7(1): 31, 2006.
3. American College of Emergency Physicians, American Academy of Pediatrics, *APLS: Advanced Pediatric Life: the Pediatric Emergency Medicine Resource*. Sudbury, MA: Jones & Bartlett Publishers; 2004.
4. Gausche-Hill M, Henderson DP, Goodrich SM, et al. *Pediatric Airway Management for the Prehospital Professional DVD*, Sudbury, MA: Jones & Bartlett Publishers and Unihealth Foundation; 2004.
5. Stockinger ZT, McSwain NE. Prehospital endotracheal intubation for trauma does not improve survival over bag-valve-mask ventilation. *J Trauma* 56: 531, 2004.
6. Wenzel V, Keller C, Idris AH, et al. Effects of smaller tidal volumes during basic life support ventilation in patients with respiratory arrest: good ventilation, less risk? *Resuscitation* 43: 25, 1999.
7. Gausche M, Lewis RJ, Stratton SJ, et al. Effect of out-of-hospital pediatric tracheal intubation on survival and neurological outcome: a controlled clinical trial. *JAMA* 283: 783, 2000.
8. Newth CJ, Rachman B, Patel N, et al. The use of cuffed versus uncuffed endotracheal tubes in pediatric intensive care. *J Pediatr* 144: 333, 2004.
9. Moynihan RJ, Brock-Utne JG, Archer JH, et al. The effect of cricoid pressure on preventing gastric insufflation in infants and children. *Anesthesiology* 78: 652, 1993.
10. 2005 American Heart Association (AHA) guidelines for cardiopulmonary resuscitation (CPR) and emergency cardiovascular care (ECC) of pediatric and neonatal patients: pediatric basic life support. *Pediatrics* 117(5): e989, 2006.
11. American Society of Anesthesiologists Task Force on Management of the Difficult Airway. Practice guidelines for management of the difficult airway: an updated report by the American Society of Anesthesiologists Task Force on Management of the Difficult Airway. *Anesthesiology* 98: 1269, 2003.
12. Barata I. The laryngeal mask airway: prehospital and Emergency Department use. *Emerg Med Clin North Am* 26(4): 1069, 2008.
13. Bogetz MS: Using the laryngeal mask airway to manage the difficult airway. *Anesthesiol Clin North Am* 20: 863, 2003.
14. Blostein PA, Koestner AJ, Hoak S. Failed rapid sequence intubation in trauma patients: esophageal tracheal Combitube is a useful adjunct. *J Trauma* 44: 534, 1998.
15. Mace SE, Khan N. Needle cricothyrotomy. *Emerg Med Clin North Am* 26(4): 1085, 2008.
16. McLeod AD, Turner MW, Torlot KJ. Safety of transtracheal jet ventilation upper airway obstruction. *Br J Anaesth* 95(4): 560, 2005.
17. Hebert RB, Bose S, Mace SE. Cricothyrotomy and transtracheal jet ventilation. In: Roberts JR, Hedges JR, eds. *Procedures in Emergency Medicine*. Philadelphia: Elsevier Publishing Co; 2008: Chapter 6.
18. Joyce S: Tracheostomy care and tracheal suctioning. In: Roberts JR, Hedges JR, eds. *Clinical Procedures in Emergency Medicine*, 5th ed. Philadelphia: WB Saunders; 2009.
19. Patel RG: Percutaneous transtracheal jet ventilation. *Chest* 116: 1689, 1999.
20. Stroh G, Braude D: Can an out-of-hospital cervical spine clearance protocol identify all patients with injuries? An argument for selective immobilization *Ann Emerg Med* 37: 609, 2001.
21. Hauswald M, Ong G, Tandberg D, et al. Out-of-hospital spinal immobilization: its effect on neurologic injury. *Acad Emerg Med* 5: 214, 1998.
22. Kwan I, Bunn F, Roberts I, WHOP-HTCSC: Spinal immobilisation for trauma patients (Cochrane Review). *Cochrane Database Syst Rev* (2): CD002803, 2002.
23. LaRocco BG, Wang HE. Intraosseous infusion. *Prehosp Emerg Care* (2003) 7: 280, 2003.
24. Babl FE, Vinci RJ, Bauchner H, et al. Pediatric prehospital advanced life support care in an urban setting. *Pediatr Emerg Care* 17: 5, 2001.
25. Engle WA. Intraosseous access for administration of medications in neonates. *Clin Perinatol* 33(1): 161, 2006.
26. de Caen AR, Reis A, Bhutta A. Vascular access and drug therapy in pediatric resuscitation, *Pediatr Clin North Am* 55(4): 909, 2008.
27. Digoy GP. Diagnosis and management of upper aerodigestive tract foreign bodies. *Otolaryngol Clin North Am* 41(3): 485, 2008.

28. Bauman B, Mcmanus J. Pediatric pain management in the Emergency Department. *Emerg Med Clin North Am* 23: 2, May 2005.

29. McManus JG, Sallee DR. Pain management in the prehospital environment. *Emerg Med Clin North Am* 23: 2, 2005.

30. Halim Hennes H, Kim MK. Prehospital pain management: current status and future direction. *Clin Pediatr Emerg Med* 7: 1, March, 2006.

CHAPTER 42

Trauma Assessment

Peter Cameron

All patients with suspected major trauma require a systematic and coordinated approach from pre-hospital care providers as part of a trauma system. This begins with Dispatch (see **Section 2, Chapter 14**, Dispatch and Communications Systems) and ends with the handover of the trauma patient to the definitive hospital.

Initial dispatch may require more than one vehicle. If injuries are anticipated to be severe, paramedics with ALS skills are needed. Accurate description from bystanders and call-taking procedures are important in dispatching the right response. Multiple paramedics may be required for assistance with extrication and scene control, advanced on-scene procedures, and to attend to multiple victims. Specialized equipment may be required to secure the scene and extricate the patient. Depending on the mechanism of trauma, scene safety and extrication of the victim may delay lifesaving procedures – in addition, **at all times, safety of the health-care provider is paramount.**

Appropriate personal protective equipment and equipment for managing the patient should be available (see **Section 2, Chapter 19**, EMS Equipment).

In general, aim for the shortest safe scene and transport times. If patients meet previously agreed triage criteria, transport them to a major trauma center, bypassing smaller hospitals.[1-3] A hospital notification to arrange a "Trauma Team" response is an essential part of this process. **Give special consideration to trauma center transport to children and the elderly, since these two age groups are often under-triaged.**[4,5] Suggested criteria for transport directly to a trauma center are shown in **Figure 42-1**.[6]

THE PRIMARY SURVEY: ABCDE

At the trauma scene, assess and manage the patient using the "**ABCDE**" approach for the primary patient survey: **Airway, Breathing, Circulation, Disability, Exposure.**

Airway Maintenance and Spine Control

Assess the airway for patency and identify potential obstruction. Clear airway debris, perform the jaw thrust, and insert an oropharyngeal airway if the patient is obtunded.

If the patient's Glasgow Coma Score (GCS) is 8 or less, consider endotracheal intubation (see ETT procedures). During all maneuvers, including airway maneuvers, stabilize the cervical spine with in line immobilization and application of a cervical collar.

Breathing and Ventilation

Assess breathing — if there is no ventilation/hypoventilation, exclude airway obstruction. If no improvement is seen, provide immediate ventilation with a bag-valve mask, followed by intubation (if the paramedic is skilled in this procedure). If the

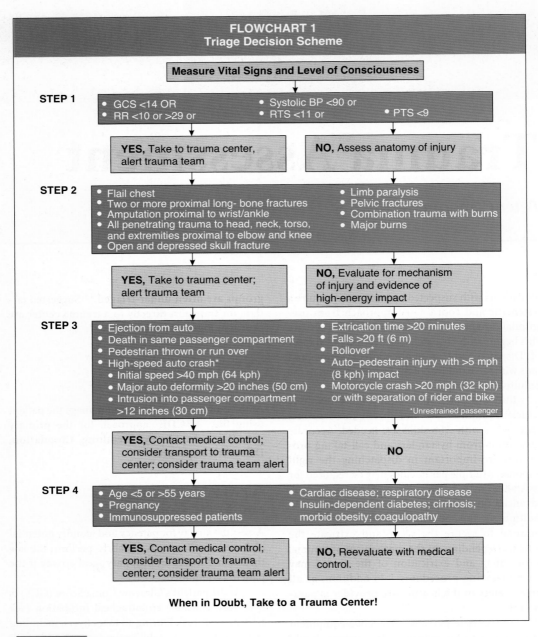

FLOWCHART 1
Triage Decision Scheme

Measure Vital Signs and Level of Consciousness

STEP 1
- GCS <14 OR
- RR <10 or >29 or
- Systolic BP <90 or
- RTS <11 or
- PTS <9

YES, Take to trauma center, alert trauma team

NO, Assess anatomy of injury

STEP 2
- Flail chest
- Two or more proximal long- bone fractures
- Amputation proximal to wrist/ankle
- All penetrating trauma to head, neck, torso, and extremities proximal to elbow and knee
- Open and depressed skull fracture
- Limb paralysis
- Pelvic fractures
- Combination trauma with burns
- Major burns

YES, Take to trauma center; alert trauma team

NO, Evaluate for mechanism of injury and evidence of high-energy impact

STEP 3
- Ejection from auto
- Death in same passenger compartment
- Pedestrian thrown or run over
- High-speed auto crash*
  - Initial speed >40 mph (64 kph)
  - Major auto deformity >20 inches (50 cm)
  - Intrusion into passenger compartment >12 inches (30 cm)
- Extrication time >20 minutes
- Falls >20 ft (6 m)
- Rollover*
- Auto–pedestrain injury with >5 mph (8 kph) impact
- Motorcycle crash >20 mph (32 kph) or with separation of rider and bike

*Unrestrained passenger

YES, Contact medical control; consider transport to trauma center; consider trauma team alert

NO

STEP 4
- Age <5 or >55 years
- Pregnancy
- Immunosuppressed patients
- Cardiac disease; respiratory disease
- Insulin-dependent diabetes; cirrhosis; morbid obesity; coagulopathy

YES, Contact medical control; consider transport to trauma center; consider trauma team alert

NO, Reevaluate with medical control.

When in Doubt, Take to a Trauma Center!

FIGURE 42–1

Trauma Triage Algorithm[6].

patient is ventilating but is in respiratory distress, consider tension pneumothorax, open pneumothorax, and multiple rib fractures and flail chest. If tension pneumothorax is suspected, perform immediate needle decompression (see procedures **Section 3, Chapter 22**, Airway and Respiratory Management). Provide appropriate analgesia if flail chest is suspected and if there are no relative or absolute contraindications to pain control with narcotics.

Circulation

Assess circulation (Table 42-1). Limit ongoing bleeding. Apply a compressive dressing to obvious

Table 42–1	**Assessment of Perfusion Status**[6]				
	Adequate	**Borderline**	**Inadequate**	**Extremely Poor**	**None**
Skin	Warm, pink, dry	Cool, pale, clammy	Cool, pale, clammy	Cool, pale, clammy	Cool, pale, clammy
Pulse	60-100/min	50-100/min	Less than 50/min or greater than 100/min	Less than 50/min or greater than 110/min	Absence of palpable pulse
Blood Pressure	Greater than 100 mm Hg	Between 80-100 mm Hg	Between 60-80 mm Hg	Less than 60 mm Hg SBP	Not recordable
Conscious State	Alert and oriented to time and place	Alert and oriented to time and place	Either alert and oriented to time and place **or may be** altered	Altered or unconscious	Unconscious

SBP = systolic blood pressure
Adapted from ATLS Manual. 8th ed. American College of Surgeons, Chicago IL, October 2008 and Ambulance Victoria protocols.

external bleeding points. Splint long-bone fractures and apply a pelvic sling to suspected pelvic fractures.

Establish two large-bore IV lines (14–16 gauge) and begin volume infusion as appropriate to circulation status. For all patients with less than adequate perfusion, begin infusion of 2 L of NS or LR (**see Table 1**). **Prehospital hypotension is one of the most important risk factors for morbidity and morality from trauma.**[7,8] The definition of prehospital hypotension ranges from ≤90 to 110 mm Hg systolic. The actual prehospital blood pressure recording should be communicated to the accepting physicians.

Disability

Assess the patient's level of consciousness state; the initial neurologic examination should include pupils (size, symmetry, response to light), level of consciousness. See **Table 42-2** and **Table 42-3** for methods of evaluating level of consciousness.

Exposure/Environment

Within limits of the environment, expose the patient and note those areas that have not been examined. If possible, examine the patient's back when log rolling him or her for transfer onto an ambulance stretcher. After the initial assessment, cover the patient with blankets during transport to minimize the development of hypothermia.

While the first paramedic assesses the patient for the primary survey above, the second paramedic or assistant applies ECG monitoring, oxygen saturation, and other monitoring if available (e.g., blood pressure cuff, End-tidal CO_2 [$ETCO_2$] monitor). If the transport is likely to be over a long time frame, such as occurs with hospital-to-hospital critical care transports, consider nasogastric tube insertion and urinary bladder catheterization.

REPEAT PRIMARY SURVEY AND SECONDARY SURVEY

A full secondary survey ("Head-to-Toe" examination) is generally not required prior to transport in the prehospital environment. The risk of time spent performing a secondary survey must be balanced against the risk of delay to obtaining definitive treatment for ongoing hemorrhage, compressive head injury,

Table 42–2	**"AVPU" acronym**[6]
A	Alert and conscious
V	Voice – responds to voice only
P	Pain – responds to pain only
U	Unresponsive

Adapted from ATLS Manual. 8th ed. American College of Surgeons, Chicago IL, October 2008.

Table 42–3	**Glasgow Coma Scale**		
A. Eye Opening	Score	**Enter best score**	
Spontaneous	4		
To Voice	3		
To Pain	2		
None	1		
		Subscore A. =_____	
B. Verbal Response	Score		
Oriented	5		
Confused	4		
Inappropriate Words	3		
Incomprehensible Sounds	2		
None	1		
		Subscore B. = _____	
C. Motor Response	Score		
Obeys Command	6		
Localizes to pain	5		
Withdraws (pain)	4		
Flexion (pain)	3		
Extension (pain)	2		
None	1		
		Subscore C. = _____	
Add subscores (A + B + C) =		_____*	

*Total GCS Maximum Score = 15
Adapted from www.paramedic-info.com/

coagulopathy, and other time-sensitive injuries. However, repeated Primary Surveys are essential for the earliest detection of preventable threats to life during transport to the major trauma service. **The most important factors for improving patient outcome are immediate attention to the "ABCs" and time to obtain definitive treatment at a major trauma service.**

INFORMATION HANDOVER FROM EMS TO THE ED

EMS providers must communicate information about the injury scene, mechanism of injury, and prehospital events as accurately as possible to emergency physicians and trauma surgeons. One study of information loss in patient handovers reported the transmission of vital information in only about 70% of incidents. Mechanism and location of injury and patient age were commonly reported, but critical information such as prehospital hypotension, patient pulse rate, and Glasgow Coma Score were reported less than 50% of the time.[9] Adding to problems with

the communication of information by EMS providers, physicians have poor recall for EMT reports, and one study reported physician recall of only about 40% of information.[10] **EMS providers must make a special effort to communicate key patient information and make sure that physicians understand and can recall the information given to them.**

References

1. MacKenzie EJ, Rivara F, Jurkovich GJ, et al. A national evaluation of the effect of trauma-center care on mortality. *N Engl J Med* 354(4): 366, 2006.
2. Haas B, Jurkovich GJ, Wang J, et al. "Survival advantage in trauma centers: expeditious intervention or experience? *J Am Coll Surg* 208(1): 28, 2009; E-pub 2008 Oct 31.
3. Twijnstra MJ, Moons KG, Simmermacher RK, et al. Regional trauma system reduces mortality and changes admission rates: a before and after study. *Ann Surg* E-pub ahead of print; PMID 20010086.
4. Chang DC, Bass RR, Cornwell EE, et al. Undertriage of elderly trauma patients to state-designated trauma centers. *Arch Surg* 143(89): 776, 2008.
5. Rivara FP, Oldham CT, Jurkovich GJ. Towards Improving the Outcomes of Injured Children. *J Trauma* 63(6 Suppl): S155, 2007.

6. ATLS Manual. 8th ed. American College of Surgeons, Chicago IL, October 2008.

7. Lalezarzadeh F, Wisniewski P, Huynh K, et al. Evaluation of prehospital and emergency department systolic blood pressure as a predictor of in-hospital mortality. *Am Surg* 75(10): 1009, 2009.

8. Bruns B, Gentilello L, Elliott A, et al. Prehospital hypotension redefined. *J Trauma* 65(6): 1217, 2008.

9. Carter AJ, Davis KA, Evans LV, et al. Information loss in emergency medical services handover of trauma patients. *Prehosp Emerg Care* 13(3): 280, 2009.

10. Scott LA, Brice JH, Baker CC, et al. An analysis of paramedic verbal reports to physicians in the emergency department trauma room. *Prehosp Emerg Care* 7(2): 247, 2003.

Part 4

Special Situations

Part

CHAPTER 43

Pediatric Care in EMS

Dagan Schwartz, Lisa Diane Amir, David Krieger, Yehezkel Waisman

KEY LEARNING POINTS

- Assess core needs of the population.
- Develop targeted medical protocols for the assessment, immobilization, and management of children, including age- and weight-specific use of equipment and delivery of fluids and drugs.
- The most common pediatric emergencies encountered in the EMS setting are trauma, respiratory problems, and seizures.
- History and physical examination techniques change based on the child's developmental age.

- Know the pediatric care capabilities of hospitals in your region and use transport accordingly.
- The care of children in mass casualty incidents needs special planning.
- Carefully allocate resources considering hourly, daily, and seasonal considerations.
- Focus training on needs, with preset educational, methodological, and performance goals.
- Evaluate time, skills, procedures, and outcomes for all EMS levels of providers.
- Assess communication, leadership, and teamwork for all EMS levels of providers.

OVERVIEW OF PEDIATRIC EMS CARE

Emergency medical services (EMS) for children constitute the emergency assistance rendered by trained emergency medical personnel at the prehospital phase, before the patient reaches a treating medical facility.[1]

Pediatric transports are estimated to account for only 5 to 10% of all emergency transports by general (not pediatric-oriented) EMS systems worldwide.[2,3] The majority of communities around the globe have formalized EMS systems that are designed and equipped to cope with children. The most common pediatric emergencies encountered in the EMS setting are trauma, respiratory problems, and seizures. Cardiac arrest is rare in children and usually has a poor outcome.[3]

The universal goal of prehospital care is to further minimize systemic insult or injury by applying the appropriate means to ensure patient safety.[1] However, the limited pediatric experience gained by general EMS systems on the one hand and the complexity of providing medical care to a wide variety of age groups on the other pose a major challenge.

This chapter defines pediatric patients as under 18 years old. However, the pediatric age group is not well defined internationally. Some EMS systems limit the pediatric age to 14 years, whereas others include adolescents and young adults up to age 21 years. Age grouping decisions are usually related to the specific organizational structure and the nature of the emergency medical response and depend greatly on local demographics and population base.

The principles of emergency prehospital care are the same for children and adults. However, children have unique anatomic, physiologic, and developmental characteristics as well as a different spectrum of diseases that need to be addressed by the EMS health care provider. For example, a respiratory rate of 13 breaths per minute in a quiet patient is within the normal range for adults but considered bradypnea in infants, and may, under certain conditions, indicate a need for assisted ventilation. Furthermore, there are also differences in the normal limits of vital signs among the pediatric subgroups of neonates, infants, toddlers, preschoolers, children, and adolescents. Therefore, EMS planning, coordination, and funding need to incorporate training in pediatric emergency care for professional staff and the adoption of targeted medical protocols for the assessment, immobilization, and management of children, including age- and weight-specific use of equipment and delivery of fluids and drugs. In addition, the ethical and legal implications of the minority status of children under international law must be taken into consideration.

This chapter addresses the different facets of EMS systems caring for children, focusing on the unique features of the pediatric age group that must be recognized in order to conduct an appropriate assessment and provide optimal management. It includes practical information on the activation of systems, scene triage, pediatric medical protocols and medical supervision, training and education, equipment for children for both routine and mass casualty events, and legal aspects.

SPECIFIC CONSIDERATIONS FOR PEDIATRIC EMS CARE

Phases of Child Development

Knowledge of key milestones in a child's physical and emotional development is a crucial aspect in the care of children. Table 43-1 summarizes milestones that are important to the prehospital provider. This knowledge will help the prehospital provider hone the approach to the ill or injured child and aid in evaluation of the child's responses. For example, a 15-month-old child should react with crying and anxiety when a stranger approaches; failure to react in this fashion may indicate a decreased level of consciousness, not an unusually cooperative child.

History

Children under the age of 4 or 5 are generally unable to provide a history, and it is usually obtained from an accompanying adult. Explicitly verify the relationship of the adult to the child: the adult male accompanying the child is not necessarily the father, nor is the adult female the mother. Also verify that the accompanying adult was indeed present at the time of injury or illness. Try to obtain the history from the child if he or she is older than 4 or 5, if only to establish a relationship with the child before performing a physical examination. Asking about the history also allows a mental status assessment. If the adult attempts to provide the history instead of the child, gently request that the child be allowed to speak. The adult can be given the opportunity to complete the history afterwards.

Past Medical History

Obtain a brief birth history in children less than 6 months of age. If the child was born prematurely, obtain a birth history in children until the age of 3 in order to verify that there are not residual complications that might impact current medical care. Common complications of preterm birth include seizures, developmental delay, chronic lung disease, and increased-susceptibility to infections in the first months of life Table 43-2 lists chronic illnesses commonly encountered in the pediatric age group. Ask about the current use of medications and allergies.

Physical Examination

Vital signs are an adjunct to assessing overall well-being. Overall appearance, rather than any particular vital sign, is the most important sign of illness. Children should be alert and responsive to voice with good eye contact. Even a 1-month old should respond to voice. Infants and children who fail to make eye contact, are not agitated when approached by a stranger, or fail to oppose being touched are not cooperative but ill.

Table 43-3 contains vital signs by age. Blood pressure measurements in the prehospital setting commonly exceed the 95th percentile. Hypertension is a rare cause of illness in children and most elevated blood pressures are due to anxiety. A shortcut for remembering minimal systolic blood pressure by age is found in Table 43-4. The formula approximates the *5th percentile* for systolic pressure and represents *hypotension* in the setting of acute illness or injury. Respiratory rate is very much dependent on the status of the child and may be elevated by fever, anxiety, or stress. Look for signs of respiratory distress in order to determine the significance of tachypnea. Oxygen saturation measured by pulse oximetry does not vary with age and is not affected by fever or anxiety. Oxygen saturation provides a more objective evaluation of a

Table 43–1	Developmental Milestones with Implications for the Prehospital Provider			
Age Group	Physiologic Changes	Motor Development	Psychosocial Development	Suggestions for Approach Patient During Examination
0–2 months	Delayed presentation of hemodynamically significant congenital heart lesions (VSD, aortic coarctation) Congenital metabolic disorders that can present with hypoglycemia, sepsis-like picture Sensitivity to hypothermia Cardiac output dependent on heart rate rather than contractility Global reaction to illness Susceptibility to dehydration	Responds to voice and light by turning head	Bonding to parents, especially voice Smile >1.5 months	Separate from parents
3–9 months	Large tongue, narrow trachea (susceptibility to upper respiratory tract obstruction) Susceptibility to dehydration persists Signs of meningitis may be subtle	Grasping, sitting, rolling over result in falls Finger-mouth behavior: foreign body ingestion and aspiration	Friendly but parental preference Displays emotion, eye contact, and vocalization	Examine in parent's arms if possible
9 months to 3 years	Plasticity of bones increases change of internal injuries in absence of fractures Large head size relative to trunk Increased risk of high level C-spine injury due to weak neck musculature, ligament laxity Increased risk of intra-abdominal and intrathoracic injury	Walking, running, and climbing result in falls	Stranger anxiety Exploratory behaviors result in falls, ingestions, and drowning Verbalization, up to short sentences Follows simple commands	Examine in parent's lap, neck down with head last Distraction techniques: talking, singing, stickers

(Continued)

Table 43–1	Developmental Milestones with Implications for the Prehospital Provider *(Continued)*		
Age Group	Physiological Changes	Motor Development	Psychosocial Development	Suggestions for Approach During Examination
3–6 years	Similar to 9 mos-3 yrs	Similar to 9 mos-3 yrs	Speaks in complete sentences, communicates complex ideas. Development of imagination' Limit testing	Examine close to or on parent, allow child to hold equipment Distraction techniques
6–12 years	Shedding of primary teeth Prominence of tonsils, adenoids may complicate intubation		Independence Street crossing Unsupervised activities	Examine on stretcher, parent close by
12 years to adult	Adult as well as pediatric diseases Sexual maturation and initiation of sexual activity Pregnancy		Belief in immortality Suicidal behavior Risk-taking behavior Drug abuse Privacy Importance of body image and fear of deformation	Examine on stretcher, may not want parent present for examination Explain all aspects of care in detail Reassure for normal findings

VSD = Ventricular Septal Defect.

Table 43–2	**Common Chronic Illnesses in the Pediatric Age Group**

Asthma
Congenital heart disease, cyanotic and acyanotic
Insulin-dependent Diabetes
Malignancy – solid tumor, leukemia, brain tumors
Metabolic disorders with hypoglycemia
Psychiatric: Attention deficit-hyperactivity disorder; depression; substance abuse; eating disorders
Seizures: febrile seizure; epilepsy
Steroid dependent diseases involving the kidneys or gastrointestinal tract

child's respiratory status than does respiratory rate. Fever, defined as a rectal temperature of 38 degrees Centigrade or above, is a common finding in acutely ill children and rarely requires treatment beyond the administration of antipyretics. Children in whom any fever may indicate severe illness include infants less than 2 months of age, immunosuppressed or compromised children, or children with evidence of poor perfusion or sepsis. Hypothermia may be a sign of severe illness, especially in infants.

Children are generally fearful of the physical examination and even adolescents may have difficulty cooperating. Try to approach every child with a smile, make eye contact, and use a calm and unhurried manner. Explain all aspects of the care that is planned, and if possible, demonstrate the equipment before use. Many adolescents have never had a medical encounter in the absence of a parent and despite their adult size, often require as much explanation and patience as a young child. Although most children (and their parents) are cooperative, some may become combative during the physical examination. The provider should clearly state appropriate guidelines governing behavior when necessary, for example, no biting or kicking. Children and adolescents should not be censored for crying. Children should be praised for *any* coopera-

tion, no matter how minimal, displayed during the physical examination.

In the case of a critically ill or injured child, consider initially separating the parents from the child until assessment and stabilization are done. As soon as it is medically feasible, allow the parent to have physical contact with the child.

Table 43-5 summarizes aspects of the prehospital physical examination that may differ from that of adults.

Pain

The emotional response to pain, namely, fear and anxiety, and the memory of pain develop in the second year of life. Children (and adults) have a great fear of pain and of needles in particular. A number of simple interventions can minimize pain and anxiety during assessment and treatment. If the situation permits, allow the parent to hold the child or to remain in physical contact by holding the child's hand. Involve the child in the process: "You hold the blood pressure cuff until I need it." *Distraction techniques*, especially in young children, are very effective – sing, talk, tell stories, use stickers. Either the prehospital provider or the parent can utilize these techniques. Adolescents may be able to "self-distract" by focusing on the explanation of the

Table 43–3	**Vital Signs by Age**		
Age	**Respirations** (Breaths per Minute)	**Resting Pulse** (Beats per Minute)	**Blood Pressure** (Systolic)
Newborn to 3 months	30–60	100–160	65–85
3–6 months	30–45	90–130	70–90
6 months to 1 year	25–40	90–125	80–100
1–3 years	20–30	80–120	90–105
3–6 years	15–25	70–110	95–110
6–10 years	12–20	60–95	100–120
> 10 years	12–18	55–85	110–135

Table 43–4	Definition of Hypotension (Fifth Percentile Blood Pressure) by Age[12]	
Age	**Systolic Blood Pressure (mm Hg)**	
Term neonates (0–28 days)	<60	
Infants (1–12 months)	<70	
Children 1–10 years	<70 + (age in years x 2)	
Children > 10 years	<90	

Adapted from: Ralston M, Hazinski MF, Zaritsky AL, et al, eds. *Pediatric Advanced Life Support Provider Manual.* American Heart Association. Dallas TX, 2006. Chapter 1, Pediatric Assessment, page 17.

prehospital provider and the surroundings rather than on himself or herself. Explain the procedure and its purpose and never lie about the pain involved.

Child Abuse

An in-depth discussion of the identification of the abused child is beyond the scope of this textbook. However, several points are important for prehospital providers in order to identify children who potentially have been abused.

History Suggesting Child Abuse

History and examination features that suggest child abuse are listed in Table 43-6.

In the case of children who are injured at home, ask to see the location of the injury and examine the surroundings to see if the environment is consistent with the injuries noted. An overall impression of the surroundings may also be helpful – that is, chaotic, unsupervised, absence of equipment for child care (bottles, bed), and level of cleanliness.

Carefully document the initial history, as the perpetrator may change the story once he or she realizes that the purported mechanism is inconsistent with the injuries sustained. Clearly communicate all concerns to the ED staff.

COMPONENTS OF EMS SYSTEMS FOR CHILDREN (EMS-C)

Most EMS systems worldwide respond to patients of all age groups, but most systems were developed with an emphasis on EMS care for adults. Children's needs are very different in many respects. The needs of EMS systems for children include preventive care, the training

Table 43–5	Physical Examination Findings in Children
Overall appearance	Smiling, eye contact, consolability by parents
Head	Anterior fontanelle (present until 9–18 months of age) should be level with skull Cephalohematoma-head trauma
Lungs	Signs suggestive of respiratory distress/failure: – Nasal flaring – Grunting: may also result from cardiac or infectious etiology – Head bobbing – Seesaw respiration: chest retraction with abdominal expansion during inspiration
Heart	Sinus arrhythmia common
Skin	Cutis marmorata (mottled appearance) – cold exposure but also infection, poor perfusion Hematomas, burns, or pattern injuries, especially in body areas covered by clothing

Table 43–6	Features of History and Examination That Raise Consideration of Child Abuse
History Items and Examples	**Physical Examination Items and Examples**
Injury inconsistent with developmental stage; 6 month old who fell while running and broke his leg	Pattern injuries: bruises or burns with a distinct pattern such as bite marks, finger marks, iron, belt buckle, cigarette
Mechanism of injury inconsistent with injury; infant with GCS 6 who fell 50 cm out of parents' arms	Extensive bruising on trunk with sparing of the extremities, especially in areas usually covered by clothing
No history in the face of significant injury; 'I just found him lying in bed', in a case of femur fracture	Injuries to the genitalia or multiple injuries without clear cause
Inappropriate delay in seeking medical attention	Children <1 year old found dead at home. Parents inappropriately unconcerned about child's injury; or parents angry with child for forcing them to seek medical attention

needs of first responders, the initial directives to be issued by the dispatch center, equipment and training of basic and advanced life support providers, care and transport protocols, and collaboration with the community and pediatric care resources in the region.[4] To adequately cater to the needs of children, an EMS system needs to focus on their requirements and make appropriate changes and enhancements in such areas as training, equipment, and protocols.

EMS System Design

EMS system design varies greatly among countries and at times even in adjacent regions within the same country. EMS systems may need to accommodate various levels of care providers and the requirements of various governmental, regional, municipal, private, and nonprofit organizations. Major components of an EMS-C (EMS for children) system need to be tailored to meet the needs of children in the region (such as its specific hazards and characteristics) and to make best use the available resources. Many of the resources needed for EMS-C are an integral part of the general EMS system (such as a medical dispatch center, a unique and publicly known access number, and telecommunication networks). EMS-C works well only when the general EMS system works well.

As an initial step to building or assessing the adequacy of the system, map the needs and resources in the service region.[5] As part of the needs assessment, institutions caring for children with special needs,

schools, and day care centers need to be identified. Mapping of regional resources includes hospitals with various capabilities to care for injured children and to care for children with life-threatening medical conditions. In many countries, great variation exists in the pediatric capabilities of individual regional hospitals. EMS-C is charged with optimizing the transport of children to the most appropriate facility in medical emergencies, trauma, and in multi-casualty incidents. Variability in pediatric care capabilities will also require the EMS-C system to perform interfacility transport of children from hospitals with limited pediatric care capabilities to pediatric specialty centers. In some regions dedicated pediatric and neonatal ground and air transport teams are available and need to be integrated into the EMS-C response plans.

The roles, responsibilities, and jurisdiction of EMS systems in general and EMS-C specifically vary widely. In some instances, the role of EMS-C may be limited solely to the rapid and effective provision of quality emergency care and transport for children, whereas in others, EMS systems are a major stakeholder in injury prevention, disaster preparedness, and other related areas.

Public Information and Education

Injury is the leading cause of pediatric death in the 1 year to adult age group.[5] EMS can play a leading role in community injury prevention programs. Training parents, caregivers, teachers, and the general public in pediatric first aid and CPR are additional tasks in which the EMS system can take a leadership role, partnering with businesses, organizations, and the community at large.

EMS-C Personnel Training

EMS personnel are usually much more confident in caring for adult injury and disease than for a child or baby with a life-threatening condition.[6-8] Therefore, theoretical knowledge and practical skills pertaining to pediatric emergencies need to be an ample part of the initial training curricula, and clinical clerkships and continuous education need to be provided. If the EMS system utilizes first responders (such as volunteers or other emergency agencies staff), it needs to teach pediatric care abilities to them as well. Adequate training and ensuring a high level of expertise for all responders in pediatric emergencies are pivotal components of the EMS-C.

EMS-C Medical Oversight

EMS-C medical oversight needs to include a physician familiar with pediatric emergencies. Medical oversight has a number of responsibilities: initial and continuing *medical education*; development of *pediatric care protocols* for dispatch, dispatcher-initiated bystander care, first responders and EMS basic and advanced life support providers; development of *transport and destination policies*; development of *procedure protocols*; the acquisition, maintenance, and periodic revision of *pediatric care equipment* to allow appropriate care for children of all ages; the provision of *on-line medical control* for pediatric emergencies; and the performance of *quality assurance* activities for pediatric care.

An additional component of EMS-C that is gaining recognition is disaster preparedness and response.[9,10] This component includes guiding needed mapping and preparation of the community so that the needs of children are recognized and an action plan for disasters is solidified. Again, as in regular emergencies, schools, daycare facilities, and households with children need to be targeted with a special emphasis on those caring for babies and children with special needs. Checklists for home and school disaster preparedness are available from EMS-C, a US Department of Health and Human Services government-sponsored program at http://bolivia.hrsa.gov/emsc/. A major issue in prehospital disaster preparedness for infants and children is mapping and augmenting surge capacity in all system components. Typically this includes both adding resources (which have to be prepared in

advance) and switching to disaster-specific standard operation procedures (SOPs). As part of such preparedness, children-specific disaster hospital resources need to be mapped, augmented, and integrated into a community plan. A large scale EMS-C disaster plan is being developed in the city of New York. This component of the US government–funded EMS-C project and some of the resources they have developed can be accessed at http://cpem.med.nyu.edu/resources/educational-resources.

EMS SYSTEM ACTIVATION GUIDELINES

All EMS systems operate according to activation guidelines, which direct all phases of the response, starting with the initial incident report. The guidelines need to address the characteristics and specific needs of all patient categories, including children, and to encompass a wide range of providers, scenarios, and special conditions. In most systems, activation is initiated by the medical dispatch center after it receives a call, usually from the patient or from a caregiver.

The guidelines should be adapted for every system's specific needs and capacities. In single patient scenarios, based on the acuity and specific nature of the emergency, this may include the activation of one or more responders. Some systems are constructed as a *one tier* system, offering a single level of provider care (EMT-B, EMT-I EMT-P, nurse or physician). Other systems are *multitiered*, with several responder levels that may include volunteer first responders with one or more levels of training, certification, equipment, and capabilities; on duty personnel from other emergency agencies such as fire or police; EMS BLS responders; EMS ALS responders ; EMS special units (such as HazMat teams, mass casualty incident (MCI) units, command and control units); specialized EMS or non-EMS units such as specialized neonatal or pediatric transport units, search and rescue units, and airborne evacuation and transport units.

Activation guidelines need to address the "how" and "when" of units' activation. They usually include checklists of required actions to be performed by the various providers and operatives in specific situations. They need to include specific guidelines for situations such as HazMat, communicable diseases in sporadic or epidemic scenarios, multi-casualty incidents, specific injury or disease processes such as burns or head injuries, and specific patient populations such as children or neonates. Guidelines need to specifically outline the minimum necessary information upon which system activation may occur (for example, a requirement for verification by an emergency agency responder prior to activation of a full Mass Casualty Incident protocol). Guidelines need to specify who needs to be notified and by whom, and if any specific precautions are necessary, such as protective gear. Additionally, guidelines need to address collaboration protocols with other emergency agencies as well as transport and destination protocols.

Guidelines should identify optimal care facilities for various conditions. In certain instances, to allow for optimal care, the patient may need to be transported for stabilization to a nearby facility (for example, a trauma patient with an unsecured airway or a hemodynamically unstable multitrauma patient), and once stabilization has been achieved, that patient may need to be secondarily transferred to a definitive care facility. In such cases the provider should notify the local receiving facility of the patient's condition so that arrangements for transfer to definitive care can begin immediately.

Guidelines also need to address the possibility that a caregiver or the on-line medical control operating in the patient's best interest may wish to override standard procedures. When this occurs, the EMS medical director should review the case with the ambulance crew to find out if the override was appropriate and to determine whether there is a need for further education or policy review.

PEDIATRIC EMS TRIAGE

Individual Triage

All individual pediatric medical cases should be transported, regardless of the lack of severity of the case, as field triage by non-physician prehospital providers has not been shown to be effective at identifying children who do not require immediate medical care. Pediatric trauma cases should be triaged to trauma centers according to established field protocols. The effectiveness of protocols for non-transport of the injured child has not been proved.[13]

Destination

Once initial stabilization has been performed in the field, a decision must be made regarding the destination of the ill or injured child. Prehospital providers must be aware of the availability and level of pediatric care that can be provided in their transport region. A stable child should be transported to the nearest facility capable of providing pediatric care, regardless of the level of care it can provide. Severely injured children should be transported to a trauma center. Studies suggest that children may have better outcomes when treated in pediatric rather than adult trauma centers and that high volume centers have better outcomes than lower volume centers.[14] In the absence of a pediatric trauma or adult trauma center, a tertiary care center with pediatric intensive care capacity may represent an acceptable alternative. Unstable children should be transported to a tertiary care pediatric facility capable of providing definitive airway and medical care; if transport times are long, it may be necessary to stop at a lower level center to stabilize the child and then proceed with definitive transport.

Parental preference may influence the prehospital provider's decision as to the final transport destination. Chronically ill or technology-dependent children may require a specific medical center, and parents may express a strong preference that the child be transported there, even if it is not the nearest center. The reputation of a particular center in the field of pediatrics may also influence parental opinion. The unstable child should be transported to the nearest center capable of stabilizing him or her, regardless of parental preference. Stable children can be transported in accordance with parental preference, provided that this does not violate prehospital provider protocols. Emergency medical systems should establish clear guidelines for situations in which conflict exists between parental preference and the child's medical needs.

Triage in Mass Casualty Incidents

Two initial issues need to be defined when discussing mass casualty incidents involving children. First, the definition of a pediatric case in a mass casualty incident may differ from that in individual events. Many protocols define an adult as over 12 or 14 years of age in these situations. However, in a mass casualty incident it may not be possible to determine a child's exact age, and therefore patient size should also be considered in triage decisions.

Second, a mass casualty incident may involve many casualties with a small percentage of children or may involve relatively few casualties with a large percentage of children. A pediatric mass casualty incident should be defined by the absolute number of children injured, regardless of the number of adults injured. When a large number of children are involved, special attention must be given to the issues discussed below. In addition to categorization by injury severity and/or injury type, a separate identification tag denoting a pediatric patient should be used. Whether or not children should receive care first in a mass casualty incident has not been clearly determined.

It is of vital importance that children be included in mass casualty incident drills to ensure that providers have proper pediatric-sized equipment, are familiar with modifications to mass casualty protocols for children, and in order to gain experience with pediatric procedures.

Initial Mass Casualty Incident Triage

There are a number of physiologic differences and developmental issues that affect the care of children in mass casualty incidents. There is a predisposition to airway obstruction in those with a depressed level of consciousness and with a relatively large tongue, increased pliability of the neck, and a relatively large head. Less mature thermoregulatory mechanisms and higher surface area-to-mass ratios make children more susceptible to heat loss and hypothermia, especially during cold weather, and during decontamination for toxicologic exposures.

Children have greater compensatory mechanisms for hypovolemia than adults and therefore hypotension is a late and ominous event. Mechanisms of injury may vary with a higher incidence of head trauma and lower incidence of torso injury and fractures in blast injuries.[15]

The first mass casualty incident protocol for children, JumpSTART Pediatric MCI Triage algorithm, shown in Figure 43-1, is a pediatric modification to the START Adult Triage algorithm; a combined algorithm also exists (Figure 43-1). This algorithm has been translated into Spanish, French, Italian, and Japanese and can be downloaded free from the web site specified at the bottom of Figure 43-1.

Combined START/JumpSTART Triage Algorithm*

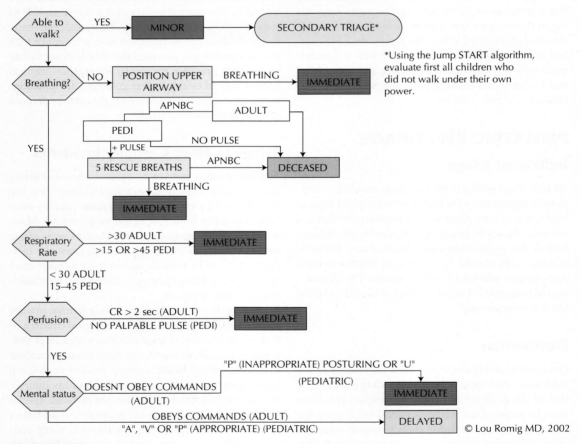

FIGURE 43-1

JumpSTART algorithm. Available at: **http://www.jumpstarttriage.com/JumpSTART_and_MCI_Triage.php**
http://www.jumpstarttriage.com/JumpSTART_and_MCI_Triage.html (revised December 2009; accessed May 2, 2010.

Table 43–7	Modifications of Field Triage for Pediatric Victims in Mass Casualty Incidents	
	Pediatric MCI	**Adult MCI**
Patient definition	Less than 12 years of age or "appears a child"	Adults only
Event definition	Children only, or more than 10 children in an event with adults	Adults only
Patient identification	Collection of identifiers and photographs of patients as soon as possible	Patients usually able to provide identifying information or have identifiers, e.g., documents
Tag identification	Tag 1: Triage category Tag 2: Pediatric case	Triage category tag only
Assessment of A, B, C	A & B: Spontaneous breathing with additional pulse assessment, respiratory rate C: Assessment of peripheral pulse only	A & B: Spontaneous respirations, respiratory rate C: Absent peripheral pulse, prolonged capillary refill
Neurologic assessment	AVPU-age dependent	Obeys commands
Secondary triage	BP measurement not critical in young children, can use assessment of perfusion	Complete vital signs as feasible
Field procedures	Not recommended; non–life saving procedures should be performed after ED admission	As dictated by protocol and availability of medical staff
Special considerations	Avoidance of hypothermia Cohorting of family members	

AVPU = AVPU scale (Alert, Voice, Pain, Unresponsive); MCI = Mass Casualty Incident; BP = blood pressure.

The Pediatric Triage Tape™ is a height-based tape system that uses a sieve system with pediatric heart rate and respiratory rate by age. Of note is the fact that none of these protocols, including JumpSTART, have been demonstrated to alter pediatric morbidity or mortality in mass casualty incidents. Triage systems that do not have pediatric modifications are not recommended.

Table 43-7 summarizes differences between adults and children in primary and secondary triage in mass casualty incidents. There are two key differences between the adult START and pediatric JumpSTART protocols. First, children who are initially apneic undergo a pulse assessment after airway opening, reflecting the high incidence of airway obstruction in severely injured children. Children in respiratory arrest but with a pulse are potentially salvageable, since airway obstruction commonly precedes cardiac arrest;

in adults, respiratory arrest is usually secondary to cardiac arrest, making a cardiovascular assessment unnecessary.

Second, mental status is assessed using Alert, Response to Voice, Response to Pain, and Unresponsive (AVPU) rather than the ability to obey commands. Children under the age of 3 and many older children when in pain or under emotional stress are unable to cooperate with paramedics. Mental status assessment using Alert, Response to Voice, Response to Pain, and Unresponsive may allow a more accurate assessment of level of consciousness. However, this assessment requires knowledge of child development (see Table 43-1) and more detailed chart documentation.

Minimize caregiver-child separation if possible during evacuation of children. If possible, transport all family members to the same trauma center. In the case of a severely injured child and minimally injured caregiver, the caregiver should be transported with the child according to the child's medical needs and the adult caregiver's injuries treated later. Preverbal and emotionally traumatized children who become separated from their families may not be able to provide identifiers. Photographs, preferably digital ones, should be obtained during secondary triage and posted at a central site or formal website along with any potential identifiers (e.g., first name, birthmarks, clothing, name of school) to enable identification and reunification in the future. This requires early involvement of social workers or hospital administrators to manage this service and to prepare for the possibility of prolonged and perhaps permanent absence of caregivers.

Secondary Triage and Interventions

Vital signs measurement is a key component of secondary triage. Blood pressure is often difficult and time-consuming to obtain, especially in young children, and may be replaced by clinical assessment using peripheral and central pulses if necessary. Consider obtaining rectal temperatures in children less than 3 years old to check for early development of hypothermia. Because of relative paramedic inexperience with pediatric mass casualty incidents as well as inexperience with performing procedures such as intubation and obtaining IV access in children, only lifesaving procedures such as airway opening and maintenance of oxygenation/ventilation should be performed in the field. Other procedures that are routinely performed in adults, such as IV access, should be delayed until arrival at the hospital.

Children under the age of 3 are often preverbal and may not be able to even follow simple commands when injured or upset. Children up to the age of 8 may be unable or unwilling to communicate with strangers. Even older children in times of injury and stress may not be able to even provide a name or other identifier. In spite of the chaotic and pressured environment that characterizes a mass casualty incident, techniques that will improve child cooperation include direct eye contact, a calm voice, and using touch to demonstrate the questions.

MEDICAL PROTOCOLS, SUPERVISION, AND QUALITY ASSURANCE/CONTINUOUS QUALITY IMPROVEMENT

Medical control is responsible for the quality of medical care rendered by the system. It exerts its responsibility through direct (*on-line*) and indirect (*off-line*) medical control. Direct medical control can be achieved through physician presence at the care site or through on-line control, by which the physician is contacted in real time and can input and contribute to the care provided to a specific patient. Indirect medical control can include such elements as basic and continuous education, choice of medical equipment and medication, and development of medical protocols and supervision, which includes quality assurance and continuous quality improvement.

Medical Protocols

Most EMS systems have developed and operate using medical protocols, which cover a variety of medical emergencies and treatment needs for adults and children. The roles of such protocols are to guide the provision of care within the EMS system in accordance with medical oversight. While protocols cannot replace sound clinical judgment, they facilitate rapid and effective treatment. Protocols standardize management actions so that prehospital providers will know how to proceed in a given patient presentation. Protocols also provide a gauge for measuring adherence to EMS practice standards. In many systems (those not utilizing a physician for on-site care provision) protocols can also serve as a legal and regulatory framework, allowing physician extenders such as nurses and EMT personnel to provide care under the legal coverage of an oversight physician.

The laws and regulations governing EMS medical oversight and treatment protocols can vary significantly among countries and even among states or regions within the same country. Despite the different system designs, needs, and resources and the fact that most systems develop their own protocols, significant similarities tend to exist. Medical oversight mostly adheres to internationally accepted care provision guidelines such as the American Heart Association (AHA) Advanced Life Support Manual, the AHA and American Academy of Pediatrics (AAP) endorsed Pediatric Advanced Life Support, and the American College of Surgeons (ACS) Advanced Trauma Life Support Manuals.[16–18]

The building of the pediatric protocols may be assisted by physicians with expertise in pediatric emergency care and in general and prehospital care in particular. Some systems also use pediatric specialty hospital physicians to aid in on-line medical control of complex pediatric emergencies. Since in some parts of the world the capabilities of community hospitals to deal with pediatric emergencies may be limited,[19,20] the transport protocols need to address the question of optimal initial hospital destination and the possible need for interfacility transport.

Each EMS system develops its own specific pediatric care protocols. The number of such protocols, the specific medical condition they refer to, and the treatment options they offer vary. In 1999 the US National Association of EMS physicians (NAEMSP) published Model Pediatric Protocols.[21] These model protocols were updated in 2003 but have not been changed to reflect the 2005 AHA pediatric resuscitation guideline updates. Nevertheless, they can serve as an example of the scope of such care protocols and the treatment options they encompass.

The "model protocols" include protocols for the following medical conditions:

1. General patient care.
2. Trauma.
3. Burns.
4. Foreign body airway obstruction.
5. Respiratory distress, failure, or arrest.
6. Bronchospasm.
7. Newborn resuscitation.
8. Bradycardia.
9. Tachycardia.
10. Nontraumatic cardiac arrest.
11. Ventricular fibrillation or pulseless ventricular tachycardia.
12. Asystole.
13. Pulseless electrical activity.
14. Altered mental status.
15. Seizures.
16. Nontraumatic hypoperfusion (shock).
17. Anaphylactic shock/allergic reaction.
18. Toxic exposure.
19. Near-drowning.
20. Pain management.
21. Death of a child and sudden infant death syndrome (SIDS).

Medical Supervision and Quality Assurance

One of the main tasks of medical oversight is to continuously monitor and measure performance using practice guidelines and validated performance measures.

Medical oversight needs to take the appropriate measures to improve the quality of medical care provided by its EMS system. Measurement and monitoring tools may include:

1. *Retrospective review* of medical EMS reports to evaluate adherence to protocols, accuracy of diagnosis and treatments, success rates of procedures, and more.
2. *Statistical analysis* using outcome measures (such as resuscitation and trauma care outcome).

3. *Direct field observation.*
4. Feedback from accepting facilities (to optimize such feedback, mechanisms need to be set through periodical written or oral reporting or through case review meetings allowing candid exchange of ideas in an open-minded atmosphere).
5. *Feedback from patient and family and customer satisfaction* surveys.
6. Some EMS systems utilize advanced command and control systems that allow the medical control to receive *real-time audio-video transmission* as well as information directly relayed from the medical monitoring devices, thus permitting real-time remote support and supervision.

The quality assurance effort must include both accountability of each and every provider in the system and an on-going search for opportunities to deploy system-wide changes (in medical protocols, equipment, operating procedures, and educational interventions).

Supervised quality assurance and improvement of the care provided for children may be aided by cooperation with a physician with expertise in pediatric emergencies or by collaboration with a pediatric specialty care center. The need to care for children with life-threatening conditions is relatively rare in most EMS systems, and therefore most EMS providers feel less comfortable and are less proficient in the care of critically ill children than in adults.[22–24] To overcome this hurdle the EMS system needs to enable pediatric proficient on-line support and stringent quality assurance for its pediatric cases. Deficiencies, if found, may be related to specific providers or reflect system-wide problems. A continuous focus for the providers on the theory and practice of pediatric prehospital emergency care is needed in most systems to ensure quality care for children. Optimally this on-going focus will include hands-on experience in a pediatric specialty center.

EMS-C RESEARCH

Medical oversight also has a pivotal role in promoting research into relevant topics. Such research may focus on local characteristics, problems, and dilemmas, or on topics that have widespread relevance. Besides the self-evident benefits of knowledge enhancement and problem identification, involving field EMS providers in such activities can boost motivation and the striving for self- and system improvement. Such activity may also help reduce burnout and improve job satisfaction, which can be major problems in some systems. Collaborative research involving EMS local hospitals and pediatric specialty centers may also improve inter-organizational communication and cooperation.

EQUIPMENT (ROUTINE AND FOR MASS CASUALTY INCIDENTS)

Equipment for EMS-C differs significantly from that used for care of adults. An EMS-C program needs to stock equipment for children of all ages. Pediatric equipment is unique in the need for a much wider range of various tubing and equipment sizes. The equipment allocated for care of sick and injured children depends on a number of factors, including level of EMS personnel training and authorization to perform various medical interventions, characteristics of pediatric emergencies in the region, geographic considerations, economic considerations, and finally regulatory and legal issues. A balance needs to be struck between commonly and rarely used equipment that has lifesaving potential. Overall, the equipment must allow EMS personnel to provide adequate care for children in various scenarios such as medical and traumatic emergencies, multi-casualty incidents, communicable diseases, natural and man-made disasters, and HazMat incidents.

EMS system design also affects the choice of pediatric equipment. A system that is tiered between BLS and ALS vehicles and responders might have two different vehicle equipment standards. Some EMS systems have incident-specific vehicles for HazMat or multi-casualty incidents. Incident-specific equipment is stored in these vehicles.

Despite the varying requirements and system designs, a template for ambulance pediatric care equipment was agreed upon by the American College of Emergency Physicians (ACEP), the American College of Surgeons (ACS), and the National Association of EMS Providers (NAEMSP) to serve as a standard for EMS services in North America.[25] This standard was published in 2009 as a position paper. It divides equipment needs between BLS ambulances and ALS ambulances and lists them according to categories.

These categories include:

1. Ventilation and airway equipment.
2. Monitoring and defibrillation equipment.
3. Immobilization devices.
4. Bandages.
5. An obstetric kit.
6. Miscellaneous, which includes, among other items, a sphygmomanometer with the various pediatric size cuffs, length/weight-based tape or appropriate reference material for pediatric equipment sizing and drug dosing, and a thermometer with low temperature recording capability.
7. Infection control equipment.
8. Injury prevention equipment.
9. Vascular access equipment.
10. Cardiac equipment.
11. Medications.
12. Other advanced equipment such as a glucometer and a nebulizer.

Disaster and mass casualty incident equipment is mostly found in specialized vehicles or in emergency storage. In some systems, local health or emergency authorities store part or all of such equipment, which is only to be distributed to EMS in emergency situations. In other systems part of the disaster equipment is found as a standard on all vehicles. It is recommended that a significant portion of the disaster response medical equipment be readily accessible, since obtaining necessary equipment from local or state authorities when disaster strikes may be time-consuming and hamper EMS disaster response.

TRAINING

Training Overview

The functions of the EMS workerare to safely access the injured or ill, understand the nature of the distress, implement stabilization techniques, and present the clinical picture to the medical center (while en route if necessary). To be effective, treatment must be focused, quick, and empathetic.

These goals may be complicated by several major factors:

1. Variable background of EMS workers: emergency medical technicians (EMTs), for example, receive 150 to 200 hours of training, whereas paramedics receive 10 times that amount.
2. Limited field conditions compared to those in the ED: poor lighting, inadequate time for a proper history and physical examination, few field diagnostic/consultative resources, and a threatening environment (crime, weather, sometimes family).[26]
3. Difficulty in transfer of information, which must rest on a commonality of prehospital/hospital procedures and medical parlance (chief complaint/assessment-based as opposed to diagnosis-based).

To overcome these problems and ensure proper care, the educational curriculum for EMS workers has to be staged and/or progressive, with clarity as to content, methods, and outcomes for each stage and verifiable short, intermediate, and long-term outcome results. The core elements of clinical practice (knowledge and skills) need to be recapitulated (in the form of continuing medical education) and, optimally, linked with job performance. Finally, an effective education should give each EMS worker the tools for self-instruction, because the knowledge base applied in clinical practice is constantly being updated.

Into the educational program of all EMS workers, including volunteers, ambulance drivers/EMTs, paramedics, and dispatchers, physicians should incorporate a subsection on pediatrics. Pediatric core content is crucial because of the small volume of pediatric transfers (5-10% in general EMS systems).[27] Due to the infrequent nature of pediatric cardiac arrest[28] and the observed deterioration of skills after formal course work training,[29-31] *content recapitulation* is essential.

Course Content

Common illnesses and acute life-threatening problems serve as the substrate for topics and skills to be learned (Table 43-8).

The skills required to manage life-threatening illnesses are covered in the Pediatric Advanced Life Support (PALS) and Advanced Pediatric Life Support (APLS) courses.

Trauma skills relevant for both adults and children are reviewed in the Pre-Hospital Trauma Life Support (PHTLS) or International Trauma Life Support (ITLS) Basic and Advanced Trauma Life Support courses. These courses, when offered, usually require biennial recertification. The course content differs by type of EMS worker.

Volunteers can be useful and cost-efficient adjuncts to care. Technically, their level of function should include basic life support (BLS) skills, knowledge of equipment, and vital sign measurements, which provide them with the ability to help the other EMS professionals with their work.

EMTs have a more limited (in hours) curriculum than paramedics, which is focused on the subjects listed in Table 43-9 and procedures shown in Table 43-10.

Paramedics should be instructed in all the subjects listed in Table 43-9. In addition, they should acquire proficiency in skills listed in Table 43-10.

Physicians active in pediatric EMS care should be regularly reassessed for knowledge and abilities in the topics and skills listed below. Their skill set should minimally be on a par with that of paramedics.

Dispatchers are frequently taken from the pool of EMTs and paramedics. They require additional course content, including EMS administrative protocols, understanding cases from aural clues and background sounds, proper ambulance allocation/dispersal, distribution of patients to hospitals in multi-casualty events, alerting other uniformed services as needed, and providing phone instruction in various emergencies (e.g., home delivery, CPR).

Training Techniques and Duration

Basic skills

Patient assessment can be taught in small groups or from videotape simulation/instruction.[33] New handheld and digital technologies can be used for self-instruction. The classic form of instruction via small groups is very dependent upon the availability of instructors and their cost.

Advanced-Integrative/Interpretive skills

These require personal instruction, notably at the debriefing section. Adler[34] has demonstrated a model for pediatric emergency medicine patient simulation. Binstadt[35] has outlined a comprehensive simulation curriculum for emergency medicine residents describing educational and testing tools useful for knowledge acquisition, decision making, skill performance, and teamwork. The concept and much of the material are applicable to EMS training. At the Israel Center for Medical Simulation,[36] Ziv has accumulated years of experience testing and certifying paramedics. The number of hours of training for each EMS worker

Table 43–8	Common Illnesses and Acute Life-Threatening Problems	
Common Illnesses		**Life-Threatening Problems**
1. Gastroenteritis and dehydration		1. Septic or anaphylactic shock
2. Febrile illness/seizure management		2. Acute traumatic injury
3. Acute respiratory illness/asthma/croup		3. Airway obstruction, respiratory arrest
4. Mental status change/hypoglycemia		4. Dysrhythmias

Table 43–9	Recommended Volunteer/EMT/Paramedic Core Content.[32,26] Lists in each column are cumulative for the most experienced provider.		
Provider	**Volunteer**	**Medic/EMT** [32]	**Paramedic** [26]
Content Area			
Patient and Provider Safety	Safety	Safety	Safety
	Transport to Chair Stretcher, Ambulance	Transport to Chair Stretcher, Ambulance	Transport to Chair Stretcher, Ambulance
	Correct Lifting	Driving regulations	Driving Regulations
		Correct Lifting	Correct Lifting
			Child Safety Seats
			Illness and Injury Prevention
		Child and Family Communication	Child and Family Communication
Patient Assessment	Vital Signs	Patient Assessment	Patient Assessment
			Growth and Development
Clinical Care	Child and Infant BLS	Child and Infant BLS	PALS, APLS
		Asthma/Epiglottitis	Respiratory Emergencies
		Hyperventilation	Hyperventilation
		Fever	Serious Infection
		Hypoglycemia	Hypoglycemia and Differential Diagnosis of Altered Mental Status
		Seizure/Syncope	Differential Diagnosis of Seizure and Syncope
			Dehydration, shock
		Stroke Signs	Stroke and Stroke Systems
			Cardiac rate and rhythm disturbances, cardiopulmonary arrest
		Basic PHTLS or ITLS	Advanced PHTLS or ITLS
			Burns
			Trauma Systems
			EMS-C Systems
			Child Abuse and Neglect Identification
			Suicide risk, aggressive behavior
		Bites and Stings	Hypothermia, hyperthermia, near-drowning, bites and stings
		Hypothermia	
		Non-medical pain management	Pain management
			Poisoning
			Newborn Emergencies
			SIDS and ALTE
			Children with special needs and with special technology and devices
Medico-Legal Issues	Emancipated Minor, Refusal of Care	Emancipated Minor, Refusal of Care	Emancipated Minor, Refusal of Care, DNR, guardianship, consent
			Reporting of abuse or assault
Self-education		Computer and library skills	Computer and library skills

BLS = Basic Life Support; PALS = Pediatric Advanced Life Support; APLS = Advanced Pediatric Life Support; PHTLS = Pre-Hospital Trauma Life Support; ITLS = International Trauma Life Support; SIDS = Sudden Infant Death Syndrome; ALTE = Apparent Life-Threatening Event; DNR = Do Not Resuscitate.

Table 43–10	**Essential Skills for Pediatric Education of EMS Workers in the Assessment of infants and children[27]**

Use of length based resuscitation tape
Airway management
  Mouth-to-mouth barrier device
  Oro/Nasopharyngeal airway
  Oxygen delivery systems
  Bag-valve-mask ventilation
  Chest decompression techniques
  Endotracheal intubation
    Use of endotracheal confirmation devices
    (end tidal CO_2 monitor)
    Rapid sequence induction
  Foreign body removal with Magill forceps
  Needle tracheostomy
  Nasogastric/Orogastric tubes
  Suctioning
  Tracheostomy management
Monitoring
  Cardio-respiratory monitoring
  Pulse oximetry
  End-Tidal CO_2 monitoring/CO_2 detection

Vascular access
  Intravenous line placement
  Intraosseous line placement
Fluid/medication delivery
  Endotracheal
  Intramuscular, intravenous
  Nasogastric
  Nebulized
  Oral rehydration techniques
  Rectal
  Subcutaneous
Cardioversion
Defibrillation, use of AED
Drug dosing in infants and children
Immobilization/Extrication
  Car-seat extrication
  Spinal immobilization
Leadership role in multi-casualty event/CPR/
  HazMat
  Teamwork

Original, adapted from: Seidel JS, Hornbein M, Yoshiyama K, et al. Emergency Medical Services and the pediatric patient: Are the needs being met? *Pediatrics* 1984;73(6),769–72.[27]

(Table 43-11) and the course curriculum/content (Table 43-9) increase progressively from volunteers to EMTs/medics to paramedics.

Continuing Medical Education

In practice, the course content and skills should be reviewed every 2 to 3 years. The professional literature and statistics relating to skill decay[37] for volunteers performing CPR/utilizing an AED suggest that a yearly review is more beneficial for skill retention. As noted above, this is particularly important in pediatric EMS, where exposure to casework is limited in number and procedure performance.

Methods for renewing knowledge and skills include:

Table 43–11	**Requisite Hours of Instruction**

Volunteer:	80 hours
Driver Medic EMT:	150–200 hours
Paramedic:	1000 hours minimum
Dispatcher:	EMT paramedic training + 40 hours

1. Emergency Department and/or hospital based rotations.
2. Simulated patients, use of sophisticated (SimMan®) mannequins and patients (actors or community-based patients).
3. Computer-based programs, including among others game-based learning and virtual reality learning.
4. On-site instruction during field work.

Optimally there should be a relationship between unsuccessful field performance and retraining. Currently this appears to be such a model only in very few EMS systems and EMS training centers.

Assessment

The pediatric skills required of an EMS member are potentially manifold. In examining the needs of an existing system or one being devised, assessment of the core needs of the population need to be made with careful allocation of resources with hourly, daily, and seasonal considerations.[38]

Once a decision is made relating to the BLS/ALS needs of the community, focused training with preset educational, methodological, and performance goals should be set. Evaluation of time, skill/procedure, and treatment outcome performance should be done for the various EMS workers. In addition, communication/leadership/teamwork components of care are crucial for efficient functioning and can be satisfactorily assessed.

The assessment of worker performance can be an important indicator of the need for content and skill renewal. This does not preclude across the board refresher courses.

Patient safety/malpractice issues have led to the development of many computer/CD/DVD–based educational tools that are used for educational and testing purposes and that with time will become more affordable.

LEGAL ASPECTS OF EMS-C

The minority status of children under international law must be taken into consideration in the formulation of rules and regulations governing the operation of EMS systems. However, local laws, by-laws, and policies vary by religion, culture, customs, and history among countries, regions, and communities, making it impossible for experts to suggest standardized universal guidelines.

In the US, federal law identifies 15 elements of an EMS system:

1. Personnel,
2. Training,
3. Communications,
4. Transportation,
5. Facilities,
6. Critical care units,
7. Public safety agencies,
8. Consumer participation,
9. Access to care,
10. Transfer of care,
11. Standardization of patient records,
12. Public information and education,
13. Independent review and evaluation,
14. Disaster linkage, and
15. Mutual aid agreements.[3]

The individual state EMS laws and regulations typically define levels of ambulance service capability and requirements for training, equipment, and physician leadership and accountability[3] applicable to both adults and children. To ensure proper emergency medical care specifically for children and to support improvements in education, advocacy, and research, the US government established the Emergency Medical Services for Children (EMSC) program under the auspices of the

Maternal and Child Health Bureau of the Health Resources and Services Administration.[1] In other countries, however, where there is no such legally funded infrastructure and no focus on quality pediatric emergency care, EMS care for children is often deficient.

In addition, elements of civil commitment, confidentiality, and mandatory reporting need to be addressed when establishing EMS systems for children[38,39] as follows:

Access of minors to emergency medical care (including the need for financial reimbursement and patient confidentiality).

Consent of parents or legal guardians for the evaluation and treatment of minors.

Initiation and termination of pediatric resuscitation decisions (including confirmation of death).

Transport decisions when no parent or guardian is available.

Refusal to transport by parents when children/minors are involved.

Mandatory reporting of suspected child abuse and duty to warn or protect third parties from harm.

Patient safety.

Confidentiality and consent for release of information.

Web Resources

1. http://bolivia.hrsa.gov/emsc/. **Emergency Medical Services for Children.**
2. http://cpem.med.nyu.edu/resources/educational-resources. **NYU Langone Medical Center, Center for Pediatric Emergency Medicine.**
3. http://www.safekids.org/safety-professionals/ **SAFE KIDS USA for professionals.**
4. http://www.jumpstarttriage.com/JumpSTART_and_MCI_Triage.php The *JumpSTART* **Pediatric MCI Triage Tool** *and other pediatric disaster and emergency medicine resources.*

References

1. Wright JL, Krug SE. Emergency medical services for children. In Kliegman RM, Behrman RE, Jenson HB, Stanton BF (eds). *Nelson Textbook of Pediatrics* (International Edition). Philadelphia, Saunders Elsevier; 2010 (in press).
2. Seidel JS, Hornbein M, Yoshiyama K, et al. Emergency medical services and the pediatric patient: Are the needs being met? *Pediatrics* 1984;73(6):769–72.
3. Lilja GP, Emergency medical services. In Tintinalli JE, Kelen GD, Stapczynski JS (eds). *Emergency Medicine A Comprehensive Study Guide.* New York, McGraw-Hill Companies, Inc; 2004.
4. *Emergency Care for Children Growing Pains, Future of Emergency Care Series.* Washington, DC: Institute of Medicine, The National Academies Press; 2007.

5. Seidel JS. A needs assessment of advanced life support and emergency medical services in the pediatric patient: state of the art. *Circulation* 1986;74(suppl 4): 129–33.

6. Federiuk CS, O'Brien K, Jui J, Schmidt TA. Job satisfaction of paramedics: The effects of gender and type of agency of employment. *Ann Emerg Med* 1993; 22(4):657–62.

7. Frush K, Hohenhaus S. *Enhancing Pediatric Patient Safety Grant.* Durham, NC: Duke University Health System; 2004.

8. Glaeser P, Linzer J, Tunik M, et al. Survey of nationally registered emergency medical services providers: Pediatric education. *Ann Emerg Med* 2000;36(1): 33–8.

9. AAP (American Academy of Pediatrics). *The Youngest Victims: Disaster Preparedness to Meet the Needs of Children.* Washington, DC: 2002;AAP.

10. Dick RM, Liggin R, Shirm SW, Graham J. EMS preparedness for mass casualty events involving children. *Acad Emerg Med* 2004;11(5):559.

11. Safe Kids USA. Report to the Nation: Trends in Unintentional Childhood Injury Mortality and Parental Views on Child Safety. Washington, DC: Safe Kids USA; 2008. Available at http://usa.safekids.org. Complete link = http://www.usa.safekids.org/content_documents/Injury_Trends_Report_FINAL.pdf

12. Ralston M, Hazinski MF, Zaritsky AL, et al, eds. *Pediatric Advanced Life Support Provider Manual.* American Heart Association; 2006.

13. Cone DC, Benson R, et al. Field triage systems: Methodologies from the literature. *Prehosp Emerg Care,* Apr-Jun 2004:130–37.

14. Centers for Disease Control and Prevention. Guidelines for triage of injured patients. *MMWR* 2009;58 (No. RR-1): 1–43. Accessed Nov 3, 2009.

15. Waisman Y, Amir L, Mor M, et al. Prehospital response and field triage in pediatric mass casualty incidents: The Israeli experience. *Clin Pediatr Emerg Med* 2006;7: 52–58.

16. American Heart Association. *Advanced Cardiac Life Support Provider Manual.* Dallas, TX: American Heart Association; 2006.

17. American Heart Association. *Pediatric Advanced Life Support Provider Manual.* Dallas, TX: American Heart Association; 2006.

18. American College of Surgeons, Committee on Trauma. *Advanced Trauma Life Support Student Course Manual.* 8th ed. Chicago, IL: American College of Surgeons; 2008.

19. Hunt EA, Hohenhaus SM, Luo X, Frush KS. Simulation of pediatric trauma stabilization in 35 North Carolina emergency departments: Identification of targets for performance improvement. *Pediatrics* 2006;117(3):641–48.

20. Isaacman DJ, Kaminer K, Veligeti H, et al. Comparative practice patterns of emergency medicine physicians and pediatric emergency medicine physicians managing fever in young children. *Pediatrics* 2001; 108(2):354–8.

21. National Association of EMS Physicians, NAEMSP model pediatric protocols: 2003 revision, *Prehosp Emerg Care* 2004;8:343–65.

22. Su E, Mann NC, McCall M, Hedges JR. Use of resuscitation skills by paramedics caring for critically injured children in Oregon. *Prehosp Emerg Care* 1997; 1(3):123–7.

23. Su E, Schmidt TA, Mann NC, Zechnich AD. A randomized controlled trial to assess decay in acquired knowledge among paramedics completing a pediatric resuscitation course. *Acad Emerg Med* 2000;7(7): 779–86.

24. Glaeser P, Linzer J, Tunik M, et al. Survey of nationally registered emergency medical services providers: Pediatric education. *Ann Emerg Med* 2000;36(1):33–8.

25. Equipment for ambulances. *Prehosp Emerg Care* 2009;13:364–69.

26. Gausche M, Henderson DP, Brownstein D, Foltin GL. Education of out-of-hospital emergency medical personnel in pediatrics: Report of a national task force. *Ann Emerg Med* 1998;31(1):58–64.

27. Seidel JS, Hornbein M, Yoshiyama K, et al. Emergency Medical Services and the pediatric patient: Are the needs being met? *Pediatrics* 1984;73(6),769–72.

28. Donoghue A, Nadkarni V, Berg RA, et al. Out-of-hospital pediatric cardiac arrest: An epidemiologic review and assessment of current knowledge. *Ann Emerg Med* 2005;46(6): 512–22.

29. Su E., Schmidt TA, Mann NC, Zechnich AD. A randomized controlled trial to assess decay in acquired knowledge among paramedics completing a pediatric resuscitation course. *Acad Emerg Med* 2005;7(7): 779–86.

30. Ali J, Howard M, Williams JI. Do factors other than trauma volume effect attrition of ATLS-acquired skill? *J Trauma* 2003;54(5); 835–41.

31. Wolfram RW, Warren CM, Doyle CR, et al. Retention of pediatric advanced life support (PALS) course concept. *J Emerg Med* 2003;24(4):475–79.

32. Ellis DY, Sorene E, Magen David Adom, EMT Course Outline Resuscitation, 2008 Jan;76(1):5–10. Epub 2007 Sep 4. PMID: 17767990.

33. Gimpel JR, Boulet DO, Errichetti A, Evaluating the clinical skills of osteopathic medical students. *J Am Osteopath Assoc 2003;* 103(6): 267–79.

34. Adler M, Mark D, Vozenilek JA, et al. Development and evaluation of a simulation-based pediatric emergency medicine curriculum. *Acad Med* 2009;84(7): 935–41.

35. Binstadt ES, Walls RM, White BA, et al. A comprehensive medical simulation education curriculum for emergency medical residents. *Ann Emerg Med* 2007;49(4):495–504.

36. Ziv A, Muntz Y, Vardi A, et al. The Israel center for medical simulation: A paradigm for cultural change in medical education. *Acad Med* 2006;81(12):1091–97.

37. Riegel B, Birnbaum T, Aufderheide H, et al. Predictors or cardiopulmonary resuscitation and automated external defibrillation skill retention. *Am Heart J* 2005;150(5):927–32.

38. Wen-Jone Chen, Shoei-Yn Lin-Shiau, Tsung-Chien LU, et al. The demand for prehospital advanced life support and the appropriateness of dispatch in Taipei. *Resuscitation* 2006;71(3);171–79.

39. Committee on Pediatric Emergency Medicine. Policy Statement. Consent for Emergency Medical Services for Children and Adolescents. American Academy of Pediatrics. *Pediatrics* 2003;111(3): 703–6.

40. Fortunati FG Jr, Zonana HV. Legal considerations in the child psychiatric emergency department. Child Adolesc Psychiatr Clin North Am 2003;12(4):745–61.

CHAPTER 44

EMS Violence

Robert E. Suter, A.J. Kirk, Gilberto Salazar

KEY LEARNING POINTS

- Violence is underestimated in the field of EMS, and its effects on personnel may not be reported.
- Injury Prevention is the mainstay of managing violence in EMS.
- The management of the violent patient by EMS personnel must be carefully considered, particularly when restraints are being considered.

- Medical Directors must be intimately involved in the development of preventive protocols and post-incident management.
- EMS documentation is an art form that serves as the first line of defense when legal action is pursued by a party in an incident involving violence.

Violence is the exertion of force resulting in physical, mental or emotional harm or injury. Violence may involve confrontation, verbal assault or physical battery and injury. Prolonged or repeated exposure to violence has subtle and insidious effects. Violence results in direct and indirect costs on EMS systems through both medical costs from injury as well as lost time available for scene response. Responders may require time to recover from non-accidental injuries suffered while on-duty. Responders may also be called upon as witnesses in legal or quality assurance proceedings.

INCIDENCE OF VIOLENCE AGAINST EMS PROVIDERS

EMS workers can experience violence at the hands of aggressive patients, families or bystanders, or can become secondary victims by witnessing to horrible and graphic accidents or conditions. There is inadequate surveillance for the identification and documentation of violence to EMS workers and few estimates are available[1]. One study reported that up to 14% of prehospital situations were associated with violence[2]. Up to 90% of EMS providers report exposure to violence and abuse in the course of their duties[3-5]. Estimates of the occurrence of violent situations during EMS runs varies from 5 to 9% of calls[6], or is as common as one in every 19 runs in some systems[7]. As many as one in five EMS providers report being threatened with a weapon at some time in their professional career[8].

TYPES OF VIOLENCE

Patients are the source of most episodes of violence against EMS personnel. In a report from southern California, nearly 50% of violent episodes involved physical aggression, 30% involved both physical and verbal aggression, and 20% involved verbal aggression only[7]. The risk of harm to EMS providers increases if weapons are encountered in the field[9]. Some societies may enable EMS workers to carry weapons, further statistically increasing the risk of weapon-related injury[5]. Risk factors for violence against EMS providers include police presence (OR 2.8, 95% CI 1.8-4.4); presence of gang members (OR 2.9, 95% CI 1.6-5.3); patients with psychiatric disorders (OR 5.9; 95% CI 3.5-9.9); and patients with alcohol or drug intoxication (OR 7.0; 95% CI 4.4-11.2)[7,10]. It is critical that the pre-hospital provider evaluate for the presence of medical or traumatic conditions which may be causative or co-existent with other conditions as a contributor to violent behavior. In the appropriate circumstances, hypoglycemia as a cause of violent behavior should be considered, diagnosed, and treated[4]. Dementia and delirium from underlying medical illnesses can also result in violent behavior, as can head injury and hypoxia.

DATA COLLECTION AND REPORTING

Two obstacles to the identification and mitigation of violence risk to EMS providers are a lack of attention to the problem of EMS provider exposure to violence and the lack of an organized method of data collection. Pre-hospital injury surveillance projects are almost exclusively focused on the management of patient injury, particularly the management of multiple trauma patients, and the identification of violence towards patients (domestic violence, child abuse, etc) rather than the identification of violence toward EMS personnel. The National EMS Information System (NEMSIS) has only one data element which could represent an episode of violence against the EMS provider (E12_01, Indication of Patient Specific Barriers to Serving the Patient at the Scene)[11].

One attempt to improve documentation of violence-related EMS encounters identified multiple barriers to data collection. Barriers included lack of organizational support; disagreement on a definition of 'violence'; documentation inconsistencies between EMS providers; and lack of documentation about violence. Concerns regarding privacy laws and policies may inhibit the reporting of violence against EMS providers. There is not only a host of federal and state legislation regarding patient privacy but, as a result of fear of reprisals in the form of fines and litigation, hospitals and EMS services have also instituted their own additional regulations based upon system-specific interpretations of the law. This yields a complex web of rules and regulations within which researchers rapidly become mired when attempting to gather the large amounts of data pertinent to violence reporting which is necessary for adequate study power and validity. The problem is further complicated by the need to gather data about multiple subjects (patient, provider, and perhaps multiples of each). EMS providers themselves may be reluctant to report their own feelings of depression, stress, or other psychological disturbances. A central reporting database documenting elements such as incident detail, type of violent exposure encountered, and its effects on the mental and physical well-being of EMS personnel could provide great insight into the problem. Such a database could be used by medical directors to develop strategies for risk mitigation and education, as well as ameliorate the rigors of gathering research data.

Even without a database, an EMS director can still draw reasonable conclusions based upon the general prevalence of violence in the system and the potential need for investigation and corrective action. A director should develop reporting mechanisms within the command structure to bring critical calls to attention and activate post-traumatic incident debriefings. Reporting should include communication between on-scene providers and mid-level personnel, such as shift duty officers and field training officers, to ensure that system-wide adaptations can be made and individuals can receive the support necessary to maintain physical, mental and emotional health. All EMS system members should be aware that the goal of reporting mechanisms is to improve the system and to protect the EMS providers. Occupational safety and health administration boards should encourage reporting of violence in the workplace.

TECHNIQUES FOR MINIMIZING RISK FROM VIOLENCE

There is no consensus in the EMS community regarding the most appropriate and effective manner of addressing violence against EMS providers. It is clear, however, that EMS systems need proactive mechanisms in place to evaluate violent exposures and to change EMS protocols to minimize risk of mental and physical injury. Mechanisms should also exist to maintain the mental and emotional health of EMS providers and to treat disorders once they develop.

The purpose of the EMS system is to assess, treat and transport the ill and injured. However, a responder's first duty is to prevent self-injury by practicing injury prevention. Injury to the EMS provider eliminates that individual as a care provider, and makes the individual a second patient requiring system resources.

SCENE SAFETY

EMS providers must take appropriate precautions and evaluate scene safety before initiating patient contact. Scene safety assessment begins with the first interaction between the individual who contacts EMS and the EMS dispatch center. In most EMS systems, a dispatcher evaluates the scene using data reported by the caller (**Figure 44-1**). Scripted questions help the dispatcher evaluate the scene. Examples of scripted questions may include "What is your emergency?", "Are there any dangers at the scene?", "Are you in a safe location?", "Are the victims in safe locations?", "Is the assailant still at the scene?" and "What types of weapons are at the scene?" Responses to such questions provide valuable information regarding the nature of a possible threat, location hazards known to the EMS system, and ongoing threat levels. A number of commercial dispatch products are available that provide this kind of scripting.[12]

Agencies may also choose to develop these scripts internally. Regardless of the source, it is imperative that appropriate questions be used to gather adequate information. If the dispatcher suspects a violent situation (gunshot, stabs, suicide, substance abuse, location associated with prior episodes of violence), public safety agencies should be dispatched simultaneously and secure the scene.[13] **EMS providers should wait until the scene is secured before beginning care.** Scene assessment and safety should be paramount in the education of a pre-hospital provider and must be practice rather than theory.

At times, scene information is limited or completely unavailable. Automated alarm systems that immediately contact rescue dispatch can create situations where no complainant or further information will be available. With alarms, the only information available to dispatch on many occasions is whether the alarm triggered is for a medical, fire or police emergency. Some cellular phone services, such as prepaid wireless services, may not provide a caller name or address, both of which may have otherwise been linked to useful information such as criminal history or a record of dispatches to that address. Telephone information may also be unobtainable if the caller is unable to speak with the dispatcher for a reason such as incapacity or imminent threat.

If EMS providers happen to be the first to come upon a scene, there will be no initial dispatch information and assessment. Danger may be present from known or unknown persons, chemicals, unfavorable weather and environmental conditions or structural instability. For all of these reasons, the first responding provider should have adequate training to evaluate scene safety and respond appropriately.

PERSONAL PROTECTIVE EQUIPMENT

Personal Protective Equipment includes gloves, masks, face shields and disposable gowns to prevent contamination of the EMS provider with the patient's bodily fluids. Personal protective

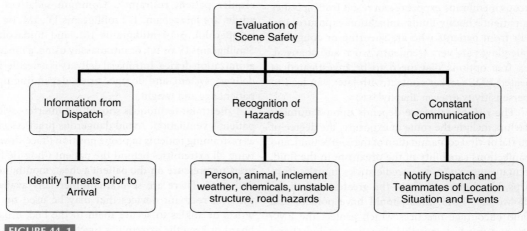

FIGURE 44–1

Basic Elements of Scene Safety.

equipment, however, cannot protect from blunt or penetrating injury. Such equipment also limits EMS provider mobility, vision and tactile sensation. Liquid- and

penetration-proof gloves designed for law enforcement and fire personnel are not thin and flexible enough to allow for reliable palpation of pulses or placement of small peripheral IV catheters. Still, EMS systems are responsible for providing education about situations that require the use of Personal Protective Equipment, and for providing the financial investment in the best protective devices available. Protocols established by local infectious disease authorities, in coordination with EMS directors, should be followed for exposures to blood and body fluid.

OCCUPATIONAL EXPOSURES

Occupational exposure is contact with potentially infectious materials during the course of performing one's professional duties. Occupational exposures can occur as a result of violence against EMS workers or during the course of normal patient care. Materials encountered by EMS workers that are potentially infectious include patient blood, blood products, or blood components; saliva; semen; vaginal secretions; and cerebrospinal, synovial, pleural, pericardial, peritoneal, and amniotic fluids.[14] EMS worker exposure can occur by contact with the worker's skin, mucous membranes (mouth, eyes, nose), or by inhalation. Skin exposure can result from percutaneous contact by needle sticks or sharp objects, from bites, or by direct skin contact with contaminated materials, especially if worker skin is abraded or excoriated. Mucous membrane exposure can result from splashes of a patient's bodily fluids. Inhalation exposures can result from patients who are sneezing or coughing. While gloves are very frequently worn and changed, latex free options may need to be investigated as repeated EMS worker contact with latex can lead to hypersensitivity or even anaphylaxis.

The risk of exposure depends upon a number of factors include the route of exposure, the degree of bacterial or viral contamination of the source fluid, and the infectious capability of the organism in the fluid. Percutaneous exposures (needle sticks, injuries from sharps, bites) generally have the greatest risk to the EMS worker. EMS units should have policies and should encourage practices which protect the EMS worker as much as possible. Practices include hand washing; use of personal protective equipment; cleaning and disinfecting equipment and environmental surfaces with patient contact; cleaning of soiled uniforms; and proper disposal of needles and other sharps and patient waste.

The first step in treatment of a potentially infectious exposure is thorough washing or irrigation of exposed sites with soap and water. **All exposures except small dermal exposures to INTACT skin need immediate medical evaluation.** Immediate medical evaluation is advised because it is best to begin postexposure prophylaxis for HIV within 1 to 2 hours, and certainly within 24 hours of exposure. For exposure to Hepatitis B virus, if the EMS worker is unvaccinated, the Hepatitis B vaccine series should be begun, and Hepatitis B immune globulin given within 24 hours of exposure[15,16].

CHEMICAL AND PHYSICAL RESTRAINT

Before using chemical or physical restraint, the EMS provider should try verbal techniques to calm the patient. At first, speak to the patient from a distance to establish rapport. Do not invade the patient's 'personal space' until you are sure the patient is comfortable with close physical contact[13]. Set explicit guidelines for the patient's behavior without being confrontational. (**Figure 44-2**).

Chemical or physical restraint may be needed to calm a patient for assessment and transport. A violent patient needs to be calmed before ground or air transport to prevent injury to EMS providers. If the patient attacks the EMS driver or pilot, a motor vehicle or aircraft crash can result. Assault on EMS personnel accounts for up to 30% of situations that require patient restraint[17]. Common sedatives for adults are lorazepam, 1-2 milligrams IV, IM, or IO; haloperidol, 5-10 milligrams IM, and midazolam, 5 milligrams IV or IO; or intranasally using, a mucosal atomization device. Intranasal delivery is a needle-free delivery system, and dosage varies depending upon patient age and weight.

Restraint techniques should not interfere with a patient's ventilation. Avoid dangerous practices such as restraining patients in prone position ('face-down'), tying all extremities behind the patient ('hog-tie'), or exerting pressure on the patient's chest, mouth, nose, and neck. There are several commercially available physical restraint devices that may be used on the wrists or ankles to secure them to the bed, a backboard or keep the extremities together (**Figure 44-3A through H**). Restraints can also be fashioned from sheets or blankets. Select restraint devices that are min-

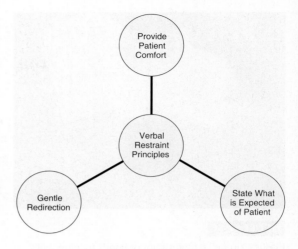

FIGURE 44–2

Diagram of the principles of verbal restraint, which should be attempted prior to chemical or physical restraint. Example of Gentle Redirection: "Please refrain from using foul language." Example of stating what is expected: "I expect you to stay seated during the ambulance ride." Example of providing patient comfort: "Can I get you a blanket to keep you warm?"

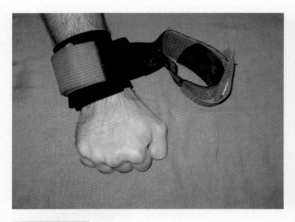

FIGURE 44–3A

Hand restraint, neoprene and Velcro, free end then attached to stabilized object. Photo courtesy of A.J. Kirk.

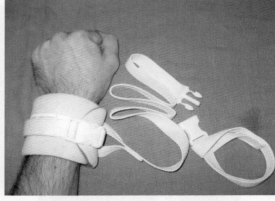

FIGURE 44–3B

Hand restraint, foam, velcro and plastic clip, free end then attached to stabilized object. Photo courtesy of A.J. Kirk.

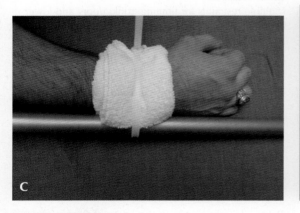

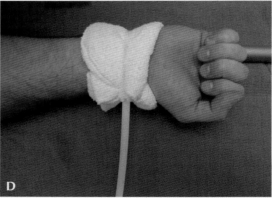

FIGURE 44–3C,D

Plastic "zip-tie" type restraint to railing with washcloth padding. Note that rigid railing is attached away from neurovascular structures. Photo courtesy of A.J. Kirk.

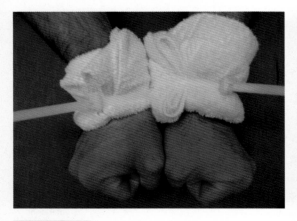

FIGURE 44–3E

Plastic "zip-tie" type restraint of hands together with washcloth padding. Photo courtesy of A.J. Kirk.

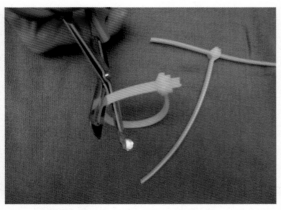

FIGURE 44–3F

Trauma shears are capable of discontinuing plastic restraints. Photo courtesy of A.J. Kirk.

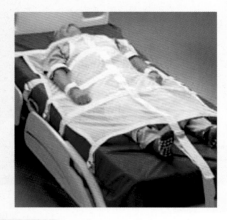

FIGURE 44–3G

Full body restraint. Photo courtesy of J.T. Posey Company, Arcadia, http://www.posey.com

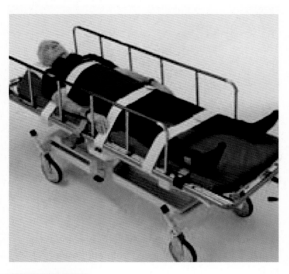

FIGURE 44–3H

Multiple restraints for limiting trunk, upper and lower extremity movement. Photo courtesy of J.T. Posey Company, Arcadia, http://www.posey.com. Permission received 2/17/10.

imally abrasive to a patient's skin, are disposable, and relatively difficult for the patient to remove. Care must be taken that restraints do not worsen a patient's medical condition, and the patient should be kept in a supine or lateral decubitus position rather than prone. Careful reassessment must be performed to ensure that the patient's condition is not worsening, that restrained extremities are distally neurovascularly intact and, if necessary, that further resuscitation/treatment is undertaken. In cases where patients have excited delirium, physical restraint may exacerbate the patient's agitation and consideration of chemical restraint should occur. If the patient is restrained by law enforcement due to legal infractions, which typically occurs via metal or plastic cuff-type devices, law enforcement personnel should accompany the patient to ensure EMS provider safety and to adjust restraint devices as necessary.

PREVENTION AND MANAGEMENT OF EMS VIOLENCE

Protocols to ensure both the safety of the patient and the provider should be in place, but not all injury can be prevented. When violence occurs in the field and a provider is injured, there must be a process in place to effectively manage the incident. The first step in this process is to involve supervising personnel. Should an EMS provider suffer an injury, medical directors and supervisors should be personally involved to ensure the medic obtains the most appropriate immediate medical care and follow-up. Second, leadership must be actively involved in reviewing the incident report to determine if protocols were followed and what can be done to prevent future occurrences. Third, the personnel involved should be debriefed. The debriefing must include discussion of the incident, a review of the protocols, a review of the documentation provided by the personnel involved, and a process to guide the medic in any legal proceedings that may follow. These quality assurance proceedings should be privileged and have a goal of improving training and education rather than of punitive action. Only egregious actions and failure to remediate should change the dynamic

The proper management of the aftermath of violence in EMS is incomplete without appropriate documentation. While thorough documentation must accompany all calls, special care must be taken when documenting calls involving violent circumstances. Providers must recognize that when charting violence-related calls that the records are more likely to be subjected to review. Documentation must be objective and without judgmental language or opinion. Medics should use simple accurate terms to avoid confusion or mis interpretation. The EMS chart provides important third party documentation of what the responding provider finds on scene, but should be limited to pertinent medical documentation. While this may involve facts which may have seemingly obvious associations, including these associations in the chart should be avoided. For instance, if an agitated, violent patient with hand lacerations is found with a bloody knife lying nearby, each fact should be documented and 'transported for evaluation of lacerations' should be used. Avoid phrases which make a conclusion such as 'cut self during murder attempt' or 'transported due to complications of violence'. Utilizing strictly fact-based charting provides a clear reference guide. Providers should be cognizant that both themselves and their charts are subject to subpoena and use care when documenting to avoid extrapolating or drawing conclusions beyond their scope of practice or above their level of expertise. Providers should be educated about appropriate documentation techniques, as well as being assisted with routine educational and quality assurance reviews.

Strong documentation is the best defense when legal action is pursued by a patient or the EMS system in legal cases involving violence against EMS personnel. Discussion of detailed legal proceedings as they pertain to EMS is beyond the scope of this chapter.

The role of the legal system in the discussion of violence in EMS is a topic of controversy. Some local or state governments have passed legislation stating that assault on a health care worker is a serious crime, often times equivalent to assault on law enforcement personnel.

EMS providers are reluctant to report symptoms of depression and post-traumatic stress disorder, such as sadness, loss of interest, poor family interaction, and hopelessness. Irritability, sleep disturbances, changed eating patterns, poor work performance, and lost time from work are other stress indicators. The medical director should be able to recognize such signs and symptoms. Part of the debriefing process after a violent incident must involve an assessment for the need for advanced professional care, from a qualified mental health provider. EMS work is a high-tension, high-stress environment. Stress debriefing (**Figure 44-4**) is an important technique for relieving the mental health strains associated with violent situations or devastating environmental or multi-casualty situations.[13]

Besides official incident debriefing, a provider involved in a violent incident should be encouraged to engage in dialogue regarding the incident. The provider should be given reassurance, and his/her family should be actively involved as a resource for the provider in dealing with the stresses of the incident. Most importantly, clinical evaluation should be arranged in instances where psychological disturbance is suspected.

Violence affects the physical and mental performance of EMS providers. Lost work time appears to be more common for EMS workers than for fire and police elements[18]. Most providers feel that the patient-provider relationship is affected when threat or violence has occurred during the EMS call[19]. Most providers (range from 59% to 89% of reporting providers) report that, to protect their personal safety, they have been forced to compromise or delay patient care. This is both tragic and worrisome, and progress must be made to decrease these interruptions of care. Multi-system and multi-national cooperation is needed to develop uniform and standardized national improvements in policies, procedures and legislation to protect EMS providers from the most corrosive complication of EMS service – exposure to violence and its sequelae.

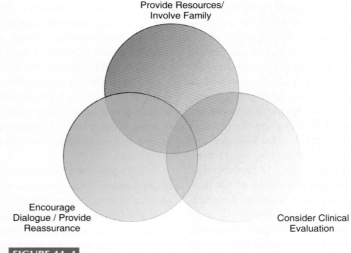

Provide Resources/
Involve Family

Encourage
Dialogue / Provide
Reassurance

Consider Clinical
Evaluation

FIGURE 44–4

Elements of a practical method of stress debriefing.

References

1. Boergerhoff LA, Gerberich SG, Anderson A et al 'Out-of-hospital violence injury surveillance: quality of data collection' Ann Emerg Med 1999 Dec; 34(6): 745-50.
2. Fowlie EJ, Eustis TC, Wright SW, Wrenn KD, Slovis CM: Prospective Field Study in Violence in EMS. Ann Emerg Med Mar 1994; 23:620
3. Pozzi C : Exposure of prehospital providers to violence and abuse. J Emergency Nursing Aug 1998; 24,4:320-323
4. Tintinalli JE, McCoy M 'Violent Patients and the Prehospital Provider' Ann Emerg Med 1993 Aug; 22(8): 1276-9.
5. Corbett SW, Grange JT, Thomas TL 'Exposure of Prehospital Care Providers to Violence' Prehosp Emerg Care 1998 Apr-Jun; 2(2):127-31
6. Mock EF, Wrenn KD, Wright SW, Eustis TC, Slovis CM: Prospective field study of violence in emergency medical services calls. Ann Emerg Med July 1998;32:33-36
7. Grange JT, Corbett SW: Violence Against Emergency Medical Services Personnel. Prehospital Emergency Care 2002; 6,2:186-190
8. Sayah AJ, Thomsen TW, Eckstein M, Hutson HR: EMS Providers and Violence in the Field. Ann Emerg Med Oct 1999;34:S16
9. Thomsen TW, Sayah AJ, Eckstin M, et al 'Emergency Medical Services Providers and Weapons in the prehospital setting' Prehosp Emerg Care 2000 Jul-Sep; 4(3):209-16
10. Flannery RB Jr, Walker AP 'Repetitively assaultive psychiatric patients: fifteen-year analysis of the Assaulted Staff Action Program (ASAP) with implications for emergency services' Int J Emerg Ment Health 2008 Winter; 10(1):1-8.
11. NEMSIS (National EMS Information System) http://www.nemsis.org/softwaredevelopers/downloads/datasetDictionaries.html Accessed Dec 14, 2009
12. Vernon, August: Responding to Violence: A Checklist of Response Considerations. EMS Magazine Nov 2009; 38 (11): 28
13. Holroyd BR, Nabors MD 'Dealing with Violence in the PreHospital Setting' Western Journal of Medicine, Nov 1993, 159(5), 597
14. US Department of Labor: Occupational Exposure to Blood-borne Pathogens: Precautions for Emergency Responders. Washington, DC. Occupational Safety and Health Administration (OSHA) 3130, 1992.
15. Centers for Disease Control and Prevention: Updated US Public Health Service Guidelines for the Management of Occupational Exposures to HBG, HCV, ad HIV and Recommendations for Postexposure Prophylaxis. MMWR 50:1, 2001.
16. Panlilio AL, Cardo DM, Grohskopf LA et al Updated US Public Health Service Guidelines for the management of occupational exposures to HIV and Recommendations for post-exposure prophylaxis MMWR 54:1, 2005.
17. Cheney PR, Gossett L, Fullerton-Gleason L, Weiss SJ, Ernst AA, Sklar D: Relationship of Restraint Use, Patient Injury, and Assaults on EMS Personnel. Prehospital Emergency Care 2006; 10,2:207-212
18. Suyama J, Rittenberger JC, Patterson PD, Hostler D: Comparison of Public Safety Provider Injury Rates. Prehospital Emergency Care 2009; 13,2: 451-455
19. Suserud BO, Blomquiest M, Johansson I: Experiences of threats and violence in the Swedish ambulance service. Accident and Emergency Nursing July 2002; 10,3:127-135

CHAPTER 45

EMS in Rural and Wilderness Areas

Lori Weichenthal, José Cabañas, Sue Spano, Brian Horan, Eric Schmitt

KEY LEARNING POINTS

- ■ Challenges for Rural and Wilderness EMS systems.
  - ■ Adapt to and minimize time delays.
  - ■ Address recruitment, training and retention of personnel.
  - ■ Seek qualified medical direction.
  - ■ Establish and maintain funding.
  - ■ Maintain adequate communication.
  - ■ Deal with unique environments.
- ■ Special Consideration for Wilderness and Rural Settings.

- ■ Access to scene.
- ■ Weather.
- ■ Day or nighttime.
- ■ Terrain.
- ■ Special transport needs.
  - ■ Special handling needs.
  - ■ Access and transport times.
  - ■ Available personnel.
  - ■ Communications.

The goals of EMS care in rural and wilderness areas are the same as those in more densely populated regions, but the capacity of EMS systems to respond to a patient is more limited (**Figure 45-1**). Response and transport time is inevitably prolonged, and the "golden hour", which is the focus of most urban EMS systems, can turn into hours or even days. Other challenges for EMS care in remote settings include: recruitment, training and retention of personnel; lack of access to qualified medical direction; funding issues; and adequacy of communication and other infrastructure. This chapter addresses some of the unique challenges that exist in providing EMS care in remote settings (**Figure 45-2**). It reviews special skills and equip-ment needed to provide prehospital care in snow and alpine environments, high altitudes, caves and marine environments

Challenges in Rural and Wilderness EMS

Time Loss in Response and Transport

In rural and wilderness settings there are delays in reaching definitive care that begin with delayed detection and notification and extend to prolonged transport times. Some of these delays can be modified by systems organization, but other delays require special training in temporizing measures during scene and transport care.

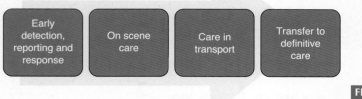

FIGURE 45–1

The goals of EMS.

Critical Incident Detection

The first delay is incident detection and reporting. Rural and wilderness areas are vast physical areas that are sparsely populated. A motor vehicle crash on a remote country or mountain road may not be detected and reported for hours or days. Land-line telephones may not be available and cell phones may not be operational. Companions can go for help, but a solo adventurer has no options other than him or herself.

The best way to decrease the time to detection of a critical incident in remote areas is *lay person awareness and vigilance*. Examples of awareness are observation for possible motor vehicle crashes, or visitation to medically fragile members of the local community. Vigilance can be promoted by public education sponsored by churches, the public sector or by community groups. Those who travel to wilderness areas need heightened vigilance to detect fellow travelers who need assistance, and should be armed with basic skills and training for survival. Education and practice in austere settings can be provided by public or private entities such as national parks or expedition services.

Critical Incident Reporting

Once critical incidents are detected, reporting is usually by calling a phone number that connects to the EMS system. Standard emergency care access numbers (**Figure 45-3**) may not be available in rural settings

In the US there are still over 400 counties and tribal nations that have no 911 access. In some remote rural areas, the only way to activate EMS may be by using emergency call boxes. In developing countries and wilderness settings it may be even more difficult

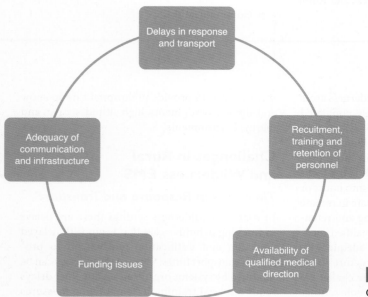

FIGURE 45–2

Challenges of EMS in Remote Settings.

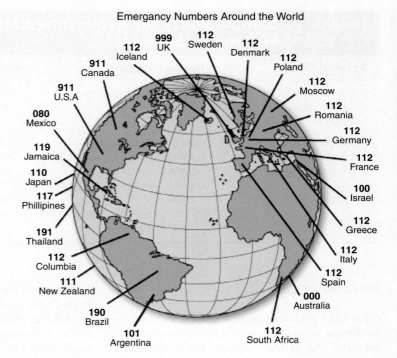

FIGURE 45–3

Some Emergency Numbers Around the World.

to report critical incidents and to activate the EMS system. If cell phone service is available, it may be intermittent or with poor reception and cannot pinpoint the call location. **The more remote the setting, the more important it is for the public to know secondary methods for EMS access.** Secondary methods include location of call boxes, ranger stations, or base camps equipped with a radio. Future US goals include insuring completed hardwire Enhanced 911 and wireless Enhanced 911 in remote areas, and the establishment of roadside call-boxes, satellite and or cellular networks to cover all rural primary roads.

EMS Dispatch and Arrival

The next challenge is getting trained personnel to the scene. If traditional ground transport is used, days or weeks can elapse due to long distances, poor roads and austere terrain. In wilderness settings, the first patient access may be by all terrain vehicle, snowmobile, pack animals, or on foot. **Rescuer safety is paramount** and may result in further delays. A full search and rescue operation may be needed **(Table 45-1)**. Thus, rural and wilderness EMS systems need alternative and rapid methods for scene access, usually helicopter or fixed wing aircraft. In very remote settings, aircraft may provide first access, and in other environments,

aircraft can be a secondary resource requested by the first responders (see **Table 45-2**). Some EMS systems have created policies that allow for simultaneous response of ground and air transport for potentially life-threatening circumstances (**Table 45-3**).

EMS personnel who work in remote settings often have less training than those who work in populated areas. This phenomenon is called the rural ALS paradox[1]. EMS aircraft can bring highly trained personnel quickly to the scene who can educate while they provide care.

Table 45–1	**Special Considerations in a Wilderness EMS Call**

- Access to scene
- Weather
- Daylight
- Terrain
- Special transport needs
- Special handling needs
- Access and transport times
- Available personnel
- Communications

Table 45–2	**Sample Policy for Requesting EMS Helicopter Services**	
Technical Criteria	**Trauma Criteria**	**Medical Criteria**
>30 mins ground transport time to an appropriate hospital	Multi-casualty incidents	Multiple or prolonged seizures refractory to medication
Helicopter transport ≥ 10 minutes faster than ground transport	Critical trauma patient(s) Spinal injuries with neurologic signs or symptoms Serious burns or environmental exposure Amputation or vascular compromise of a limb	Seizures in pregnancy Cardiovascular instability Any injured or ill patient in an inaccessible area or with an extended time for arrival of local care

Provision of Care

Once EMS personnel reach a patient in a rural or wilderness setting, the focus turns to providing care on scene and during transport. EMS personnel in more remote settings many spend hours or even days with their patients before reaching definitive care. Thus, special training, standard orders and written policies should be in place for the management of lengthy scene and transport times. Standing orders are important in the event of radio failure, which occurs frequently in remote settings. The recently modified US National Park Service (NPS) Field Manual has several examples of polices adapted for remote settings. The manual not only breaks down policies for the different levels of training of EMS personnel, but also has time considerations and orders in the event of radio failure. EMS in the National Parks is mainly provided by first responders, EMTs and Paramedics (Park rangers who are trained as intermediate EMTs with special skills that pertain to the wilderness setting). Examples of standing orders include options for repeat boluses during prolonged patient contacts and orders for antibiotics to be given for serious wounds if the transport time to definitive care is greater than three hours (**Table 45-4**).

Table 45–3	**Sample Policy of Simultaneous Dispatch of EMS Ground and Air Medical Transport**	
Technical Criteria	**Medical Criteria**	
Primary EMS helicopter for the zone is available for immediate response	Burns >18% BSA	
Incident is outside a metropolitan area	Unconscious	
Large scale multi-casualty incidents	Severe dyspnea	
Incident site is not within the city where an available ambulance is stationed	Seizures in pregnancy Diving accident Industrial accident (status questionable or caught in machinery) Gunshot wound or stab (not alert, central wound, multiple wounds, multiple victms) Major motor vehicle accident or serious mechanism of injury	

Table 45–4	**Sample Protocol for Major Trauma in a Wilderness Setting**

EMT Standing Orders
1. ABCs: Protect airway, assist ventilations and suction as needed
2. Spinal immobilization
3. Primary assessment: Check vital signs, check the back for penetrating trauma, calculate trauma score
4. Control bleeding: Direct pressure and elevation, three-sided dressing to open chest or neck wounds, and bandage non life/limb threatening injuries in route
5. Transport/ALS back-up: On scene time <10 minutes when transport available. Consider air transport for altered level of consciousness or unstable vital signs
6. Oxygen: Low flow for stable patients; high flow or Bag-Valve-Mask ventilation for unstable patients as indicated
7. Prevent hypothermia: Remove wet clothing and apply blankets
8. Secondary Assessment: Repeat vital signs and mental status, perform secondary survey and determine medical history, medications and allergies
9. Base contact
10. Splint/bandage injuries: Immobilize and splint fractures in route. Reduce fractures/dislocations with deformity affecting ability to splint/transport or if decreased distal pulses exist

Parkmedic Standing Orders
All that are included in EMT standing orders plus:
1. ABCs: Secure airway with ALS airway (Combitube/King or Endotracheal tube)
2. IVs: Establish one 14-16 gauge IV for stable patients. For unstable patients establish two 14-16 gauge IVs. For SBP >100 and HR <100 give LR/NS at maintenance (120 mL/hour); If SBP 80-100 or HR >100 give a 500 mL bolus; If SBP<80 then bolus 1 Liter (L) under pressure

Parkmedic Base Hospital/Communication Failure Orders
1. Needle Thoracostomy: If not in arrest, must have severe respiratory distress, hemodynamic compromise, decreased breath sounds on one side and distended neck veins/tracheal deviation
2. Intravenous Fluid (IVF): After 3 L of IVF, continue boluses per standing orders based on SBP
3. Cefazolin: Consider for serious wounds if >3 hours between injury and arrival at hospital

ALS = Advanced Life Support; SBP = systolic blood pressure; HR = heart rate; LR = lactated Ringer's; NS = normal saline.
Adapted from NPS EMS Field Manual Protocol 2150. http://nasemso.org/documents/FRFieldManual.pdf.

Recruitment, training and retention of EMS Personnel

In most urban settings, EMS call volumes are high which makes it easy to attract private agencies to provide EMS services, and may allow for adequate salaries to attract and retain personnel. In rural and wilderness settings, calls are sporadic and there may be no ability to collect payment for care. Thus, most EMS care in remote areas is provided by public agencies that rely largely on volunteers or by lay persons with some form of basic medical training. The exception to this is austere settings that are managed by government agencies, such as national park services, or situations where private companies or expeditions access the wilderness. In such circumstances, paid and more highly trained personnel are frequently available.

Regardless, training and re-training is more difficult in rural and wilderness settings, due to lack of access to training institutions, and lack of training in special wilderness situations. Even if initially well-trained, skills maintenance is difficult because patient contacts are less frequent and continuing education is not as available.

These challenges make the recruitment, training, and retention of personnel difficult. Many EMS volunteer personnel have other responsibilities including full time jobs and families, and they have little time for additional training in skill maintenance. Concerns about personal liability, and a lack of community understanding and appreciation can also result in low retention rates for volunteer EMS personnel.[2]

Community awareness and support are needed for rural and wilderness EMS systems to recruit, train, and retain adequate personnel. This support can take many forms, including but not limited to: using local schools to help develop a culture of volunteerism and community service; fundraising to support EMS personnel with on-call pay; asking local businesses to provide paid time off for employees who serve as EMS volunteers so that they can further their training and education; encouraging communities to recognize the volunteers who serve in their community.

Personnel need to be cross-trained in more patient rich settings (i.e. spend time in urban settings, with high call volumes) or they must have access to continuing education to assure skill maintenance. Some rural communities can integrate EMS personnel into the local health care systems, serving as physician or nurse extenders in primary care offices or local hospitals setting.

Availability of Qualified Medical Direction

Distance and financial disincentives make it difficult to find physicians willing to provide medical direction to remote EMS systems.

These difficulties convinced the United States National Highway Traffic Safety Administration (NHTSA) to co-sponsor the development of a "Guide for Preparing Medical Directors" through the National Association of EMS physicians and the American College of Emergency Physicians. Still, it is hard for many rural physicians who have the interest and desire to access these courses. Thus communities in remote settings need to decide to support EMS medical director training for local physicians, or otherwise to seek medical direction from developed EMS systems. Both options have their advantages and disadvantages. Local physician oversight assures that the medical direction has an understanding of local issues and impediments to EMS care. Use of medical direction from other EMS systems provides experienced medical direction but not always a clear understanding of the special local circumstances, and community support is less likely.

Funding Issues

Providing adequate financial support for EMS services is an issue in even the most developed urban EMS system. In rural and wilderness settings, due to few patient encounters, funding is often very limited, and even when available, does not take into consideration the time that EMS personnel invest in patient care on scene or in transport. Because of a limited ability to generate revenue, many EMS agencies in remote settings do not put time or energy into billing and collections. If the EMS role is a public service the concept of billing may not exist.

One option is the formation of small agency EMS collectives so that billing tasks can be shared. This collective approach not only helps smaller agencies develop a broader geographic basis for financial support, but it can also allow sharing of other services such as alternative forms of advanced life support transport, medical oversight, and continuing education and quality improvement[1]. Some public agencies in wilderness settings, such as the National Park Service, who traditionally did not charge for their EMS care, are now doing this. In many very austere settings, such as Mt. Everest, individuals entering the environment are now required to have medical and rescue insurance.

While rural and wilderness EMS systems have fewer calls in any particular time period, the personnel tend to spend more time with each patient and to provide more care on scene and in transport. Reimbursement models need to take this into consideration.

Communications and Infrastructure

Many remote EMS service providers depend on Very High Frequency (VHF) and Ultra High Frequency (UHF) radio frequencies for communication. This aging infrastructure has resulted in crowded radio frequencies and unreliable radio equipment. More remote settings must rely on radio repeaters where an initial weak radio transmission is received and retransmitted at a higher or more powerful level. Such transmission requires extra personnel and adds an element of time delay in on-line medical control. Cellular and satellite technology is unreliable for the same distance and topography related reasons as radio. Thus, technology updates must be investigated to provide better and more innovative communication options in remote settings.

Unique Settings in Rural and Wilderness EMS

Snow and Alpine Environments

Injuries in snow and alpine environments are common. The National Ski Areas Association reports an average of 38 deaths per year in the US from skiing and snowboarding, and non-lethal injuries are common. Worldwide the current incidence of ski injuries is 2/1000 skier days. Traumatic brain injury is the leading worldwide cause of ski and snowboarding morbidity and mortality. Other alpine illnesses are due to exposure (hypothermia, frostbite, etc.) altitude (mountain sickness, pulmonary or cerebral edema), or exacerbations of underlying medical illness. The concentration of individuals in dangerous locations also creates the opportunity for multi- or mass-casualty incidents, for example resulting from an avalanche or ski lift collapse.

Work within the snow environment requires special equipment. Warm clothing in removable layers is needed for provider comfort and safety. The minimum standard includes hat, gloves, a base layer, a middle insulation layer, and a waterproof shell. Patients are often cold, wet, or inadequately prepared for the environment, so rescuers should carry extra clothing for patient use. Sleeping bags or blankets are useful for hypothermic patients or to protect frostbitten extremities. If there is *any* risk of avalanche or unstable snow conditions, then *every* provider should carry a shovel, avalanche probe, and transceiver. Patient care equipment should include a variety of bandages for dressing wounds, materials for splinting orthopedic injuries, and equipment for spinal immobilization. Standard resuscitative aids should also be available (oxygen delivery apparatus, IV catheters and fluids, monitor/defibrillator or AED, etc.). Specially designed sleds or toboggans are available for patient transportation over snowy terrain and work well in areas that are rugged or difficult to access. All providers should be able to assess for hypothermia, frostbite and altitude sickness and provide appropriate treatment when these conditions are encountered. Rescue teams need members who can assess snow stability and avalanche risk. Team members should know how to use an avalanche transceiver and practice with it frequently. Travel over snow requires skis or snowshoes. Steep or icy terrain requires experience in the use of crampons, ice axes, and/or ropes and belaying techniques. Belaying consists of a variety of techniques used in climbing, to exert friction on a climbing rope to prevent a climber from falling. Snowmobiles, toboggans or sleds facilitate patient transport over snow.

High Altitude and Mountain Settings

Travel to high altitude is popular, and environments that were formerly accessed by professional mountaineers are now available to casual outdoor enthusiasts. About one in ten who summit Mt. Everest die.[3]

Caring for patients in high altitude settings commonly requires all the equipment, knowledge and skills described in the snow and alpine environment section. The ability to perform high angle rescue is frequently required. The level of training needed to perform high angle can require over 100 hours of instruction. Some examples of skills that providers need to perform high angle rescue include the ability to assess the rescue operation; the ability to work with ropes and related equipment; and the capability to belay and rappel and to set up lowering, ascending and tensioned rope systems. Basic equipment needed for

| Table 45–5 | **Sample list of basic personal and team equipment needed for high angle rescue**[4] |

Personal Protective Equipment
- Gloves
- Helmet
- Hiking or high top duty boots
- Protective Clothing
- Lighting
- Harness

Team Equipment
- Static rescue rope
- Locking D carabiners
- 2 inch pulleys
- O ring or steel rigging ring
- 7 mm Prusiks (friction hitch)
- Daisy chains
- Eight plates with ears
- Brake bar rack
- Münter hitch carabiners
- Webbing
- Line gun
- Radios
- Edge rollers
- Cliff pickets
- Stokes Litter basket/stretcher

high angle rescue include personal protective equipment and team equipment, in addition to necessary medical supplies (see **Table 45-5**)[4].

Air rescue at high altitude creates special challenges, as the displacement of enough air to keep rotary wing aircraft airborne in low density atmosphere limits the altitude for safe operation. Patient and equipment weight restrictions are significant considerations as is finding an adequate landing zone.

Proficiency in rapid recognition and treatment of High Altitude Sickness (HAS) is also required. HAS is a spectrum of disease. Acute mountain sickness (AMS), which is characterized by symptoms including headache, nausea, vomiting, malaise, insomnia, anorexia, and shortness of breath on exertion is quite common at elevations above 10,000 ft (3000 meters) **(Figure 45-4)**[5,6]. The more severe presentations of HAS are high altitude pulmonary edema (HAPE) or the combination of ataxia, confusion, nausea and vomiting, and headache of high altitude cerebral edema (HACE). With HACE or HAPE victims, immediate descent is the top treatment priority. Several pharmacologic adjunctive measures are available to mitigate

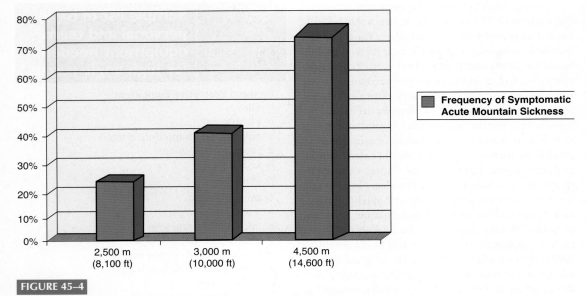

Relationship Between Altitude and Acute Mountain Sickness.

symptoms including: Acetazolamide for the prophylaxis and treatment of HAS; Nifedipine to treat HAPE, and Dexamethasone to treat HACE. Specialized equipment, such as a portable hyperbaric chamber, can also help in the treatment of more life threatening forms of HAS when decent is not an option. Although in-depth discussion of high-altitude pathophysiology and treatments are outside of the scope of this text, the appropriate resources should be available to rescue personnel both in their training and via on-line or off-line medical control. The National Park Service's policy for the treatment of HAS is a good example of how off-line medical control can be provided in this austere setting (**Table 45-6**).

Cave Rescue

Cave rescue is a highly specialized field within wilderness medicine in which wounded, trapped and on occasions, lost explorers are medically treated and extracted from a subterranean environment. The number of cave rescue incidents around the world is small compared to other common wilderness emergencies. For example, in the US the average number of reported cave related incidents is usually between 40-50 per year. Generally, caving accidents are attributed to poor judgment, combined with little or minimal caving experience. **Common causes of injuries are falls, becoming pinned in cracks, injuries from falling rocks, and hypothermia.** Fatalities are rare and vary according to geographical regions and the

type of caves in those areas. For instance, in Puerto Rico fatalities are very low, approximately 1 every 6 years in average and most are related to drowning.

Responding to caving incidents is a huge challenge for wilderness emergency care providers because of the extreme environmental conditions they may encounter. Being a cave rescuer is like a mountain rescuer except the cave rescuer usually works upside down, with limited visibility and in mud. Cave rescuers are confronted with darkness, dust, mud, and water currents. Temperature extremes are common and will have a direct impact on patients and rescuers. Temperature illnesses (e.g. hypothermia, hyperthermia) are frequent and rescuers must be skilled in their identification and management. Temperature differentials can exist within a single cave, as a result of exposure, orientation, and water flow. Usually, US continental caves run from cool to cold. In tropical and warm environments caves can be hot, and cavers must wear lightweight clothes. All of these environmental conditions will slow down the goal in a cave rescue operation, which is to safely extricate the patient.

A significant number of caves around the world are formed by flowing water through rocks. There is a significant hazard every time water currents exist in a cave. Rescuers must understand local water current flows because small streams can become powerful torrents in response to an unexpected rain. Cave rescue teams can be caught unexpectedly while crossing water streams. Therefore, planning is very important before entering a cave.

Table 45–6	**Sample Protocol for HAPE**

EMT Standing Orders
1. ABCs
2. Assessment: Vital Signs, respiratory distress at rest, lung sounds, sputum, mental status, rapid ascent to altitudes >8,000 feet (2438 meters)
3. Oxygen: per procedure oxygen administration
4. Rapid descent: Assist patient with rapid descent. Consider air transport
5. Transport/ALS back up: do not delay descent for ALS arrival
6. Base contact: For all patients

Parkmedic Standing Orders
All that is included in EMT standing orders plus:
1. ABCs: ALS airway if indicated
2. Intravenous (IV) fluids: Saline lock or TKO per protocol

Parkmedic Base Hospital/Communication Failure Orders
1. Nifedipine: If severe symptoms:
   a. Adults: 10 milligrams capsule chewed until capsule is broken and swallowed
   b. 6-12 years: Squeeze $^1/_2$ capsule under tongue
   c. <6 years: Squeeze $^1/_4$ capsule under tongue
   d. All ages: Repeat every 20 minutes up to 3 doses, unless symptoms resolve or SPB drops by 20 mm Hg and SBP <100
2. Gamow Bag: If descent not possible, go to procedure on Gamow Bag (inflatable pressure bag)
3. IV fluids: Consider maintenance fluids for prolonged transport per procedure

ALS = Advanced Life Support; TKO = to keep vein open; SBP = systolic blood pressure.
Adapted from US National Park Service EMS Field Manual Protocol 2030. http://nasemso.org/documents/FRFieldManual.pdf.

Vertical hazards are very dangerous in a subterranean environment. Many caves have multiple vertical passages that represent a potential for falls, falling rocks and rescue team fatigue. Inexperienced rescuers in an unfamiliar cave can encounter unexpected drops while walking, which could be fatal.

Biologic hazards are present in a number of caves around the world. Water contamination, histoplasmosis, and rabies are some of those potential hazards. For instance, inhaled urine droplets from bats infected with rabies have been linked to outbreaks in humans. In Central America, exposure to soil-born organisms can cause lung and skin irritation. Therefore, cave rescuers must take all the necessary precautions in areas that are suspected for contamination.

Cave rescuers tailor rescue techniques from firefighting, confined space rescue, high angle mountaineering and rope rescue and develop their own set of special skills. When a caving incident occurs, regular prehospital care providers are rarely deployed in the cave extraction phase. Generally cave rescue is undertaken by specially trained experienced cavers. Traditional, emergency care providers and managers must understand that cave rescue operations are slow and require high level of organized teamwork. A network of international cave rescue units is organized under the banner of the Union International de Spéléologie (UIS) - Cave Rescue Commission. In the US the leading cave rescue training is taught by the National Cave Rescue Commission (NCRC), which operates as a division of the National Speleological Society (NSS). The NCRC is not an operational unit, but the organization is comprised of members of regional and local rescue squads. The NCRC provides a number of weeklong seminars that consist of extensive classroom and fieldwork in all elements of a cave rescue operation.

Marine Environments

The earth's oceans cover approximately 70% of the earth's surface. More than half of this area is over 3000 meters (9800 feet) deep. Seawater has an average salinity of 35 parts per thousand and temperatures that range from -2 to 30 degrees Celsius. Much of the earth's population lives within a few hundred miles of the coastline and the oceans are used for recreation and professional endeavors. EMS agencies whose catchment area includes oceans must be prepared to deal with this special environment including having the knowledge and skills to perform water rescue, manage immersion injures and exposure, deal with marine envenomations and treat illness related to dysbarism.

Water rescue is a specialized skill that requires training and continuous maintence of abilities. Water rescue in the marine setting can vary depending on the situation: open water, surf and swift water, or dive rescue. The International Life Saving Federation (ILS) has set basic standards for all levels of water rescue. The focus of water rescue is always to rescue the endangered person while preventing the rescuers from becoming victims. Thus the focus is on attempting rescue first without having the rescuer enter the water. **A common algorithm is "Talk, Reach, Wade, Throw, Hello, Row, Go, Tow".** All water rescue personnel, at a minimum, require a personal flotation device (PDF). Depending on the rescue situation other specialized equipment may be utilized including throw bags, flotation canisters, personal water craft, paddle boards wet and/or dry suits and SCUBA gear.

In addition to skills in water rescue, EMS personnel who work in a marine environment must be able to recognize and treat the illnesses and injuries common to the setting. Immersion injures and exposure is quite common. Near drowning victims and individuals suffering from hypothermia first must be removed from the marine environment. Then the focus is on airway stabilizations, resuscitation, re-warming and timely transfer to definitive care.

Envenomations are also frequently encountered in this setting. The ocean is home to over 200,000 species of animals, some of which are the most toxic on the planet. Marine animals use venoms as both a means to acquire food and for defense. **Most of the common marine venoms are heat labile and are denatured in hot water.** There are antivenins for only a few specific toxins. The first goal of rescue from toxic envenomation is removal from the ocean environment to prevent drowning. Then, proper wound care, with cleaning and removal of foreign bodies and hot water as tolerated, are general care guidelines until transfer to definitive care is possible.

If EMS personnel work in a marine environment where SCUBA diving is common, they need training in dysbarism and complications of diving. Dysbarism refers to medical conditions resulting from changes in ambient pressure. These conditions can simply be painful and irritating (mask squeeze, middle ear squeeze) or they can be life-threatening (decompression sickness, arterial gas embolism). The focus is again on rescue from the ocean environment, stabilization and resuscitation and recognition of the condition. If a serious form of dysbarism is suspected, transportation to a facility with a hyperbaric chamber may be of benefit. **EMS personnel who work in a marine setting should be aware of the closet hyperbaric facility and have policies and procedures which support transportation of victims with severe forms of dysbarism to these facilities.** The Divers Alert Network (DAN) is a good resource for identifying where hyperbaric chambers are located.

Web Resources

1. http://www.equipped.com. Equipped to Survive: Contains sections on survival in different austere settings and has a list of schools and course available in wilderness medicine. Accessed & verified 02/12/09.
2. http://www.wms.org. Wilderness Medicine Society which has lists of conferences in wilderness medicine as well as educational and research resources. Accessed 06/23/09, 02/13/10
3. http://www.nols.org. National Outdoor Leadership School which offers a wide range of courses in wilderness medicine skills throughout the world. Accessed 07/12/09, 02/13/10
4. http://www.ilsf.org. International Lifesaving Federation which provides education and resources on water safety, lifeguard training and drowning facts and prevention. Accessed 08/17/09, 02/13/10
5. http://ismmed.org. International Society of Mountain Medicine that contains information on high altitude illness and a bookstore. Accessed 08/18/09, verified 02/13/10
6. http://www.caves.org. National Speleological Society (NSS) offers information on caves and cave safety. Accessed 08/20/09, verified 02/13/10
7. http://www.diversalertnetwork.org Divers Alert Network (DAN) offers emergency hotlines, dive medicine frequently asked questions, training information and more. Accessed 09/19/09, verified 02/13/10

Selected Readings

1. McGinnis KK. Rural and Frontier Emergency Medicine Services: Agenda for the Future. *National Rural Health Association* 2004.
2. Auerbach PS. *Wilderness Medicine.* 5th edition. Mosby, Inc. 2007.
3. Bledsoe G, Manyak MJ, Townes DA. *Expedition and Wilderness Medicine.* First Edition. Cambridge University Press 2008.
4. Greyman JP, Norris TE, Hart LG. *Textbook of Rural Medicine.* First Edition. McGraw-Hill 2001.
5. Yawn BP, Bushy A, Yawn RA. *Exploring Rural Medicine: Current Issues and Concepts.* SAGE Publications Inc. 1994.

References

1. McGinnis KK. Rural and Frontier Emergency Medicine Services: Agenda for the Future. *National Rural Health Association* 2004; 6–7.
2. Erisman G. Rural Emergency Response-the Safety and Health Safety Net. *National Ag Safety Database* 2001; 5–6.
3. Mt. Everest History, Facts: at http://www.mnteverest.net/history.html. (accessed 11/09).
4. Soderstrom M, Hogan M, Turnbull P et al. Technical Rope Rescue: Technician Level. *Rescue Three International* 2001; 47–49.
5. Hackett PH, Roach RC. High Altitude Illness. *N Engl J Med* 2001; 345:107–114.
6. Honigman B, Theis MK, Koziol-McLain J, et al. Acute mountain sickness in a general tourist population at moderate altitudes. *Ann Intern Med* 1993; 118: 587.

CHAPTER 46

Military EMS Systems

Robert A. De Lorenzo, Julio Lairet, Jerry Mothershead, C. James Holliman

KEY LEARNING POINTS

- Unique aspects of military EMS include the need to provide care and evacuation in battlefield environments and to manage sudden large numbers of casualties.

- Many of the most important components of civilian EMS, including aeromedical evacuation, resuscitation techniques for shock, and tiered trauma referral developed from military medical innovations and experience.

Military forces in different countries have developed structured and organized systems of early medical care and evacuation to deal with the high numbers of battlefield casualties in their armed conflicts and have often developed prehospital care systems to care for military personnel who reside on military bases. Of note, many of the key innovations in modern civilian EMS came as a direct result of information and experience gained through medical support of military operations. Progressive military organizations have recognized the effectiveness, efficiency, and morale boosting of having reliable EMS services for both the battlefield and garrison environments.

HISTORY OF MILITARY EMS DEVELOPMENT

Throughout much of history, the care of wounded soldiers was neglected or poorly administered. Military commanders were more concerned with tactics, troop movements, and supplies. Before the

18th century, surgeons accompanying armies usually served only the nobility. Troops had to depend on nonmedical comrades or family for medical care. Queen Isabella of Spain was possibly the first monarch to organize field help for wounded soldiers. In 1487 at the siege of Malaga, wounded soldiers were carried in bedded wagons to large tent hospitals in safe rear areas. These ambulances were unwieldy, requiring up to 40 horses to pull them, and were initially stationed miles from the battlefield. The limited available surgical care for the wounded troops was then typically delayed many hours. Thoughtful military leaders recognized that this recurrent poor medical care wasted military manpower and was demoralizing to the soldier.[1]

Routine organized collection of the wounded from the battlefield began during the Napoleonic Wars. Napoleon's surgeon Jean Larrey developed what became known as the ambulance volantes or "flying" field hospitals. These lightweight carriages and medical facilities moved quickly to collect, transport, and care for the injured, even as the fighting continued.[2]

The earliest major development of US military emergency medical care came during the US Civil War (1861 to 1865). More than 600,000 soldiers died in this conflict, making it the US's most costly life conflict (by comparison there were about 400,000 US military deaths in the Second World War). The first major battle of the war, (First) Bull Run in 1861, was a disaster by most military and medical standards. The Union Army entered the battle with few ambulances or medical personnel. Many litter bearers were untrained bandsmen who laid down their musical instruments and then picked up litters. Civilian ambulance drivers reportedly often drank the alcohol in their medicine chests and stayed near the battlefield only long enough to rob the wounded. Uninjured but panicking, Union soldiers commandeered some ambulances near the end of the battle that had not broken down or been already taken over by officers for their personal use. In the Union Army's panicked retreat, reportedly not a single wounded soldier was directly transported to safety. Three days after the battle, over 3000 wounded men still lay on the battlefield unprotected from the elements. Some were without care for 6 to 7 days. Many died from lack of food, water, and basic medical care.[3]

As a result of the Bull Run fiasco, the Union Army restructured its initially haphazard wartime emergency care services. William Hammond, Surgeon General of the Union Army, and Jonathan Letterman, medical director of the Army of the Potomac, were two of the most active proponents in improving the Army's delivery of organized medical care and field evacuation. Letterman is credited with developing the first Army-wide ambulance service in 1862.[4] In 1887 the Hospital Corps was established, which is the forerunner of the modern enlisted medical corps. Men who volunteered from line units were given training in first aid and litter bearing. After a one-year apprenticeship, candidates could take an examination for selection as privates in the Hospital Corps. Following one year of probationary training and passing another examination, they could be appointed "Hospital Stewards."[5]

The military EMS system relies on the training of individual nonmedical soldiers in basic preventive medicine and first aid, prepositioned more advanced care providers ("medics"), adequate numbers of appropriate ambulances, and a system of graduated care. Rapid transport and early hospitalization and surgery made a tremendous impact on military preparedness by preventing disease, boosting morale, and conserving manpower. Through evolving technology and individual creativity, the military medical system

Table 46–1	**Overall Mortality of Battle Casualties Reaching Treatment Facilities**[19]
War	**Mortality (%)**
World War I	8.0
World War II	4.5
Korea	2.5
Vietnam	2.0

Adapted from: [19]Baxt W.G., Moody P. The impact of rotorcraft aeromedical emergency care services on mortality. *JAMA.* 1983; 249:3047–3051.

has continually improved wartime military casualty survival rates (Table 46-1). An estimated 22,000 lives were saved in Vietnam as a result of advances developed during or after the Korean War.[6]

Lessons learned and innovations developed in Vietnam were brought to the United States by returning military care providers during the 1960s and early 1970s. Elements of the US military's systems approach to emergency medical care were integrated into the civilian community. Contributing to civilian EMS improvements were military influences such as aeromedical evacuation, centers specializing in the care of trauma victims, provision of advanced life support care, and tiered levels of providers.[7,8] Civilian EMS services enjoyed tremendous growth during the 1960s and 1970s, in part due to the role the military played in laying the groundwork for prehospital care and also to the knowledge of the many military personnel who returned from the war to civilian life having received relatively advanced military medical training.

CURRENT MILITARY EMS

The modern military EMS system exists as a result of both military wartime and peacetime requirements. The goal of each of these requirements is to accomplish a specified mission. The military medical system's overall mission is to conserve the forces' fighting strength.[9] During peacetime the mission is accomplished much as it is in the civilian EMS community, but it is drastically modified during conflict. The wartime medical system can best be understood by describing its personnel, organization, transportation, equipment, communications, and control.

Military Medical Personnel

The military services provide medical assistance through a spectrum of trained personnel. From battlefield medics with basic skills to sophisticated nursing, physician, administrative, and logistical support personnel, individuals are assigned a specific job with associated training and skills that are divided into different levels of care providers.

All nonmedical military personnel receive basic first-aid training in procedures such as bleeding control and simple splinting. The military uses the terms "self-aid" and "buddy-aid" to describe this "first line" of emergency medical defense. In the Army, selected nonmedical soldiers (usually one per vehicle crew or operating team) are given an additional 40 hours of training to include intravenous insertion, advanced splinting, and other more complex first-aid measures. This level is termed "combat lifesaver" and approximates the civilian certified first-responder program, with an expanded scope of practice.[9]

Up until the year 2000, the Army Military Occupational Specialty (MOS) 91B Medical Specialist (combat medic) received ten weeks of training that roughly correlates with the civilian basic emergency medical technician (EMT-B) training. Additional training is provided in intravenous insertion and the care of patients with military-related problems such as nuclear, biological, and chemical warfare injuries.[5] Medical noncommissioned officers (sergeants) then received ten weeks of further training, roughly equivalent to the EMT Intermediate (EMT-I) level. Skills covered included intubations, intravenous access, and advanced cardiac life support (ACLS).

Beginning in 2001, the Army embarked on a major overhaul of the combat medic program that included increased initial training (to 16 weeks), expansion of skills, and increased emphasis on preventive medicine and weapons of mass destruction casualty management. Increased medical oversight, clinical practicums in initial training, and a minimum requirement for EMT-B certification by the National Registry of EMTs have become standard.[10,11] These individuals are assigned to a redesignated MOS of 68W (91W was used as an interim designation and is now obsolete).

Medical direction of Army medics is generally conducted by the unit surgeon (note that "surgeon" is a designation reflecting the traditions of the medical corps and does not necessarily connote surgery in an invasive medical procedure sense or in terms of prior specialty training). Unit surgeons are often generalist physicians with variable experience and education in EMS and prehospital care. Physician assistants are often utilized at the unit level and can assist the unit surgeon. Efforts to strengthen medical direction are ongoing but are constrained by the relative shortage of emergency physicians in the military and the demands of the current Iraq and Afghanistan wars. The Air Force's version of the Army identification system is the Air Force Specialty Code (AFSC). The 4N0X1 medical technician receives 14 weeks of in-house training, including an EMT-B curriculum. They are required to pass the US national registry exam to complete the didactic portion of their training. This 14-week block is followed by 6 weeks of clinical exposure in different departments of military medical teaching hospitals. Medical technicians progress to the 4N051 level or "Journeyman" by completing self-study Career Development Courses (CDC) while enrolled in on-the-job training. The 4N071 or "Craftsman" level is achieved by completing one year in upgrade training time and additional CDCs. The next step within the career field is accomplished when personnel reach the level of "Superintendent" or 4N091. This level cannot be accomplished until the medical technician reaches the rank of SMSgt (E8).

To maintain currency and keep up-to-date, it is a requirement that all 4N0X1s maintain their national registry EMT-Basic certification. While it is not required by the career field, many 4N0X1s have chosen to further continue their prehospital education, obtaining their national registry certification at the EMT-Intermediate and EMT-Paramedic levels.

Navy enlisted hospital corps personnel provide the vast majority of the medical personnel for operational (deployment, shipboard, or combat) prehospital emergency care for both the Navy and the Marine Corps. (Recent policy changes as a result of the Iraq and Afghanistan conflicts and the global war on terrorism have resulted in the nearly complete transfer of EMS functions at fixed site Navy and Marine Corps installations to those services' respective Fire Departments.) Prior to 2000, hospital corpsmen received all didactic material and practical skills training in accordance with the EMT-B National Standard Curriculum as part of Hospital Corpsman Basic "A" School. Some of this material has since been removed, but the majority of the information is still presented. Following completion of "A" School, corpsmen are classified as "general duty," or 0000. Corpsmen assigned to deployable Fleet Marine Force Units are provided further training as Field Medical Technicians (8404). This training, approximately 12 weeks in length, includes the equivalent of prehospital trauma life support, treatment of chemical, biological, and nuclear agent casualties, and other medical skills. Additional training for shipboard hospital corpsmen is primarily "on-the-job" but includes those skills necessary to assist shipboard medical officers or Independent Duty Hospital Corpsmen (see below). There is no Navy equivalent to the Army 91W.

The military contains another level of health-care provider that has no real counterpart in the civilian system. This is the "independent duty medic" and is represented by the Navy Independent Duty Hospital Corpsman, Air Force Independent Duty Technician, and Army Special Operations Medic. Although their training is slightly different, each shares the common experience of extensive (1000 to over 2000 hours) training in limited primary care to include diagnosis and treatment of minor ailments and limited laboratory and radiographic interpretation.[12,13] Individuals assigned duty with special operations forces are additionally registered with the National Registry of EMTs as paramedics. Independent duty medics exist in limited numbers and have a practice generally restricted to active-duty service members. Most serve in locations such as on ships or at remote bases where an on-site physician would be impractical. They have the training, skills, and a scope of practice somewhat equivalent to that of a physician assistant. They have often provided basic health-care services to indigenous populations in conflict or disaster areas.

The service branch medical corps provides medical oversight for military advanced health-care practitioners. Military physicians are required to be state-licensed, and the majority are specialty board eligible or certified. Unique military requirements necessitate that physicians be proficient in medical problems specific to their patient populations. Physician assistants also play an important role in bridging the gap between physicians and the ever-mobile and widely dispersed soldiers, sailors, and airmen.

Many nurses in the Air Force, and a more limited number in the Navy, are trained as Flight Nurses. These personnel are provided additional training to allow them to serve, independent of direct medical oversight, during fixed-wing air evacuations. All are certified in Advanced Cardiac Life Support and receive additional training in advanced life-support procedures as well as specific training in the physiologic effects of flight on patients.

All military health-care providers receive training in emergency care specific to military needs, including treatment of chemical and radiation casualties and handling mass casualty incidents. Military hospitals and EMS systems are mandated to exercise their mass casualty capabilities several times a year;

deployable assets such as ships and special support facilities have these exercises on an even more frequent and mission-specific basis to maintain efficiency and readiness.

TIERED ORGANIZATION OF MILITARY HEALTH-CARE DELIVERY

The military Levels of Care (formerly referred to as "Echelons of Care") system describes a graduated hierarchy of combat medical care and facilities (Table 46-2).[14,15] Treatment capabilities are roughly standardized for each level of care across the services, in compliance with the Joint Chiefs of Staff doctrinal directives.

Level I is located closest to the fighting, and thus Level I care is austere and its elements are light and mobile. It includes four levels of care: (1) self- and buddy-aid, (2) combat lifesaving, (3) combat medic care, and (4) "aid station care." The first three of these were described above. For the US Army and Marines, the battalion aid station is the first medical "facility" casualties will encounter and may be staffed by physicians or physician assistants. It is challenging and highly mobile, with Advanced Trauma Life Support (ATLS) capabilities, including endotracheal intubation, tube thoracostomy, intravenous medication, and other physician-directed medical care. Navy ships have a rough equivalent in various satellite "battle dressing stations" located remotely from the primary shipboard medical department.

Level II is a divisional level "clearing station" that is staffed by a medical company of physicians, nurses, and medics. Casualties are examined to determine treatment needs and evacuation triage priority. Emergency medical treatment, including initial comprehensive resuscitation, is provided and is supported by limited radiographic, dental, and laboratory services with whole-blood transfusion capacity. The "clearing station" provides limited duration patient-holding capability for sick or injured personnel, roughly at the "general ward" level. Ship medical departments approximate this capability, as do the Marine Fleet Surgical Support Groups. In the case of casualties generated by a shipboard incident, response by the ship's medical department is designed to be rapid and effective. Patients with injuries or illnesses beyond the capabilities of the ship's sick bay are evacuated to a rear-area facility or major hospital ship.

Level III is the first true "full-service" medical facility a casualty will encounter on the battlefield. At

Table 46–2	The Five "Levels" of Military Medical Care		
Level	Military Hierarchy	Personnel/Facility	Type of Care
I	Unit	Self/Buddy Aid	First Aid
		Combat Lifesaver	First Aid, Beginning Emergency Treatment
		Combat Medic	Emergency Medical Treatment
		Battalion Aid Station	Advanced Trauma and Medical Management
II	Division	Medical Company (Clearing Station)	Initial Resuscitation
		Field Surgical Support Group	
III	Corps	Combat Support Hospital	Resuscitative Surgery and Medical Care
		Fleet Hospitals	
		Augmented Amphibious Ships	
IV	Echelons above Corps	Combat Support Hospital	Definitive Care
		Host Nation Hospitals	
		Hospital Ships	
V	Out of Theater Continental US	Fixed Medical Facilities	Restorative and Rehabilitative Care

present, this is US Army "combat support hospitals," the Air Force Theater Hospitals or Expeditionary Medical Support (EMEDS) facilities, the Navy fleet hospitals, and the major amphibious assault ship medical departments if augmented by surgical support teams. These amphibious vessels are capable of converting several hundred marine berthing spaces into medical wards of various capabilities. Level III hospitals provide comprehensive resuscitative surgery and medical care. Medical providers at them include general surgeons and both surgical and medical subspecialists, with comprehensive anesthesia and nursing support. Patients who are unlikely to return to duty are evacuated as soon as possible from these facilities after stabilization.

Level IV has been traditionally represented by comprehensive theater hospitals variously designated as General, Field, Theater Area, or Station Hospitals. These large and generally poorly mobile facilities provided definitive medical and surgical care and were equipped with a broad array of support services. Since today's operational requirements call for a more flexible and mobile medical facility, it is unlikely that a true Level IV hospital capability will exist in future war fighting theaters of operation. Instead, enhanced Combat Support Hospitals in the theater, plus direct evacuation of "stabilized" patients to the US will meet

this Level IV requirement. Two key exceptions to this continue to exist: the Navy's two 1000-bed hospital ships (the USNS Mercy and the USNS Comfort), and any host nation hospitals with which these services may have developed official relationships. Both of these Level IV capabilities were in use and in theater during Operation Desert Storm in 1991. During current operations in the Middle East and Central Asia, Landstuhl Army Regional Medical Center (LRMC) in Germany has been serving as the Level IV facility for both Operation Iraqi Freedom (OIF) and Operation Enduring Freedom (OEF).

Level V represents fixed hospitals located outside the theater of operations and in the continental US These are primarily military medical facilities, augmented within the US by Veteran's Administration and civilian hospitals as part of the National Defense Medical System. Definitive and rehabilitative care of all types may be found in Level V facilities, and most have extensive medical education training programs.

The numerical sequence of these levels may appear to imply a rigid stepwise movement of patients from Level I to Level II and upward. This may have been true in the system's earliest conception, but is too inflexible for the dynamic operational environments of modern warfare. A strict hierarchy of units and levels is unlikely to be efficient on the modern battlefield.

Another major change in military medical doctrine is the increased forward availability of medical expertise and technology. The Army "Forward Surgical Teams," and Marine "Forward Resuscitative Surgical Systems" are now able to provide a Level II trauma surgical capability for rapidly advancing forces and provide care extremely close to the site of injury.[16] This addition of surgical capability so close to the front lines has been instrumental in saving the lives of many soldiers who would have been too unstable to survive the evacuation to a Level III facility.[16] A key component that makes these teams so versatile is that they are 100% mobile and capable of setting up operations quickly.[17]

Reflecting the rapid shift in doctrine resulting from the wars in Iraq and Afghanistan, the military is considering changing the term "level" to "role." This terminology change is an effort to help remove any vestiges of hierarchy, or further still, sequence of care. The blurring of the front lines and the availability of advanced care, including surgery in far forward locations, is driving this line of thinking.

MILITARY PATIENT TRANSPORTATION

The goal of combat medical evacuation (MEDEVAC) is the safe and effective movement of the casualties to health-care facilities. As used by the military services, MEDEVAC refers to the transportation of casualties on a dedicated or specially outfitted vehicle. Inherent in the definition is the assumption of some degree of care en route. In contrast, casualty evacuation or CASEVAC is the transportation of casualties on vehicles of opportunity (e.g., a truck) with limited or no care capability beyond that of "buddy first aid."[18] Transportation modes might include manual carries, ground vehicles, aircraft, watercraft, or any combination of these.

In many military operations, the manual carry is the primary means of moving casualties from the point of injury or illness to a point of safety where the medical evacuation can begin. Despite tremendous advances in many other areas of evacuation, manual carries remain almost unchanged over the centuries. Manual carries can be exhausting work and necessarily have a range limited to a few hundred or thousand meters.

Litter transportation offers some modest improvements over manual carries. Some support and comfort are afforded the patient, and spinal immobilization, fracture splinting, oxygen therapy, and other static treatments can often be maintained during movement. Airway management, ventilation, and other dynamic care remain difficult to perform. Litter carries have the additional advantage that the work of transporting a patient can be shared by two to four persons (but this also takes these persons away from being actively involved in supporting combat operations). The shipboard environment poses additional constraints of difficult extraction and hazardous operating conditions. These are overcome by training, drills, a pervasive emphasis on safety, and innovations such as specialized stretchers and backpack transport of medical supplies to incident locations.

Specially protected and equipped ground vehicles are the most common platform used to move casualties over relatively long distances on the battlefield. Current US military doctrine places dedicated ambulances in the war fighting maneuver units. In most scenarios, battlefield casualties are carried or dragged several hundred meters to a casualty collection point where ground ambulances can pick them up. As a result, ground ambulances can be expected to get fairly close to the scene of injury. Some countries such as Israel have developed specialized armored ambulances to allow safer pickup and transport in combat zones (Figure 46-1).

The helicopter ambulance has been a valuable component of the MEDEVAC system since its introduction for this role during the Korean War. By the end of the Vietnam War, MEDEVAC helicopters offered speed and versatility unmatched by ground vehicles.[19] They are largely unaffected by terrain and can reach remote areas inaccessible to ground vehicles. Disadvantages include their cost and vulnerability to small-arms fire, especially in open terrain environment. This latter factor accounts for the doctrine of keeping helicopter pickup points a safe distance from direct hostile fire. Helicopter evacuation is also very weather-dependent, and some helicopters have altitude-related takeoff weight restrictions. Most casualties will still need to be carried to a point of safety by a combination of manual or litter carry and ground vehicle transportation.[20] The Army provides all dedicated helicopter MEDEVAC services for military units, and Army helicopter squadrons are designated as transportation assets for the Navy hospital ships. Navy helicopters can and have conducted Combat Search and Rescue (CSAR) operations, but these airframes are all dual use for other purposes.

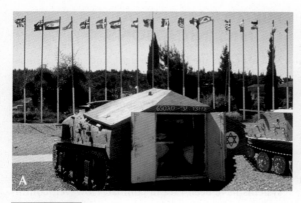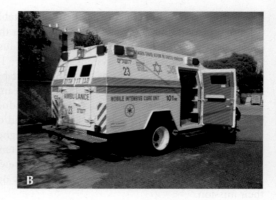

FIGURE 46–1

A, Armored ambulance at the Israeli Armor Museum at Latrun, Israel. **B**, New Israeli armored ambulance. Photo courtesy of Jim Holliman, MD.

MEDEVAC shares two significant limitations: availability and limited patient care en route. Battlefields and disasters are fluid and dynamic situations, making it challenging to anticipate where air ambulances will most be needed. Field medical providers must be capable of improvising transportation when ambulances are not available. Using nonmedical vehicles and personnel for casualty evacuation (CASEVAC), including trucks, buses, and nonmedical helicopters, is a well-recognized part of military contingency and disaster planning.[21]

The second limitation of tactical MEDEVAC is the difficulty in providing en route or ongoing care. Ground and air vehicles are usually cramped, noisy, poorly illuminated, and prone to vibration, jarring, and sway. Patient access, assessment, monitoring, and interventions are difficult at best. Only in the most modern ground and aeromedical platforms are there provisions for onboard oxygen and suction.[8] Airway, breathing, and monitoring equipment are not built in and thus must be brought separately. An attempt to compensate for this deficiency may be seen with the development of the Life Saving Treatment and Transport module (LSTAT) (Figure 46-2). The LSTAT is a state-of-the-art patient stretcher that allows more sophisticated patient monitoring and treatment than has been possible in the past. Complementary to this push for advanced equipment is a drive to improve the training of care providers aboard helicopters, especially for the growing intratheater (between field hospitals within the war zone) movement of casualties. The term "en route care" has begun to denote this phase of evacuation care.

The mode of movement of casualties within the area of responsibility (AOR) is largely dependent on the terrain and battlefield constraints. During OIF and OEF the MEDEVAC system has been a key component for the reduction of mortality on the battlefield.

After patients arrive at a Level III facility where fixed-wing aircraft are able to conduct operations, their transport is continued by the Air Force and the Aeromedical Evacuation (AE) system. This is a regulated system in which all the patient transports must be preapproved by a validating flight surgeon. The Aeromedical Evacuation crews (AECMs) are made up of Flight Nurses and Aeromedical Evacuation Technicians (AETs). Patients ideally must be hemodynamically stable prior to being transported by AE crews.

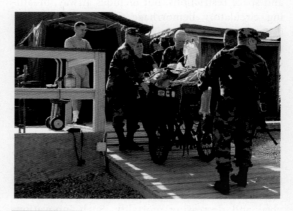

FIGURE 46–2

Life Saving Treatment and Transport (LSTAT): a state-of-the-art patient stretcher. From http://student.ttuhsc.edu/mmsa/home.htm.

While it would be ideal for all patients to be stable prior to transport, this is not always possible. After the experiences encountered during Operation Just Cause in Somalia, a void within the system was noted.[22] To fill the doctrinal requirement of transporting "stabilized" patients, the Critical Care Air Transport Teams (CCATT) were created. Their mission is to conduct seamless ICU level care to critically ill/injured and/or burned patients while transporting them to a higher level of care. While CCATTs are part of the AE system, they do not function independently from AE crews. They augment established AE crews as they carry out their mission.

The composition of CCATTs includes a critical care physician, who may be a general surgeon, pulmonary/critical care physician, anesthesiologist, emergency medicine physician or cardiologist. The other two members of the CCATTs are a critical care nurse and a respiratory therapist. CCATTs have the capability of caring for up to three ventilator patients or six less acute patients.[23] This capability can be expanded up to five ventilator patients by augmenting the primary CCATT with a Medical CCATT-Extender Team.[23] The Medical CCATT-Extender Team is composed of two critical care nurses and has been employed during OIF/OEF to transport larger numbers of casualties from LRMC to the Level V facilities in the United States.

MILITARY MEDICAL EQUIPMENT

Forward medical equipment is often limited by weight and space restrictions, but includes airway, breathing, circulatory, hemorrhage control, and splinting devices. Intravenous or intraosseous circulatory support and basic invasive procedures, including needle and tube thoracostomies, may be performed at the aid station. Simple lifesaving surgery may be performed at the forward support surgical team collocated with the medical company (clearing station, Level II), but definitive procedures are reserved for the hospitals further "rearward" in the evacuation chain. Rear-area evacuation hospitals are capable of modern, comprehensive, and sophisticated services. Military research commands continue to experiment with sophisticated technology aimed at improving survival and decreasing mortality. Such innovations as electronic "dog tags" that include important medical information, physiologic monitoring vests, and collagen-impregnated battle dressings are but a few of the useful items that have evolved from focused military medical research.

MILITARY MEDICAL COMMUNICATIONS

Much of the medical oversight and many clinical or logistical decisions affecting patient care and movement take place from afar during combat operations. Medical communications networks are vital to these requirements. The direct radio supervision of field providers through radio communications in the tactical setting must be minimized for security reasons.[24] Because of communications bandwidth limitations, dedicated, sole-use medical communications systems have been rare in combat. However, continued research and development in audio, video, and data transmission technology or "telemedicine" show promise to link far-forward enlisted care providers with physicians farther in the rear who can then direct the in-field providers to perform more difficult or advanced medical care procedures. Pilot programs aboard ships and in remote outposts have demonstrated this potential. Again, many of these innovations have direct applicability to the civilian sector. The now common practice of digitizing radiographs and transmitting these data to remote radiologists for interpretation was developed and field tested beginning in the late 1970s and early 1980s by the military for use in such places as forward deployable clinics or ships at sea. Because of weight, bulk, reliability, and cost concerns, we will likely see only modest deployment of advanced communications equipment in the far-forward field environment in the foreseeable future.

MILITARY MEDICAL DIRECTION AND CONTROL

Control of tactical prehospital personnel and other medical resources is generally under the direct supervision of the unit commander, who is usually not a medical officer. This situation is analogous to the incident command system (ICS), where the medical sector is under the control of the Incident Commander, often a nonmedical fire department officer.[25] The reasons are again parallel to the civilian ICS example: the medical mission is often subordinate to the overall tactical mission. In this regard, the military command-and-control format is not unfamiliar and in fact underscores another aspect of modern civilian EMS that draws its origins from the military. Although overall control of military medical units rests with the unit commander, day-to-day medical oversight and operational control are directed by the medical officers and noncommissioned officers (sergeants and petty officers) within the medical section or element.

Owing to the dispersed nature of combat units, intervening independent-duty medics or physician assistants are often called upon as delegated representatives of the physician.

Lessons Learned from OIF/OEF

A large focus of modern casualty care research has centered on the prehospital arena. This can be attributed to the fact that most combat-related deaths occur prior to definitive (hospital) care. Types of injuries that medics have encountered in Iraq and Afghanistan have been unique in many ways. This is primarily a result of the devastating and evolving nature of the Improvised Explosive Devices (IEDs) used by the insurgents.

As the conflicts of OIF and OEF have evolved, it has been learned that one of the largest groups of casualties that is potentially salvageable includes those with compressible hemorrhagic injuries.[26] This knowledge has led the military to change the way it approaches casualties on the battlefield. When a medic encounters a patient with a compressible hemorrhagic injury, the first priority becomes gaining control of the active hemorrhage. The rationale for this paradigm change in priorities is a simple one. In many cases these casualties could hemorrhage to death while a medic is taking time to establish an airway, and many more soldiers injured on the battlefield have hemorrhage than have airway problems. Because of this challenge, medics treating casualties now follow the pneumonic MARCH (Table 46-3).[27]

Another paradigm change that has occurred in recent years has been in the use of tourniquets. While the traditional model in the US places the tourniquet at the end of the algorithm of hemorrhage control, in the battlefield, combat doctrine dictates that tourniquets be used as a "first-line treatment for casualties who have suffered from extremity hemorrhage when care is administered under hostile fire."[22] Preliminary

reports have demonstrated that early and liberal use of tourniquets has resulted in a significant decrease in mortality on the battlefield.[28] The goal when using a tourniquet should be to remove it within 2 hours of application. This practice will limit the possibility of damage to neuromuscular structures and has been deemed a safe practice.[29] In an Israeli study performed by Lackstein and colleagues, they used >90 tourniquet applications and noted complications only after the tourniquet had remained on for >150 minutes.[30] Experiences in Iraq have been similar. Between 2003 and 2004, the tourniquet time at the 31st Combat Support Hospital in Baghdad averaged 70 minutes. Their experience showed no complications related to tourniquet application.[26]

Another major advance in the management of severe hemorrhagic injuries has been in the development of hemostatic agents.[31] Over the past few years several products have come into the market, assisting in the care of critically injured patients. The two products that are currently used by the United States Military in Iraq and Afghanistan are the Chitosan® dressing and QuikClot®. The primary mechanism of action of the Chitosan® dressing appears to be tissue adherence and mechanical sealing of the injury.[31] As of 2004 over 103,000 dressings had been distributed into combat operations in Iraq and Afghanistan.[32] QuikClot® is a granular zeolite powder. When placed on a bleeding wound, it adsorbs water, thereby concentrating platelets, erythrocytes, and clotting factors at the site of application.[31] While QuikClot® has been effective in animal models, it has the drawback of causing an exothermic reaction in humans.[32]

To date there have been numerous animal studies involving hemostatic agents, including the two discussed above. Unfortunately, prospective controlled hemostatic agent studies involving human subjects are limited. Wedmore and coworkers published a case series under combat conditions in which the Chitosan® dressing was successful in 42 of 44 cases.[32] The best potential benefit of the hemostatic dressings appears to be in complex wounds on the trunk or proximal extremities that are not treatable with tourniquets.

Table 46–3	**MARCH Mnemonic for Directing Treatment Priorities**
M	Massive hemorrhage
A	Airway
R	Respiration
C	Circulation
H	Head injury/hypothermia

MILITARY EMS DURING PEACETIME

Each military installation is generally responsible for its own medical care under the guidance of a centralized military medical command. The medical services of each installation are linked to the overall military medical care system. At smaller or more isolated locations, patients are referred to larger military hospitals at other locations for secondary care. These in turn are linked to a series of more sophisticated tertiary-care medical centers, each with special capabilities, consultants, and equipment. However, referral is not restricted to military systems. A patient may be referred to the closest appropriate hospital, whether military or civilian. Occasionally, civilian patients may be referred to a military facility when appropriate resources are not otherwise available.

Prehospital care at military installations has historically been the function of the supporting medical treatment facility, whether an outpatient clinic or a full-service military hospital. Over the past few years there has been a diversification within military installations as to who delivers EMS. Currently, military installation EMS is delivered through a number of different structural models. At some installations military personnel under the auspices of the medical installations still provide this service. At other installations EMS could be delivered by the Fire Department, by contracts with civilian companies, or through civil service employees under the leadership of the Fire Department or the medical installation.

Installation needs and overall medical requirements drive levels of care and system design at military installations. The combined total population (US military personnel and their dependents) requiring EMS services at these sites approaches 3.5 million (more than each of the US territories and 26 of the states). However, with over 800 worldwide military installations, the majority of military locations have populations, including resident dependents and civil servants, of less than 20,000. With its younger, healthier population, superficial inspection would suggest the incidence of significant medical problems requiring EMS would be low. This does not seem to be the case—one study revealed BLS and ALS level requirements similar to those of civilian communities, and this was borne out in a service-wide survey conducted in the Navy in 1998.[34,35]

Most states provide general exemptions for military base EMS services from statutes and administrative codes for federal EMS services. Each of the three services (Army, Navy, Air Force) has regulations governing installation EMS operations. In general, wide latitude is provided to base/installation commanders in the provision of these services, but commanders are directed to meet community standards of care. Additionally, although not binding, the Government Services Chapter of the American College of Emergency Physicians, composed primarily of active duty, reserve, and retired military medical officers, has recommended that installation EMS

services meet or exceed community standards.[36] Difficulties arise in that no two communities are identical, standards of care may be insufficient or nonexistent at overseas locations, and none of the services has specifically identified the various standards with which to comply (e.g., response times, equipment, levels of providers). At a time of shrinking budgets and manpower, the services are struggling to ensure the optimal quality of this service for all beneficiaries without escalating costs at the expense of other medical services.

In general, access to services is through an installation-specific phone number, usually not through the national emergency number 9-1-1. The area of responsibility is normally restricted to federally owned land, although at many overseas locations beneficiaries reside in the local community, often without community EMS. At these locations, the catchment area may be extended. Dispatch may occur from a centralized location or through the installation Fire Department or medical treatment facility. At most locations, Fire Department personnel (who are trained at either the First Responder or EMT-Basic level) perform nontransport first response functions. Provision of primary EMS response services is usually at the EMT-Basic level, although an increasing number of installations have upgraded to the EMT-Intermediate or EMT-Paramedic level. Ambulance service providers include supporting military hospitals or federal Fire Departments, contracted ambulance agencies, or community municipal agencies. Patients are delivered to the installation medical treatment facility, or, if the patient's condition exceeds the capabilities of that facility, they are directly transported to area hospitals.

MILITARY MEDICAL INTERACTION WITH THE CIVILIAN COMMUNITY

Military-civilian interactions may be considered in two parts: those occurring in the course of daily, routine operations and those that may occur in response to disasters or other emergency situations.

At overseas locations, cooperative sharing of resources occurs under the auspices of written agreements between the US and the host nation governments, referred to as Status of Forces Agreements (SOFA). SOFAs allow for utilization of each of the parties' capabilities to the mutual benefit of both. In the United States, this cooperative sharing arrangement occurs less frequently because of issues of competition between local vendors and the federal government. There are notable exceptions, however.

Military hospitals occasionally provide the only resources or augment scarce resources in the civilian community. Many serve as specialty care centers for large geographic areas: for example, Madigan Army Medical Center in Tacoma, Washington; Brooke Army Medical Center in San Antonio, Texas; William Beaumont Army Medical Center in El Paso, Texas; and Wilford Hall Air Force Hospital in San Antonio, Texas, all serve as trauma centers in their communities. Madigan is an important provider of paramedic ambulance services for an otherwise underserved portion of Washington state; it also serves as an EMS direct medical control facility. Darnall Army Community Hospital in Killeen, Texas, is the only hospital providing sophisticated emergency services in a large area of central Texas. Brooke Army Medical Center is an important international resource for burn victims.

The Military Assistance to Safety and Traffic (MAST) program exemplifies the use of military resources for community services.[36] Since 1969 the MAST program has provided military aeromedical evacuation capabilities to civilian communities. MAST pilots have flown thousands of missions and transported tens of thousands of patients. This service has been accomplished safely and without expense to the patients; the military has benefited by maintaining aeromedical evacuation skills. Such services were the forerunners to the now prevalent civilian air medical programs. In developing civilian programs, much was learned from military air medical evacuation experience. Since the development of civilian helicopter systems throughout the United States, the number of MAST missions has declined dramatically, primarily because of the non–compete requirement placed on the military. Where civilian aeromedical systems exist, they must be accessed first and decline a mission before MAST may participate.[37]

In the event of a large-scale emergency or disaster situation, military response, including medical and EMS, is governed under a concept referred to as Defense Support to Civil Authorities (DSCA). There are two levels of response. Under the DSCA doctrine, commanders, including medical commanders, may utilize existing military resources to assist local communities to preserve life or to mitigate or prevent major property loss. This may be done without higher-level authority and is known as the "Immediate Response" clause of DSCA. In the case of a disaster of the magnitude requiring a larger force or more prolonged assistance, all military actions are governed by the Stafford Act. Under the Stafford Act, each of the various federal agencies is assigned Lead Federal Agency responsibilities to assist the states and local communities in disaster response. The military is assigned a supporting role only but has this role in all emergency support functions of disaster relief as described by the National Response Plan. For most disasters, ultimate coordination of the federal response is assigned to the Federal Emergency Management Agency. Medical support is assigned to the Department of Health and Human Services.

For overseas disasters or other humanitarian assistance missions, appropriate arrangements and details of provided support and services are developed by the Department of State and the supported nation.

THE MILITARY AND THE NATIONAL DISASTER MEDICAL SYSTEM

The Department of Defense is a prime initiator, planner, and current participant in the National Disaster Medical System (NDMS). Military resources are the transportation backbone for many NDMS missions. Military personnel and facilities assist in the coordination of participating hospital networks. Department of Defense leadership, medical personnel, and logistic groups may assist in relief efforts.[38-40]

The NDMS concept has been tested, primarily in the prehospital setting, and military medical providers have assisted other federal agencies in hurricane relief or other humanitarian assistance missions within the continental United States. For domestic disaster medical support, the Office of Preparedness and Response within the DHHS has operational authority over the NDMS. DHHS unfortunately possesses few facilities and even fewer personnel in comparison to the Department of Defense and the Veteran's Administration. Military personnel, physical resources, and facilities are crucial to the overall success of the NDMS.

SUMMARY

The military pioneered systematic emergency care. Both the military and civilian sectors have come a long way in adapting wartime lessons to peacetime EMS. The sharing of resources and responsibilities by civilian and military communities can improve these services even more. Because much can be learned from each other, open professional exchanges and planning to meet the needs of the ill and injured must take priority over issues of jurisdiction, sources of payment, and patient eligibility. Working from these premises, the mission and goals of both the civilian and military sectors may be accomplished.

References

1. Boyd D, Edlilch R, Micik S, eds. Systems approach to emergency medical care. Norwalk, CT: Appleton-Century-Crofts; 1983.
2. Richardson RG: *Larrey: Surgeon to Napoleon's Imperial Guard.* London: John Murray, 1974.
3. Adams GW. *Doctors in Blue, The Medical History of the Union Army in the Civil War.* New York: Collier Books: 1961.
4. Stewart MJ. Moving the Wounded: Litters, Cacolets and Ambulance Wagons, US Army 1776–1876. Fort Collins, CO: The Old Army Press; 1979.
5. Summers MB, Bryan DN, De Lorenzo RA. The US Army Medical Specialist. In On-line supplement to American Academy of Orthopedic Surgeons. Emergency Care and Transportation of the Sick and Injured. 7th ed. Sudbury, MA: Jones and Bartlett; 1999.
6. Bellamy R. The causes of death in conventional land warfare: implications for combat casualty care research. *Military Medicine.* 1984;1495:55–62.
7. De Lorenzo RA. Improving combat casualty care and field medicine: focus on the military medic. *Military Medicine.* 1997;162(4):268–272.
8. De Lorenzo RA. Military and civilian emergency aeromedical services: achieving common goals with different approaches. *Aviation, Space and Environmental Medicine.* 1997;68(1):56–60.
9. Department of the Army. *Field Manual 8-10: Health Service Support in a Theater of Operations.* Washington, DC; 1 March 1991.
10. De Lorenzo RA. 91W: Force XXI combat medic. *US. Army Medical Department Journal (AMEDD Journal).* 1999; Oct–Dec: 2–6.
11. De Lorenzo RA: 91W Health Care Specialist: Medic for the Millennium. *Military Medicine,* 2001; 166(8): 685–688.
12. De Lorenzo RA. Military medic: the original expanded-scope EMS provider. *JEMS.* 1996; 21(4): 50–54.
13. De Lorenzo RA. Special Training for Special Missions. Sidebar to accompany Military Medic: The Original Expanded-Scope EMS Provider. *JEMS.* 1996;21(4):52.
14. Department of the Army. *Field Manual 8-10-5. Brigade and Division Surgeon's Handbook.* Washington, DC; 1991.
15. Duggan B. Organization of military medical units. In Burkle F, ed. *Disaster medicine.* New York: Medical Examination Co.; 1984.
16. Beekley AC. United States Military Surgical Response to Modern Large-Scale Conflicts: The Ongoing Evolution of a Trauma. *Surgical Clinics of North America.* 2006; 86, (3) 689–709.
17. Hetz SP. Introduction to Military Medicine: A Brief Overview. *Surgical Clinics of North America.* 2006; 86: (3) 675–688.
18. Hurd WW, Montminy RJ, De Lorenzo RA, Burd LT, Goldman BS, Loftus TJ: Physician Role in Aeromedical Evacuation: Current Practices in USAF Operations. *Aviation, Space and Environmental Medicine* 2006; 77(6): 631–638.
19. Baxt W.G., Moody P. The impact of rotorcraft aeromedical emergency care services on mortality. *JAMA.* 1983; 249:3047–3051.
20. Dorland P, Nanney J. *Dust Off: Army Aeromedical Evacuation in Vietnam.* Washington, DC, Center of Military History, United States Army; 1982.
21. Department of the Army. *Field Manual 8-10-6. Medical Evacuation in a Theater of Operations.* Washington, DC; 2000.
22. Beekley AC, Starnes BW, Sebesta JA. Lessons Learned from Modern Military Surgery. *Surgical Clinics of North America.* 2007 Feb; 87(1): 157–184.
23. United States Air Force. Air Force Tactics, Techniques, and Procedures 3-42.51. Critical Care Air Transport Teams. 7 September 2006.
24. Bowen TE, Bellamy RF, eds. *Emergency War Surgery,* 2nd ed. Washington, DC, Department of Defense; Government Printing Office; 1988.
25. De Lorenzo RA, Porter RS. Tactical Emergency Care. Upper Saddle River, NJ: Brady (Prentice Hall); 1999: 384.
26. Sebesta JA. Special Lessons Learned from Iraq. *Surgical Clinics of North America.* 2006; 86 (3): 711–726.
27. Tactical Combat Casualty Manual. First edition. Washington, DC Dept. of Defense; 2005.
28. Fox CJ, Starnes BW. Vascular Surgery on the Modern Battlefield. *Surgical Clinics of North America.* 2007; 87 (5): 1193–1211.
29. Walters TJ, Mabry RL. Issues Related to the Use of Tourniquets on the Battlefield. *Mil Med.* 2005 Sep; 170(9):770–5. PMID: 16261982
30. Lakstein D, Blumenfeld A, Sokolov T, et. al. Tourniquets for Hemorrhage Control on the battlefield: a 4 year accumulated experience. *J Trauma.* 2003 May;54(5 Suppl):S221-5. PMID: 12768129
31. Pusateri AE, Holcomb JB, Kheirabadi BS et. al. Making Sense of the Preclinical Literature on Advanced Hemostatic Products. *J Trauma.* 2006 Mar; 60(3): 674-82. PMID: 16531876
32. Wedmore I, McManus JG, Pusateri AE, Holcomb JB. A Special Report on the chitosan-based hemostatic dressing: Experience in current combat operations. *J Trauma.* 2006 Mar; 60(3):655-8. PMID: 16531872
33. Alam HB, Burris D, DaCorta JA, Rhee P. Hemorrhage control in the battlefield: Role of new hemostatic agents. *Mil Med.* 2005 Jan; 170(1):63–9. Review. PMID: 15724857
34. Leonard F. Ambulance use in a military population: epidemiology and implications. *Mil Med.* 1992, May; 157 (5):239–243. PMID: 1630655

35. Author (J. Mothershead) personal correspondence. (December 2009)

36. American College of Emergency Physicians: Military emergency medical services systems. Policy Statement. Dallas TX (Revised and approved by the ACEP Board of Directors June 1997 and October 2009 Reaffirmed by the ACEP Board of Directors October 2002) avail able at: http://www.acep.org/practres.aspx?id=29576

37. Gerhardt RT, McGhee JS, Cloonan C, Pfaff JA, De Lorenzo RA. "US Army MEDEVAC in the new millennium: A medical perspective." *Aviation Space and Environmental Medicine* 72(7) :659-64, July 2001.

38. Dolicker GJ; Preparing for the worst. The challenge facing NDMS (National Disaster Medical System), *JEMS* Aug 1991, 16(8), 94–101.

39. Heaton LD. Army medical service activities in Vietnam. *Mil Med.* 1966; 131:646.

40. Knouss RF National disaster medical system. *Public Health Reports.* 2001;116 (Suppl 2):49–52 PMID: 11880672

CHAPTER 47

Disasters and HazMat

Pinchas Halpern

KEY LEARNING POINTS

- EMS is a critical component of disaster response.

- The relative rarity of major events in some parts of the world and the lack of resources in other parts may make investment by EMS in disaster preparedness a difficult decision.

- Hazards and vulnerability assessment will guide optimal resource allocation.

- Policies must be developed to cope with all likely disasters.

- Protocols and operating procedures must be written in order to permit policy implementation.

- Integration and cooperation with other relevant agencies is critical.

- Communications, command, and control for disasters must be in place and utilized in daily operations.

- Training and drilling of staff, with appropriate positive and negative incentives, must be carried out.

- Actual response to disaster should be standardized per policy but with sufficient flexibility to account for expected differences in each event.

- Documentation and debriefing are critical for quality improvement.

This chapter will review:

1. Disaster planning for EMS systems.
2. EMS operations in disasters (natural disasters, mass casualty incidents [MCIs]), and terrorist events).
3. Comparisons of EMS disaster response systems and performance in different countries.
4. EMS's roles in hazmat incidents.

It will also describe the preparations for and actions of emergency medical services and systems (EMS) in the management of disasters. In modern times, the specter of disaster seems to be increasing. Whether it is a real increase or partly a perceived increase due to better information sharing, the

medical response to disasters has become a major issue for planners of medical systems in general. Medical management of complex situations such as disasters requires extensive preparation, training, and coordination. It seems intuitively clear (although not much comparative literature exists for obvious reasons) that in most disasters, the quality of the response of EMS at the site of the disaster has a major impact on the mortality and morbidity of casualties.

Disasters come in many shapes and forms and vary among locations on the globe; they may be predictable but often are not. Unpredictability in this context may mean that an accurate pre-event hazards and vulnerability analysis (HVA)

has not been done. Disasters often strike poorly prepared and poorly resourced communities, where
even prior correct HVAs may not elicit a systematic
and efficient preparation or response by the medical
systems. Appropriate EMS preparation for disasters
depends on at least these components:

1. High-level management (national, regional, and
   local) decisions.
2. EMS top management decisions to invest in disaster preparedness and long-term commitment.
3. An accurate, up-to-date hazards and vulnerability
   analysis.
4. Allocation of the appropriate resources.
5. Integration of EMS into the overall ideally coordinated response.

DISASTER TYPES

There are obviously many types of disasters. They
may also be classified according to EMS response
(Table 47-1). The relevant variables affecting EMS

preparation and response include likelihood (risk)
and magnitude, type, location(s), rate of onset, duration, and effect on infrastructure relevant to EMS.

PREPARATION AND PLANNING

Preparing the EMS system to cope with disaster consists of the basic good governance of any EMS organization, with the addition of specialized components
listed in Table 47-2.

1. **Hazard and vulnerability assessment** (HVA) is
   critical in determining the likelihood, distribution,
   and type and magnitude of potential disasters,
   which will largely determine the required preparations. Such assessment needs to be repeated
   periodically, as conditions change. For example, the
   building of a new factory or a seaport with chemical
   storage facilities that is subject to changing geopo-
   litical conditions or changing weather patterns
   will require reanalysis of the entire risk/response

Table 47–1	Disaster Variables and Their EMS Considerations	
Relevant Variable	**Details, Severity**
Type	Man-made, natural, complex humanitarian emergency
Onset	Sudden versus gradual (e.g., earthquake, tsunami, bombs versus bioterrorism, radio terrorism, pandemic)
Number of casualties	Small, moderate, large, overwhelming. Definition needs to be local, based on resources, and may vary among different types and severities of injuries and different regions in same country
Severity of casualties	Mix of severity among total number
Type of casualties	Special injuries (e.g., burns, respiratory failure), children, pregnant women, elderly
Geographical extent	Size of affected area in relation to EMS assets
Location	Distance from EMS base stations, quality of roads and weather
Infrastructure condition	Roads, communications, fuel supplies, electricity, oxygen, medical supplies
Effect on EMS personnel	Injuries to EMS staff or their families, ability to travel to workplace
Effect on EMS resources	Need for decontamination of ambulances, provision of PPE, espe- cially for repeat or prolonged operations, damage to base stations
Risk to EMS personnel	Contagious bioagents, radiologicals, weather, human violence
Injuries requiring specialized equipment	Respiratory failure requiring ventilators and oxygen, crush injuries requiring dialysis, burns, children requiring specialized units, hazmat requiring field antidote administration
Context	Warfare or civil strife, complex humanitarian emergencies, large natural disaster, focal event
Existing EMS capacity	Level of development of national and/or regional medical and EMS, resources and training

PPE = personal protective equipment.

Table 47–2	**Components of EMS Preparation for Disasters**

1. Hazards and vulnerability assessment
2. Infrastructure assessment
3. Relevant equipment and supplies
4. Communications, computers, command, and control (C^4)
5. Disaster protocols and operating procedures
6. Staffing
7. Training
8. Interagency coordination

equation. A structured approach to HVA is important, since realistically few EMS organizations will repeat their assessments frequently enough to maintain currency. Coordination with all relevant agencies (e.g., fire brigade, environmental protection agencies, health bureaus, epidemiology units, police, transportation authorities, and armed forces) should produce a standard of interagency communications and notification regarding any new relevant hazard, whereby each agency updates all other relevant agencies of any new potential threat.[1]

2. **Infrastructure assessment:** By definition, EMS functions in the field and is therefore largely dependent on the quality and functionality of the road system, including the effects of weather.

While EMS operators are the experts on such matters in daily operations, clear plans must be in place to cope with extremes of weather in the context of natural disasters and with the loss of major roads and refueling stations. Prolonged operations, such as in natural disasters, will entail resupply with fuel, spare parts, and maintenance support, medical equipment, and oxygen.

3. **Relevant equipment and supplies:** EMS agencies staff and equip for daily operations. The quantity and type of assets needed for disaster response vary with disaster type and with the baseline of each organization. For example, the proportion of all-terrain vehicles, of ALS units, of specially protected units (e.g., bullet proof), of water rescue assets, and of personal protective equipment (PPE) varies in different countries and regions, producing different gaps between daily operations and disaster response capabilities. The need for specific equipment for response to specific disasters must be defined and such equipment stocked and maintained appropriately. (see Table 47-3 for hazmat response equipment) For other checklists useful both for hospital and EMS see http://www.apic.org/bioterror/checklist.doc and http://www.nnepi.com/pdf/VIID_Hospital_Nursing1_Prepare.pdf).

A clear knowledge of the available assets within the EMS organization as well as resources available after such in-organization resources are exhausted or rendered unavailable by circumstances is critical. Contingency agreements may need to be signed with other organizations. Directives may need to be promulgated by relevant authorities

Table 47–3	**Disaster-Specific Equipment for EMS**
Conventional MCI	Stretchers, tourniquets, thorax needle decompression sets, basic and advanced airway equipment, analgesics, oxygen, blankets, triage tags, documentation charts, splints, bandages, IV cannulas and fluids
Hazmat	PPE, antidotes and antagonists, relevant medications (e.g., benzodiazepines), oxygen, dry decontamination equipment, protective covers for stretchers and ambulances
Major natural disaster	
Casualty transfer	All-terrain ambulances and/or motorcycles, and/or helicopters
C^4 (see below)	Alternate means of communications assuming most conventional means will fail. Alternate command and control center. Access to overhead imagery (e.g., satellite, aircraft)
Medications	Large supply of EMS-relevant medications (e.g. fluids, venous access equipment, oxygen, analgesics)
Equipment	Stretchers, fracture casts, dressing material, skin disinfectants, blankets

C^4 = Command, control, communications, and computers.

ahead of time (e.g., by armed forces commanders to provide fuel and depot maintenance to EMS ambulances, ministry of health to provide oxygen and medications, environmental protection agencies to provide PPE and decontamination capabilities). In Israel, since the national EMS organization Magen David Adom (MDA) is the nationally designated EMS agency for both daily operations and disaster management, there are clear procedures for the resupply of MDA with relevant supplies in case of need, both from the armed forces and emergency supply centers of the ministry of health.

4. **Communications, computers, command, and control (C^4):** a well-designed C^4 system that integrates with similar systems of other relevant agencies is a critical component for disaster management. Lessons learned from recent disasters indicate that obtaining timely, relevant, accurate information regarding the victims and the management of disasters is one of the most important unsolved issues (Table 47-4).

The larger the incident, geographically and in number of victims, the more numerous the caregivers and care-giving organizations involved, and the more important information becomes. In the end, the actual specific patient-oriented medical care of victims of disaster and mass casualty incidents (MCI) is relatively simple and easily mastered by competent health professionals. However, the success or failure of incident management and consequently, the prognosis of the victims, will largely depend on effective and timely command and control (C&C).

Effective command and control is largely dependent on information: Information regarding the event, the scene, the available response, the effectiveness of the response, and required real-time changes in plans. Without such information, any event outside of a continuous line of sight and hearing of a single incident commander becomes difficult to manage effectively.

Evolving technology has made the application of informatics in the field feasible. The miniaturization of electronics, the availability of wireless communications, including satellite-based, unlimited location and unlimited range communications, has for the first time made it possible to achieve effective data collection and dissemination in disasters. The advent of cellular telephones, usually with photographic capability, has improved availability tremendously, assuming cellular infrastructure is intact (which unfortunately has not been the case in many disaster situations to date). It is incumbent upon every EMS organization to look into available technologies and available resources and determine which if any information technology (IT) it wishes and can afford to adopt for its disaster plans. Components to be addressed include casualty flow control, care-team management, resource management, communications and automated data linking, data retrieval, analysis and reporting, easy and timely access to current relevant literature and databases, algorithms and local literature, and decision support tools (e.g., specific protocols, differential diagnoses, telephone numbers, and drug administration software).

Table 47–4	**Difficulties with Disaster Information Management for EMS**
Multiple players	Involvement of multiple persons and agencies
Information availability	Gradual availability of information. In geographically distributed events, lags may be days, weeks, or months
Information accuracy	Often inaccurate information at first, sometimes intentionally misleading, often initially transmitted by untrained observers
Information sources	Information is gathered by persons with varying backgrounds and there is varied access to the information
Information type	Mix of important information with voluminous but irrelevant information
Information managers	Caregivers are stressed, have limited time, and often feel that information gathering other than that directly relevant to operations is an imposition by management and therefore they fail to utilize available informatics equipment
Lateral and longitudinal portability and continuity	The need to transfer the information along the casualty care path and also disseminate it among agencies

Off the shelf systems are becoming available, although few, if any, have been fully implemented or certainly tested in real disasters. Some examples are the (British) semi-automatic casualty tracking system available at: http://www.ists.dartmouth. edu/docs/ists_v2_3_05.pdf. Also see http://www. upmc-cbn.org/report_archive/2007/04_April_2007/ cbnreport_04262007.html for information regarding US "RxHistory," which provides Internet access to medication histories of patients who are displaced in a disaster. The British Disaster Communications Recovery Unit available at: http://www.standardsglobal.com/british-standards-bs-257772008/ may also be useful.

5. **Disaster operating procedures and protocols:** EMS personnel and systems are geared toward lifesaving and often rescue of an individual, or at most small groups of victims. The transition to the rescue and care of large numbers of victims is far from trivial. Adequate concepts must be developed based both on universal principles as well as on specific requirements stemming from locally relevant hazards and existing capabilities. Concepts are then developed to fit the national or local philosophy of disaster management. Systems in different nations and even regions may differ in their staffing and patient care philosophy (e.g., physicians versus EMTs, ALS versus BLS). Sadly, economic realities may be the most important determinant of the amount of resources a nation or region may wish to invest in disaster preparedness, but political imperatives and public opinion may also have much to do with such resource allocation. For example, systems may elect not to invest in hazmat management or in radiologic event management or to prepare for natural disasters beyond a certain magnitude. In some countries the armed forces step in early following major disasters (e.g., Russia, Israel, and many Asian countries). While few individual nations can prepare adequately for all types and all magnitudes of disasters, most can and do selectively prepare for what they deem to be the most cost-effective response.

6. **Staffing:** personnel needs in disasters are different from those of daily operations. EMS systems normally determine their manpower needs according to their daily operations and their concept of operations, with little if any regard for disaster situations. However, planning and preparing for contingencies is part of the duties of any EMS manager. For example, the French and German systems rely largely on doctors to provide advanced life support (ALS) in the field. Such a system may not work very well in disasters (because of the limited number of available prehospital doctors), and a personnel mix for disaster management may need to be different, with more emphasis on use of emergency medicine technicians (EMTs) and on a BLS concept.

Disasters may pose two distinct challenges in as far as EMS staffing. For local, limited disasters, such as terrorist bombings, fires, or a building collapse, there is a need for immediate surge capacity with mobilization of existing and possibly some permanent standby staff, which will permit adequate although short-term response. For large-scale or prolonged disasters, there is a need for a preplanned, possibly prolonged, surge in staffing. Such a surge can only be achieved if it is planned for and if specific potential personnel are identified, trained, and incorporated into day-to-day EMS operations or at least during multiple drills. Options include a volunteer corps (e.g., Israeli MDA has 1500 permanent staff and 11,000 volunteers), retired EMS personnel, armed forces, police, university students, or even high school students.

A preplanned system must be in place to support EMS personnel and their family members during prolonged disaster operations. Safe shelter, food, communications, spare clothing, transportation to and from home, child-care facilities, and family support (e.g., psychological, financial, transfer to safe areas) are the most important if one is to rely on the continued presence and motivation of EMS personnel.

A well designed *call-up system* is important. One must assume that most existing means of communications will fail, at least initially. Many available options exist (e.g., cellular voice, cellular data, land telephone lines, Internet, beepers, two-way radios, satellite radio, or mobile telephone). At least two redundant communications technologies must be in place, based on local resources and regularly tested.

7. **Training:** training of EMS varies internationally, to some extent based on the local concept of operations (e.g., physician-based or EMT-based). Some nations are barely beginning to set up EMS systems, while most developed nations already have such systems in place. However, in many countries, especially the larger ones, there may be a multiplicity of agencies providing field care, each with its own training philosophy and contents. This may work well in daily operations but will be highly detrimental to disasters operations in which coordination and unified protocols and training are extremely important.

It is therefore incumbent upon each nation or region to decide on the appropriate training for disaster operations and to ensure that a unified approach exists, similar contents, training materials, and certification requirements. Having staff from different EMS and non-EMS agencies train and drill together will also enhance personal intercommunication during the actual event, an extremely important power multiplier in the chaotic world of disasters. Training for disaster operations should include both the "all hazards" approach as well as type-specific training. Realistic drilling is much more effective than classroom or Internet-based learning (although these methods have their place). Periodic retraining is a must because retention is usually poor and the "it won't happen here" syndrome is easily embraced. Financial remuneration for time spent training for disasters as well as other means to enhance both participation and retention must be in place.

8. **Interagency coordination:** disaster management is never a single-organization incident. To varying degrees in different nations and also in different types and magnitudes of disasters, EMS is only part of the overall (ideally, coordinated) response. Thus, police often are in command of the scene initially, ensuring safety, crowd control, transportation lanes, and coordination. In other events, especially very large natural disasters or complex humanitarian catastrophes, armed forces, international agencies, and nongovernmental organizations (NGOs) will likely be involved. EMS must liaise and coordinate with them all. Only an agreed upon common philosophy of operations, clear protocols, shared communication means, training and drilling together, and finally personal relationships among senior staff at different agencies will ensure effective coordination.

DISASTER OPERATIONS

1. **Notification:** false alarms are common in many places, sometimes as pranks or personal idiosyncrasies, sometimes as deliberate acts of social disruption. A predefined balance must be struck between the need to ascertain reliability of initial notification and the need to respond quickly. Procedures may include crosschecking information, callbacks, and recording calls.

2. **Event protocol activation:** clearly defined authority to declare an emergency must be in place. Protocol activation must be drilled frequently. Multiple protocols may be needed as part of the generic, all-hazards protocol. Protocols for different disaster "sizes" are needed.

3. **Dispatch:** Number and type of ambulances and personnel must be clearly spelled out in protocols. Casualty number, type, severity, geographic distribution as well as hospital distances, road conditions, and thus expected travel times dictate response magnitude. Many EMS systems have GPS tracking devices on their ambulances, permitting effective prioritization and distribution of vehicles to the closest incident sites, and even selective call-up of ambulances and personnel based on their proximity to the incident site.

4. **Surge capacity activation:** Call-up of staff requires effective means of communications. In the Israeli system we rely on one-way beepers and on data channels in the cellular network. However, the media often have excellent resources and provide what is probably the best picture of the event in initial stages. Staff members should be advised to listen to the media for information not forthcoming from their own system. When risks are elevated, such as due to severe weather or civil strife, drivers may take their ambulances home and save valuable time when they respond.

5. **C⁴ system activation:** Although ideally C^4 (communications, computers, command, and control) systems should function during day-to-day operations, some of the components of the complete system are likely to be used only during drills. Still, the entire system in its disaster mode should be ready to function in the field within literally minutes. This probably requires that most of the hardware be permanently located on ambulances or on specialized vehicles able to reach the scene of the incident at the same time as ambulances. The ideal system will be automatic, seamless, intuitive to use, and robust.

   An example of such a system might include the following:

   a. the immediate establishment of a wireless communications capability on site, performed by non-EMS personnel.

   b. immediate availability of video coverage of the disaster area for the benefit of command centers.

   c. electronic tags for casualties, which automatically relay GPS data to command centers and may incorporate severity, triage priority, and special circumstances (e.g., need for decontamination) information.

   d. GPS-enabled electronic tags for personnel and ambulances.

e. real-time tracking of casualties, ambulances, critical equipment such as ventilators, PPE, and of EMS personnel by command center.

f. information transfer to hospitals and any other care centers.

g. report generation in real-time and also for debriefing. Not many such complete systems are already in place. The Swiss have invested in an electronic system called Coordinated Medical Service (Rudolf Junker MD, personal communication, October 2009), operated by the armed forces. The German government is developing a similar system.

6. **Initial scene survey:** the greatest temptation and basic instinct of a medical person upon seeing casualties is to treat as many of the injured as possible to the best of his or her ability. However, in large incidents the most effective function of the first medical person on site is to survey the site, estimate the numbers, severity, and type of casualties, find a suitable staging area for patient care and for ambulances, determine the best ingress and egress lanes for ambulances, liaise with police or other relevant authorities already present, establish a communications line with the EMS command room, and provide the best estimate of the situation to authorities. Subsequently, it will be his or her job to direct EMS units as they arrive at the designated staging area. Upon arrival of senior EMS personnel, a fast but structured handover should be performed. Clear visual marking of the scene commander (e.g., a unique colored hat or vest) is very useful.

7. **Safety:** Ambulance personnel and EMTs must liaise with the local commandant from police, fire, armed forces, and others, as relevant. Simultaneously, the EMS command center should also open communication lines with relevant agencies, trying to obtain information relevant to scene safety. Hazmat, radiologic, or bioagent involvement may need to be ruled out either via dedicated detection equipment available in a few countries (and there, too, not universally available and subject to significant false-positive ratios) or via clinical detection of relevant symptoms (relevant only to hazmat, not radiologic or bioagents). Crowd control staff, PPE, bulletproof vests, and bioprotection may be required for EMS personnel safety. Whether a particular piece of equipment is permanently located in ambulances or not must be determined by local EMS authorities based on threat assessment and quantity of available equipment.

The issue of how much risk should an EMS operative take in providing medical care in disas-

ters is difficult to define in a protocol. Generally speaking, EMS personnel have a duty to provide care even under adverse conditions, balancing their personal safety against the urgency of the situation. It is the duty of EMS management to appropriately train and equip their staff so they are able to provide the most timely care possible, while they achieve the most personal safety.

In tactical situations, especially terrorist incidents, some simple principles apply. Mobilize a bomb disposal unit (police, fire, or military) if there is any suspicion of a bomb at the scene. The first responding unit should always follow the "2 in: 2 out" rule: in entering a potentially dangerous area, personnel must remain in direct contact with each other and exit together. The second unit should wait outside the danger zone (it may need to rescue the first unit).

The "LACES" Principle for Responding EMS units should be applied: *Lookout:* safety officer views overall scene from a safe distance; *Awareness:* all must maintain situational awareness; *Communications:* primary and secondary communications are needed; *Escapes:* all must have a preplanned escape route from the scene; *Safety Zones:* an upwind and uphill distant safe zone must be set up.

8. **Communications:** As was discussed in the preparations section, communications is a critical tool in disaster management. Increasingly, technology permits more efficient communications with the advent of satellite communications, wireless "bubbles" that may be quickly set up at the incident site, GPS tracking of assets and patients, agile software driven by two-way radios, and robust cellular infrastructure. Simple means such as megaphones work effectively in small sites (up to as much as several hundred meters or 600 feet). Two-way radios using dedicated frequencies work well unless there too many radios on the same frequency and call discipline is not maintained. Cellular telephones may be used to deliver still or video pictures to the command center. Whether continuous information must be provided to receiving hospitals is debatable and depends on how likely any of them is to be overcome with unmanageable numbers and severity of casualties. In my experience, a seasoned EMS operative is assigned to every hospital ED, serving as an effective liaison with his or her EMS colleagues on site, filtering raw information, and distilling it into useful data for hospital and ED managers.

9. **Liaison with other agencies on site:** since there may be multiple agencies responding to the event,

there must be a single event commander, and he or she must periodically physically gather senior staff from all agencies for briefings, coordination, and decision-making. Working on the same radio frequency may be useful in theory, but reality indicates that overcrowding of the ether quickly occurs and a Tower of Babylon effect is rapidly achieved.

10. **Care and evacuation plan:** evacuation plans based on the actual event must be formulated as early in the event as possible. The organization must have a clear chain of command, indicating which authority is empowered to formulate the plan. It may be the commander on site or a senior person in the command center, but it must always be the same chain of command. Unless the plan is formulated and also quickly disseminated to all units, personal initiative or work by the day-to-day operations protocol may result in many casualties being triaged and evacuated inappropriately. Generally, the most severely injured victims are the first to be evacuated to a hospital. If stable enough, they are transported to the nearest designated trauma center. When the nearest trauma center is far and the patient is unstable (such as with a partially compromised airway), he or she may be transferred to the nearest hospital for initial stabilization and later transferred to a regional trauma center.

   Minor injury cases are usually spread out among more distant hospitals. On many occasions, an ambulance transferring a critical patient will also take some "walking wounded" patients to facilitate evacuation. Use of a bus (rather than an ambulance) can facilitate transport of ambulatory, less injured patients to more distal facilities.

11. **Casualty rescue:** another instinct of EMS caregivers arriving at the site may be to participate in the rescue of trapped victims. This would be a significant waste of their capabilities. Rescue must be performed by the designated agencies and specifically trained personnel, while EMS personnel must focus on medical care.

12. **Triage:** "The art of sorting." Triage represents a method of quickly prioritizing victims with immediately life-threatening injuries AND who have the best chance of surviving in a situation where needs outstrip resources; it aims to save as many lives and limbs as possible under the circumstances and forego administration of treatment to hopeless casualties when it may impact the care of salvageable victims. Several primary and secondary triage tools have been developed, including Simple Treatment and Rapid Transport (START), JumpSTART, Care Flight Triage, Triage Sieve, Sacco Triage Method, Secondary Assessment of Victim Endpoint (SAVE), and Pediatric Triage Tape. Evidence to support the use of one triage algorithm over another is limited, and the development of effective triage protocols is an important research priority.[2] The most widely recognized mass-casualty triage algorithms in use today are not evidence-based, and no studies directly address these issues in the mass-casualty setting. Furthermore, no studies have evaluated existing mass-casualty triage algorithms regarding ease of use, reliability, and validity when biological, chemical, or radiologic agents are introduced. Currently, the lack of a standardized mass-casualty triage system that is well-validated, reliable, and uniformly accepted remains an important gap. In Israel we use a "gestalt" type triage termed the "look-listen-feel" method. Simply put, the assessor asks a question of the victim, listens to the answer (or lack of) and at the same time looks for obvious signs of severe injury and palpates the radial pulse for a qualitative evaluation.

    Triage is both a medical and a management decision: *Medical triage* entails the decision of how urgent it is to treat each patient. *Organizational triage* entails the decision of which patients should be treated and what resources are assigned to each patient, if any. Triage is an ongoing process and varies at different stages of the event: from initial evaluation to determine who should not be given care at all (not very sick or too sick) to who should be transported to the hospital first (or not at all). Casualties are re-triaged in the ED, usually more than once. Then triage is again applied for scarce resources in the hospital and beyond.

    There are many difficulties in disaster field triage. The most experienced personnel may not be available; stress may affect performance; weather and lighting conditions may be bad; there may be interference by onlookers or media. Physical risks may exist (e.g., secondary devices, chemicals). Not surprisingly, accuracy of field triage is not very high. In the study by Askenazi significant under-triage was found to occur when two actual mass casualty incidents (MCI's) were reanalyzed post hoc.[3]

13. **Casualty treatment:** perhaps the most controversial aspect of EMS operations is the extent of evaluation and treatment performed on site prior to evacuation to medical facilities. Various

philosophies of care are implemented in different countries, and there exist few if any relevant data to support one method over the other. Briefly, there are five main options.

a. *"Scoop and run, no on-site care:"* in underdeveloped nations there may be no EMS system as such or it may be very rudimentary. EMS serves as literally mechanized "scoops" bringing casualties and ill patients to hospitals with no care provided either on site or en route.

b. *"Scoop and run, on-site BLS:"* in other nations EMS may have BLS capacity but early evacuation is the norm.

c. *"Save and run:"* a compromise between BLS and ALS, practiced in the US, Canada, Israel, and elsewhere. Lifesaving procedures are performed, such as airway management (see later on), pleural cavity decompression, and external hemorrhage control. The patient is then evacuated as soon as possible.

d. *"Stay and play:"* full ALS applied in the field, often by physicians with varying degrees of expertise in field care.

e. *"Treat and discharge:"* practiced mostly in eastern Europe. Patients are evaluated, treated and – if appropriate – discharged by the ambulance crew. The EMS team essentially functions as a mobile clinic.

The correct technique for on-site disaster medical care varies with the type and extent of the disaster. Thus, conventional explosive terrorist bombs may result in tens to hundreds of casualties, located in one or at most several sites, usually in an urban location. ALS is available in most western EMS systems, and how much care is delivered on site depends on available resources and local protocols. Appropriate casualty distribution becomes the major concern. In Spain (2004 Madrid bombings)[4] and the UK (2005 London bombings), a significant amount of care was delivered on site. In Israel, experience from a large number of events has resulted in the "save and run" philosophy.[5] A similar event occurring in an underdeveloped location will likely result in "scoop and run" evacuation, mostly by non-EMS means, with little control over destinations. The very role of ALS in the field has repeatedly been challenged. At the very least, one should carefully balance the pros and cons of an ALS policy in disaster situations when its place in unrestricted daily operations is being challenged.[6]

14. **Airway management:** An ongoing debate currently exists regarding the place of field advanced airway management in trauma. A number of studies have documented worse or not improved outcomes with field endotracheal intubation.[6,7]

In the context of a disaster, this issue becomes much more significant because of the existing severe time and manpower constraints. It seems prudent to suggest that victims of major disasters, especially natural catastrophes, who require intubation and ventilatory support are unsalvageable in this context and should be treated expectantly. Conversely, in moderate sized, localized events such as terrorist bombings, tornadoes, avalanches, or other disaster events when hospital infrastructure is intact and the burden on EMS is not excessive, the same principles that the organization uses for daily operations should apply.

In major natural disasters, such as tsunamis and earthquakes, there is usually a period of recovery and stabilization (1 to 3 days), during which there may be little coordinated EMS activity, and local organizations may need to function as best they can. Factors such as area hospital conditions, EMS staff injuries (or injuries to their family members or their property), and road conditions will modify the response. Thus, a well-functioning EMS may need to evacuate to distant hospitals because the ones at the epicenter of the event were rendered nonfunctional by the event itself. ALS then becomes critical for some casualties, given prolonged evacuation times. On the other hand, alternate care sites may become available in the disaster zone, obviating this consideration and mitigating rapid transfers to such sites with little if any on-site care. The important thing in such situations is that EMS personnel are taught the relevant options and empowered to take responsibility beyond that of day-to-day conditions. Thus they are given the tools needed to make informed decisions on their own when centralized command and control are not yet available.

15. **Casualty evacuation and distribution:** Although every EMS organization has protocols and procedures in place for most if not all disaster types, the reality is that there are large differences even among events of the same type, often requiring minor or even major adjustments to protocol. For example: a terrorist bomb goes off 10 minutes away from a community hospital, 30 minutes from a Level II trauma center and 60 minutes from a Level I hospital. Does uniform distribution of casualties to many hospitals constitute the best

response in this scenario? Perhaps very severely injured victims should be taken to the nearest hospital, stabilized, and then transferred onward to Level 1 centers? Emergency personnel have learned to utilize bystanders to help care for the injured, and there is even some data showing improved survival of severely injured casualties transported by laypersons.[8] Bystanders can be used to help carry stretchers, apply pressure to bleeding limbs, and even manually ventilate patients with a bag-valve mask while waiting for additional medical back-up. Victims with minor injuries can also be transported to distant hospitals by willing bystanders. In fact, even in well-functioning systems, up to 50% of terrorist-bomb casualties arrive at hospitals in non-EMS vehicles. This ratio is higher in countries with less well-developed or limited-resource EMS.

16. **Casualty holding:** in very large events, or when infrastructure has been severely damaged or hospitals damaged or overwhelmed with patients, it may be necessary to hold patients on site or rather in the nearest safe location. Plans must be made for such an eventuality, with operating procedures for holding areas being developed, equipment and staffing determined, and secondary evacuation modes planned. In the New Orleans hurricane Katrina disaster, many victims were held at the airport, awaiting stabilization and transportation to health-care facilities at more distant locations.

17. **Documentation, identification of victims:** many victims lose their identification (ID) documents in the event, and some are confused, in shock, or truly unconscious. Attempts to identify victims in the field may lead to unnecessary and sometimes tragic errors, unless victims are clearly identified by family or friends (and even then, errors may still occur with facial injuries, with blood and soot often present). Documentation is important both for patient care and for the learning process of the organization.

18. **Analgesia:** Analgesia is part of medical management. Much literature indicates insufficient analgesia administration ("oligo analgesia") in trauma, while little if any exists regarding analgesia in the context of disaster and MCIs. What are the special risks of analgesia in the setting of an MCI? The two potential risks are respiratory depression with opiate administration and obscuration of symptoms. When should analgesia be administered to an MCI victim? As soon as is practically possible, except if it delays transfer and transportation times. What analgesic drugs are better suited for the specific environment of an MCI? Such drugs must have the features shown in Table 47-5.

A triage scheme for choice of analgesics in disasters is shown in Figure 47-1.

19. **Hazmat:** Some disasters may involve or primarily consist of hazardous materials. Good communications with agencies capable of detection and characterization of risks is key. Realistically, in a mass casualty event, EMS and other agencies will not be able to meet the immediate needs of all or most of the victims. If several sites are attacked or affected, personnel and equipment shortages will immediately become manifest. While manpower surge capacity for conventional incidents may be feasible as discussed earlier, such staff mobilization for a chemical incident may be impossible (compliance) or ineffective and dangerous (surge staff not properly trained and equipped). The major goal of EMS is to deploy to the closest safe (usually upwind) location to the event site and receive victims who either do not require decontamination or have at least taken their clothes off.

Decontamination may or may not be needed, and this is a critical decision to be taken early in the event by experts in toxicology. In fact, most toxic agents are so volatile and nonpersistent as to not require decontamination at all. If decontamination is required, disrobing the victims down to their underwear will remove >95% of the offending agent.[9] An ongoing debate exists regarding where the location of decontamination should be, either near the incident site or at the receiving hospitals.

Asymptomatic casualties may be transferred to alternate care sites if available or more distant hospitals. Severely affected casualties are provided initial specific or nonspecific treatment, respiratory support, and then transportation. If site decontamination facilities are erected, casualties may be decontaminated by fire fighters or other agencies, while EMS provides care before and after decontamination. If such facilities are not available in a timely manner, triage and evacuation to hospitals are carried out. However, casualty distribution is not necessarily based on the hospital's trauma designation but on its ability to decontaminate and treat hazmat-exposed patients. Figure 47-2 shows the increasing complexity of EMS response related to increasing toxicity and time of notification in events with hazmat agents.

Table 47–5	**Requirements for Analgesics in Disasters and Suggested Medications**

Drug Characteristics	
	Onset: rapid
	Duration: moderate
	Cardiorespiratory side effects: minimal
	Cost: low (large quantities must be stocked)
	Delivery: via multiple options (e.g., IV, IM, PO, nasal, buccal)
	Ready to use, i.e., no reconstitution required for delivery
	Shelf life: long, even at high/low temperatures
	Permits delivery by many personnel (e.g., EMT-P or even EMT-B)
Specific Drugs for Disaster Analgesia	
	Ketamine: rapid onset, stable hemodynamics, no respiratory depression, no reconstitution, may be given IV, IM, and even PO Depresses consciousness at high doses
	Suggested dosing: 0.25–0.50 milligram/kg IV bolus or 2 milligrams/kg IM and PO
	Morphine: rapid onset, may depress blood pressure if patient is hypovolemic, may depress respirations, consciousness
	Suggested dosing: 0.15 milligram/kg IV bolus in divided doses (start at 0.05 mg/kg), 0.15–0.25 milligram/kg SC or IM. Monitor consciousness, respirations
	Buprenorphine: moderately rapid onset, has "ceiling effect" and unlikely to depress blood pressure and respirations
	Suggested dosing: Tablet 0.2–0.4 milligrams SL
	Tramadol: moderately rapid onset, moderate efficacy, fairly frequent nausea and vomiting. Flexible dosing IV, IM, PO
	Suggested dosing: 1.0–1.5 milligrams/kg IM (IV requires unrealistically prolonged drip). "Flashtabs" or solution is also effective
	NSAIDs: rapid-acting "gelcaps," IM, IV, oral solutions of various drugs May exacerbate bleeding (and therefore are not recommended by the US military)

NSAIDs = Nonsteroidal anti-inflammatory drugs.

EMS personnel should not, as a rule, be used for rescue from the "hot zone" except if no other option exists. Their capabilities are put to best use after rescue from the hot zone has been achieved by specialized personnel from other agencies.

My personal bias, based on the Tokyo sarin incidents and much discussion with experts, is that most victims will not wait at the event site for mobile decontamination units to be brought and activated but will either go home to shower or to the nearest hospital ED.[9] Equipment needed for on-scene hazmat management is shown in Table 47-6.

20. **Ethics:** Preparing for and responding to major emergencies threatens the ethical underpinnings of routine, individualized, patient-centered, emergency health care. The exigency of a critical incident can instantly transform resource-rich environs to those of austerity. Health-care workers, who only moments earlier may have been seeing one to three patients at a time, are instantly thrust into a sea of casualties and more basic "lifeboat" issues of system overload and the thornier determinations of who will be given every chance to live and who will be allowed to die. Given time constraints, safety issues, uncertainties, and personal issues, EMS functioning in disasters must promulgate a clear but concise set of ethics rules to be applied in disaster situations. Issues to be addressed include:

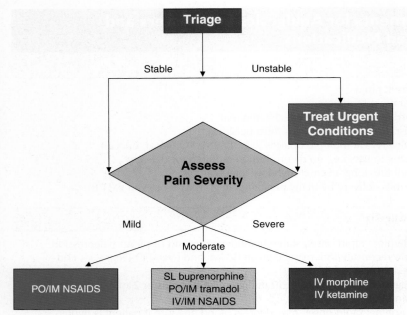

FIGURE 47–1

Magen David Adom field analgesia algorithm. Reprinted with permission of Magen David Adom, Israel.

- unbiased *triage* and prioritization of care and resource allocation, regardless of age, gender, nationality, social status. The International Federation of Red Cross and Red Crescent Societies' code of conduct for disaster relief states that "aid priorities are calculated on the basis of need alone."

- balancing the rescuer's own *safety* and that of the victim's (see above).
- patient *autonomy* (e.g., refuses care or wishes to be transported to a specific hospital against current policy), and.
- patient *privacy* (may resist exposure or transfer of personal details).

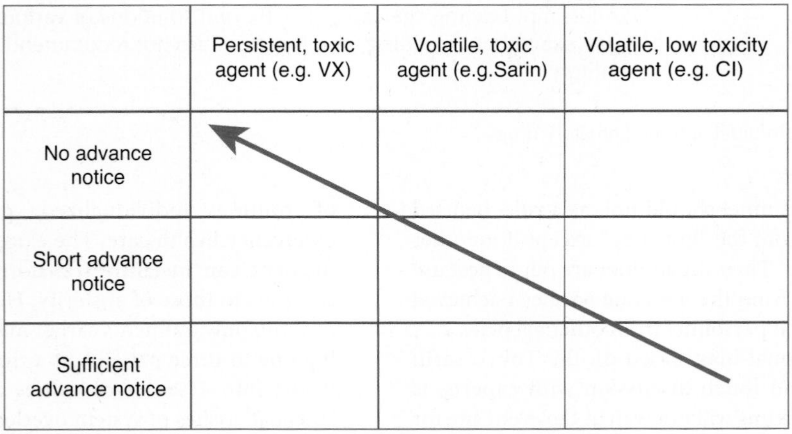

	Persistent, toxic agent (e.g. VX)	Volatile, toxic agent (e.g.Sarin)	Volatile, low toxicity agent (e.g. Cl)
No advance notice			
Short advance notice			
Sufficient advance notice			

FIGURE 47–2

Vertical axis shows increasing complexity of EMS response. Note: This diagram shows the increasing complexity of response occurring with progressively more toxic and persistent agents versus advance notice to the medical system. The worst scenario entails a very toxic, very persistent agent (such as VX) and no advance notice.

Table 47–6	**Equipment for Hazmat Response**	
Function	**Equipment**	**Quantity and Remarks**
Initial response for suspected but undeclared event	Level B or C PPE	May be stored in ambulances with extra kits at base
Identification of agent	Sensors, clinical training	Sensors may produce too many false-positive results and be rendered untrustworthy
Decontamination of staff and ambulances after initial response	Decontamination facility at base camp suitable for both personal and vehicle decontamination	Alternate site in case primary one is affected
Repeat cycle responses	PPE for multiple rounds of response, effective and rapid ambulance decontamination. Monitoring and other life support equipment protected or suitable for decontamination	
Casualty treatment	Antagonists and antidotes, supportive medications and equipment, as per hazards analysis	
Staff treatment in case of exposure	Personal antidote kits	

PPE = personal protective equipment.

21. **Debriefing:** immediately after event termination in the case of short-term emergencies or periodically during prolonged emergencies, the organization must look at its documented and also undocumented functions and learn lessons for the future or even for the same event. Memories fade and become distorted, and special interests come into play if such debriefing is postponed. A structured tool must be provided as an integral part of disaster manuals and protocols. A transparent, "no fault" organization approach will facilitate timely and accurate reporting, which will permit ongoing improvement of the system. Figure 47-3 demonstrates an unfortunately all too common type of event requiring post-event management analysis and debriefing.

A summary of the sequence of events and considerations for EMS response to disasters is presented in Table 47-7.

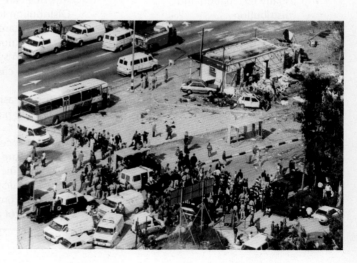

FIGURE 47–3

Two suicide cars exploded in this Israeli bus station. Reprinted with permission of Magen David Adom, Israel.

Table 47–7 | Sequential Components of EMS Disaster Operations

1. Notification	Including cross-checking reliability
2. Protocol activation	Organization must have clear protocol regarding who is authorized to declare a disaster situation and how such a decision is immediately communicated to the entire organization
3. Dispatch	Number and type of ambulances and personnel must be clearly spelled out in protocols
4. Surge capacity activation	Communications with surge capacity staff must be effective and redundant
	Coordination with neighboring EMS organizations for surge support established
5. C^4 (Command, control, communications, and computers)	Equipment may need to be brought in, technical staff may be required, protocols and hardware activated in multiple locations
6. Initial scene survey	First EMT does not treat but surveys scene and reports back to command center
7. Safety	EMT liaises with local commandant from police, fire, and armed forces, as relevant
	Hazmat, radio, or bioagent involvement ruled out
	Crowd control, staff PPE, bullet-proof vests, bioprotection may be required
8. Communications	Scene commander vis-à-vis command post, in coordination with other agencies on site
9. Liaison with other agencies on site	Brief face-to-face meeting of scene commanders
	Establishment of communication lines
10. Care and evacuation plan	Scene commander briefly discusses type and magnitude of event with command center, and a plan is formulated and then communicated to all participants
11. Casualty rescue	Usually not a job for EMS
	Other organizations should rescue while EMS concentrates on medical care
12. Casualty triage	Triage concepts and methods may be different than during day-to-day operations
13. Casualty treatment	According to protocol (i.e., on scene ALS/BLS)
14. Casualty evacuation and distribution	ALS/BLS care during transportation?
	Distribution to multiple hospitals
	Alternate care sites if hospitals damaged
15. Casualty holding on site	Very large numbers of casualties, damaged transportation system, damaged or distant hospitals
16. Documentation, identification of victims	Tagging of casualties, care documentation
17. Analgesia	Even in disasters, do not lose sight of the need to alleviate pain as best possible under the circumstances
18. HazMat	Special procedures, equipment, and training and drilling are required for proficiency in managing hazmat incidents
19. Ethics	Special ethical difficulties arise in disasters
20. Debriefing	Learning from each mass event is imperative for quality control and improvement

SUMMARY

All EMS organizations must recognize their critical role in the management of MCIs and disasters. Based on appropriate hazards and vulnerability assessment, EMS leaders must define appropriate policies, dedicate appropriate resources, and ensure development of appropriate protocols and operating procedures and their incorporation into the training and drilling routine of the organization. The decision to activate a mass casualty event response is often made with little information using a very low threshold. The first EMS person to arrive at the scene becomes the temporary medical site commander, relaying vital information back to the command center. Medical care is rendered only after additional medical teams arrive. Bright hats and jackets may identify the scene commander and EMS personnel. Communication at the scene may be with megaphones, while multiple modes of communication may need to be employed vis-à-vis the EMS command center and other agencies.

The primary casualty survey focuses on basic airway and external hemorrhage control. Evacuation is based on injury severity; however, ambulances transporting critical patients also may transport more minor casualties. Bystanders are utilized when appropriate. Documentation is important both for patient care and for the learning process of the organization.

References

1. Garwin TM, Pollard NA, Tuohy RV, eds. Project Responder National Technology Plan for Emergency Response to Catastrophic Terrorism. Prepared by Hicks and Associates, Inc. for The National Memorial Institute for the Prevention of Terrorism and the United States Department of Homeland Security; April 2004.
2. Jenkins JL, McCarthy ML, Sauer LM, et al. Mass-casualty triage: time for an evidence-based approach. *Prehospital Disaster Med* 23(1): 3, 2008.
3. Ashkenazi I, Kessel B, Khashan T, et al. Precision of in-hospital triage in mass-casualty incidents after terror attacks. *Prehospital Disaster Med* 21: 20, 2006.
4. Peral-Gutierrez de Ceballos J, Turégano-Fuentes F, Pérez-Díaz Mercedes Sanz-Sánchez D, et al. 11 March 2004: The terrorist bomb explosions in Madrid, Spain – an analysis of the logistics, injuries sustained and clinical management of casualties treated at the closest hospital. *Crit Care* 9: 104, 2005.
5. Liberman M, Mulder D, Sampalis J. Advanced or basic life support for trauma: meta-analysis and critical review of the literature. *J Trauma* 49: 584, 2000.
6. Davis DP: Should invasive airway management be done in the field? *Can Med Assoc J* 178(9): An, 2008.
7. Lecky F, Bryden D, Little R, et al. Emergency intubation for acutely ill and injured patients (Review) 2008; http://www.thecochranelibrary.com, http://www.mrw.interscience.wiley.com/cochrane/clsysrev/articles/CD001429/frame.html (accessed 02/14/10).
8. Demetriades D. Paramedic vs. private transportation of trauma patients. Effect on outcome. *Arch Surg* 131(2): 133, 1996.
9. Levitin W, Siegelson HJ, Dickinson S, et al. Decontamination of mass casualties—re-evaluating existing dogma. *Prehospital Disaster Med* 18(3): 200, 2003.

CHAPTER 48

Tactical EMS Medicine

Jimmy T.S.Chan, Yuk-yin Chow

KEY LEARNING POINTS

- Provision of medical care in the tactical environment requires special training and ongoing skills maintenance.

- Some EMS clinical care protocols need to be modified for use in the tactical environment.

- There are significant differences between civilian and tactical EMS.

- Special training for medics is needed for TEMS.

- There are different phases of care in the TEMS environment.

- The three zones concept is used in managing Chemical, Biological, Radiologic, and Nuclear (CBRN) environments.

- EMS personnel need to know about management of injuries from less lethal weapons.

On many battlefields soldiers continue to die just as they did in the Civil War of the United States from 1861 to 1865. The civilian prehospital care components such as Emergency Medical Technician (EMT), Basic Trauma Life Support (BTLS), and Advanced Trauma Life Support (ATLS) may not work well in austere and unsafe environments. It has been discovered that patient outcomes in these environments can be improved by better immediate control of hemorrhage and early use of fluid resuscitation, analgesics, and antibiotics. In the continuum of combat casualty care, the application of a correct intervention but with the wrong timing could cause additional damage to the patient. To provide medical care in a tactical environment is very different from conditions in the ordinary prehospital environment. Medical personnel may be required to work in an unsafe tactical environment with minimal outside support. In the urban areas of Hong Kong, police medics may need to provide emergency medical care before the arrival of the

civilian EMS personnel in situations such as riots, hostage-taking, and chemically dangerous areas. With the increasing threat of terrorism, tactical EMS personnel need to have good knowledge of how to provide care in hazmat environments.

In the US, the concept of tactical EMS was first developed in the special operations forces of the US Army and by US Navy Hospital Corpsmen.[1]

Later, the system was further incorporated by Special Weapons and Tactics (S.W.A.T.) police units in the evolution of tactical emergency medical support. In 1996, the Military Medicine Supplement published the guidelines for Tactical Combat Casualty Care (TCCC) in Special Operations.[1] The important guiding principles of trauma response in the combat environment were presented. As these guidelines were tactically and medically sound, the recommendations were endorsed by the American College of Surgeons and the National Association of EMTs. The TCCC was also published in the 5th edition of Pre-Hospital Trauma Life Support (PHTLS) in 2003.[2]

In Hong Kong, the first tactical EM care course was launched by the Accident and Emergency Medicine Academic Unit of the Chinese University of Hong Kong in 2000.[3] The response from the police officers of different grades was excellent. Since then the medical personnel have had many opportunities to provide medical training to different units of the police, such as the Special Duties Unit (SDU), Airport Security Unit (ASU), Witness Protection Unit (WPU), Very Important Person Protection Unit (VIPPU), and the Emergency Unit (EU). In the 6th World Trade Organization Ministerial Conference in 2005, tactical first-aid training was also provided to more than 200 officers in the Police Tactical Units (PTUs). This was the first time in Hong Kong that witnessed large-scale cooperation between the Hong Kong Hospital Authority and the Hong Kong Police for medical response in a planned major operation. After this event, many doctors, nurses, and police officers thought that there was a need for Hong Kong to further develop tactical emergency medicine, as the area would host many additional international events in the future. Therefore, a Police-Oriented Tactical Emergency Medicine (POTEM) program was jointly developed by the Hong Kong Police College and the Hong Kong Association for Conflict and Catastrophe Medicine[4] (Figure 48-1).

DEFINITIONS

Tactical EMS (TEMS): the provision of prehospital or out-of-hospital care in austere and unsafe police situations. Tactical EMS encompasses patient care

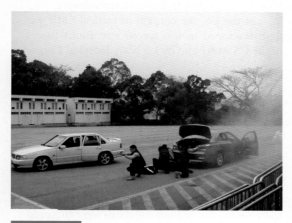

FIGURE 48–1

Police-oriented tactical emergency medicine program.

rendered to victims who are in unsafe areas such as riots or areas where ongoing gunfire is occurring. The target patient group includes tactical team members, victims, hostages, spectators, bystanders, and perpetrators.

Hazmat (Hazardous Materials): Any substance posing a significant risk to human, animal, and plant life when released, including chemical, biological, radiologic, and nuclear (CBRN) agents.

Basic Trauma Life Support (BTLS), Pre-hospital Trauma Life Support (PHTLS), Advanced Trauma Life Support (ATLS), and Advanced Hazmat Life Support (AHLS) are standardized courses that may be useful in tactical EMS training.

DIFFERENCES IN TACTICAL EMS AND CIVILIAN EMS

Civilian EMS training is well structured and standardized in many countries. However, there is no national standard for tactical EMS (TEMS) training in either the US or in Hong Kong. Police medics need to provide care in hostile and unsafe environments with limited resources in equipment, personnel, and patient evacuation. The comparisons between in-hospital, prehospital, and tactical EMS care are summarized in Table 48-1.

THE THREE PHASES OF CARE IN TEMS

According to the guidelines stated in Tactical Casualty Combat Care, there are three phases of tactical care: Care Under Fire, Tactical Field Care, and Combat Casualty Evacuation Care. The working principles in these different phases of care are very different. The main objectives are treatment of victims, prevention of additional casualties, and completion of the mission.

Care Under Fire ("Hot Zone")

This is the most dangerous phase of care. The medics need to work in an austere and unsafe environment and very often under fire. The objectives in this phase of care are avoidance of being shot, protection and treatment of team members, victims, and bystanders, treatment of perpetrators, and rapid evacuation of victims to cover areas. In the phase of care under fire, return fire by both medics and victims (if possible) is important to prevent further injury (Figure 48-2). Victory is the best medicine in this phase. Smoke

Table 48–1	**Comparison of Tactical EMS and Civilian EMS**	
In-Hospital Care	**Civilian Prehospital Care**	**Tactical EMS**
Advanced Trauma Life Support (ATLS)	Basic Trauma Life Support (BTLS)	Mainly penetrating trauma
Safe environment	Safe environment	Austere and unsafe environment
Access to full range of specialist physicians	Well equipped and supported	Minimal support in austere environment
Rapid response time	Rapid response time	May be delay in response time
Communication is very good	Communication is good	Communication may not be possible
Resources intensive	Resources adequate	Resources limited
Timely advanced trauma care facilities with intensive care support	Rapid access to ambulance and short evacuation time	Unknown access to ambulance and evacuation time

grenades, flash bangs, tear gas, and armored vehicles are good tools to help the scoop and run process.

In this phase of care, not much in the way of first-aid procedures can be done with respect to airway, breathing, and circulation. Besides returning fire, rapid evacuation to nearby cover and reassurance of the victims are the priorities. For more than 2500 prehospital deaths in the Vietnam War, the cause of death was uncontrolled hemorrhage from extremity wounds. Control of severe bleeding from extremity wounds by the combat application tourniquet (CAT) has been shown to be important as a lifesaving procedure. Although many emergency physicians are very reluctant to use tourniquets in the prehospital environment, their use in the phase of care under fire is very important to save lives (Figure 48-3).

The probability of ischemic damage from the tourniquet is rare within 90 minutes of application. It is important to write down the time of application on the tourniquet area skin or on a dressing. Usually when under fire there is no immediate direct management for the airway and breathing, and evaluation and care for these are deferred to the warm zone care. Protection of the cervical spine when under fire (with immobilization utilizing a stiff collar or other device) should only be considered for severe neck injuries, as might occur from falls greater than 5 meters (16 feet) (as from fast roping accidents or parachuting). Even with a patient with highly probable neck injury,

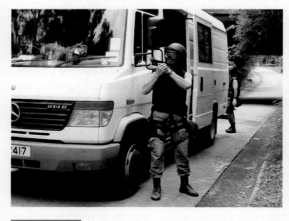

FIGURE 48–2

Return fire in care under fire phase.

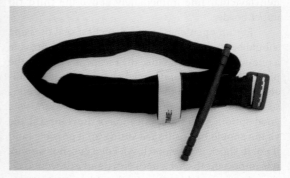

FIGURE 48–3

Combat application tourniquet (CAT) used to control massive bleeding.

the risk/benefit for cervical spine protection and the chance of being shot should be considered.

Tactical Field Care ("Warm Zone")

Working in this phase is still unsafe. Resources are still limited. Although gunfire has stopped, return of enemy fire may happen at any time. Therefore only simple stabilizations can be done, and the victims evacuated to medical treatment facilities as soon as possible. However, the evacuation time is unpredictable and may range from 30 minutes to several hours' time. Simple procedures for airway, breathing, and circulation should be done according to the special circumstances of each situation.

For airway management for an unconscious patient, simple hand-held suction, jaw thrust, and putting the victim in the recovery position should be done. An oropharyngeal airway or nasopharyngeal airway can be used to hold the airway open. For victims with a completely blocked airway, emergency cricothyroidotomy should be considered. Adjunct airway equipment such as the Combitube or laryngeal mask airway (LMA) can be considered. However, the use of the laryngoscope for endotracheal intubation should be avoided because the white light of the laryngoscope may incite shooting from different sources.

Tension pneumothorax is the second leading cause of death on the battlefield. The classic signs and symptoms are severe shortness of breath, engorgement of the neck veins, hyperinflation of one side of the chest, and, rarely, deviation of the trachea from its central position to the unaffected side. The insertion of a needle catheter to release the air under tension in the thoracic cavity is important. The needle catheter can be inserted in the second intercostal space, the midclavicular line immediately above the third rib upper border.

For an open chest wound, a chest seal dressing should be applied (Figure 48-4). The idea is to provide a one-way valve to enhance the escape of air from the pleural space. If a commercial chest seal is not available, the application of a plastic sheet with three ends sealed and one end opened around the wound is a good option. After the application of the chest seal, the victim should be positioned sitting up if possible (and if not in shock from blood loss). For a gunshot wound, it is important to check both entry and exit wounds.

Control of bleeding is also important at this stage. Tourniquets and pressure dressings are both acceptable. However, a tourniquet used for bleeding control should be changed to a pressure dressing

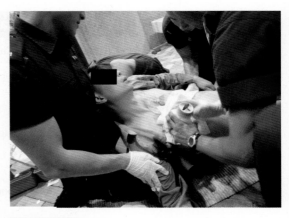

FIGURE 48–4

Application of chest seal in open chest injury.

whenever possible. IV infusion can be considered if the patient has severe bleeding. If the bleeding is controlled and the victim is not in shock, IV infusion is not required. If the victim is in shock and the bleeding is controlled, IV infusion should be considered. However, if the victim is in shock and the bleeding cannot be controlled, such as in internal bleeding, IV infusion should be withheld, as more infusion will enhance more bleeding. Wide-bore IV catheters (at least 18 gauge) should be used, and the intravenous site should be selected in areas proximal to major wounds or suspected fractures. Crystalloid such as NS or LR solution or a colloid such as hetastarch (e.g., Hespan®) can be used; 1000 mL of LR will expand the intravascular volume by 250 mL within 1 hour and 500 mL of 6% hetastarch will expand the intravascular volume by 800 mL within 1 hour and will sustain this expansion for 8 hours. Because of the concern about its effect on the coagulation system, usually not more than 1000 mL of hetastarch should be given at one time. For trained medics, an IO needle can be placed in the leg or humerus to provide fluid resuscitation.

As in care under fire, immobilization of the cervical spine is usually not done unless there is probable severe neck injury, as occurs from falls greater than 5 meters (16 feet). All suspected major fractures should be splinted, and wounds covered with dressings. It is important to check the distal pulse after splinting or application of a pressure dressing. Minimal clothing should be removed in order to prevent hypothermia. In this stage, use of pain control agents such as acetaminophen 1000 milligrams orally (PO) or injection of morphine 5 milligrams IV may be helpful. Fentanyl 400-microgram lozenges may be as effective as morphine injection for pain treatment. Use of fentanyl is simple, safe, effective, and does not require an IV line.

However, the use of nonsteroidal anti-inflammatory drugs (NSAIDs) such as aspirin or ibuprofen should be avoided because these may interfere with the hemostatic process. Broad-spectrum antibiotics can be considered for open fractures and penetrating abdominal trauma if evacuation is expected to be prolonged. Gatifloxacin 400 milligrams PO and slow IV or IM injection of cefotetan 2 grams are options.

As the successful outcome of cardiopulmonary resuscitation (CPR) is only minimal, CPR for nontraumatic cardiac arrest in this phase is usually not performed except for those who have experienced hypothermia, near drowning, or electrocution. Moreover, weapons such as grenades, pepper spray, or pistols should be removed from mentally confused victims. All victims should be disarmed before the application of lifesaving procedures.

Combat Casualty Evacuation Care ("Cool Zone")

In this phase of care, medics are working in a transport environment such as a vehicle, boat, or helicopter (Figures 48-5 A, B and C). The main objectives in this phase are to further stabilize the patient and facilitate the safe transfer of victims to medical treatment facilities as soon as possible. However, the evacuation process can range from minutes to hours. In the cool zone, special attention should be given to medics, as they may be dehydrated, injured, hypothermic, or exhausted.

The medical care in the cool zone is more advanced as more resources are available (medical personnel and equipment). The BLS care in the cool zone is essentially similar to that in the warm zone, but the care is enhanced. Oxygen can be given to victims if indicated. Most combat casualties do not require oxygen except for those with low pulse oximeter readings, unconscious patients, or those with thoracic blast injury. However, it is still important to watch out for the development of tension pneumothorax. Spinal immobilization should be done if required. Electronic monitoring equipment can be used to measure blood pressure, pulse, and oxygen saturation (pulse oximetry). Continuing monitoring of the victims to include the vital signs, pulses distal to splint sites, and the

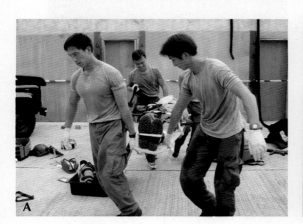

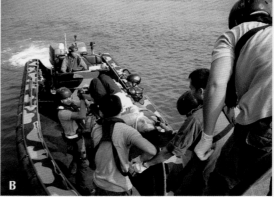

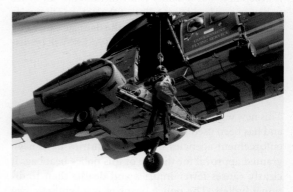

FIGURE 48–5

A, B, C Land, boat, and air transport of victims.

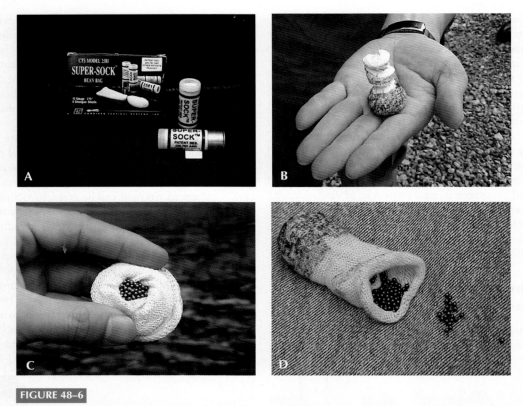

FIGURE 48–6

A, B, C, D Police bean bag round (four parts).

level of consciousness of the patient is very important throughout the journey to medical treatment facilities.

FEWER LETHAL WEAPONS

In modern police departments, less lethal weapons such as the "police bean bag" ammunition and the TASER® stun gun have been developed for law enforcement personnel in situations where armed force is acceptable but lethality is unwarranted.[5,6] In order to have a good understanding of the nature of injuries inflicted by these new weapons, the damage caused by the police beanbag round and the TASER® will be discussed.

Police Bean Bag Ammunition

This new weapon was first developed in the early 1970s and has been used in the US since 1994. Currently law enforcement agencies in many countries have been granted approval for the use of this police beanbag. It clearly causes fewer injuries and deaths than traditional bullets. The police beanbag is a synthetic bag filled with lead pellets and is fired from a shotgun (Figures 48-6A, B, C & D). The bag is designed to exit the shell, separate from the wadding, and unfold so that the largest area of the bag will hit and transmit all the kinetic energy to the target, usually resulting in knocking down the struck person. The manufacturer alleges that this weapon will usually only cause bruises, skin abrasions, and minor injuries in incapacitating the violent suspect.

The police beanbag delivers its kinetic energy over an area of approximately 40 mm in diameter to impart a less lethal impact to the target. It may cause bruises, skin abrasions, and other injuries associated with blunt trauma. The optimal firing ranges are between 3 and 15 meters (10 to 49 feet), with a projectile velocity of 70 meters (230 feet) per second. However, it is stressed that shot placement rather than the deploying range is the critical factor in determining the extent of injuries. Shots to the head, neck, thorax, or spine can result in fatal or serious injuries. Cases have been reported where the beanbag penetrated a body cavity.

In an experiment done in Hong Kong using a pig model, it was shown that all shots of the police bean bag could produce injuries, ranging from minor

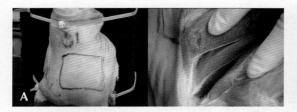

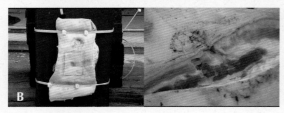

FIGURE 48-7

A, B Effect of police bean bag on pork target (five).

indentation to laceration of soft tissues (Figure 48-7A, 7B).[5] The degree of trauma was greatly diminished if the target was protected with heavy clothing (Figure 48-8). Moreover, the trauma produced in the rib region was more severe than that on the thigh region. The larger the volume of soft tissue, the better the absorption of kinetic energy expected, resulting in a lesser degree of injuries. According to the experience of Los Angeles County and the University of Southern California in the US, the trauma produced by the police beanbag might range from minor injuries to

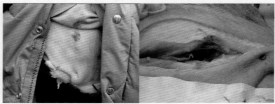

FIGURE 48-8

Effect of police bean bag greatly diminished by clothing.

fatality. Serious injuries like penetrating wounds, massive hemothorax, pneumothorax, pulmonary contusion, ruptured globe, splenic rupture, subcapsular hepatic hematoma, pneumopericardium, and compartment syndrome have been reported. The manufacturer advises that the shots should avoid the regions including the head, neck, anterior thorax, or spine.

TASER®

TASER® (the word comes from the comic book name "Thomas A. Swift Electric Rifle") was originally designed for law enforcement as a "less lethal" weapon.[6] The shape and size are similar to a handgun (Figure 48-9). When fired, the two shooting-out electrodes will penetrate the skin of the suspect and deliver high electrical voltage (up to 50,000 volts). The shock will immediately incapacitate the victim. The

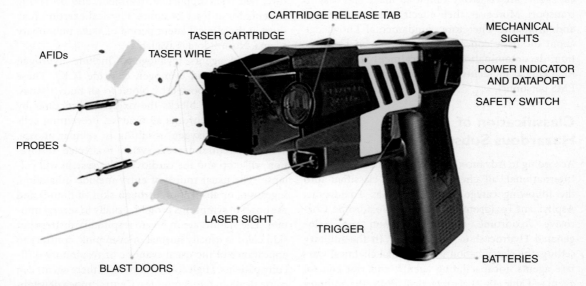

CARTRIDGE RELEASE TAB

TASER CARTRIDGE

MECHANICAL SIGHTS

AFIDs   TASER WIRE

POWER INDICATOR AND DATAPORT

SAFETY SWITCH

PROBES

LASER SIGHT   TRIGGER

BATTERIES

BLAST DOORS

FIGURE 48-9

TASER® with two electrodes. Image provided Courtesy of Ryan Karpilo, Owner, RKDefense at *http://www.RK Defense.com*.

TASER® is available in civilian and law enforcement models. The shooting range is about 4 to 5 meters (13 to16 feet). Although the manufacturer claims that the use of the TASER® is safe, deaths related to its use have been reported since its first utilization in 2001. Head injuries from the sudden fall to the ground and burns from petroleum-contaminated clothing catching on fire have been reported. There have also been some deaths reported apparently due to the TASER®'s causing cardiac dysrhythmias.

Chemical, Biological, Radiologic, and Nuclear (CBRN) Incidents

Hazmat (hazardous material) refers to substances posing a significant risk to human, animal, and plant life when released, which includes chemical, biological, radiologic, and nuclear (CBRN) agents. Chemical agents are the most likely choice for a terrorist attack because of their easy availability and their immediate effect on alarming the population. A chemical warfare agent is a chemical that is intended for use in military operations to kill, seriously injure, or incapacitate humans (or animals) through its toxicologic effects. Military chemical weapons were used in relatively recent military conflicts in Afghanistan, Iraq, and Iran. It was not until the sarin attack in the Tokyo Subway on 8th March 1995 that attention was drawn to this issue of use of chemical weapons by terrorists against civilian populations. Many dangerous chemical agents are relatively simple to make and easy to transport. Moreover, their effects may be immediate and dramatic. Therefore, fundamental knowledge about the basic concepts, toxicity, personal protection, decontamination, and treatment with respect to chemical incidents is very important for tactical EMS personnel.[7]

Classification of Hazardous Substances

According to Advanced HazMat Life Support (AHLS) International, all chemicals can be classified into the following categories: Irritant Gas Toxidrome, Asphyxiant Toxidrome, Cholinergic Toxidrome, Corrosive Toxidrome, and Hydrocarbon and Halogenated Hydrocarbon Toxidrome.[8] In the military setting, the classification used is lethal chemical warfare agents, incapacitating agents, and riot control agents (Table 48-2). For tactical EMS, the military classification is more relevant.

Pulmonary agents (choking agents) include phosgene (CG), diphosgene (DP), chlorine (CL), and

Table 48–2	Classification of Hazardous Materials
AHLS classification	Military classification
Irritant gas toxidrome	Pulmonary agents
Asphyxiant toxidrome	Blood agents
Cholinergic toxidrome	Nerve agents
Corrosive toxidrome	Blistering agents
Hydrocarbon and halogenated hydrocarbon toxidrome.	Incapacitating and riot control agents

AHLS = Advanced HazMat Life Support.

chloropicrin (PS). These agents damage the lungs and irritate the eyes and respiratory tract. The route of entry is mainly through inhalation. Phosgene, for example, can cause delayed onset of pulmonary edema following a clinical latent period (usually 4 to 6 hours, but may be up to 24 hours). Initially victims present with shortness of breath and later develop hypoxia, cyanosis, and hypotension as a result of acute pulmonary edema. Irritation of the larynx by very high concentrations of the agent may lead to sudden laryngeal spasm and death. Death can occur within 24 hours. The treatments include termination of exposure, bed rest, supportive treatment, and observing patients for at least 24 hours. Physical exertion may shorten the clinical latent period of acute pulmonary edema. No antidote is available.

Blood agents (cyanogens) include hydrogen cyanide (AC) and cyanogen chloride (CK). These agents are transported by blood to all body tissues, where the agent blocks the oxidative processes by binding to cytochrome a3 oxidase, preventing cells from utilizing oxygen, resulting in cellular anoxia. When the central nervous system is affected, respiration will stop and the cardiovascular system will collapse. The usual routes of entry include inhalation, ingestion, or absorption through skin (if liquid) and the onset of symptoms is rapid, usually in several minutes. The victims are in severe respiratory distress but skin color is usually normal or even pink, contrary to appearance of the usual cyanotic or respiratory difficulty patients. High concentrations of these agents can cause death in 6 to 8 minutes. Central apnea develops in 2 to 5 minutes after high-dose exposure, resulting in opisthotonus, trismus, decerebrate posture, bradycardia, dysrhythmias, hypotension, and eventually

Table 48–3	**Antidotes for Cyanogen Poisoning**				
Antidotes	**Packing**	**Starting Dose**	**Injection Speed**	**Repeat Dose**	**Remarks**
Amyl nitrite	Vial	1 Vial	–	–	Gauze + Mask
Na nitrite	3% 10-mL ampule	10 mL 3% solution IV (300 milligrams) Pediatric dosage: 0.33 mL/kg 3% solution IV	3 minutes	50% original dose if signs recur	Displacement, (<40% MetHb) Beware of hypotension
Na thiosulfate	25% 50 mL vial	50 mL 25% solution IV (12.5 grams) Pediatric dosage: 1.65 mL/kg 25% solution IV	10 minutes	50% original dose if signs recur	May induce nausea and vomiting
Other sulfur donor Hydrox-ycobalamin	2.5-gram vial	2.5 to 5 grams	15 minutes	<15 grams in total	Expensive

cardiac arrest. The treatments include termination of exposure, supportive treatment, and observation for at least 24 hours. Treatment with 100% oxygen is beneficial. Antidotes are available but are not a must for survival. Many victims can survive with vigorous supportive treatment alone. The antidotes for cyanogen poisoning are given in Table 48-3.

Nerve agents (anticholinesterases) such as Tabun (GA), Sarin (GB), Soman (GD), and V-agent (VX) inhibit the cholinesterase enzymes. The cholinesterase enzymes are responsible for the hydrolysis of acetylcholine, a chemical neurotransmitter. This inhibition creates an accumulation of acetylcholine at cholinergic synapses, which leads to overstimulation and transmission of nerve impulses. The usual routes of entry are inhalation or skin and eye contact. Nerve agents produce rapid onset of symptoms (seconds to minutes for vapor exposure). The signs and symptoms are similar to those of organophosphate insecticide poisoning. The classic signs of "DUMBELS" (Diarrhea, Urination, Miosis, Bronchospasm/Bronchorrhea, Emesis, Lacrimation, and Salivation) may occur. Death can occur within minutes. The treatments include termination of exposure and basic life support for airway, breathing, and circulation, decontamination, and treatment with antidotes. Rapid decontamination is extremely important for patients to reduce the absorption and improve medical team safety. The administration of antidotes should be done as soon as possible before the "aging" process occurs, an irreversible binding between the acetylcholine esterase and the nerve agent (Table 48-4).

In the tactical environment, auto-injectors for tropine and pralidoxime (2-PAM chloride) are available in the Mark I kit (see Figure 48-10). For critically injured victims of nerve agents, two to three injections of Mark I components may be required. Note that the antidotes may be given by the IO route if an IV line is not available.

Blistering agents (vesicants) include sulfur mustard (H/HD) and nitrogen mustard (HN), lewisite (L), and phosgene oxime (CX). Blister agents produce initial irritation to the eyes and skin, with subsequent formation of blisters. When inhaled, these can damage the mucous membranes of the respiratory tract, resulting in pseudomembrane formation. The main route of entry, however, is usually through the skin. Other routes of entry include the eyes, airway, and ingestion. Blister agents cause a high incidence of eye and lung damage. From skin contact, they cause erythema, vesicles, bullae, and eventually necrosis. In the respiratory system, they cause necrosis and hemorrhagic edema of the mucosa of the airway. Pseudomembrane formation may lead to sudden death. Death can occur as a result of damaged airway, infection, depressed immune system, and sepsis. Blister agents may affect the stem cells in the bone marrow and may produce cancer. The treatments for blister agents include termination of exposure, early decontamination, and supportive treatment. No antidote is available.

Table 48–4 | Antidotes for Nerve Agent Poisoning

Antidotes	Packing	Starting Dose	Injection Speed	Repeat Dose	Remarks
Atropine	2-milligram ampule or autoinjector	2 milligrams IM/IV/IO Avoid IV in case of hypoxia because it will induce cardiac arrhythmia Pediatric dosage 0.05 mg/kg	–	5 to 10 minutes	Usual range: 15 to 20 milligrams until secretions dry up and there is ventilation improvement; atropine will not help miosis
Pralidoxime (2 PAM-CL)	500 mg/20-mL vial or 600 milligram autoinjector	1gram IV <12 years 20 to 50 mg/kg IV >12 years 0.5 to 1 gram IV	20 to 30 minutes	1 hour later may require 1 to 2 repeat doses	Useless if aging occurs GD: 2 minutes GB: 3 to 4 hours
Diazepam	10-milligram ampule	10 milligrams IM/IV Pediatric dosage 0.25 to 0.4 mg/kg IV	–	Repeat as required	Usual range: 10 to 20 milligrams

GB = sarin; GD = soman.

Riot Control Agents

In modern cities, civic demonstrations may sometimes get out of control and may require use of riot control agents by law enforcement personnel. Tear gas and pepper spray are two commonly used agents by law enforcement to get the riot under control. The main effect of tearing agents is to irritate exposed skin and mucous membranes so as to produce temporary incapacitation in recipients. In Hong Kong, the tearing agent adopted is Corson Stoughton (CS) (Figure 48-11). CS has a high safety profile. For example, in 1989, the Hong Kong Police had fired about 30,000 rounds of CS to control a riot in a Vietnamese boat people's camp. There were no reported permanent injuries or deaths. Tearing agents are aerosols and the onset of symptoms is within minutes. They cause pain and severe irritation to the eyes, skin, and respiratory

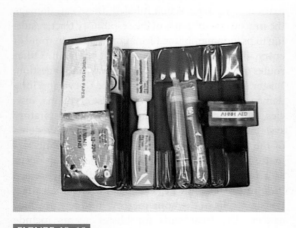

FIGURE 48–10

Mark I kit.

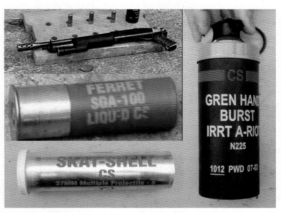

FIGURE 48–11

Tearing agent used in Hong Kong: Corson Stoughton (CS).

tract but there is no permanent damage to chronic lung disease patients. The effect of tearing agents is usually self-limiting to 15 to 30 minutes. Less than 1% of exposed people have effects severe or prolonged enough to cause them to seek medical care. There is no special treatment for tearing agents except decontamination by wind or water before going into the ambulance. Small vesicles on the skin should be left intact. Only symptomatic treatment is needed and no antidote is required. Tearing agents may have no effect on psychotic patients and those people under the influence of drugs or alcohol.

Pepper spray is derived from chili pepper. It contains a powerful alkaloid called capsaicin. In Hong Kong, oleoresin capsicum (OC) is used for riot control (Figure 48-12). Its strength ranges from 0.5 million up to 5 million Scoville heat units (SHUs). Pepper spray is an inflammatory agent and has painful effects on the mucous membranes. It can cause immediate dilation of the capillaries in mucous membranes, leading to temporary blindness and irritation of the airway. The effects last from 15 to 60 minutes. Pepper spray is a relatively safe agent. The main treatment is decontamination by copious amounts of cool water. Warm water may intensify the burning and inflammation. Oleoresin capsicum is fat-soluble and therefore oil-containing soap and lotions should not be used. It is important to wash the hands thoroughly before helping with the removal of contact lenses. Infants are very sensitive to riot control agents and should be taken to a doctor immediately. Some people may have violent allergic reactions to pepper spray. Usually only symptomatic treatment is needed. Some manufacturers advocate special decontamination agents (such as Sudecon® and Arm II), but the beneficial effect of these has not yet been confirmed. In Hong Kong, Arm II has been tried and the initial emulsification of OC seems promising.

Personal Protective Equipment (PPE)

There are four levels of protection for dealing with hazardous substances. They are described as level A through level D chemical protective clothing in combination with different types of respiratory protection (Figure 48-13A). In the tactical situation, the PPE commonly used by the military or law enforcement personnel will be different (Figure 48-13B).[9] Level A protection should be worn when the highest

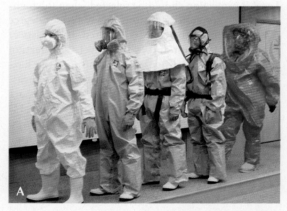

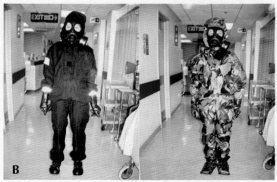

FIGURE 48-13

A, Civilian Level A through D personal protective equipment (PPE). Level A is on the far right, and Level D on the far left. **B**, PPE for military or law enforcement personnel.

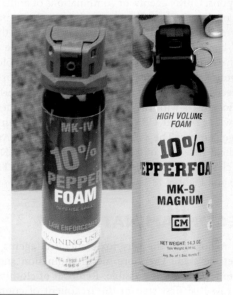

FIGURE 48-12

Pepper spray used in Hong Kong: oleoresin capsicum.

Table 48–5	**Vital Signs Before and After Working in PPE for 45 minutes**						
Team Members	Time Out	Pulse (per Minute)	BP (mm Hg)	Time In	Pulse (per Minute)	BP (mm Hg)	Temp (°C)
Member #1	10:25	120	171/88	11:18	148	157/86	38.4
Member #2	10:25	98	120/80	11:20	154	141/73	38.3
Member #3	10:25	102	161/93	10:50	109	150/47	37.9
Member #4	10:25	102	125/87	10:50	111	150/60	37.6
Member #5	10:45	112	137/80	11:15	92	141/73	38.2
Member #6	10:45	96	131/70	11:15	125	171/82	37.1

level of respiratory, skin, eye, and mucous membrane protection is needed. It consists of a fully encapsulated, vapor-tight, chemical-resistant suit together with a self-contained breathing apparatus (SCBA). Level B protection should be selected when the highest level of respiratory protection but a lesser degree of skin and eye protection is required. It consists of chemical splash suit and SCBA. Level C protection should be selected when the type of airborne hazardous substance is known, its concentration is measured, criteria for using air-purifying respirators are met, and skin and eye exposures are unlikely. Level D protection is primarily a work uniform. It provides no respiratory protection and minimal skin protection. It should not be worn on any site when respiratory or skin hazards exist. Level C and level D protection cannot work in oxygen-deficient environments.

PPE Complications

Personnel wearing PPE are likely to encounter a number of potential problems, including limited visibility, reduced dexterity, claustrophobia, restricted movement, insufficient air supply, dehydration, and the effects of heat and cold. According to Hong Kong experience, eight staff members working in a local ED had tried level A and B PPE during a Hazmat Medical Life Support workshop that was held in Singapore on September 25 to 26, 2001. Only one of them could successfully perform intubation and intravenous access after wearing level A or B PPE. Moreover, in a hazmat disaster drill in Hong Kong on 27 April 2000, six staff dressed in level C PPE working outdoors for 45 minutes experienced dehydration and heat exhaustion. On that day the environmental temperature was 28° C and relative humidity was 89%. Before fully removing their PPE, all their body temperatures were normal

but many of them had abnormal physical signs after working in level C PPE for the 45 minutes (Table 48-5). Therefore, the decontamination team leader should maintain close monitoring of the team members. In hot and humid environments, they should not work more than 60 minutes and the second team should take over the work.

TRIAGE CATEGORIES

It is important to note that in a terrorist attack there may initially appear to be a large number of victims. However, in fact only a minority of the people at the scene of an event are usually injured by conventional weapons, CBRN agents, or combinations of both. The rest of the people at the scene who may be in panic may experience symptoms that may resemble those of a chemical attack. These symptoms may be due to their inappropriate psychological or physiologic response. Therefore, field triage is very important to recognize the true victims and not to overload the local EDs with the "worried well." Fundamental knowledge about CBRN agents is important in the triage process. The same as the United States Army Medical Research of Chemical Defense, Hong Kong has classified victims into four categories (see Table 48-6 and Figures 48-14 and 48-15).

DECONTAMINATION

The majority of the very toxic chemical agents can penetrate skin. Therefore, decontamination should be done as soon as possible. Removal of clothing is the essential first step in the treatment of contaminated victims. Once the clothing has been removed, then about 80% of the contaminant after liquid

Table 48–6	**Triage Categories in CBRN Incidents**	
Hong Kong Classification	**US Classification**	**Meaning**
Red	Immediate	Abnormal vital signs, requires immediate intervention
Yellow	Delayed	Care can be delayed but there is no change in outcome
Green	Minimal	Walking and talking victims with minor injuries
Black	Expectant	Survival unlikely even with optimal treatment

CBRN = Chemical, Biological, Radiologic, and Nuclear.

contamination and nearly 100% after vapor contamination are removed. Removal of clothing is also important because of the possibility of "trapped vapor" in the clothing. This may be the only decontamination procedure that is required for those victims exposed to only a chemical gas or vapor or some biological exposures. Although some centers advocate 0.5% hypochlorite solution as the universal decontamination agent, it is generally accepted that copious amounts of water and soap are equally effective for decontamination, since the majority of contaminants can be removed by physical means. All suspected victims are considered contaminated until proven otherwise. Decontamination Team members should watch and ensure that the decontamination process is thorough and adequate.

The decontamination site should be set up in a three-zone arrangement: hot, warm, and cold zones. It is important to ensure the wind and water flow from cold (clean) to hot (contaminated) zones. The hot zone is the incident site zone. The highest level of PPE

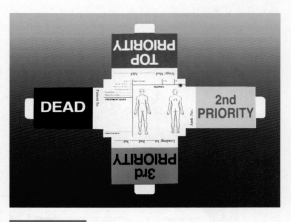

FIGURE 48–14

Triage tag used in Hong Kong.

protection should be used for unknown chemical agents in the hot zone. The main objectives in the hot zone are to rescue and bring patients out into the

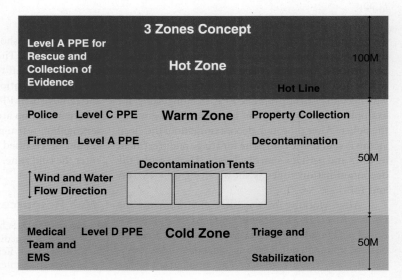

FIGURE 48–15

Decontamination three zones concept: hot, warm, and cold zones.

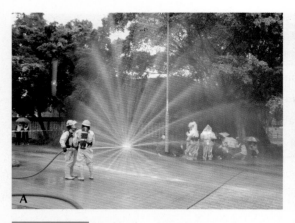

FIGURE 48–16

A, B Decontamination zones in civilian setting.

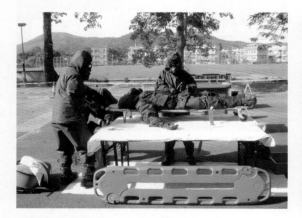

FIGURE 48–17

Decontamination of nonambulatory police officers in PPE.

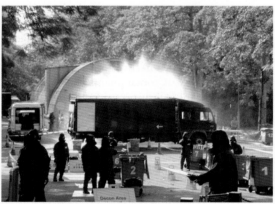

FIGURE 48–18

Decontamination of ambulatory police officer in PPE.

decontamination zone and the collection of evidence by the police. The warm zone is for the decontamination process. Ambulatory and nonambulatory victims will be decontaminated by the decontamination team, who need to be in appropriate PPE. In Hong Kong, for example, property collection from victims is done by the police. After thorough decontamination, the clean victim is sent to the cold zone for triage and treatment by EMS and perhaps a medical team. The layout of the decontamination zones is shown in Figures 48-16A and 16B.

After working in a CBRN environment, the police officers in PPE should undergo decontamination. The injured nonambulatory police officers should be decontaminated first by a special police decontamination team (Figure 48-17). The ambulatory police officers in PPE should disarm their weapons in the unloading areas. The weapons will be decontaminated by a separate staff team. Police officers should know the decontamination procedures and how to put on and remove their PPE (Figure 48-18). The layout of the decontamination areas is similar to that of the civilian setting: hot, warm and cold zones. All police officers should be certified "clean" before allowing them to enter the cold zone.

Web Resources

1. International School of Tactical Medicine: http://www.tacticalmedicine.com (accessed on 1 Oct 2009).
2. Casualty Care Research Centre: http://www.casualtycareresearchcenter.org (accessed on 1 Oct 2009).

References

1. Butler F Jr, Hagmann MC, Butler G. Tactical combat casualty care in special operations. *Mil Med* 161: Suppl 1, 1996.
2. Tactical Combat Casualty Care, Committee on Tactical Combat Casualty Care, Government Printing Agency, Feb 2003.
3. Chan JTS. Disaster medicine: The development of Tactical Medicine in Hong Kong. In: Wong TW, Kan PG, Lau CC, Lo CB, Ong KL, Rainer TH, et al., editors. From "casualty" to emergency medicine: half a century of transformation. 1st ed. Hong Kong: *Hong Kong College of Emergency Medicine*; 2006. pp. 193-196.
4. Police Oriented Tactical Emergency Medicine (POTEM) Training. http://www.police.gov.hk/offbeat/835/eng/n14.htm (accessed on 1 Oct 2009).
5. Chan TS, Yeung SD. A study on police bean bag injuries in a pork model. *Hong Kong J Emerg Med* 10(2): 124, 2003. http://www.hkcem.com/html/publications/Journal/2003-2/124-129.pdf (accessed on 1 Oct 2009).
6. TASER: http://www.taser.com (accessed on 1 Oct 2009).
7. Chan TS, Yeung SD, Tang YH. An overview of chemical warfare agents. *Hong Kong J Emerg Med* 9(4): 201, 2002. http://www.hkcem.com/html/publications/Journal/2002-4/201-205.pdf (accessed on 1 Oct 2009).
8. Advance HazMat Life Support Provider Manual. 3rd ed. University of Arizona Medical Research Center, American Academy of Clinical Toxicology http://www.ahls.org (accessed on 1 Oct 2009).
9. Yeung SD, Chan TS, Lee LY, Chan YL. The use of personal protective equipment in HazMat incidents. *Hong Kong J Emerg Med* 9(3): 171, 2002. http://www.hkcem.com/html/publications/Journal/2002-3/171-176.pdf (accessed on 1 Oct 2009).

Additional References

1. Hogan DE, Burstin JL, eds. Disaster Medicine. Philadelphia, PA: Lippincott Williams & Wilkins; 2002.
2. Hagmann J. Operational Emergency Medical Skills Course Manual; 2004. Powerpoint presentation by US Army Board Study Guide Posted Thursday, November 10, 2005. at: http://www.armystudyguide.com/content/powerpoint/First_Aid_Presentations/tactical-combat-casualty–2.shtml (accessed on 1 Oct 2010).
3. Emergency War Surgery NATO Handbook: Chemical Injury. United States Department of Defense; 2004.

4. Field Management of Chemical Casualties Handbook by US Army Medical Research Institute of Chemical Defense (USAMRICD), Chemical Casualty Care Division; July 2000.
5. FM 21-11 First Aid for Soldiers: Decontamination Procedures by Headquarters, Department of the Army, Washington, D.C.; Oct 1988.
6. FM 21-11 First Aid for Soldiers: First Aid in Toxic Environments by Headquarters, Department of the Army, Washington, D.C.; Oct 1988.
7. Medical Management of Chemical Casualties Handbook by United States Army, Medical Research Institute of Chemical Defense Chemical Casualty Care Division; July 2000.
8. NATO Handbook on the Medical Aspects of NBC Defensive Operations by Department of the Army, the Navy, and the Air Force; Feb 1996.
9. NAVEDTRA 13119 Standard First Aid Course—Chemical, Biological, and Radiological Casualties by Department of the Navy, Bureau of Medicine and Surgery; Feb 2005.
10. Textbook of Military Medicine: Medical Aspects of Chemical and Biological Warfare by Office of the Surgeon General, Department of the Army; 1997.
11. Treatment of Chemical Agent Casualties and Conventional Military Chemical Injuries by Departments of the Army, the Navy, and the Air Force, and Commandant, Marine Corps; Dec 1995.
12. Chan JT, Yeung RS, Tang SY. Hospital preparedness for chemical and biological incidents in Hong Kong. *Hong Kong Med J* 8(6): 440, 2002. Review. PMID: 12459601.
13. Chan J. Management of HazMat incidents in hospitals. Business Briefing of Hospital Engineering Facilities Management; 2005. *Touch Briefings, Saffron House. London, UK*, pp 26–27. available at: http://www.touchbriefings.com/cdps/cditem.cfm?NID=1140 (accessed on 1 Oct 2009).
14. Chan JTS, editor-in-chief. Police Oriented Tactical Emergency Medicine. Alice Ho Miu Ling Nethersole Hospital A&E Department ISBN: 962-8741-06-3 Copyright © 2006 by *AHNH A&E.*, all rights reserved. July 2006. (This is a classified document by Hong Kong Police Medical Panel. For Authorized readers only)
15. Chan JTS. Disaster medicine: the development of a hazardous material plan for Hong Kong. In: Wong TW, Kan PG, Lau CC, Lo CB, Ong KL, Rainer TH, et al., editors. From "casualty" to emergency medicine: half a century of transformation. 1st ed. Hong Kong: Hong Kong College of Emergency Medicine; 2006. pp. 173–175.

CHAPTER 49

Aeromedical Programs

Robert Anthony Cocks

KEY LEARNING POINTS

- Safety requirements are critically important components of aeromedical programs and need to be in place prior to initiation of a program.
- Special training beyond that of ground ambulance personnel is needed for aeromedical program personnel.

- Aeromedical programs need to be integrated with and cooperate with the other components of the regional health-care system.

Aeromedical programs (also known as "air medical services") provide a vital service within the EMS system, offering rapid delivery of medical care to sick or injured patients and timely delivery of patients to definitive care at higher capability facilities (rather than just the nearest facility). However, many aspects of this work are inherently dangerous. 2008 was the deadliest year in the history of Helicopter Emergency Medical Services (HEMS) operations in the US with 29 fatalities in 8 separate fatal accidents.[1] This chapter will place strong emphasis on all aspects of operational safety and discuss the training necessary to maintain that safety. Safety does not come cheap, but the cost of the alternative – cutting corners and losing crew and patients – is too great to bear.

This chapter briefly discusses the origin and history of airborne EMS, the influences on its development, and its present situation and status in various areas of the world. It is hoped that the international view offered on current operational aspects and training will allow anyone given the

task of establishing a new aeromedical program to plan that program safely and efficiently.

DEFINITIONS FOR THIS CHAPTER

ADAC – Allgemeiner Deutscher Automobil-Club. Europe's largest automobile association which, for many years, has provided a comprehensive HEMS roadside rescue program (first in the former West Germany and subsequently for the whole of unified Germany).

AMPA – Air Medical Physician Association.

Casevac/Medevac – Literally, casualty evacuation or medical evacuation by air. These were originally military terms (the original use of the term "casevac" was for basic medical care rendered during patient transport by military nonmedical personnel in combat areas, and the term "medevac" was for medical care rendered during patient transport in the field environment by military trained medical personnel).

CBD – Criterion-Based Dispatch System.

Coast Guard – The government department of each coastal nation responsible for maritime security and emergencies occurring within that nation's coastal waters.

ELT – Emergency Locator Transmitter. This is a device attached to an aircraft or a person that emits a specific radio signal, allowing rescue services to locate the position of the casualty. One well-known variety is known as **SARBE** – Search and Rescue Beacon Equipment. ELT fitted to the aircraft can be designed to deploy automatically following a crash on land or at sea – otherwise known as **ADELT** (Automatically Deployed Emergency Locator Transmitter).

FAA – Federal Aviation Administration. The government regulator of civil aviation in the US.

Fixed Wing – This term means any aircraft that obtains its lift from integral, stationary wings. It encompasses unpowered gliders, piston-engined aircraft, and jet aircraft. As forward motion is required to create lift, these aircraft need a longer, prepared runway for take-off and landing, although some types (Vertical/Short Take Off and Landing – or VSTOL) are designed to avoid this need.

GFS – The Government Flying Service of the Hong Kong Special Administrative Region of China.

GPS – Global Positioning System.

GPWS – Ground Proximity Warning System. A system fitted to some aircraft offering an audible/verbal warning of height above terrain. This system may employ RADALT data.

HEMS – Helicopter Emergency Medical Services.

HUET – Helicopter Underwater Escape (or Egress) Training.

IMO – The International Maritime Organization.

MPDS – Medical Priority Dispatch System.

NVIS/NVG – Night Vision Imaging System/Night Vision Goggles. Technology designed to enhance the vision of pilots and air crew in the dark.

RADALT – Radar-Altimeter. Equipment fitted to aircraft that registers height above ground by means of a radar pulse return.

RAF – The Royal Air Force of the United Kingdom.

Rotorcraft – in our EMS context, this term is synonymous with "helicopter" and describes any aircraft for which lift is provided by a rotary wing. Generally, these aircraft can take off and land vertically or from a short airstrip. The term rotorcraft is used by regulatory authorities such as the FAA, CASA, and JAA/EASA and also covers other aircraft such as autogyros.

SAMU – Service d'Aide Médicale. France's prehospital care system consisting of ground-based vehicles and helicopter assets covering France's approximately 100 "Departments" or administrative regions. Paris SAMU also covers in-flight advice for emergencies aboard Air France aircraft.

SAR – Search and Rescue. In military terms, this usually means the rescue of pilots who have been shot down over enemy territory or who have been involved in aircraft mishaps on land or at sea. In civilian terms, the term means the airborne search for and rescue of any lost or distressed persons on land (including mountain rescue) or at sea.

SOLAS – The International Convention on the Safety of Life at Sea.

STASS/SEA/HEED – Short-Term Air Supply System Survival Egress Air/Helicopter Emergency Egress Device. Personal survival equipment designed to provide emergency breathing air during escape from a ditched aircraft submerged in water.

TAWS – Terrain Awareness and Warning System.

Transponder – An electronic beacon fitted to commercial (and some military) aircraft that broadcasts the unique identity of that aircraft. Air Traffic Control can use this beacon to track the position and height of each aircraft.

A BRIEF INTERNATIONAL HISTORY

Much effort has been expended by EMS historians in trying to find the earliest recorded event of a patient being carried by aircraft. Despite tantalizing reports of the use of air balloons in the very early days of aviation,[1] there seems to be little evidence of the widespread use of air transport dedicated to the needs of casualties until the end of the Second World War (1939–1945). By the time of the Korean War (1950–1953), the use of helicopters to evacuate injured troops from forward battle areas was becoming routine, and it is felt that this means of rapid transport to Mobile Army Surgical Hospitals (MASHs) reduced the mortality rate. This trend of reduced mortality from survivable injury continued throughout the Vietnam War (1959–1975), in which a well-planned system of early aeromedical evacuation and trauma care ensured the delivery of definitive care within minutes of injury.[2]

MODERN AEROMEDICAL SYSTEMS – A COMMENTARY

The controversy surrounding the safety of HEMS should not detract from discussion of the very real benefits afforded by aeromedical systems. It is possible to achieve an operational system with a minimal (even zero) accident rate provided that vested interests are put aside and all parties work toward a safe system.

At present, within the debate on civilian HEMS operations at least, there appear to be two main camps that are at loggerheads. On one side of the fence, accident investigators see recurring features of mishaps that are preventable. Many of these involve human and organizational factors for which there are ready solutions, although at a cost. On the other side, HEMS operators are interested in cost-efficiency as well as operational efficiency. Companies that have never experienced an accident within their operation tend to resist any suggestion of tighter regulations on safety, partly because they believe that they are already safe and partly because higher standards cost more money.

Civil aviation regulators may also be reluctant to enact further rules as a result of lobbying and pressure from the industry, and it is notable that some of the key recommendations of the 2006 US National Transportation Safety Board (NTSB) Aviation Special Investigation Report on Emergency Medical Services Operations[3] have yet to be addressed by the FAA. In February 2009, the NTSB held a four-day public hearing to address the issues of HEMS safety.[4] It was noted that three of the recommendations from the year 2006 were still open, and the FAA response had been unacceptable. First, positioning flights with no patients on board was still being allowed under less stringent Federal Aviation Part 91 Regulations rather than the Part 135 regulations normally applicable to EMS flights (this had previously been identified as the riskiest element of HEMS operations, appearing as a factor in 64% of accidents). Second, recommendations regarding the implementation of flight risk evaluation programs had not been addressed – such programs would protect the pilot from pressure to accept a mission by relieving him or her of the final decision in marginal safety conditions. Third, a recommendation requiring the installation of terrain awareness and warning systems (TAWS) on EMS aircraft had not been addressed.

CONSTITUTION OF AN AEROMEDICAL SERVICE: GOVERNMENT, PRIVATE, OR CHARITABLE?

The need to establish an aeromedical EMS program may arise from a wide range of considerations. These affect governments, health services, private operators, and charitable organizations alike.

In the case of government, there may be a statutory requirement under local, national, or international law to provide a service. Examples of this would include obligations to meet a public EMS response time standard that could be met only by using air assets, or an international obligation to rescue mariners shipwrecked around the coastline.

Health services, both governmental and nongovernmental, vary in their structure around the world. However, citizens in rural or remote areas should have equal rights to timely and efficient health care as do city dwellers, and in such situations air transport may be the only way to achieve such equity. This may involve delivering doctors, nurses, and/or paramedics to these areas to provide health clinic sessions as well as transportation of sick or injured patients to regional hospitals.

Private EMS operators are perhaps the most varied of all provider sectors. Some exist purely for commercial gain, functioning in the same way that an airline or air taxi company would operate. Some provide statutory services on behalf of government under a contract, and others exist as assets of large hospitals for retrieving or transferring patients. Still others operate as highly specific services, such as the service run by the German Automobile Association (ADAC) to provide roadside rescue and international repatriation for its members following accidents or critical illness.

Charitable and humanitarian organizations have always played a prominent part in providing prehospital emergency care worldwide, exemplified by the St. John Ambulance and Red Cross. Although most of the work of these two voluntary aid societies centers on terrestrial emergency care, both organizations provide staff for aeromedical services in many countries.

DECIDING ON THE PROGRAM'S PURPOSE AND MISSION

Far too often in the past, aeromedical programs have been established on grounds unrelated to genuine need. Helicopters can be an impressive sight, and their advertising potential is considerable. Owing to television and film, they are part of popular culture and this has led to a "must have" attitude among the public and some administrators, sometimes in the face of opposing economic and safety realities.

The main bases of genuine need are

1. Geographical isolation of a population from major hospitals.

2. Inaccessibility by road, for example, in mountainous terrain, or on islands.
3. Casualties occurring at sea.
4. "Situational entrapment" such as a predictable traffic gridlock.
5. A need for speed due to patient's clinical condition.
6. Search and rescue efforts.

Geographical Isolation

The vast country of Australia has many geographically isolated communities located hundreds of kilometers from the nearest hospital. Some are too remote for helicopter transport to be feasible. Most civilian helicopters have unrefueled range limitations of about 200 kilometers (125 miles), and fixed-wing aircraft are commonly used, both to deliver health-care staff for routine clinics and to evacuate sick or injured patients. The Royal Flying Doctor Service of Australia (RFDS) was formed in 1928 to provide care to these isolated communities, and the following text from the RFDS illustrates very well the problems faced prior to its formation.[5] The story is attributed to the Reverend John Flynn, first Superintendent of the Australian Inland Mission, and the incident took place in 1917 (story is also available at http://www.eurekacouncil.com.au/ Australia-History/History-Pages/1928-royal_flying_ doctor_service.htm).

"Darcy was a stockman in Western Australia. After being found injured, with a ruptured bladder, by some friends, he was transported over 30 miles (12 hours), to the nearest town, Halls Creek. Here, Darcy was met by FW Tuckett, the Postmaster, and the only man in the settlement trained in first aid. Tuckett said there was nothing he could reliably do for injuries so serious, and tried unsuccessfully to contact doctors at Wyndham, and then Derby, by telegraph. He eventually got through to a doctor in Perth. Through communication by Morse code, Dr Holland guided Tuckett through two rather messy bladder operations utilizing the only sharp instrument available, a pen knife. Due to the total absence of any medical facilities, Darcy had been operated on strapped to the Post Office counter, having first been made insensible with whisky. Holland then traveled 10 days to Halls Creek on a boat for cattle transport, a Model T-Ford, a horse-drawn carriage, and even on foot, only to find that Darcy had died the day before. To rub salt in the wound, the operations had been successful, but the stockman had died from an undiagnosed case of malaria and ruptured abscess in his appendix."[5]

As of January 2009, the RFDS operates 56 fixed-wing planes, comprising 34 Beechcraft King Air and 22 Pilatus PC-12 aircraft, covering vast areas of Australia.

Inaccessibility

Inaccessibility is a somewhat different problem from the geographical isolation described above (Figure 49-1). Hiking is a popular pastime in Hong Kong, and it is common for hikers to be injured on hillsides and mountainous terrain within direct sight of the city, yet the nearest road may be inaccessible. In these circumstances, the Hong Kong Government Flying Service may transport mountain rescue team members to the scene by helicopter, or alternatively achieve rescue by winching the injured victim into the aircraft by strap or stretcher (Figure 49-2).

Casualties at Sea

In addition to search and rescue at sea described below, serious illness or injury may occur on board ocean-going vessels (Figure 49-3 and Figure 49-4). It may not be possible for the vessel to reach a port to offload the casualty, and many nations have rescue services capable of taking the patient off the ship by helicopter. While large ships may have marked helipads, these are not rated to a defined international standard and may not be suitable for large helicopters because of the weight and rotor disk diameter of the aircraft. Therefore, it is common to use winching to first land an aircrew member onto the ship to assess the patient and to then remove the patient by stretcher (Figure 49-5 and Figure 49-6).

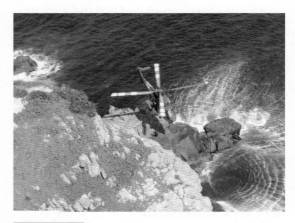

FIGURE 49-1

Inaccessibility – a cliff rescue in progress. Photo courtesy of Government Flying Service, Hong Kong (GFS), www.gfs.gove.hk.

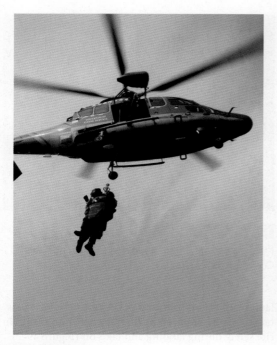

FIGURE 49–2

Single strop winching. Photo courtesy of Government Flying Service, Hong Kong (GFS).

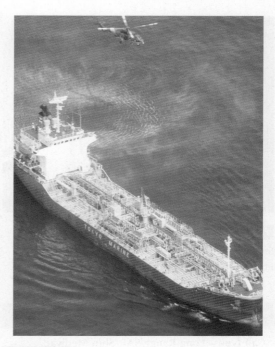

FIGURE 49–3

Approach to ship. Photo courtesy of Government Flying Service, Hong Kong (GFS).

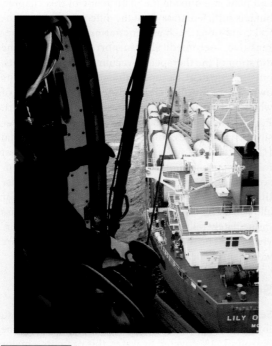

FIGURE 49–4

Difficult approach to ocean-going ship. Photo courtesy of Government Flying Service, Hong Kong (GFS).

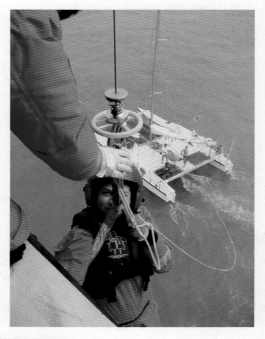

FIGURE 49–5

Winching onto a catamaran. Photo courtesy of Government Flying Service, Hong Kong (GFS).

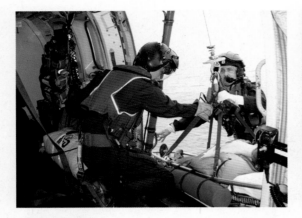

FIGURE 49–6

Stretcher winching. Photo courtesy of Government Flying Service, Hong Kong (GFS).

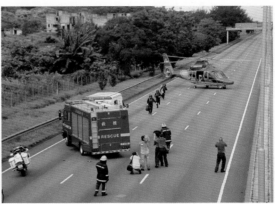

FIGURE 49–7

Roadside rescue. Photo courtesy of Professor Robert Cocks.

Case History

Call Type – Long-Range SAR/Ship Medivac

A 50-year-old woman developed abdominal pain on a fishing vessel 80 nautical miles southeast of Hong Kong on 06/08/2003.

Call Time 16:50, takeoff 17:14, patient contact 18:00. Arrival at hospital by helipad 18:35.

Female patient, age 50 years, developed right-sided abdominal pain and vomiting 3 days ago.

On examination: appears dehydrated – minimal saliva output. Temperature = 37.7°C, pulse = 80 bpm, BP = 154/66 mm Hg, Sa_{O2} = 99%. Alert and talking, but in pain. Tenderness over right kidney area.

Actions: Establish IV line, give 500 mL NS over next hour. Administer morphine, 10 milligrams, by slow IV push. Monitor vital signs.

Diagnosis: Large right kidney calculus with acute pyelonephritis.

Situational Entrapment

Many large cities worldwide experience regular traffic congestion and even gridlock, making rapid EMS transport on the ground difficult or impossible to achieve. One solution to this difficulty is to survey and designate potential helicopter landing sites around the city, utilizing wide roads, parks, sports fields, schoolyards, and fire station yards for landing and pick-up. Some means of communication with these sites is needed to forewarn occupants of the imminent landing of the aircraft, and police or fire service assistance may be required to clear the area and maintain site safety during landing and take-off (Figure 49-7).

Need for Speed

The arguments for "swoop and scoop" versus "stay and play" are outside the main scope of this chapter, but it is sufficient to say that the outcome of some clinical conditions, such as penetrating trauma, is time-sensitive. Aeromedical transport can shorten the duration of the therapeutic vacuum for such patients, but this element cannot influence outcomes on its own. There must be an integrated trauma system of which aeromedical transport forms a component part. Perhaps the most spectacular example of what is possible is the success of the Royal London Hospital HEMS team in successfully treating cardiac arrest following penetrating cardiac injury by means of on-scene thoracotomy.[6] In this series, short response times to the scene by helicopter or rapid response car allowed an HEMS physician to perform the procedure immediately following cardiac arrest, with a 10% survival rate. The majority of survivors of the procedure were neurologically intact.

Search and Rescue (SAR)

Search and rescue includes operations to locate lost, injured, or sick persons on land or at sea. As the globe is around 71% covered by water, this presents a major challenge.

The International Convention for the Safety of Life at Sea (SOLAS) is the most important treaty protecting the safety of merchant ships.[7] The sinking of the RMS Titanic in 1912 led to the first convention in 1914 of SOLAS, and there have been four subsequent revisions. Administration of the treaty is the responsibility of the International Maritime Organization (IMO–www.imo.org), which maintains a Joint Search and Rescue (SAR) Working Group with the International Civil Aviation Organization (ICAO–www.icao.int). Both are specialist agencies of the United Nations.

While each coastal nation is responsible for SAR within its national waters, SOLAS divides international waters into regions. Certain nations with specific capabilities are assigned to coordinate SAR within those regions, many of which are too large to cover with air assets alone. For example, Hong Kong is responsible for a vast area occupying the northern half of the South China Sea, extending along the South China and Vietnamese coasts, across to the Philippines and back up to Taiwan. Within helicopter range (including the extended range afforded by refueling aboard oil rigs), the search and rescue operation can result in direct rescue of victims. Farther out, fixed-wing aircraft can conduct grid search patterns. If victims are located in open water, the aircraft can drop lifesaving dinghy packs and direct nearby shipping vessels to complete the rescue.

FLIGHT OPERATIONS

Alerting

Tasking of the aeromedical service is crucial for the safety and efficiency of the operation. Selection of appropriate cases is a skilled task requiring specific training and secures appropriate use of a scarce and expensive resource. In most areas of the world, the public access emergency operator (e.g. 911 in the US, 999 in the UK) is the first filter for the mobilization of an EMS response. Calls for Police/Fire/Ambulance services are generally passed to a secondary operator at the appropriate emergency service, and rapid identification of tasks appropriate for aeromedical/HEMS services at this stage may allow the mission to be activated as a primary response rather than awaiting assessment by ground crews. At an early stage in the launch of the London HEMS scheme in 1990 to 1991, a dedicated HEMS desk was set up at the London Ambulance Service control center, manned by a paramedic who monitored incoming tasks for selection of serious trauma cases. At that stage, tasks were recorded in paper format, but the widespread introduction of the Criterion-Based Dispatch System (CBD)

and Medical Priority Dispatch System (MPDS) potentially allows a protocol-based set of selection criteria to partially replace human surveillance.

Flight Dispatch

Flight dispatch is the single most critical stage in ensuring the safety of aeromedical operations. Inappropriate acceptance of a task that is mismatched to the skill level of the flight crew, aircraft technological capability, or environmental operating conditions lays the foundation for disaster. Studies of aviation human factors show that once a mission has been accepted and launched, there is a tendency to press on with the task even when safety parameters have been breached. This is particularly the case with HEMS operations when the pilot and crew believe that a patient's life might be at stake, and it proves difficult or impossible to abort the mission when new developments indicate an objective need to abort it.

According to data derived from the US National Aviation and Space Administration Aviation Safety Reporting System, patient condition was cited in 44% of EMS accident or incident reports as a contributing factor to time pressure leading to inaccurate or hurried preflight planning. A report by Air Medical Physician Association (AMPA) in 2002 further identified that accidents occurred more often while flight crews were en route to pick up a patient.[8]

Robust risk management governing flight dispatch can protect operating crews from the pressures described above. Key concepts described in the 2006 NTSB Special Investigation Report include an overriding concept that the pilot's authority to decline a flight assignment is supreme but that his or her decision to accept an assignment is subject to review:

1. The pilot's decision to decline, cancel, divert, or terminate a flight overrides any decision by other parties to accept or continue a flight.
2. The pilot's decision to accept a flight may be overridden by other personnel by use of operational control procedures and policies of the certificate holder (i.e., the operator), including the use of risk assessment and management tools and techniques.

Furthermore, once a pilot has declined a flight, no other party is entitled to continue with a risk assessment. This removes any pressure on the pilot to change the decision.[3]

The objective of risk management tools is precisely to manage risk. In some situations there are significant risks, such as extreme weather conditions during SAR operations at sea, and many mitigating techniques can be introduced with that objective. For example, thresholds can be built including mandating two-pilot rather than single-pilot operation of the aircraft, the use of IFR-equipped aircraft for a task, or the use of real-time satellite weather mapping to identify a window of opportunity to launch an operation.

On-Line Control and Monitoring

Once a mission has been launched, flight crews need to be able to maintain two-way communication with their control center or dispatcher. A considerable number of aircraft accidents have occurred in which no such communication was possible, and the accident has only been suspected when the aircraft was reported overdue by the receiving hospital. This inevitably results in delays in mounting rescue operations, particularly in remote areas where a local population might not have observed the accident from the ground.

On-line control and monitoring allow the progress of the flight to be plotted and for up-to-date weather conditions for the route ahead to be communicated to the pilot. In particular, when deteriorating conditions at the destination become obvious, communication of the situation to the pilot allows diversion to be planned under nonemergent conditions and before the aircraft enters hazardous conditions.

NVIS/NVG

Night vision imaging systems (NVIS) are widely used in military operations but may also enhance safety in civilian operations when properly used. A 1994 FAA study found that Night Vision Goggles (NVGs) could help pilots maintain situational awareness and reduce pilot workload and stress during night operations.[9] Night hours are over-represented in HEMS accident statistics according to the AMPA study, with 49% of HEMS accidents occurring at night, whereas only 38% of operations took place at night.

Advantages of NVGs include the enhanced ability to distinguish contrast between features of terrain and to view obstructions such as poles and wires. Grass has a reflectivity of about 14%, sand 35%, and snow 70 to 80%, making it possible to distinguish between media on the ground. Acuity with NVGs is much better than that of the naked eye at night because of the exploitation of high-resolution cones; in addition, the need for full dark adaptation (which may take 15 to 20 minutes) is removed.

However, acuity is never as good as during the daytime and **20/30** (6/9 **metric**) is the best that may be achieved. Vernier acuity (the ability to distinguish straight lines) is reduced, and there is still an increased risk of wire strikes compared to daytime operations despite the advantages of night vision systems being cited by the NTSB and FAA reports. Peripheral vision is severely limited by NVGs, with a field of vision limited to about 40 degrees. Most types are helmet-mounted, and the combined weight of the helmet, goggles, and power pack may lead to considerable strain on the pilot's neck with prolonged use. Saturation of the retinal green cones leads to an after-effect on color vision known as "magenta eye."

Overall, NVGs carry significant advantages during night operations as long as the operator is properly trained in their use and their limitations are understood.

Hospital Helipads and In-Hospital Arrangements

Thomas has described the important role of hospital helipads in enhancing EMS efficiency and eliminating the risks of additional ground transfer by ambulance.[10] In addition to the advantages of delivering patients to definitive care more quickly, the use of hospital helipads reduces the difficulties inherent in maintaining patient care and performing interventions within a transport vehicle, and ground ambulance resources are freed up for other missions. However, the in-hospital logistics must be considered, as significant hazards may be introduced by having the hospital helipad placed remotely from the ED or other designated critical care units.

For ground level helipads, there should be minimal distance required for stretcher (gurney) transfer to the definitive care area; for rooftop helipads, there should be direct lift (elevator) access to the definitive care area, which should be placed within the same building (Figure 49-8). Rearranging in-hospital facilities to service a new helipad may sometimes be as challenging as planning the helipad itself.

Deciding on Aircraft Type

Deciding on the type of aircraft most suitable for an aeromedical scheme is not straightforward. A thorough analysis on the type of operations likely to be conducted should precede the acquisition of any specific model. The choice of helicopter will depend largely on the tasks it will perform, and an aircraft suitable and equipped for the critical care transfer of a

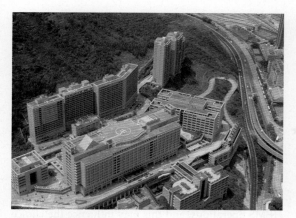

FIGURE 49-8

Hospital rooftop helipad. Photo courtesy of Professor Robert Cocks.

single patient may not be appropriate for the transport of large numbers of casualties from, for example, the scene of a natural disaster.

In light of the excess risk of accidents associated with HEMS operations, safety features must take a high priority and can act as the starting point in designing an HEMS service.

In the case of long-range operations, a fixed-wing aircraft would clearly be required, as the speed and fuel range of helicopters are limited. Where scheduled air services exist, it is often possible and more economical to fix stretchers within a regular commercial aircraft. Where no scheduled transport exists, a chartered business jet or dedicated air ambulance may be required. The choice of aircraft is important, as many smaller types have cabin doors and internal configurations that will not admit or accommodate a stretcher.

When dealing with commercial airlines, it is probable that the transfer team will need to comply with airline medical clearance procedures before travel. These procedures exist to ensure that the transfer is conducted safely and with proper equipment and preparations. Up to 48 hours may be required to position and load stretchers and supplementary oxygen cylinders and to clear electrical monitoring equipment as flight-safe. The International Air Transport Association (IATA–www.iata.org) produces a medical manual and also a standard form and checklist termed the "MEDIF" clearance form to assist patients and doctors in obtaining clearance. Specialist nurses or aviation medicine physicians employed by the airline normally handle this clearance process.

Crash-worthiness— Certification Basis

Crash-worthiness refers to the ability of a vehicle to protect its occupants from injury in the event of a crash, and both road vehicles and aircraft are subject to regulation regarding expected performance. The prerequisites are that all occupants must be using the restraints and systems provided.

The following principles of crash-worthiness (mnemonic CREEP) apply to EMS helicopters:

1. **Container** – is the cabin strong enough to withstand deforming forces and to protect the occupants from intrusion of external objects?
2. **Restraints** – are the harnesses effective in restraining the occupants and absorbing crash energy?
3. **Environment** – are there any hard surfaces, sharp objects, loose objects, or protrusions that might cause injury to the occupants? This is particularly relevant in aeromedical operations because of the considerable amount of heavy medical equipment carried that must be secured.
4. **Escape** – are occupants able to escape from the aircraft in the event of a crash? Are doors and windows removable?
5. **Post-crash factors** – does the aircraft have robust fuel tanks to prevent a post-crash fire and features that will prevent other secondary mishaps? Is the aircraft fitted with an automatically deployed emergency locator beacon (ADELT)?

An egg-box (Figure 49-9) exemplifies a good design incorporating the first three features.

Transport helicopter crash-worthiness is certified under (US) Federal Aviation Regulation (FAR)

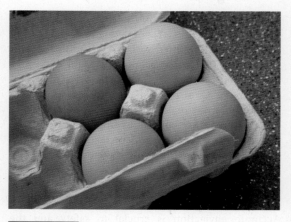

FIGURE 49-9

Principles of crash-worthiness. Photo courtesy of Professor Robert Cocks.

27.562 or its European equivalent for the majority of current models. A crucial initial action when choosing an aircraft is to discover whether the model is certified to 1965[11] or 1997[12] standards regarding its performance under Emergency Landing Conditions.

FAR 29.561 (1965) standards are still used under "grandfathering" concessions for many currently built transport helicopter models whose forerunners existed before the enhanced 1989 and 1997 standards were adopted. In applying for certification of a new variant of one of these older models, the manufacturer simply has to demonstrate to the regulatory authority that the improved standards are "not necessary as the changes are not significant," "not practical," or "would not materially change the level of safety." Under "not practical," justifications regarding avoidance of additional cost and weight penalty may be taken into account. The 1965 standards demand only the most basic protection designed to give each occupant a reasonable chance of escaping serious injury in the event of a minor crash landing. The maximum forces that the standards offer occupants protection against are 4G downward, 4G forward, 2G sideward, and 1.5G upward.

FAR 29.562 (1997) mandates considerably higher crash protection standards with air frames being tested to protect occupants against a minimum 30G vertical deceleration over 0.031 seconds and an 18.4G forward deceleration. It is recommended that all new EMS helicopters should be certified to this more stringent standard.

Terrain Awareness and Warning Systems (TAWS)

The National Transportation Safety Board has repeatedly made specific recommendations that EMS aircraft should be fitted with TAWS equipment, in recognition that such technology could have prevented 17 out of the 55 accidents studied in the NTSB 2006 report.[3] Controlled Flight Into Terrain (CFIT) is a common factor in EMS accidents, usually due to adverse weather conditions impairing the visual references available to the pilot on take-off, landing, or during transit over hilly or mountainous terrain.

Navigation Aids

Accurate navigation is crucial to safety and the avoidance of dangerous terrain and adverse weather conditions. While Global Positioning System (GPS) equipment may be useful and gives a good two-dimensional plot, height readings may be inaccurate or misleading.

Engine Power

All EMS helicopters should have the capability of operating under twin-engine conditions and have sufficient power to operate in all circumstances without the need to offload key personnel or equipment.

Size/Utility/Configuration Aspects

Access to all parts of the patient is important during HEMS operations, and this may influence the choice of aircraft. The first consideration is whether the aircraft will be used solely for HEMS operations, thereby offering the possibility of permanent, fixed installation of medical equipment. While it is desirable, this feature is by no means essential, and utility helicopters can be rapidly fitted with a medical panel, including stretcher, oxygen supply, and integral medical monitoring and therapy equipment (Figure 49-10 and Figure 49-11). Even in planes in which no medical panel is fitted, utility helicopters still offer the possibility of carrying one or more patients on stretchers using the hand-carried equipment of a skilled EMS practitioner.

Communication in the noisy environment of a helicopter is difficult. Crew helmets with a connection to an aircraft intercom system allow good communication between EMS staff, air crew, and pilots, but communication with the patient is frequently problematic (Figure 49-12). Few schemes allow the patient to be included in the main intercom

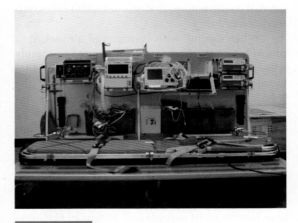

FIGURE 49-10

Removable EMS panel. Photo courtesy of Professor Robert Cocks.

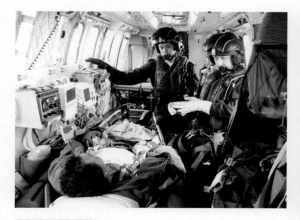

FIGURE 49–11

EMS cabin environment. Photo courtesy of Government Flying Service, Hong Kong (GFS).

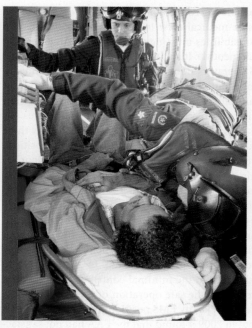

FIGURE 49–12

Difficulties in patient communication. Photo courtesy of Government Flying Service, Hong Kong (GFS).

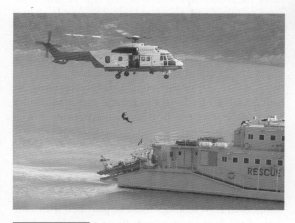

FIGURE 49–13

Winch training. Image provided Photo courtesy of Professor Robert Cocks.

communication system because of the potential for distraction of the pilot and crew, but it is possible to use a separate, partitioned channel for EMS crew-patient dialogue.

Winch

A winch is not required for most EMS operations but is an essential feature for all SAR and mountain rescue applications. Where the winch is fitted, all personnel who will be deployed by the winch for the purpose of delivering medical care or rescue must receive safety training and practice (Figure 49-13).

Deciding on Crew

While the eyes and ears of every crew member contribute to the overall safety of a flight, the most crucial sensory and motor skills are those of the pilot. Basic flying skills become second nature to a pilot, but proficiency and judgment in aviation require constant practice, and this is particularly true in difficult flying environments. "Taxi" style EMS operations in good weather between prepared landing sites do not require the pilot to exercise the highest levels of skill, but a sudden and unpredictable deterioration in flying conditions is an ever-present hazard, and these circumstances demand experience and higher levels of competence.

It is essential when planning an EMS scheme to accurately predict what level of pilot skill will be required in the worst of circumstances, whether the operation will provide pilots with enough ongoing experience to keep skills sharp, and what recurrent training will be required. Aviation fuel and aircraft servicing may be expensive, but some non-operational flying time must be invested in actual training activity designed to stretch the skills of all crew members.

Dedicated nonmedical flight crew members are essential to the safety of EMS operations, and while it is possible to cross-train operational crew in medical skills or medical crew in operational skills, the two responsibilities must never rest with a single person simultaneously. It has been noted in the past that some EMS operators train and assign medical personnel to perform duties that loosely relate to the operation of the aircraft, including looking outside the aircraft for possible obstructions and evaluating landing sites.

This policy permits the operator to classify these personnel as flight crew members, allowing positioning flights to be operated under the less rigorous requirements of Part 91.[3] The NTSB has categorically stated that medical personnel cannot be expected to meaningfully participate in the decision-making process to enhance flight safety or to significantly contribute to operational control of the flight without specific flight training, and that such personnel generally do not receive such training. In 2006, the NTSB concluded that the minimal contribution of medical personnel to the safe operation of EMS flights is not sufficient to justify EMS positioning flights under Part 91, but in 2009 it found that the FAA had not satisfactorily addressed this recommendation.

The job of a non-medical operational flight crewmember includes safety procedures during start-up of the aircraft, the safe boarding of passengers, medical crew, and patients, checklist completion with the pilot, assistance with navigation, identification of landing sites, acting as a lookout on landing, and the safe disembarkation of occupants. In the event of an emergency, these skills extend to onboard fire fighting, the emergency landing or ditching of the aircraft, and responsibility for survival equipment and procedures. All of these skills require training, practice, and avoidance of competing interests, and it is therefore important to board sufficient crew of this nature who will not primarily be involved in the medical management of the patient.

The debate regarding the ideal medical crew composition for EMS operations continues, with various valid arguments for and against the inclusion of physicians, nurses, or paramedics in the crew. A number of permutations and combinations have been studied. In their analysis of 5275 HEMS missions in the UK, Roberts and colleagues (2009)[13] found that, contrary to the views of critics concerning the contribution of air ambulance doctors, such physicians did not increase their time on the scene even when advanced medical procedures such as rapid sequence intubation, chest drainage, or nerve blockade for femoral shaft fractures were used. Furthermore, these physicians were significantly more likely to declare death at the scene or discharge patients directly from the scene after treatment than non-physician crews, potentially reducing the number of patients transported to a hospital.

Dissman and colleagues (2007)[14] conducted a much smaller study (203 cases) comparing physician-paramedic partnerships (PPPs) with conventional paramedic crews (CPCs) and found no significant differences in on-scene times between the groups despite advanced medical interventions having been employed in a third of the PPP cases. They did, however, comment on a trend toward reduced on-scene times for PPPs dealing with medical emergencies and patient entrapments.

In Australia, similar debates exist concerning the value and role of physicians as part of HEMS teams.[15]

Two areas in which part-time physicians, nurses, or paramedics may not be suitable for all operations are airborne search and rescue and mountain rescue. The access and rescue skills required in some of the more hazardous operations of this type require constant training and practice. Unless the medical staff can devote the time to do this training and serve regularly in an operational role, there is a good alternative argument for selecting suitable helicopter SAR crew members for training in emergency medical care to the EMT or paramedic standard. If necessary, the health-care professional can remain in the helicopter pending the rescue of the patient and continue care en route to the hospital.

Safety Equipment

Where any part of the operation takes place over open water, each crew member must be provided with a life vest of the highest standard. Basic vests carried for emergency passenger use on commercial aircraft are not adequate for this purpose, and crew vests that are fully securable and adjustable are required. The vest should be fitted with pockets for a short-term emergency air supply bottle, emergency radio beacon, and survival equipment, including a mirror and flares. The equipment illustrated in Figure 49-14 used by the Government Flying Service in Hong Kong is termed a special operations vest (SOV).

The basic standard of a life vest includes the ability of the garment to maintain an unconscious wearer in a face-up 45-degree attitude with the mouth and nose at least 12 cm (5 inches) above the water level. In order to achieve this, the center of buoyancy is designed to sit in front of the wearer's upper sternum.

Where operations are planned to travel over extensive areas of cold water, crew members must be provided with an immersion suit and suitably

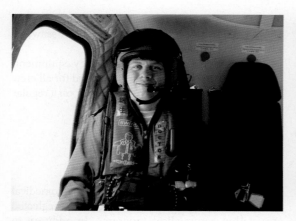

FIGURE 49-14

SOV life vest. Photo courtesy of Government Flying Service, Hong Kong (GFS).

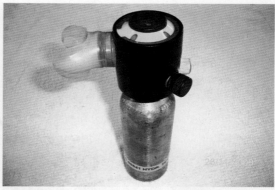

FIGURE 49-15

STASS bottle. Photo courtesy of Government Flying Service, Hong Kong (GFS).

insulated undergarments. Such combinations exploit the trapping of layers of warm air between the skin and a watertight suit to reduce heat conduction to the cold water. The shock of entering very cold water (<10° C) causes uncontrolled gasping in most people and a rapid inability to assist in their own rescue. Hypothermia will occur rapidly in these conditions. Even in warmer subtropical waters, hypothermia resulting from prolonged immersion is a significant risk.

Where operations are conducted over sea or over remote areas, each crew member should be provided with a personal locator beacon. Most designs require activation by a switch or toggle, but some autoactivate on contact with water. The device transmits a radio signal on specific emergency frequencies that can be detected by passing aircraft, satellites, or ground receiving stations, allowing the position of the wearer to be fixed and rescue services to be directed accordingly.

Flares carried for alerting rescuers come in two main types: personal mini-flares carried as part of life-vest equipment and larger flares carried on the survival dinghy (lifeboat).

Mini-flares are launched from a pen-like device containing a spring, firing pin, and trigger mechanism. Each red flare is typically projected to a height of around 50 meters (164 feet) with a burn duration of 5 to 6 seconds and an intensity of 10,000 candela (cd). The flares may be seen in clear weather from up to 5 nautical miles (9 km, 6 miles) in daylight and 10 nautical miles at night.

Larger distress flares carried on board the dinghy may be constructed with the dual purpose of generating

orange smoke (day use, at one end) and a red flare (day or night use, at the other end). The orange day smoke is typically generated for around 20 seconds, and the night flare (hand-held) burns at 15,000 cd for 20 seconds. A ribbed end-cap distinguishes the smoke end from the flare end of the device.

When operations are conducted over water, each crew member should be provided with and receive regular practical training to use a short-term air supply in the event of the aircraft's ditching in the water (Figure 49-15, Figure 49-16, and Figure 49-17). Typically, this equipment has a demand-actuated mouthpiece attached to a small compressed air cylinder providing around 30 surface breaths of air. With increasing depth in the water, the usable delivered air volume decreases due to increased pressure. If used by a person undertaking moderate escape

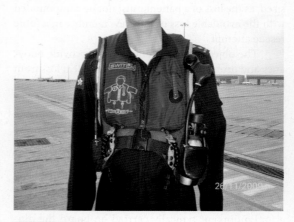

FIGURE 49-16

SEA bottle in life vest. Photo courtesy of Government Flying Service, Hong Kong (GFS).

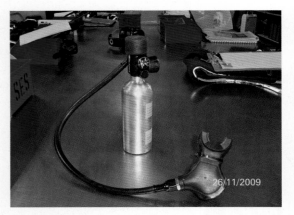

FIGURE 49–17

SEA bottle and regulator/mouthpiece. Photo courtesy of Government Flying Service, Hong Kong (GFS).

activity submerged under 3 meters (10 feet) of water, the volume of air in the bottle should sustain consciousness for an extra two minutes. However, panic and excessive physical activity would severely reduce this survival opportunity, and regular practical training in a pool or helicopter underwater escape trainer (HUET) is essential to build confidence in the equipment and drills.

All aircraft operating over water must carry one or more survival dinghies and equipment appropriate to the number of crew and passengers carried. While medical crew would obviously do their best to rescue their patients and preserve life, the situation of aircraft ditching is an extreme and life-threatening event for all occupants. This eventuality must be discussed as part of training and personal safety must be emphasized, as the loss of a patient must not be compounded with the avoidable loss of the crew member in a futile rescue attempt.

The objective of the dinghy is to provide buoyancy and protection from the elements. Heat loss from an unprotected body is rapid during immersion in water, and the dinghy allows survivors to avoid major conductive heat loss. However, heat loss by convection and evaporation continues while out of the water and is exacerbated by wind. This means that the erection of the dinghy canopy is a priority. Dinghies are provided with a bailer to remove water that inevitably enters the vessel resulting from the initial ditching and subsequent wave action.

Equipment typically carried on board the dinghy may include limited emergency water supplies, glucose tablets, seasickness medication, mirror and flares, repair kit, and basic first-aid supplies. More

sophisticated equipment such as a reverse osmosis pump (ROP) to generate fresh water from seawater may also be included.

As with the use of other emergency equipment, recurrent dinghy drill training is required for all crew likely to undertake operations over water on a regular basis.

CLINICAL ASPECTS OF AEROMEDICAL CARE

Establishing patient selection criteria for aeromedical transport is an important and frequently neglected area within aeromedical programs. In addition to cost-effectiveness considerations, aspects of clinical safety and operational safety must be considered.

Considerations include:

1. How stable is the casualty? If unstable, is the speed of transfer to definitive hospital care justified when balanced against the risk of deterioration or cardiac arrest in flight?
2. Does the casualty victim have any trapped air inside his or her body (e.g., pneumothorax or air in the skull). If so, drain the air if possible (e.g., via thoracentesis) or restrict the flight to low altitude (often operationally impossible). Any entrapped air will greatly expand in volume as the altitude increases.
3. Is all of the necessary equipment for transfer available (e.g., defibrillator, airway gear)?
4. Remember that the medical escort's ability to monitor the condition of the casualty in flight is limited by noise and cramped conditions. Electronic monitoring (e.g., using a pulse oximeter) should be done if possible.
5. If there are doubts about the patient's ability to survive the flight, are there alternatives (e.g., fly in more advanced medical assistance or seek on-line medical advice)?

Conditions/situations that may cause problems in flight:

1. Pneumothorax.
2. Pneumoperitoneum (e.g., abdominal injury or following surgery).
3. Pneumocranium (gas in the head, e.g., after gunshot/penetrating injury).
4. Penetrating eye injury (or recent eye surgery); patients should not fly unless other injuries have priority, and then the flight should be restricted to under 1000 meters (approximately 3300 feet).
5. Air in the cuff of an endotracheal tube will expand and stretch the trachea, causing pain and a risk of

rupture. Water or saline should be used to inflate the cuff before flight.

6. Plastic IV fluid bags are satisfactory, but closed rigid IV bottles (e.g. glass) containing air are not suitable for air transport.

7. During flights at high altitude or long-distance transfers on airliners or military transports, hypoxia of **any cause** may worsen, even at normal cruising altitudes. Supplemental oxygen may be needed.

Checklists are an integral part of the aviation world and are similarly recommended to cover all stages of the aeromedical flight planning process, whether for a scene-hospital transfer lasting 20 minutes or for a long intercontinental secondary transfer lasting perhaps 20 hours.

Most complications occurring during transfer of patients by air can be predicted, and it falls within the duty of care of all aeromedical programs to anticipate what may go wrong, to identify clinical "red flags," and to plan appropriate staffing and equipment for the mission. The days of volunteer amateurs "doing their best" are over. Preventable harm occurring to patients during transfer caused by failure to anticipate likely complications may be considered negligent by the courts.

CLEARANCE FOR TRAVEL WITH COMMERCIAL AIRLINES

Scheduled services of commercial airlines are frequently used for long-distance aeromedical transfers, and many airlines have adopted rules and guidelines regarding the acceptance of passengers with special needs beyond normal service, including medical passengers. It is essential that aeromedical transport teams understand these rules in order to make sure that the correct clearances are achieved and the airline's full assistance is gained in ensuring the safety of the transfer.

By way of example, the OneWorld Alliance (which includes American Airlines, British Airways, Cathay Pacific Airways, and Qantas) has established a consensus set of aeromedical requirements known as MEDA ("Medical Emergency Disability Assessment") Fitness Guidelines (a MEDA case means that the potential traveler has to be examined by a certified physician to be potentially cleared to go on the flight): Some medical conditions that are covered are listed below.

Pregnancy

1. The mother may travel until the end of 36th week of gestation (singleton) or the 32nd week (multiple pregnancy).
2. Newborn babies are accepted after 48 hours, but 7 days of age before travel is recommended.
3. OneWorld consensus: Healthy babies may travel after 48 hours without MEDA clearance.

Myocardial Infarction

1. Any cardiac failure?
2. Any arrhythmia?
3. Any post-MI anginal pain?
4. All dealt by MEDA guidelines at <21 days.
5. If NO, uncomplicated; patient may travel 7 days after symptom, event.
6. If YES, complicated; decision depends on individual assessment (e.g. stability, success of stenting, escort proposed).

Angioplasty/Stenting

1. Elective, uncomplicated cases may travel 3 days after angioplasty, 5 days after stenting.

Open-Chest Cardiac surgery

1. May travel after 10 days if uncomplicated. All treated as MEDA during the 10 to 21 days of the postoperative period.

Anemia

1. Cut-off hemoglobin level: 7.5 g/dL.
2. Treat as MEDA assessment if level is between 7.5 and 10.0 g/dL.
3. Sickle cell crisis: passenger accepted after 10 days if otherwise stable.

Pneumothorax

1. If chest drain is in situ, patient may travel with medical escort at any time if other injuries/conditions permit and equipment including spare drain is carried.
2. May not travel until 14 days after full lung inflation if chest drain is closed, where trapped air may be present.

Abdominal Surgery

1. General: accepted after 10 days if uncomplicated.

2. Laparoscopy (investigation): accepted after 24 hours if all gas absorbed.
3. Laparoscopic surgery: MEDA assessment required if traveling between 1 and 10 days postoperatively.

Gastrointestinal Bleeding

1. Bleeding must have stopped.
2. Hemoglobin limits must be met.
3. Risks of rebleeding must be assessed and be acceptable.
4. No travel for any case <24 hours after bleed.
5. MEDA assessment required if patient is 1 to 10 days post-bleed.

Stroke

1. No case, however minor, may travel <3 days after a cerebrovascular accident.
2. OneWorld consensus: may travel after 10 days if uncomplicated.
3. 3 to 10 days: treat as MEDA, possibly may travel with escort.

Intracranial Surgery

1. May only travel when cranium is free of air.
2. May not travel within 10 days of surgery.

Psychiatric Cases

1. Must be stable and appropriately escorted.
2. Escort may range from correctional officers, friends/relatives, to medically trained personnel with appropriate medications.
3. MEDA assessment required in all cases.

Fractures

1. Splints/casts must be bivalved if traveling within 48 hours of injury or surgery on the fracture.

No-Divert Agreements (not all airlines will allow)

1. In cases of serious or terminal illness, where fitness guidelines are not met but passenger or relatives still request transport.
2. Exceptional cases only.

TRAINING

The expense of crew, fuel, and air time makes realistic training difficult within aeromedical programs, but

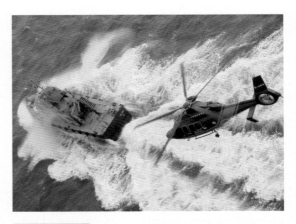

FIGURE 49–18

Situational EMS training. Photo courtesy of Government Flying Service, Hong Kong (GFS).

nevertheless it is essential that time be devoted to both ground and airborne training activity (Figure 49-18). Some of the latter can be situational training during actual operations, provided that the aircraft payload can accommodate additional crew members.

Essential training includes:

1. Training for dispatchers and controllers in appropriate task selection and in overseeing the mission from beginning to end.
2. Training for all staff in operational safety (including coverage of human factors).
3. Training for all staff in the operation of an effective flight risk management system applicable to the specific service offered.
4. Operational orientation training for all new pilots, irrespective of experience and seniority.
5. Crew resource management (CRM) for all pilots and crew members, undertaken together rather than as discrete groups.
6. Theoretical and practical training in the use of all safety, emergency, and survival equipment carried.
7. Helicopter underwater escape training (HUET) for all crew who undertake regular missions crossing open water.
8. Dinghy (lifeboat) and survival training as appropriate to the scheme's mission.

AUDIT

An operational and clinical audit is essential for the maintenance and development of aeromedical programs. While imperfect performance and outcomes are an embarrassment at best and a tragedy at worst, true failure lies in an organization's inability to learn from the suboptimal result and to avoid recurrence.

Wherever possible, an audit should take place in an atmosphere that concentrates on learning and remedy rather than on establishing blame; however, where deficiencies in individual performance are identified, these should be addressed by supervision and training. Whenever individual crew members (including pilots and medical personnel) find themselves in a situation that they are not trained to handle, there are organizational issues to address.

SUMMARY

Well-planned aeromedical programs, whether established for primary scene responses or for secondary patient transfers, are effective elements within EMS systems. It is essential when establishing a new program to be clear about the objectives to be met and to make certain that other elements of the EMS and hospital system are adapted to ensure maximum efficiency.

Multidisciplinary advice regarding the suitability of the proposed aircraft for the tasks at hand, personnel selection and training, and risk management systems are further important planning elements. Once established, the program should be subject to rigorous audit. As all members of the program are dependent on one another for safety and effectiveness, training should involve all professional groups using crew resource management principles.

Web Resources

1. Allgemeiner Deutscher Automobil-Club (ADAC) HEMS www.adac-hems-academy.de.
2. Air Accidents Investigation Branch, UK (AAIB) www.aaib.gov.uk.
3. Air Medical Physician Association (AMPA) www.ampa.org.
4. Australian Transport Safety Board (ATSB) www.atsb.com.au.
5. Federal Aviation Administration (FAA) www.faa.gov.
6. Government Flying Service, Hong Kong (GFS) www.gfs.gov.hk.
7. International Air Transport Association (IATA) www.iata.org.
8. International Civil Aviation Organization (ICAO) www.icao.int.
9. International Maritime Organization (IMO) www.imo.org.
10. National Transportation Safety Board (NTSB) www.ntsb.gov.
11. Royal Flying Doctor Service of Australia (RFDS) www.flyingdoctor.net.

Selected Readings

1. National Transportation Safety Board. Special Investigation Report on Emergency Medical Services Operations. NTSB/SIR-06/01; 2006.
2. Rainford D, Gradwell DJ, eds. Ernsting's Aviation Medicine. 4th ed. Hodder Education, London, UK 2006.

References

1. Coker, WJ. Aeromedical evacuation: medical aspects. In: Ernsting's Aviation Medicine. Fourth edition 2006;56:813–823. Hodder Education, London, UK.
2. Committee on Trauma and Committee on Shock, Division of Medical Sciences, National Academy of Sciences, National Research Council; Accidental death and disability; the neglected disease of modern society. 1966; p 12. National Academies Press, Washington, DC.
3. National Transportation Safety Board. Special Investigation Report on Emergency Medical Services Operations. Washington, DC, NTSB/SIR-06/01. 2006.
4. Fiorino F. NTSB Plans New Emergency Medical Helo Rules. *Aviation Week* 28 Aug 2009. McGraw Hill Companies, New York, NY, available at: http://www.aviationweek.com/aw/generic/story_channel.jsp?channel=busav&id=news/HEMS082809.xml.
5. Royal Flying Doctor Service of Australia; available at http://www.eurekacouncil.com.au/Australia-History/History-Pages/1928-royal_flying_doctor_service.htm) accessed 2/12/10.
6. Coats TJ, Keogh S, Clark H, Neal M. Prehospital resuscitative thoracotomy for cardiac arrest after penetrating trauma; rationale and case series. *The Journal of Trauma: Injury, Infection and Critical Care: April* 2001;50(4):670–673.
7. International Maritime Organization. Convention for the Safety of Life at Sea (SOLAS). 1974, entry into force 25 May 1980. Web version and map at http://www.imo.org and http://www.imo.org/Conventions/contents.asp?topic_id=257&doc_id=647 (accessed 23 Dec 2009, verified 2/15/10).
8. Blumen IJ, UCAN Safety Committee. A safety review and risk assessment in air medical transport. In *Supplement to the Air Medical Physician Handbook, eds. Salt Lake City, UT,* Air Medical Physician Association: November 2002.
9. Sampson WT, Simpson GB, Green DL. Night vision goggles in the Emergency Medical Services (EMS) helicopter. FAA Report DOT/FAA/RD-94/21. 1994. Federal Aviation Administration, Washington, DC.
10. Thomas SH. On-site hospital helipads. Resource document for the NAEMSP position paper on on-site helipads. *Prehosp Emerg Care.* 2009 Jul-Sep; 13(3):398–401. PMID: 19499480.
11. Emergency Landing Conditions. Federal Aviation Regulations; 14 CFR Part 29, 561. Federal Aviation Administration; Washington, DC, 1965.

12. Emergency Landing Conditions. Federal Aviation Regulations; 14 CFR Part 29, 562. Federal Aviation Administration; Washington, DC 1997.

13. Roberts K, Blethyn K, Foreman M, Bleetman A. Influence of air ambulance doctors on on-scene times, clinical interventions, decision-making and independent paramedic practice. *Emerg Med J*, Feb;26(2):128–34. PMID: 19164630.

14. Dissman PD, Le Clerc S. The experience of Teesside helicopter emergency services: doctors do not prolong prehospital on-scene times. *Emerg Med J* 2007 Jan;24(1):59–62. PMID: 17183051.

15. Garner AA. The role of physician staffing of helicopter emergency medical services in prehospital trauma response. *Emergency Medicine Australasia* 2004 Aug; 16(4):318–23. Review. PMID: 15283719.

Web Links and Resources

Sergey M. Motov

NATIONAL EMS ORGANIZATIONS

Associations

1. http://www.naemse.org/ – The National Association of EMS Educators, (accessed on 10/12/09).
2. http://www.naemsp.org/ – The National Association of EMS Physicians, (accessed on 101/2/09).
3. http://www.nasemsd.org/ – The National Association of State EMS Officials, (accessed on 10/12/09).
4. http://www.emsvillage.com/resources/associations.cfm – The National Association of Emergency Medical Technicians, (accessed on 10/16/09).
5. http://www.naemt.org/ – National Association representing and serving all emergency medical services practitioners through advocacy, educational programs and research, (accessed on 10/16/09).
6. http://www.the-aaa.org/ – American Ambulance Association, (accessed on 10/16/09).
7. http://www.aams.org//AM/Template.cfm?Section=Home –Association of Air Medical Services, (accessed on 10/16/09).
8. http://www.nemspa.org/ – National EMS Pilot Association, (accessed on 10/16/09).
9. http://www.fapep.org/ – The Florida Association of Professional EMTs and Paramedics, (accssed on 10/20/09).

10. http://www.naemse.org/ – The National Association of EMS Educators provide excellence in EMS education and lifelong learning, (accessed on 10/20/09).

Centers/Services

11. http://www.nhtsa.dot.gov/ – The National Highway Traffic Safety Administration, (accessed on 10/12/09).
12. http://www.colorado.edu/hazards/ – Natural Hazards Center, (accessed on 101/2/09).
13. http://www.emsc.net/ – Emergency Medical Services Corporation (EMSC) is the leading provider of emergency medical services in the United States (accessed on 10/15/09).
14. http://www.nemsmf.org/ – National Emergency Medical Services Museum Foundation (accessed on 10/16/09).
15. http://nationalregistryemts.com/ – National Registry EMTs, (accessed on 10/16/09).
16. http://www.nremt.org/Content/NREMT_Home.nremt – National registry of emergency medical technicians, (accessed on 10/16/09).
17. http://www.nassauems.com/ – The Nassau Regional EMS Council (accessed on 10/16/09).
18. http://www.nycremsco.org/ – The Regional Emergency Medical Services Council of New York City, (accessed on 10/16/09).
19. http://www.wemsi.org/ – Wilderness Emergency Medical Service Institute-provides

medical care to patients in the specialized prehospital situations of wilderness, (accessed on 10/16/09).

20. http://www.caas.org/ – The Commission on Accreditation of Ambulance Services (CAAS), (accessed on 10/16/09).

21. http://www.emsc.net/ – Emergency Medical Service Corporation, (accessed on 10/22/09).

22. http://www.nemsms.org/ – National EMS Memorial Service-to honor and remember those men and women of America's Emergency Medical Services who have given their lives in the line of duty, and to recognize the sacrifice they have made in service to their communities and their fellow man, (accessed on 10/16/09).

23. http://www.emergencycareny.com/ – EMT Training by Emergency Care Programs of New York, (accessed on 10/16/09).

24. http://www.fema.gov/ – Federal Emergency Management Agency (FEMA), (accessed on 10/19/09)

25. http://bolivia.hrsa.gov/emsc/ – Emergency Medical Services for Children, (accessed on 10/19/09).

26. http://www.naems.org/ – Northern Arizona Emergency Medical Services, (accessed on 10/20/09)

27. http://www.ncemsf.org/ – The National Collegiate Emergency Medical Services Foundation (NCEMSF), (accessed on 10/20/09).

28. http://www.ncemsf.org/resources/links/showlinks.ems?category=999 – Campus EMS Organizations (USA), (accessed on 10/20/09).

29. http://www.jibc.ca/paramedic/ – The Paramedic Academy is committed to building and supporting innovative training programs that shape both traditional and emerging career paths, (accessed on 10/20/09).

30. http://www.volunteerems.org/ – The directory of Emergency Medical Services Volunteers, (accessed on 10/20/09).

31. http://www.emergencydispatch.org/ – The National Academies of Emergency Dispatch-NAED is a non-profit standard-setting organization promoting safe and effective emergency dispatch services world-wide, (accessed on 10/22/09).

INTERNATIONAL EMS ORGANIZATIONS

Associations

1. http://www.iaemsc.org/ – The International Association of Emergency Medical Service Chiefs (IAEMSC) (accessed on 10/15/09.

2. http://www.iafc.org/ – The International Association of Fire Chiefs represents the leadership of over 1.2 million firefighters and emergency responders, (accessed on 10/15/09).

3. http://www.iaep.org/ – The International Association of EMTs and Paramedics (accessed on 10/15/09).

4. http://www.isips.org/iaep.php – International Association of EMT's and Paramedics, (accessed on 10/15/09).

5. http://www.paramedic.ca/ – Paramedic Association of Canada (accessed on 10/15/09).

6. http://www.britishparamedic.org/ – British paramedics association, (accessed on 10/16/09.

7. http://www.ontarioparamedic.ca/ – Paramedic Association of Ontario, (accessed on 10/16/09).

8. http://www.acert.ca – The Association of Campus Emergency Response Teams of Canada (ACERT) is a federally incorporated, charitable organization in place to support, promote and advocate emergency care on Canadian post-secondary campuses, (accessed on 10/20/09).

9. http://www.peelparamedics.com/ – Canadian EMS forum and blog and Paramedics Ambulance Union (accessed on 10/22/09).

10. http://www.internationalems.net/ – World Class Care, (accessed on 10/15/09).

11. http://news.ciems.org/ – International EMS News, (accessed on 10/22/09).

12. http://www.paramedic-community.com/ – Paramedics around the world, (accessed on 10/15/09).

13. http://paramedicresearch.ca/ – The Canadian research resource for EMS and paramedics (accessed on 10/15/09).

14. http://www.emsindex.co.uk/ – Worldwide Emergency Medical Services List, covering air, road and sea EMS ambulance services for paramedics (accessed on 10/16/09).

15. http://emsconnect.ems1.com/ – Paramedics of the World (accessed on 10/16/09).

16. http://emt.co.za/ – Emergency Medical Training, South Africa, is a national medical training institution offering a range of courses, (accessed on 10/16/09).

17. http://www.phecit.ie/DesktopDefault.aspx – The Pre-Hospital Emergency Care Council (PHECC) is the Irish EMS regulator, (accessed on 10/16/09).

18. http://www.isic.ie/about.html – The Irish Society for Immediate care (ISIC), (accessed on 10/16/09)

19. http://gmr.net/ – Global Medical Response (GMR) offers emergency ambulance and emergency department medical services to the international community, (accessed on 10/20/09).

20. http://www.iemsr.org/ – International EMS Registry offers testing and skill verification to all EMS personnel all over the world,(accessed on 10/20/09).

21. http://www.eeii.org/ – Emergency and Investigative Educational Institute, (accessed on 10/20/09).

22. http://www.rallye-rejviz.com/ – Emergency Medical Service of Czech Republic, (accessed on 10/20/09).

23. http://www.unimed.org.au/ – UniMed is a unique new non-profit organisation providing first aid to the community of Australia,(accessed on 10/20/09).

24. http://www.ambulance.act.gov.au – This is the highest level of pre-hospital clinical care provided by any ambulance service in Australia, (accessed on 10/20/09).

25. http://www.ambulansforum.se/forum/englishpage. shtml – Internet forum for the Pre-hospital Emergency Care in Scandinavia, (accessed on 10/20/09).

10. http://www.highbeam.com/Prehospital+ Emergency+Care/publications.aspx – Prehospital Emergency Care articles, (accessed on 10/20/09).

11. http://www.who.int/violence_injury_prevention/ publications/services/39162_oms_new.pdf – Pre-hospital trauma care systems (WHO Publications), (accessed on 10/20/09).

12. http://whqlibdoc.who.int/publications/2005/ 924159294X_chap4.pdf – Prehospital Trauma Care for First Responders, (accessed on 10/20/09).

13. http://www.jephc.com/ – Journal of Emergency Primary Health Care, a peer-reviewed, international journal to advance and promote the science and the art of prehospital care research, education, (accessed on 10/20/09).

14. http://www.iaff.org/tech/PDF/Monograph1.pdf – Department of Emergency Medical Services International Association of Fire Fighters, (accessed on 10/20/09).

15. http://www.iaff.org/Tech/PDF/Monograph6.pdf – Paramedics Extended Scope of practice monograph, (accessed on 10/20/09).

EMS JOURNALS/MAGAZINES

1. http://www.emsresponder.com/ – The online home of EMS Magazine. Our online publication provides EMS news and training for paramedics and EMTs, as well as other prehospital practitioners and public safety responders (accessed on 10/15/09).

2. http://www.jems.com/index.html – Journal of Emergency Medical Services, (accessed on 10/16/09).

3. http://www.advancedrt.com/ – Advanced Rescue Technology Magazine, (accessed on 10/16/09).

4. http://www.prenhall.com/mistovich/ – Pre-hospital Emergency Care Books, (accessed on 10/16/09).

5. http://informahealthcare.com/pec?cookieSet=1 – Pre-hospital Emergency care journal, (accessed on 10/16/09).

6. http://www.emergency.com/ennday.htm – Emergency Net News-World Watch Desk, (accessed on 10/19/09).

7. http://www.ispub.com/journal/the_internet_ journal_of_disaster_medicine.html –The Internet Journal of Disaster Medicine, (accessed on 10/20/09).

8. http://journals.lww.com/jtrauma/ – The Journal of Trauma, (accessed on 10/20/09).

9. http://www.sciencedirect.com/science/journal/ 1067991X – Air Medical Journal, (accessed on 10/20/09).

EMS Transport

1. http://usairambulance.net/ – US Air Ambulance provides domestic and international medical transport of patients requiring various levels of assistance, (accessed on 10/16/09).

2. http://www.flightparamedic.org/ – International Association of Flight Paramedics (accessed on 10/15/09).

3. http://airambulanceinternational.blogspot.com/ – The Air Ambulance Professional for folks who travel (accessed on 10/16/09).

4. http://www.emtambulance.com/ – Emergency medical transport corporation (accessed on 10/16/09).

5. http://www.americanairambulance.com/ – American Air Ambulance and its emergency air care service is the trusted leader for medical air transportation internationally (accessed on 10/15/09).

6. http://www.aerocare.com/ – AeroCare provides Air Ambulance services and is recognized throughout the world as a leader in medical air transportation (accessed on 10/15/09).

7. http://www.flightweb.com/index.php – FlightWeb is dedicated to Air Medical Professionals around the world-EMS Pilots, Flight Nurses, Flight Medics, Flight RTs, Flight MDs. (accessed on 10/16/09).

8. http://www.johngodwin.net/1195/ax0007gr/1201. html – Emergency Vehicles online, (accessed on 10/20/09).

9. http://www.medwayairambulance.com/ – Medway Air Ambulance, (accessed on 10/20/09).

10. http://ambu-care.com/ – AMBU-CARE provides long distance ambulance transportation to patients traveling interstate along the East Coast of the United States, (accesed on 10/20/09).

11. http://www.ambunet.com/ – Ambulance Network, a worldwide industry leader in New and Used Ambulance sales, (accessed on 10/20/09).

12. http://www.peacefulpalate.com/results.phtml? dtvr5=Ambulance – The ultimate ambulance vehicles and transportation site, (accessed on 10/20/09).

13. http://www.ambulance.co.uk/ – Worldwide EMS Services indexed by Air, Road or Sea, (accessed on 10/20/09).

14. http://www.airmed.com/ – AirMed is the ultimate air ambulance company,(accessed on 10/20/09)

15. http://ampa.org/ – The Air Medical Physician Association, (accessed on 10/20/09).

16. http://www.ambulanceforum.nl/forum/   – Translation required, (accessed on 10/20/09).

EMS PRODUCTS AND EQUIPMENT

1. http://www.progressivemed.com/   – Medical equipment and emergency care supplies (accessed on 10/15/09).

2. http://www.wildernessmedical.com/ – Wilderness Medical Systems provides you with the highest quality medical kits available to adventure travelers (accessed on 10/16/09).

3. http://www.emtcatalog.com/ – unique collection of merchandise for EMTs and Paramedics, EMT Departments and anyone in the EMS profession, (accessed on 10/16/09).

4. http://www.emergencystuff.com/ – One stop shopping for your Emergency Medical Service needs, (accessed on 10/16/09).

5. http://www2.mooremedical.com/index.cfm   – The easiest way to order medical supplies, medical equipment and pharmaceuticals online, (accessed on 10/16/09).

6. http://www.eventmedical.com/ – The ultimate EMS Medical products site, (accessed on 10/16/09).

7. http://www.aedsuperstore.com/ – AED superstore, (accessed on 10/16/09).

8. http://www.medicplanet.com/ – EMS supplies online store, (accessed on 10/16/09).

9. http://www.acidremap.com/index.html   – Purchase Paramedic Protocol Provider for your

iPhone or iPod Touch (links to and requires iTunes)., (accessed on 10/20/09).

10. http://www.rescuestat.com/ – Emergency Medical Services Products, (accessed on 10/20/09).

EMS Educational Sites

1. http://teexweb.tamu.edu/esti/ – Emergency Services Training Institute, (accessed on 10/15/09).

2. http://www.fire-publications-dvd.com/ – Emergency Books and Training Materials, (accessed on 10/15/09.

3. http://www.open-er.com/ – Open Bank EM Questions, (accessed in 10/15/09).

4. http://www.templejc.edu/dept/ems/Pages/Power Point.html – EMS Power Point Presentations of various topics, (accessed on 10/15/09).

5. http://www.rescuehouse.com/ – The ultimate first responders site (accessed on 10/15/09).

6. http://www.thelancetstudent.com/2009/09/17/ models-of-international-emergency-medical-service-ems-systems/ – Models of International Emergency Medical Service System, (accessed on 10/15/09).

7. http://www.emtt.org/ – Provides professional tactical medic training to professional medics (accessed on 10/15/09).

8. http://www.ems1.com/ – The leading online EMS resource (accessed on 10/15/09).

9. http://www.emtlife.com/ – The #1 Online Forum for EMS-Related Discussion (accessed on 10/15/09).

10. http://www1.emsjane.com/ – Cutting edge online continuing education for firefighters and EMS professionals (accessed on 10/16/09).

11. http://www.ssrsi.org/911.htm – Covers Medical Practices and Emergency situations, providing a wealth of information on illness & wound treatment (basic to advanced) and what to do when confronted with hazardous situations (accessed on 10/16/09).

12. http://r.webring.com/hub?ring=paramedicsring – This ring provides information and links to EMS and other prehospital care sites. It includes educational, chat and informational links (accessed on 10/16/09).

13. http://www.nhtsa.dot.gov/people/injury/ems/ pub/emtbnsc.pdf   – EMT-Basic: National Standard Curriculum,(accessed on 10/16/09).

14. http://www.emsdr.com/ – Rare and valuable domain name for an Emergency Medical Physician or an EMS Corporation desiring to have

a professional image and a more meaningful presence on the internet (accessed on 10/16/09).

15. http://www.fyrfytr.com/home/ – This site was developed to provide Firefighter, EMT, Paramedic, and other FIRE/EMS Professionals a place to share Articles, News Stories, Photos, Links, Classified Ads and More. (accessed on 10/16/09).

16. http://www.idsemergencymanagement.com/ – IDS-Emergency Management is an online conference, exhibition, and trade show for the industry, (accessed on 10/16/09).

17. http://www.defrance.org/ —This site is dedicated to all who so caringly provide EMS, (accessed on 10/16/09).

18. http://www.emsbest.com/ – Best Practice Resources for EMS Providers, (accessed on 10/16/09).

19. http://www.emsvillage.com/ –EMS at the tip of your hands,(accessed on 10/16/09).

20. http://www.lessstress.com/ – Basic Resuscitation Tools, (accessed on 10/16/09).

21. http://orise.orau.gov/reacts/ – Radiation Emergency Assistance Center/Training Site (REAC/TS), (accessed on 10/16/09).

22. http://www.24-7ems.com/index.htm – Training courses for EMS providers, (accessed on 10/16/09).

23. http://www.theemsinstitute.org/ – This web site is dedicated for all EMS and health care colleagues, (accessed on 10/16/09).

24. http://www.emergency.com/ –Crisis, Conflict, and Emergency Service News, Analysis and Reference (accessed on 10/17/09).

25. http://www.paramedic.com/ – Online gateway to prehospital emergency medicine, (accessed on 10/17/09).

26. http://www.ncemi.org/cse/contents.htm – Common Simple Emergencies, (accessed on 10/19/09).

27. http://www.firehouse.com/ –Firefighters, Rescuers, EMS, (accessed on 10/20/09).

28. http://www.pcrf.mednet.ucla.edu/pcrf/ – Pre-hospital Care Research Forum at UCLA, (accessed on 10/20/09).

29. http://www.emslive.com/ – EMSLive.com is a resource by paramedics, for paramedics- it is a weekly Podcast EMS radio show that delivers interviews with industry experts, and allows listeners to send in their questions via email or live chat, (accessed on 10/20/09).

30. http://www.paramedic-network-news.com/ – Paramedic Network News (PNN) is a daily news and information source on the EMS industry, (accessed on 10/20/09).

31. http://cpem.med.nyu.edu/files/cpem/u3/trippals.pdf – Teaching Resource for Instructors in Prehospital Pediatrics for Paramedics, (accessed on 10/20/09).

32. http://emsresource.net/ – The Ultimate EMS site, (accessed on 10/20/09).

33. http://www.mediccast.com/ – The MedicCast programs target busy medical medical and rescue personnel, providing up-to-date news, commentary, and reviewing patient care standards, (accessed on 10/20/09).

34. http://www.thelunatick.com/ems/ – The EMS Humor, (accessed on 10/20/09).

35. http://www.medicalmnemonics.com/ – World Database for Medical Mnemonics, (accessed on 10/22/09).

Advanced Life Support

1. www.americanheart.org –American Heart Association, (accessed on 10/15/09).

2. http://www.facs.org/dept/trauma/atls/ – Advanced Trauma Life Support, (accessed 10/15/09).

3. http://www.aplsonline.com/ –Pediatric Advanced Life Support, (10/15/09).

4. http://www.acls.net/ – ACLS Algorithms (accessed on 10/15/09).

5. http://www.itrauma.org/ – International Trauma Life Support, (accessed on 10/16/09).

6. http://www.netmedicine.com/cyberpt/cyberptframe.htm – These highly interactive patient-care simulators are designed to help emergency care providers to practice their skills at ACLS/PALS, (accessed on 10/17/09).

7. http://www.nrcpr.org/ – The National Registry of CardioPulmonary Resuscitation (NRCPR®) is an international database of in-hospital resuscitation events, (accessed on 10/17/09).

8. http://www.cpr.net/ – Online CPR training directory listing,(accessed on 10/19/09).

9. http://www.naemt.org/education/PHTLS/phtls_a.aspx – Pre-hospital Trauma Life Support (PHTLS), (accessed on 10/20/09).

10. http://www.eacls.com/ – Convenient and Affordable Online ACLS Training, (accessed on 10/20/09).

11. http://www.profirstaid.com/ – ProFirstAid is a nationally recognized online e-learning company offering lay rescuer/general workplace CPR & First Aid certification and training, (accessed on 10/20/09).

Airway Management

1. http://magicanimation.com/intubation/   –   Animated Intubation Skills, (accessed on (10/15/09).
2. http://airwayinstitute.com/ – The Airway Institute is focused on delivering material relevant to the management of airway issues in an effective, new and exciting way, (accessed on 10/16/09).
3. http://enw.org/AirwayHell.htm – Action-Plan for Airway Problems From Hell, (accessed on 10/16/09).
4. http://airwayeducation.homestead.com/ – Airway Education Web Resource (accesses on 10/17/09)
5. http://www.theairwaysite.com – The definitive site for Airway management education (accessed on 10/17/09).
6. http://magboul.multiply.com/ – designed for Physicians, CRNAs, Physician Assistants, Registered Nurses, Medical Students, EMS providers, (accessed on 10/17/09).
7. http://www.meduniwien.ac.at/combitube/ – The Ultimate Combitube Site, (accessed on 10/17/09).
8. http://www.slamairway.com/ – Street Level Airway Management-offers basic through advanced airway management training that is useful wherever emergency or difficult airway situations occur (accessed on 10/17/09).
9. http://www.airwaycarnival.com/ – Animated Airwaymanagement Site, (accessed on 10/17/09)
10. http://www.chems.alaska.gov/EMS/Assets/EMSC/pediatric_airway.pdf – Pediatric Airway Management self study module, (accessed on 10/17/09).
11. http://www.airwaycam.com/ – The best way to teach intubation, (accessed on 10/19/09).

EKG's for EMS

1. http://www.emedu.org/ – Emergency EKG Online Training Module, (accessed on 10/15/09).
2. http://ecg.bidmc.harvard.edu/maven/mavenmain.asp – EKG Heaven-Self-assessment tutorial for health professional, (accessed on 10/15/09).
3. http://www.ecglibrary.com/ecghome.html   –   Library of the EKG's, (accessed on 10/15/09).
4. http://library.med.utah.edu/kw/ecg/index.html EKG's Learning Center, ((accessed on 10/15/09).

Obstetrics for EMS

1. http://www.obgyn.net/ – vast, an ever growing and expanding universe with over 1,000,000 pages of educational content, discussion forums, videos, educational tutorials, images, (accessed on 10/15/09).
2. http://ems-ceu.com/courses/184/index_ems.html – The Obstetric Course for EMTs and first responders, (accessed on 10/16/09).
3. http://www.gov.mb.ca/health/ems/guidelines/docs/M10.04.05.pdf – Obstetrical Emergencies for EMS Providers, (accessed on 10/16/09).
4. http://www.emtlife.com/showthread.php?p=181549 – EMT's forum on Obstetrics Emergencies, (accessed on 10/16/09).
5. http://www.jbpub.com/catalog/9780763769611/ – Paramedic Interactive Module: Obstetrics, (accessed on 10/16/09).
6. http://www.perinatology.com/exposures/druglist.htm – Drugs in Pregnancy and Breast feeding, (accessed on 10/17/09).
7. http://ec.princeton.edu/ – All you need to know about emergency medicine, (accessed on 10/20/09).
8. http://connect.jems.com/forum/topics/prehospital-medications-in – EMS Forum-Pre-hospital Drugs in Pregnancy, (accessed on 10/20/09).

Pre-Hospital Pain Management

1. http://www.hcmcems.org/ems/QA/Prehospital_Pain_Management.pdf – POSITION STATEMENT on Pre-hospital Pain Management.

INTERNATIONAL EMS

1. http://www.03.ru/ – Russian Emergency Medical Service Blog, (accessed on 10/15/09.
2. http://www.international-ems.com/forum/ – EMS forum all over the world, ((accessed on 10/15/09).
3. http://www.emergency.com.au/ – First Aid Training and Kits in Australia, (accessed on 10/19/09.
4. http://www.wiems.net/ – Worldwide International EMS provides quality EMS training to medical professionals around the world, (accessed on 10/20/09).
5. http://www.parasolemt.com.au/index.php   –   PARASOL EMT is Australia's premier commercial provider of first aid and OHS training courses, (accessed on 10/20/09).
6. http://www.qldwaterpolice.com/links.html   –   Australian Emergency Services Links, (accessed on 10/20/09).
7. http://www.paramedic.com.ar/htm/index.htm – Paramedics Service in Argentina, (translation required), (accessed on 10/20/09).
8. http://www.falck.com/emergency_medical_services –Emergency Medical Services in Europe,(accessed on 10/22/09).
9. http://www.emagister.co.uk/pre_hospital_emergency_care_training_agency-en170003638.htm   –   Pre-Hospital Emergency Care Training Agency, (UK based), (accessed on 10/16/09).

PEDIATRIC EMS

1. http://www.pemdatabase.org/ems.html – Pediatric protocols & practice guidelines, (accessed on 10/16/09).
2. http://www.peppsite.com/ – Pediatric Education for Prehospital Professionals. Developed by the American Academy of Pediatrics, PEPP is an exciting curriculum designed specifically to teach prehospital professionals how to better access and manage ill or injured children, (accessed on 10/16/09).
3. http://www.paramedicsforchildren.com/ – Contributions to children from all over the world, (accessed on 10/20/09).
4. http://www.childrensnational.org/EMSC/ – The Emergency Medical Services for Children (EMSC) National Resource Center (NRC) helps to improve the pediatric emergency care infrastructure throughout the United States and its territories, (accessed on 10/20/09).
5. http://www.pemdatabase.org/ – Pediatric Emergency Medicine Ultimate database, (10/20/09).

GERIATRIC EMS

1. http://www.gemssite.com/ – Geriatric Education for Emergency Medical Services-an exciting curriculum designed specifically to help EMS providers address all of the special needs of the older population. (accessed on 10/16/09).

ORTHOPEDICS FOR EMS

1. http://www.wheelessonline.com/ – "the premier website for EMS orthopedics".

TRAUMA FOR EMS

1. http://www.trauma.org/ –Trauma.org is an independent, non-profit organization providing global education, information and communication resources for professionals in trauma and critical care, (accessed on 10/17/09).
2. http://www.ssgfx.com/CP2020/medtech/procedures/protocols.htm – Trauma Team EMS Prehospital Medical Protocols & Standing Orders, (accessed on 10/20/09).

ON-LINE CME FOR EMS/PARAMEDICS

1. http://www.webcme.com/home1.html – On-line CMA for EMS, EMT and paramedics, (accessed on 10/17/09).

2. http://www.fireandemstraining.com/onlinece.html – A variety of online and classroom CE for both Paramedics and EMT's approved by the National Registry for EMS, (accessed on 10/17/09).
3. http://www.onlineaha.org/index.cfm?fuseaction=info.healthcare – The American Heart Association is the trusted leader in emergency cardiovascular care training and education for healthcare professionals, (accessed on 10/17/09).
4. http://ems-safety.com/seminars.htm – The EMS Professional offers unique seminars to EMS professionals that are targeted to increase knowledge in areas such as specific field operations, vehicle operations, unusual call types etc., (accessed on 10/17/09).
5. http://www.emspic.org/documents/PDF/Online12LeadECGInterpretationCourseFAQand Instructions.pdf – Online 12 Lead ECG Interpretation Course, (accessed on 10/17/09).
6. http://www.stroke.org/site/PageServer?pagename=EMS – National Stroke Association's *Stroke Rapid Response*™ is a new innovative program that teaches EMS and prehospital providers basic and advanced stroke information, (accessed on 10/17/09).
7. http://www.geocities.com/nyerrn/ems/tests.htm – A variety of free pre-hospital emergency care tests and CME credits for Emergency Medical Technicians and Paramedics, (accesed on 10/17/09).
8. http://www.aplsonline.com/ – The Pediatric Emergency Medicine Resource, a continuing medical education program developed by the American Academy of Pediatrics and the American College of Emergency Physicians, (accessed on 10/17/09).
9. http://www.aclsonline.us/ – The nation's largest free-standing provider of ACLS and PALS education since 1984 presents online ACLS provider course certification and recertification, (accessed on 10/17/09).
10. http://www.procpr.org/ – Online CPR Certification by ProCPR, (accessed on 10/19/09).
11. http://www.ems-ce.com/ – Continues Education for EMS (accessed on 10/15/09).
12. http://www.mywebce.com/ – Unparallel continuing education programs for EMS personnel, (accessed on 10/16/09).

PREHOSPITAL MEDICATIONS USE (EMS PHARAMCOLOGY)

1. http://www.bffire.org/File_Cabinet/downloadable_info/EMS_protocols/CH8%20Medications.pdf –

EMS Pre-hospital Medications Overview, (accessed on 10/20/09).

2. www.defrance.org/EMSER/prehospital_medications_glotfelty.ppt – Power Point Presentation on Pre-hospital Medication, (accessed on 10/20/09).

3. http://www.flashcardexchange.com/tag/medic – Essentials of Paramedics pharmacology, (accessed on 10/20/09).

PREHOSPITAL ULTRASOUND (EMS ULTRASOUND)

1. http://www.sonoguide.com/ems_pre-hospital.html – Introduction to Pre-hospital Ultrasound, (accessed on 10/20/09).

2. http://www.drf-luftrettung.de/sonography.html?&L=1 – German and Austrian Prospective on Pre-hospital Ultrasound Use, (accessed on 10/20/09).

EMS TOXICOLOGY

1. http://acmt.net/ – American College of Medical Toxicology, (accessed on 10/20/09).

2. http://www.aapcc.org/DNN/ – The American Association of Poison Control Centers, (accessed on 10/20/09).

3. http://toxnet.nlm.nih.gov/ – Databases on toxicology, hazardous chemicals, environmental health, and toxic releases, (accessed on 10/20/09).

4. http://toxtown.nlm.nih.gov/ – Environmental health concern and toxic chemicals where you live, work and play, (accessed on 10/20/09).

5. http://www.911emergency.org/links.html – EMS, Poison Control and Ground Ambulance Links, (accessed on 10/20/09).

6. http://www.emsvillage.com/articles/index.cfm?Cat=43 – Great Source of case-based scenarios for EMS Providers, (accessed on 10/20/09).

7. http://www.ahls.org – Premiere HAZMAT training for the healthcare professional (10/15/09).

DISASTER MEDICINE FOR EMS

1. http://wadem.medicine.wisc.edu/ – The World Association for Disaster and Emergency Medicine (WADEM),(accessed 10/12/09).

2. http://www.who.int/hac/en/ – World Health Organization (WHO)-Division of Emergency and Humanitarian Services,(accessed 10/12/09).

3. http://www.adpc.net/v2007/ – Asian Disaster Preparedness Center, (accessed 10/12/09).

4. http://www.cdera.org/ – Caribbean Disaster Emergency Management Agency, (accessed on 10/12/09).

5. http://www.coe-dmha.org/ – Center for Excellence in Disaster Management & Humanitarian Assistance, (COE-DMHA). (accessed on 10/12/09).

6. http://www.cne.go.cr/ – Costa Rica National Emergency Commision (accessed on 10/12/09).

7. http://www.disaster-medicine.de/ – German Institute for Disaster Medicine and Emergency Medicine, (accessed on 10/12/09).

8. http://www.medbc.com/ – the Mediterranean Council for Burns and Fire Disasters (MBC), (accessed on 10/12/09).

9. http://www.savan.org/ – Save Accident Victims Association of Nigeria, (accessed on 10/22/09).

10. http://www.homeland1.com/ – Welcome to the ONE resource for domestic preparedness, (10/15/09).

11. http://www.medicalcorps.org/ – Medical Corps' Combat/Field Medicine School, (accessed on 10/20/09).

12. http://www.operationalmedicine.org/ – Operational Medicine is the healthcare provided in unconventional settings where important resources may be significantly restricted, (accessed on 10/20/09).

13. http://www.emdat.be/ – Emergency Events Database, (accessed on 10/20/09).

14. http://www.ndcrt.org/ – The Emergency Response and Logistical Information Network, (accessed on 10/20/09).

15. http://www.emedprofessional.com/ – a comprehensive resources for emergency medical professionals, first responders, and anyone concerned with disaster prevention and preparedness, (accessed on 10/20/09).

16. http://disastermgmt.org/ – DisasterMgmt.org provides detailed information on type of disasters, how to prepare for them, and how to respond to them, (accessed on 10/22/09).

17. http://www.ipred.co.il/english/ – International Preparedness & Response to Emergencies and Disasters 2010 aims to provide a platform for networking and sharing ideas, experiences and lessons learned from preparedness and response to emergencies and disasters, (accessed on 10/20/09).

18. http://www.hazmatforhealthcare.org/ – Providing emergency planning, exercising, training for hospitals and healthcare, (accessed on 10/20/09).

19. http://orise.orau.gov/reacts/ – the Radiation Emergency Assistance Center/Training Site (REAC/TS), (accessed on 10/20/09).

20. http://www.atsdr.cdc.gov/ – Agency for Toxic Substances and Disease Registry (ATSDR)- serves the public by using the best science, taking responsive public health actions, and providing trusted health information to prevent harmful exposures and diseases related to toxic substances, (accessed on 10/20/09).

21. http://www.reliefweb.int – the global hub for time-critical humanitarian information on Complex Emergencies and Natural Disasters, (accessed on 10/12/09).

Index

Page numbers followed by *f* and *t* indicate figures and tables